Milady's Standard Textbook for Professional Estheticians

Delmar Publishers' Online Services

To access Delmar on the World Wide Web, point your browser to:

http://www.delmar.com/delmar.html

To access through Gopher: gopher://gopher.delmar.com

(Delmar Online is part of "thomson.com", an Internet site with information on
more than 30 publishers of the International Thomson Publishing organization.)

For information on our products and services:

email: info@delmar.com

or call 800-347-7707

Milady's Standard Textbook for Professional Estheticians

Joel Gerson

Seventh Edition

Milady Publishing Company
(A Division of Delmar Publishers Inc.)

NOTICE TO THE READER

Publisher does not warrant or guarantee any of the products described herein or perform any independent analysis in connection with any of the product information contained herein. Publisher does not assume, and expressly disclaims, any obligation to obtain and include information other than that provided to it by the manufacturer.

The reader is expressly warned to consider and adopt all safety precautions that might be indicated by the activities described herein and to avoid all potential hazards. By following the instructions contained herein, the reader willingly assumes all risks in connection with such instructions.

The publisher makes no representations or warranties of any kind, including but not limited to, the warranties of fitness for particular purpose or merchantability, nor are any such representations implied with respect to the material set forth herein, and the publisher takes no responsibility with respect to such material. The publisher shall not be liable for any special, consequential or exemplary damages resulting, in whole or in part, from the readers' use of, or reliance upon, this material.

Credits:
  Supervising Editor: Catherine Frangie
  Developmental Editor: Joseph Miranda
  Project Editor: Andrea Edwards Myers
  Production Manager: John Mickelbank
  Art Manager: Rita Stevens
  Art Supervisor: John Lent
  Design Supervisor: Susan C. Mathews

  Artists: Shiz Horii
          Robert Richards
          Judy Francis
          Cynthia Saniewski
          Randy Tibbot
          CEM
          Nelva Richardson
  Photographers: Michael A. Gallitelli, on location at the Austin Beauty School,
                  with Dino Petrocelli
                Steven Landis, with direction from Vincent and Alfred Nardi
                  of Nardi Salon
                Gillette Research Institute
                New Image's Salon System

  Cover courtesy of *Dermascope Magazine*
  Cover Photographer: Christopher Mann
  Cover Director: Elayne Mayes
  World Wide Phone Number: 1-214-526-0752

Hardcover ISBN 1-56253-129-8

Library of Congress Cataloging-in-Publication Data

Gerson, Joel.
    Standard textbook for professional estheticians / Joel Gerson. --
7th ed.
        p.   cm.
    Includes index.
    1. Beauty culture. 2. Skin -- Care and hygiene. 3. Cosmetics.
  I. Title.
  TT957.G47   1992
  646.7'26 -- dc20   91-18525
                                                            CIP

Printed in the United States of America
10 9 8 7

DEDICATION

I dedicate this book to my father, Ben Gerson, who encouraged me to continue my studies in cosmetology when I wanted to drop out of school. He said, "Finish school, and get a license, and no matter where you go, you will always be able to find work." And he was right!

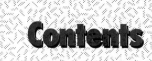

Contents

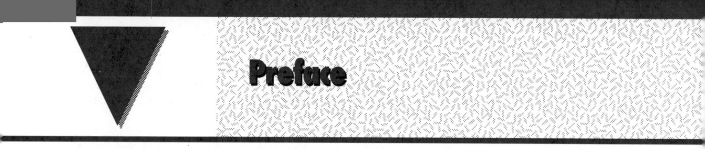

Preface

Milady's Standard Textbook for Professional Estheticians fully explains and illustrates the knowledge and skills the professional esthetician must possess. The overall objective of this text is to prepare students for careers in the diversified areas of skin care, including the cosmetic industry.

• This textbook has been designed to provide students with the skills required to render professional services and pass State Licensing Examinations. It gives students a thorough understanding of both the theory and practice of all pertinent subjects dealing with skin care, and provides special emphasis on the application of cosmetics.

• The complete course of study allows for flexibility so that instructors and students can adapt the material to the system they find to be most practical and effective.

• Headings and sub-headings are highlighted in red and prominently displayed to provide the instructor with an outline to facilitate the presentation of subject matter.

• Students can use the topic headings to locate and identify subject matter more readily, and to isolate specific subjects for concentrated study.

• Each chapter in the text is a complete unit of study that can be shortened or lengthened to meet the needs of the instructor's personalized lesson plans.

• Students will derive maximum benefit from the text by practical performance, demonstrations, and practice employed in conjunction with the study of the theory. Students will achieve the physical dexterity and manipulative skills required of the professional esthetician.

• To further aid the instructor and student, the text contains an extensive glossary/index of terms, illustrations (with some highlighted in red for added emphasis and instructional value), and charts. Objectives are listed at the beginning of each chapter, and each chapter is followed by suggested questions and topics for discussion and review. These elements are of great value when utilized as a means of summarizing the main topics of each chapter.

• The content of the text is arranged in a sequence generally preferred by professional estheticians. Detailed, step-by-step procedures, and up-to-date information has been included to keep pace with industry trends.

• An attractive and instructional four-color section is included. The pages are arranged by topic to follow the sequential order of the text. The four-color illustrations and photographs depict some of the more important subject areas covered in the text, such as: anatomy and physiology, disorders of the skin, cleansing and massage, machines and apparatus for professional skin care, advanced topics in esthetics, and color theory.

• Graduating students will be better qualified to enter the job market and to realize their career goals.

• A selection of supplementary materials is available for the student and for the instructor to accompany this text. They include: *Milady's Standard Workbook for Professional Estheticians, Milady's State Exam Review for Professional Estheticians, Lesson Plans for Milady's Standard Textbook for Professional Estheticians,* and *Professional Skincare Techniques* (8 videocassettes featuring Joel Gerson).

A Message from the Author

It was more than a decade ago that I sat at this same desk to write the first edition of *Milady's Standard Textbook for Professional Estheticians*. I gave up my position as vice president of a cosmetics firm so that I could devote my time and energy to writing this book. At the time, our industry was in desperate need of a basic text, and I am proud to say that this book has become the most widely used esthetic skin care textbook in the world today, and has helped set the industry standard. It is used in such countries as Australia, South Africa, the United Kingdom and Japan.

Writing this text has also been richly rewarding for me because I was able to share with you, the future esthetician, cosmetician and makeup artist, the techniques, methods, and knowledge based on my many years of experience. As an esthetician you will work closely with your clients. It is rewarding to know that the improvement the client sees in his or her skin has been brought about by your knowledge and skill as a professional esthetician. To experience success, knowing this principle is not enough; you must put it into practice every day.

Milady's Standard Textbook for Professional Estheticians will show you the way to become confident as a professional esthetician. This course of study and the guidance of your instructor will help you to achieve your goals in the exciting, lucrative, and rewarding field of esthetics. I congratulate you on the profession you have chosen. Have no doubt that if your mind is set on success, if you have feelings of concern and well-being for others, use your creative imagination, love what you are doing, and "dare to be different," then you too, will be successful.

GOOD LUCK!

Joel Gerson

New York, New York
1992

Acknowledgments

We wish to thank the following people and organizations for their various contributions to this textbook. These contributions include photographs, illustrations, permissions, and much valued advice.

Contributors and editors: Patricia Borcik, H.J. Gambino, Tama Kieves, Bobbi Ray Madry, Alfonso Peña-Ramos, and Patricia Roberts.

Reviewers: Rafael E. Acosta, Jonell Baldwin, Edwina Bogosian, Vicki Lynn Hummell, Dorothy Lemstrom, Kim Litzenberger, Gail E. Mangold, Florence A. March, Renee Poignard, Michael Prevette, Wallace A. Roberts, and Judy Thelen.

Sherrell J. Aston, M.D., F.A.C.S., New York, NY, for the photographs of cosmetic surgery reprinted by permission.

Robert Dorr, color specialist, author of *The Color Key System*, Woodland Hills, CA, for the color chart reprinted by permission.

Elizabeth Fong, Elvira B. Ferris, and Esther G. Skelley, authors of *Body Structures & Functions*, Seventh Edition, for illustrations on anatomy and physiology reprinted by permission.

Karl Laden, Ph.D., bio-chemist/author; Fellow of the Society of Cosmetic Chemists; for technical information.

Lydia O'Leary, Inc., for photographs of corrective makeup, permission of Lydia O'Leary, New York, NY.

Norman Orentreich, M.D., P.C., Orentreich Medical Group, New York, NY, for photographs of Dermabrasion reprinted by permission.

Simona Morini, author of *Encyclopedia of Health and Beauty*, permission of publisher Bobbs-Merrill Company, Inc., Indianapolis, IN, for illustrations and technical information.

Gerd Plewig, M.D., and Albert M. Kligman, M.D., Ph.D., authors of *Acne Morphogenesis and Treatment*, permission of publishers Springer-Verlag, New York and Berlin, for photographs and technical information.

Mark Richard, for photographs of chemical peeling reprinted by permission.

Ellis Rottman, Director, Communications Staff, Food and Drug Administration, U.S. Department of Health, Education and Welfare, Rockville, MD.

Dr. Lee SaintMartin, for photographs of chemical peeling reprinted by permission.

J. Bedford Shelmire, Jr., M.D., author of *The Art of Looking Younger*, permission of publisher, St. Martin's Press, New York, NY, for photographs.

Genevieve Love Smith, Phyllis E. Davis, and Jean Tannis Dennerll, authors of *Medical Terminology—A Programmed Text*, 6th Edition for illustrations on anatomy and physiology reprinted by permission.

Barbara Snelling, Departments Editor, *The Body Forum Magazine*, Atlanta, GA, for permission to use "The Complete Vitamin Chart," and for information about human nutrition.

Superintendent of Documents, Metric Information, U.S. Government Printing Office, Washington, DC.

Edward J. Tezak, Ph.D., author of *Salon Management for Cosmetology Students*, published by Milady Publishing Company, Albany, NY.

Ungerer and Company, New York, NY, for the introduction on aromatherapy.

Charles W. Whitmore, M.D. and William H. Young, Ph.D., authors of *A Complete Guide to Skin and Hair for the Cosmetologist*, permission of Educational Research Foundation, Lynchburg, VA, for technical information and quotation.

Jacob J. Yahm, consultant for Milady Publishing Company, Albany, NY.

Jonathan Zizmor, M.D. and John Foreman, authors of *Dr. Zizmor's Skin Care Book*, permission of publisher, Holt, Rinehart & Winston, Inc., New York, NY, for technical information and quotation.

Career Opportunities for the Professional Esthetician

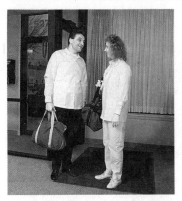

Welcome to the world of esthetics.

How would you like to perform a facial on a movie star or apply his or her makeup? Or how about a career where you travel frequently and demonstrate up to the minute cosmetic products to audiences around the country? When you complete your training and acquire the license to practice as an esthetician and makeup artist, exciting and unlimited opportunities await you. Buckle up. With your license in hand, you're on your way to a lifetime career in a dynamic and prestigious industry.

As an esthetician or makeup artist you can exercise your creative abilities in a stable career that rewards talent. Best of all, for the amount of preparation time and expense you put in, no other field offers as many job opportunities.

Growing Interest in Skin Care

In recent years, the public has grown more interested in the health and beauty of their skin than ever before. Skin care salons and new beauty services have cropped up to satisfy the public's rising interest. As the demand for these new services soars, more positions await licensed professionals.

The sale of grooming products for men and women has grown rapidly into a multi-million dollar a year business. As men and women spend more money on how to look and feel their best, they also require professional advice as to how to use the products they purchase. For example, women, especially, want to know how to apply facial makeup. And both sexes desire guidance on keeping their skin looking healthy and youthful.

The sale of new cosmetics and new grooming services has boosted the profits and growth of the personal care and beauty culture industry. This means salons earn more than ever and so do licensed estheticians.

In the past, salons offered only traditional services such as haircare, hairstyling, and caring for wigs and hairpieces. Today, modern salons offer some or all of the following special services:

1. Skin care (esthetics) and facials
2. Makeup application for daytime, evening, and special occasions
3. Corrective and therapeutic skin care and makeup
4. Eyebrow shaping, eyelash application
5. Manicuring (care of the hands and nails)
6. Pedicuring (care of the feet and legs)
7. Removal of unwanted hair on the face and body
8. Consultations to coordinate colors of hair, makeup, and fashions

Defining Our Terms

Here are some terms commonly used to refer to various professionals in the professional esthetics field:

ESTHETICIANS *Estheticians* specialize in skin care rather than hairstyling. They may also manufacture, sell, or apply cosmetics. As highly trained specialists, estheticians provide preventative care for skin and offer treatments to keep skin healthy and attractive. Unless the esthetician is also a licensed dermatologist, he or she does not prescribe medication or give medical treatments. However, the esthetician is trained to detect skin problems that require medical attention.

The name esthetician comes from the French "Esthétique," a branch of philosophy relating to the nature and forms of beauty. In many states estheticians must have a cosmetology license before specializing in skin care, facial massage, and makeup application.

COSMETICIANS *Cosmeticians* have cosmetology licenses and perform a variety of personal services in salons.

BEAUTY THERAPISTS *Beauty therapists* perform services that are intended to remedy or alleviate a disorder or undesirable condition.

PRACTITIONER The term *practitioner* refers to anyone who practices a particular art or profession.

MAKEUP ARTISTS *Makeup artists* have been trained to embellish or beautify the facial features by the skillful application of cosmetics. They work in salons or can expand into theatrical (character) makeup. Many makeup artists are also cosmetologists and/or estheticians. The makeup artist assists clients in selecting and applying skin care and beauty products, attempting to create the best look for the individual. Makeup artists specializing in television and theatrical makeup often serve an apprenticeship under a master makeup artist.

DERMATOLOGISTS A *dermatologist* is a physician who specializes in dermatology, the branch of medical science that relates to the skin and its diseases. A dermatologist acquires the necessary qualifications to prescribe internal and external medication and to apply mechanical apparatus for the benefit of the skin.

PLASTIC SURGEONS *Plastic surgeons* perform surgery that restores or heals lost, wounded, or deformed parts of the face, head, and body. Plastic surgeons often work on victims of accidents or those who suffer from diseases, burns, or birth deformities. A plastic surgeon may specialize in cosmetic surgery, the art of improving and/or restoring physical attractiveness.

Estheticians and makeup artists often work with the patients of plastic surgeons at the recommendation of the surgeon. Estheticians and makeup artists teach patients preventative and maintenance skin care and/or how to use makeup skillfully to conceal scars and imperfections.

RESTORATIVE ART SPECIALISTS *Restorative art specialists* restore the facial features of the deceased. They have been trained in the scientific aspects of cosmetology and mortuary science. Cosmetologists and estheticians sometimes work as assistants to morticians and restorative art specialists. (In some states only a licensed mortician may work on the deceased.)

Opportunities for Licensed Estheticians in the Cosmetic Industry

MERCHANDISING The merchandising field offers many opportunities to licensed estheticians. Salons, department stores, boutiques, and specialty businesses employ estheticians as salespersons and sales managers, who often work their way up to top management positions and ownership of businesses.

Manager or Salesperson As a salesperson, your duties would include keeping records of sales and stock on hand, demonstrating products, selling to clients, and cashiering. You must have thorough product knowledge and be able to answer questions authoritatively and help clients select cosmetics that suit their individual skin types and colors. In many cases, you might answer the telephone and schedule appointments. Since salespeople serve the public, a polished appearance, pleasant manner, and good communication skills are definite assets.

The sales manager must have the same qualities as the salesperson, but he or she assumes more responsibility. The sales manager runs the entire cosmetic department and trains and directs salespersons.

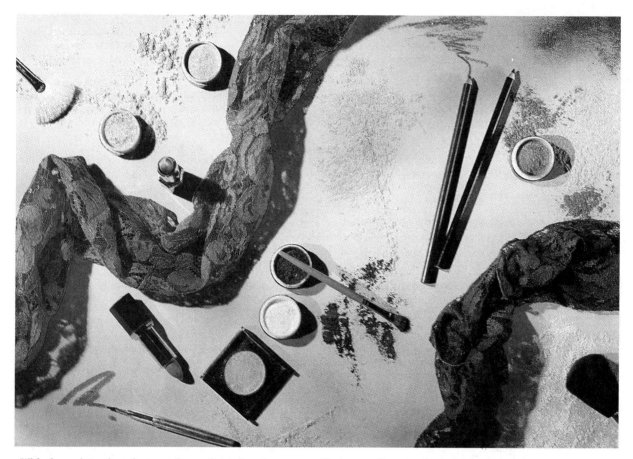

With the variety of products on the market today, the opportunities are endless for the licensed esthetician in the cosmetics industry.

Cosmetic Buyer or Assistant Buyer   As a buyer of cosmetics in a department store, salon, or specialty business, you must keep up with the latest products advertised in the industry. Buyers travel frequently, visiting markets, trade shows, and cosmetic manufacturer's showrooms. As a buyer, you must estimate the amount of stock your operation will need for a period of time, and you must keep records of purchases and sales. The buyer's assistant places orders, keeps records of inventory, and assists the buyer in any way necessary.

Manufacturer's Representative   Manufacturers employ men and women as representatives to explain and/or demonstrate how to use the company's products. As a representative, you call on salons, drug stores, department stores, and specialty businesses to build new clientele and increase product sales. For this position, you must have a neat appearance, an outgoing personality, and sales ability. As a representative, you can expect to travel a great deal, exhibiting products at trade shows and conventions.

Direct Sales, Demonstrations, Sales Presentations

As a licensed esthetician, you may sell directly to consumers as owner of a new cosmetic and toiletry line, or you may become a distributor for an already established cosmetic firm.

When selling cosmetics by way of party plans (one form of direct selling), the director stocks the cosmetic line to be distributed and supervises his or her managers and consultants. The consultant carries a sample kit and calls on clients at home. As a consultant, you would demonstrate products, help customers select specific items, take orders, and see that those orders are filled and delivered. You would also keep records of total sales and money received.

Managers direct consultants and directors supervise managers. Directors, managers, and consultants are usually paid on a commission basis and those who exceed their sales quota may win incentive prizes. While selling cosmetics, these professionals often sell other items such as jewelry and fragrances.

Home party or professional presentations for clubs and organizations are other forms of direct selling. In every avenue of direct selling, the beauty professional aims to help consumers select appropriate items to encourage regular clientele who will purchase their cosmetics from local or regional studios or outlets.

SCIENTIFIC

Manufacturers constantly compete with one another to produce newer and better products. That's why an esthetician with an additional background in science, such as cosmetic chemistry, will usually find opportunities in this field. Some positions, though, require advanced scientific training. But you can look for job opportunities that offer on-the-job training.

Research and Research Assistants

Research and development of cosmetic and grooming products is an active and ongoing process. Most directors of cosmetic research have backgrounds in chemistry, physics, biology, and other subjects of value to a scientist. As a research director or assistant, you run laboratory tests (often on animals) to determine the safety of products before the company distributes them.

Facial treatments, cosmetics, and practically all new products undergo extensive testing before they reach the public. Sometimes products are tested on volunteers for allergic reactions. The Food and Drug Administration (FDA) requires that products labeled "hypoallergenic" be thoroughly tested and manufacturers document whatever claims they make about their product.

As a research director or assistant, you may also conduct consumer reports and surveys. You must be able to write and prepare accurate reports for scientific journals. Since performing research often requires telephone work, a pleasant speaking voice is a plus. The research director or assistant who can lecture or present his or her findings to interested groups will increase his or her value to the company.

Trade Technicians and Technical Supervisors

General technicians are usually responsible to a technical supervisor or advisor who works in the home office of the manufacturer. Technicians must know the formulas and ingredients used in the company's products and be especially familiar with business operations. As a technician, you will often introduce new products and demonstrate their uses. You may appear at trade shows and call on salons and department and drugstores.

The technical supervisor handles customers' inquiries and complaints. The supervisor may also be involved in public relations and promotional activities.

Specialist in Restorative Art or Assistant to a Mortician

If you wish to pursue a career in mortuary science, a background in cosmetology and esthetics will benefit you immensely. As part of a mortuary education, you will learn restorative art, the preparing of the deceased. Many people believe that viewing the deceased has a comforting psychological effect on bereaving family and friends and the custom is widely practiced. Restoration work requires a high degree of skill and must be performed under the direction of a mortician. The esthetician or cosmetologist works only on cosmetic preparation and application.

COMMUNICATIONS Beauty Editor of a Newspaper, Magazine, or Journal

If you have talent and training in journalism, you may wish to pursue a career as a beauty editor or editor's assistant. As a beauty editor, you might write about manufacturer's products to stimulate readers' interest and boost product sales. You may write a daily or weekly column, a "question and answer" column, feature articles, or educational books and brochures distributed to teachers. The beauty editor may also lecture, do fashion coordination and commentary, and make media appearances.

Advertising and Sales Promotion

Cosmetics and grooming products are heavily advertised on television and radio and in magazines and newspapers. As an advertising and sales promotion writer, you must design ads and commercials that will make your products highly desirable to the public. You must also write the materials enclosed in packages and the information on labels. You must write clearly so that consumers understand the information you wish to communicate. Advertising and sales promotion writers often work with photographers and television technicians to create commercial messages. They may be involved in the production of audio-visual programs used in classrooms to educate the consumer.

Freelance Writing and Lecturing

Many magazines accept articles for publication written by freelance writers. If you can write and you also know the field of cosmetics, you may be hired by a number of manufacturers and advertising agencies. In these positions, you write informational booklets, brochures, ads, and articles. The freelance writer may also lecture and appear as a guest speaker at conventions, clubs, schools, and other organizations.

Personnel Manager   Large cosmetic and grooming products companies generally staff a personnel manager. The personnel manager knows about the company's products as well as the scope of job requirements throughout the company. As a personnel manager, you must be able to interview people for various job openings that arise within the company and hire competent people who will benefit your team of professionals.

Opportunities for Experienced, Licensed Estheticians in Education

PUBLIC, VOCATIONAL, AND TECHNICAL SCHOOLS Teacher of Skin Care and Makeup   If you want to teach cosmetics or esthetics in a public, vocational, industrial, or technical high school, you must meet the same requirements as other teachers of career prep courses. You must be trained in curriculum and lesson planning, classroom management, and presentation techniques.

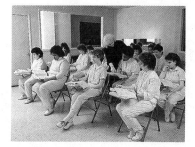

There are opportunities for licensed estheticians in the educational field.

Teacher of Related Subjects   As a licensed esthetician, you may find that you wish to acquire additional certification in order to teach subjects related to the field of cosmetology such as home economics, health, nutrition, or mortuary science. Many subjects relate to a career in cosmetology.

Substitute or Part-Time Teacher   You might prefer to do substitute or part-time teaching while pursuing other areas of interest. Contact your local Board of Education to register for substitute and part-time teaching jobs.

Department Head or Assistant   As a licensed cosmetologist or esthetician, you may be interested in acquiring the necessary degree of certification to head a department of cosmetology or esthetics in a public or private school. These positions require administrative and supervisory skills.

As an assistant to the department head, you must be highly qualified. You would assist in managing the department, planning curriculums, keeping records, preparing examinations and cooperating with the school guidance counselor. This department also works closely with the State Department on licensing and curriculum requirements.

PRIVATE COSMETOLOGY SCHOOLS
Teacher of Skin Care

Many private cosmetology schools or schools for estheticians and makeup artists have a teacher training program for promising graduates. Some states require a teacher to train in teaching all subjects, while others require teachers to specialize in one area. Some teacher training courses are prescribed by the State Department. As a teacher, you must keep up with developments in the educational field and new beauty products entering the market. Many teachers attend workshops and conferences to keep up to date on their knowledge. As an esthetician, you may specialize in teaching skin care, makeup styling, eyelash application, and the removal of unwanted hair.

Teacher of Related Subjects

The job market is limited to professionals wishing to specialize in the fascinating and highly technical field of theatrical makeup. You may have to do an apprenticeship in addition to extensive training in order to become a teacher of advanced theatrical makeup. As an esthetician, you may find job opportunities to investigate while teaching skin care, makeup styling, and advanced makeup artistry. All teachers must know their subjects thoroughly and be able to impart their knowledge to students.

School Director or Owner

A large number of private school owners and directors started their careers as general practitioners, while others became directors of departments in public schools. The director of a school or a department within a school has many duties, including preparing the curriculum and making certain that the physical qualifications of the school meet state standards. As the director, you would work with teachers and counsel students with respect to licensing and placement. You would also work with trade and school organizations and other educational authorities.

To be a successful teacher, supervisor, dean, director, registrar, or school owner requires a good sense of commercial operations, a thorough knowledge of the business, and the ability to direct people and get along with them. These professionals dedicate themselves to improving the beauty culture industry by working together in associations on national, state, and local levels. They help establish, amend, and repeal state laws and regulations, improve and standardize curriculums, and insure the professionalism of the entire industry.

OUTSIDE COSMETOLOGY SCHOOLS
State Licensing Inspector or Examiner

Most states have laws governing cosmetology and personal services and give examinations periodically for cosmetology and related licenses. As a licensed, experienced cosmetologist and/or esthetician, you may become a state inspector or examiner. As a state examiner, you prepare and conduct examinations, announce and enforce rules and regulations, investigate complaints, and conduct hearings. To insure that rules and regulations are enforced and ethical practices are maintained, each state employs a team of inspectors to cover specified territories throughout the year. These teams inspect salons to see that managers and employees are conforming to official rules and regulations. For example, individual licenses must be on display and all sanitary practices must be strictly observed.

State Licensing Member

Members of state licensing organizations must be highly qualified and experienced in their specific professions. They conduct examinations, grant licenses, and inspect schools to see that certain physical standards, such as space and equipment, are maintained. In addition, they see that educational materials meet certain specifications. The chairperson of the board is usually a full-time employee, but other members may be school owners or people in related professions.

Education Director for a Manufacturer

Manufacturers of cosmetics and other products frequently employ licensed cosmetologists and estheticians as education directors. As an education director, you would educate the public about the manufacturer's products and conduct seminars for teachers of consumer education. As part of the manufacturer's consumer education program, education directors appear at conventions to display products, talk with teachers about the merits of the products, and distribute educational materials for classroom use. Education directors may also be workshop or seminar directors, lecturers, and/or writers.

Guest Artist or Demonstrator

As a professional esthetician, you may find that some jobs require traveling to conventions and other events to demonstrate products, techniques, and/or equipment to prospective buyers and the general public. As a guest artist or demonstrator, you would demonstrate skin care and makeup techniques. You might appear in the cosmetic section of a department store to promote a new line of products or to promote existing products and services.

Some manufacturers of products hire trained estheticians and makeup artists as directors of home party plans. The director supervises the managers, and the managers supervise salespersons. The salespersons make contacts (usually women) who act as party hostesses. The hostess receives a gift and sometimes a profit on the total sales made to guests. Guests usually receive samples of cosmetics and lessons in how to apply makeup artfully. The salespeople aim to entice guests to become regular clientele.

Opportunities in Specialized Careers and Salons for Licensed Estheticians

SALONS
Esthetician—
Skin Care Specialist

As an esthetician, you perform as a skin care consultant and specialist. You perform facials and facial massage, manually and with the aid of machines. You must keep records of the services you provide and the products you use. You must always behave pleasantly towards clients and you must sell products. You may also apply makeup artfully when clients request personal application.

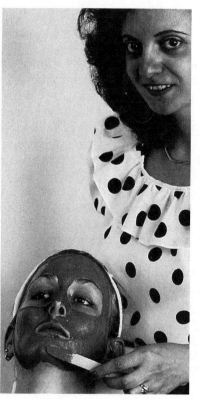

Skin care specialist/esthetician

Makeup Artist

As a makeup artist, you may offer facials and facial massage as part of your services, or concentrate only on makeup application. You must have a keen eye for color and color coordination in order to select the most becoming cosmetic shades for the individual's personal coloring of hair, skin, and eyes. Makeup artists in salons work on a sales commission basis and/or salary.

Salon Manager, Supervisor,
or Owner

As an esthetician or makeup specialist, you can work your way up to management and/or supervisory positions. After some success and experience, you may open your own salon or buy an established business.

There are also opportunities to acquire franchises and establish one of a chain of name salons. Most private salon or franchise owners have multiple responsibilities. In addition to running the business, you may perform any one or all of the services your business offers. However, as an esthetician or makeup artist, you may prefer to limit your services to the areas of skin care and makeup.

Department stores and hotels generally operate full service salons.

SPECIAL ASSISTANTS
Assistant to a Dermatologist or Cosmetic Surgeon

In addition to other related subjects, cosmetology and esthetics include the study of the structure and function of the skin. This gives the esthetician a better understanding of the nature of a dermatologist's and cosmetic surgeon's services. An assistant to a dermatologist or to a cosmetic surgeon may work as a receptionist and/or secretary. A knowledge of advanced skin care and makeup techniques will prove invaluable. For example, following cosmetic surgery, a female patient may need to know the type of makeup, if any, she should use while her skin heals.

Research Specialist or Assistant

A research specialist or assistant is employed by a cosmetic manufacturer to research and test new products. This type of job appeals to professionals who enjoy working in a laboratory or research environment. This position usually requires a background in cosmetic chemistry.

MAKEUP ARTISTS
Makeup Artist for Portrait or Commercial Photography

A photographer may have need for a full-time makeup artist, or the artist may combine his or her work with secretarial and bookkeeping duties. The makeup artist may also be a photographer's assistant, helping with set designs and makeup, or assisting with bridal photographs. For fashion photography, the makeup artist may be needed to apply special makeup on the featured models. Magazine advertising layouts often call for ultra-fashionable hairstyles and makeup to call attention to the product or fashion being photographed.

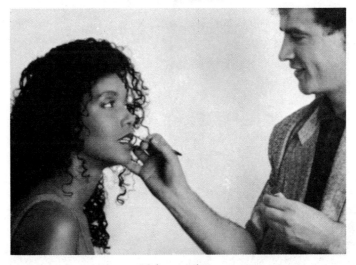

Makeup artistry

Makeup Artist for Television, Stage, Motion Pictures, and Fashion Shows

For this highly competitive field, you may need a lengthy apprenticeship and acceptance by a makeup artist's union. Most major television and motion picture productions are shot on the east or west coast and this may limit the number of jobs available. The same holds true for theatrical productions and large fashion shows; however, many cities support a community theater, and most large department stores produce fashion shows. In many cases when full-time work as a makeup artist is not available, the makeup artist can combine his or her position with other duties in the department store or theater.

Esthetician and Makeup Artist for Resorts, Cruise Ships, and Health Spas

Resorts, cruise ships, and beauty and health spas operate full service salons that offer full or part-time employment. Services include facials, facial massage, and makeup and related services, such as eyebrow shaping, manicuring, pedicuring, and unwanted hair removal. In addition to offering personal services, these companies provide special demonstrations in skin care and makeup techniques to interested groups.

Note: Some jobs require more extensive training in scientific and medical subjects.

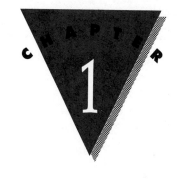

Your Professional Image

LEARNING OBJECTIVES   *After completing this chapter, you should be able to:*

❶ Discuss the importance of personal and public hygiene.
❷ Explain the importance of correct posture for standing and sitting.
❸ Demonstrate good human relations and a professional attitude.
❹ Define professional ethics.

INTRODUCTION

Your professional image is your credibility, and your success as an esthetician will depend on the credibility that you build with clients. Although many people think of image as only the exterior, in reality it is a projection of our innermost self. When you cultivate a good, professional image, you are developing those inner traits that will make you valuable to your clients and others. In this chapter we will ask you to look at yourself, and then at how you relate to other people, with an emphasis on the things you *do*, rather than simply on what you think or believe. After all, you project an image by *doing*, not simply by being.

Hygiene

Hygiene is the branch of applied science that deals with healthful living. It includes both personal and public hygiene.

PERSONAL HYGIENE   *Personal hygiene* concerns the intelligent care taken by the individual to preserve health by following the rules of healthful living, especially as they relate to such aspects as:

1. Cleanliness
2. Oral Hygiene
3. Posture
4. Exercise
5. Relaxation
6. Adequate Sleep
7. Balanced Diet
8. Healthy Attitude

PUBLIC HYGIENE   To protect the health of the public, people suffering from an infectious or contagious disease must not be allowed to attend a school for cosmetologists, estheticians, or makeup artists. Nor should they work in a salon or department store where there may be danger of infecting other persons. A thorough physical examination is required of all persons seeking to be licensed to work in any area of the cosmetology field.

HYGIENE AND GOOD GROOMING   *Appearance*—Present a clean, neat, and attractive appearance.

Daily Bath or Shower and Use of Deodorant—Bathe or shower daily. Use cologne and other fragrances sparingly.

Oral Hygiene (Teeth and Breath)—Brush your teeth regularly, especially after meals and at bedtime. Use mouthwash to help eliminate unpleasant breath odor. Have regular dental and physical checkups.

Hairstyle and Facial Makeup (Women)—Keep your hair clean and lustrous. Wear an attractive, up-to-date hairstyle that flatters your face and features. Keep your eyebrows well groomed. Use cosmetics that enhance your natural beauty—never over or poorly apply.

Hairstyle, Beard and/or Mustache (Men)—Keep your hair clean and lustrous. Wear an attractive and up-to-date hairstyle. Trim excess hair from nostrils, if necessary. If you choose to wear a beard or mustache, keep it styled and trimmed.

Clothing and Shoes—Uniforms, or whatever clothing you wear to work, should be neat, clean, and properly fitted, selected to project a conservative, professional image, rather than a sexy or super-stylish one.

Hands and Nails—Hands should be clean at all times and nails well cared for. A woman who prefers colored polish should be sure that it is never smeared or chipped.

A HEALTHFUL WAY OF LIFE A healthy person will usually have a clear complexion, luxuriant hair, and bright, clear eyes. Guard your health by allowing yourself sufficient exercise and recreation with fresh air and sunshine, and by keeping a healthful diet through well-balanced meals.

Exercise and Recreation—Whether through walking, dancing, sports, or gym activities, exercise and recreation keep the muscles firm and strong and help you stay alert and energetic by enhancing the flow of nutrients and oxygen throughout your body. As with anything, exercise can be overdone, and care should be taken to avoid overexposure to the sun.

A Healthful Diet—A diet is not an attempt to lose weight; it's whatever you eat! Eating well-balanced meals and drinking sufficient water helps us stay healthy by avoiding malnutrition. Both over- or undereating can cause serious health problems. Read up on good nutrition, and consult your doctor if you make any major changes in your diet.

FATIGUE *Fatigue or tiredness,* resulting from work, exercise, mental effort, or the strain caused by hurry and worry tends to drain the body of its vitality. Therefore, an adequate amount of sleep, not less than seven hours, is necessary. This allows the body to recover from the fatigue of the day's activities and replenish itself with renewed energy. A refreshed body and mind contribute to a sense of well-being.

A HEALTHY ATTITUDE *The mind and body operate as a unit.* A well-balanced condition of body and mind results in good health. This enables them to perform all their functions normally. A healthy attitude can be cultivated by self-control. In place of worry and fear, the health-giving qualities of cheerfulness, courage, and hope should be encouraged. Outside interests and recreation relieve the strain of monotony and hard work.

THOUGHTS AND EMOTIONS *Thoughts* and *emotions* influence body activities. An angry thought may cause the face to turn red and increase the heart action. A thought may either stimulate or depress the functions of the body. Strong emotions, such as worry, anger, and fear, have a harmful effect on the heart, arteries, and glands. Mental depression weakens the functions of the organs, thereby lowering the resistance of the body to disease.

> **Note:** Good grooming adds to self-esteem. Observing the rules of hygienic living, cultivating positive attitudes, and keeping emotions under control, help you to project yourself as a successful esthetician.

Posture and Visual Poise

Correct posture is vitally important to your body because it helps to prevent fatigue, improves your personal appearance, and permits graceful movements in relation to your everyday work as an esthetician.

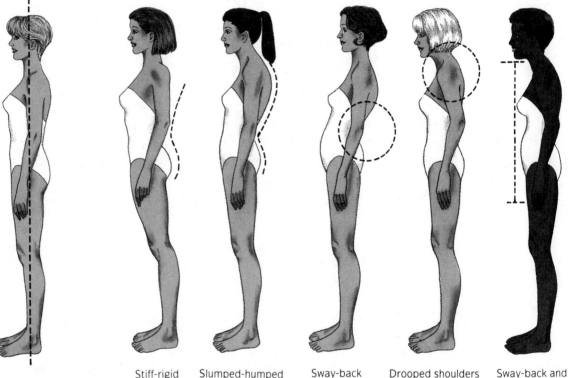

Stiff-rigid (poor posture)   Slumped-humped (poor posture)   Sway-back   Drooped shoulders   Sway-back and drooped shoulders

1.1—Good posture

1.2—Five defective body postures

Good posture is an important part of personal care. Its continued practice assists in the prevention of many physical disturbances. In addition, it is a self-disciplinary factor which contributes to the development of other good habits. These are determining elements of a gracious and pleasing personality. When present, they indicate a poised, well-ordered individual (Fig. 1.1).

Consult your doctor if you suffer from severe or chronic pain in your back, joints, or muscles. "Toughing it out" will only lead to exhaustion, and may cause permanent injury.

Salon owners consider appearance, visual poise, and personality to be almost as important to the esthetician as technical knowledge and manual skills.

STANDING   *Regular exercise* keeps the muscles of the body in good condition and assists in forming the habits of good posture. Practice trains the muscles to hold the body correctly. Avoid slouching, humped shoulders, and spinal curvature (sway-back) while working (Fig. 1.2).

To *walk and stand* correctly, and to attain good body balance, distribute your body weight properly.

People who are on their feet for long hours should stand with their feet close enough together so that the body weight is distributed onto the balls of the feet rather than onto the heels. When one foot (either the left or right) is placed slightly ahead of the other, it is easier to balance the body weight. Good balance, muscle control, and coordination of the hands and feet help to prevent fatigue.

This is the basic (at ease) stance for men and women:

1. Turn the left foot out at a forty-five degree angle.
2. Point the right foot straight ahead with the heel at the instep of the left foot. The right foot may also be placed several inches ahead of the left. This is usually more comfortable.
3. Keep both knees slightly flexed (flexed knees act as shock absorbers when walking or standing) with the right knee bent inward.

The basic stance enables you to shift your weight from one foot to another easily. Place the left foot forward with the right foot angled when it is more practical to do so.

CORRECT YOUR POSTURE   Use a mirror to note the defects that need to be corrected, then observe the following good posture rules:

1. Carry the weight on the balls of your feet, not on the heels. Imagine a plumb-line falling from your shoulder, and stand so that it falls just forward of the ankle.
2. Keep your knees flexed.
3. Keep your shoulders back. You don't have to stand at attention, but you should be close to it.
4. Hold your abdomen in. Even if you're not overweight, poor posture can give you a protruding abdomen.
5. Hold your head high. This gives you the appearance of confidence and reduces aching shoulders as well.

Benefits of Good Posture   It is important to maintain good posture.

1. It gives a feeling of confidence.
2. Good posture helps build good health by allowing the inner organs room to function properly.
3. "Standing tall" helps to improve your speech by freeing the power-source of your voice, the diaphragm.
4. Proper body alignment contributes to a dynamic personality.

CORRECT SITTING POSTURE   Just as there is a mechanically correct posture for standing, so is there one for sitting.

1. Place your feet on the floor directly under your knees.
2. Have the seat of the chair even with your knees. This will allow the upper and lower legs to form a ninety-degree angle at the knees.
3. Allow your feet to carry the weight of your thighs.
4. Rest the weight of your torso on the thigh bones, not on the end of your spine.
5. Keep your torso erect.
6. Make sure your chair is at the correct height so that the upper and lower parts of your arm form a right angle when you are working.
7. Sit well back in the chair.
8. Never slouch.

CORRECT LIFTING TECHNIQUE   When you lift something heavy, be sure to use the weightlifter's method, or you may cause a rupture or a slipped disk. Lift with your back straight, pushing with the heavy thigh muscles, never the back muscles. Further, know how heavy the object you are lifting is. You can hurt your back just as severely by lifting a light object your muscles expected to be heavy as you can by lifting a heavy object incorrectly.

CORRECT STOOPING OR BENDING TECHNIQUE   To pick up an article from the floor:

1. Place your feet close together.
2. Keep your back perpendicular to the floor as you bend your knees.
3. Lift with the muscles of your legs and buttocks, not with the back.

Hand and Nail Grooming

People who represent the beauty industry are expected to practice what they teach. A client will rarely expect perfection from the esthetician, but there is no excuse for bitten nails, ragged cuticles, and rough, red hands. Follow these suggestions for everyday handcare:

1. When you must place your hands in harsh solutions, wear plastic or rubber gloves.
2. Use a protective hand cream or lotion after washing your hands and at bedtime.
3. Keep the cuticles pushed back. Use a cream or oil to keep cuticles soft. Push back the cuticles with a soft cloth after washing your hands.
4. Nail enamel, colored or clear, should never be smeared or chipped.
5. Nails should not be too long and never pointed. They can scratch your client or interfere with your work if they are too long.
6. If you bite or pick your nails, you must break this habit. Your bad habit will be noticed by the client.

Care of Feet

Poorly fitted shoes are often responsible for poor posture, malformed feet, and aching backs. Women should avoid extreme high heels because the weight of the body is thrown forward, exerting an extra strain on the feet and back.

Well fitted shoes give the body support and balance which help to maintain good posture and comfort (Fig. 1.3).

Keep the toenails filed smooth.

Corns, bunions, or ingrown nails should receive care from a chiropodist.

Giving the feet a few minutes of daily care is essential to good posture and good health.

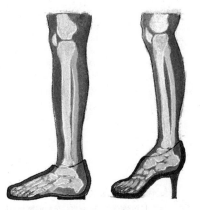

1.3—For comfort and to help maintain good posture, wear well-fitted, low-heeled shoes.

Personality and Human Relations

Your personality is the key to a successful career in the professional world. You can build a personality that helps to open doors to a life full of happy experiences.

Only you can draft the pattern of the "ideal you," who can step through these doors. No one can make you over—*no one but yourself*.

People develop their personalities according to the way they meet their everyday problems. Both the good and the bad situations that affect their lives can be used to strengthen their personalities.

ATTITUDE   Attitude has a great deal to do with personality. It influences your likes and dislikes and your response to people, events, and things. People who meet difficult situations with calmness and who are cheerful, pleasant, and easy to get along with are said to have a healthy attitude toward life.

EMOTIONAL STABILITY   Practice self-control. Realize what a great beautifier serenity is and strive for emotional balance. Develop the qualities of character that command respect, chief among them being emotional stability. Learn to suppress the signs that betray unpleasant emotions: facial grimaces or gestures of anger, impatience, envy or greed. *Always control your temper.*

GRACIOUSNESS   Learn to display pleasant emotions. A smile of greeting and a word of welcome, the willingness to assume the responsibilities of friendship, the ability to fit into new situations and to meet new people with friendliness, all are part of professionalism. A sincere smile sets the mood for warm human relations.

POLITENESS   The root of politeness is thoughtfulness of others. It includes all the little things, such as saying "Thank you," and "Please," treating people with respect, exercising care of other people's property, being tolerant and understanding of other people's efforts, and being considerate of those with whom you work.

SENSE OF HUMOR   Cultivate your sense of humor. Take yourself less seriously. When you can laugh at yourself, you have gained the ability to evaluate realistically your relative personal importance.

Voice and Conversation

Tone of voice, conversational skills, and good language skills equal success. The use of proper grammar and intelligent conversation will serve you well as a professional esthetician.

Remember that success is not made within the salon alone, but depends also on personal contacts, associations, and active participation in many social and business functions.

A PLEASANT SOUND   Cultivate a voice that sounds pleasant and cheerful. Try tape recording yourself and listening for any harshness, whining or sarcastic intonations in your everyday conversations, then focus on replacing these with more positive, friendly speech mannerisms. Speak clearly and loudly enough to be heard without overwhelming.

PLEASANT CONVERSATION   Now is perhaps when you wish you had paid more attention to your English teacher. Relax. You don't have to sound like a college professor. Avoid using slang, vulgarisms, and poor grammar. You will find that speaking correctly becomes a habit, just like good posture.

When speaking with clients, avoid negative statements or topics. Don't ridicule or condemn anything or anybody. Be polite and pleasant. Always stay away from controversial or negative topics.

WHAT YOUR VOICE SHOULD SAY

Your voice is you. That is what it should convey about you.

1. Sincerity—honesty of mind or intention
2. Intelligence—the act of understanding
3. Friendliness—friendly behavior
4. Vitality—vigor and liveliness
5. Flexibility—pliable, not rigid voice tones
6. Expressiveness—the expression of your individuality

Topics to Discuss

Topics to discuss in conversation:

1. Client's personal interests, personal grooming and cosmetic needs
2. Client's own activities
3. Fashions
4. Literature
5. Art
6. Music
7. Education
8. Travel
9. Civic affairs
10. Vacations

Try to understand the client's state of mind and fit your conversation to the client's mood, temperament, and interests.

Conversational Ease

To acquire conversational ease:

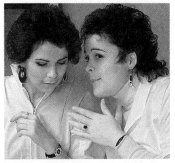

1.4—Nobody likes a person who gossips.

1. Guide the conversation.
2. Do not be argumentative.
3. Be a good listener.
4. Do not monopolize the conversation.
5. Do not become personal by prying into private affairs.
6. Talk about ideas rather than people.
7. Use simple language that all can understand.
8. Never gossip (Fig. 1.4).
9. Be pleasant.
10. Use good language skills.

Topics not to Discuss

Never discuss the following topics:

1. Your own personal problems
2. Religion
3. Other client's poor behavior
4. Your personal affairs
5. Your own financial status
6. Poor workmanship of co-workers
7. Your own health problems
8. Information given to you in confidence

Project Professionalism

Being professional means attending to all the details about yourself and your business. You must be punctual. Your work area must be tidy and clean. You must be prepared for each client and each question. You must genuinely care that each client receives the very best service and products possible.

We've all heard the old saying about never getting a second chance to make a first impression. That's true, but every time a client sees you or speaks with you, whether in the salon or elsewhere, you make another impression. Strive to make sure that it is always a good one.

EVERY CLIENT IS A V.I.P.   Treat all your clients as "Very Important Persons" and you will be rewarded with their loyalty and business. Giving V.I.P. treatment is as simple as following a few basic rules:

1. Be honest but tactful.
2. Be alert, cheerful, and enthusiastic.
3. Be patient and courteous.
4. Be orderly and punctual.
5. Be honest, dependable, and loyal.
6. Be concerned about your clients' needs.
7. Be diligent about educating yourself, so that you can better serve your clients.

Professional Ethics

Ethics deals with the study and philosophy of human conduct, with emphasis on the determination of right and wrong. Simply stated, living by standards of *good ethics* will assure that you are doing what is right as an esthetician, whether personally, socially, or in business. A set of high moral principles and values is a prerequisite for building confidence and developing increased clientele.

GOOD ETHICS   Ethical behavior is a simple, straightforward matter.

1. Be honest, but tactful, with all your clients.
2. Treat all clients fairly and with equal respect.
3. Be dependable in all your dealings with co-workers, clients, and others.
4. Take the initiative in solving problems for your clients and for your salon.
5. Practice the highest standards of professionalism at all times.

POOR ETHICS   Questionable practices, extravagant claims, and unfulfilled promises violate the rules of ethical conduct. These acts cast an unfavorable light on your profession, teachers, and on the entire beauty industry.

Laws, Rules, and Regulations

The successful esthetician must know the laws, rules, and regulations governing esthetics, and must comply with them. By such compliance, the esthetician is contributing to the public's health, welfare, and safety.

STATE LICENSING MEMBERS AND INSPECTORS

The state licensing members and inspectors are charged with maintaining professional standards for competence and ethics. Develop a respectful relationship with them by knowing what their duties, rights, and responsibilities are, and by always dealing with them on a professional level.

QUESTIONS DISCUSSION AND REVIEW

YOUR PROFESSIONAL IMAGE

1. Define hygiene.
2. Define personal hygiene.
3. Define public hygiene.
4. List eight basic requirements for good personal hygiene.
5. How do attitude, thoughts, and emotions affect the body?
6. Name five rules of good posture the esthetician should remember, when giving a service while standing.
7. What are the three rules for standing in the basic stance position?
8. What are three benefits of correct posture?
9. What constitutes good sitting posture?
10. Describe the proper way to lift a heavy object.
11. List six suggestions for hand and nail grooming.
12. List three ways to take good care of your feet.
13. List four desirable qualities to cultivate in your personality.
14. Describe the qualities of a pleasant voice.
15. What are six good topics for conversation between an esthetician and a client?
16. What topics should be avoided when conversing with a client?
17. What are some ways to project professionalism as an esthetician?
18. List the eight rules for treating each client as a V.I.P.
19. Define ethics.
20. List five rules for ethical behavior.
21. How should one deal with state licensing members and inspectors?
22. What is an esthetician's responsibility toward the laws, rules, and regulations governing esthetics?

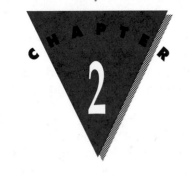

A History of Skin Care and the Use of Cosmetics

2

LEARNING OBJECTIVES

After completing this chapter, you should be able to:

❶ Discuss the different cosmetics used by earlier cultures.
❷ Explain how we have benefited from the health and beauty habits of past cultures.
❸ Discuss and compare the different cosmetic practices, from ancient times to modern day.

INTRODUCTION

The practices of self grooming and cosmetology have their origins in the most ancient culture known, when they were allied with the practice of medicine. Ancient ruins and archeological excavations have given us proof that even in prehistoric times men and women were interested in improving their appearances. Paintings, sculpture, photographs, and the written word are just a few of the means we have of journeying back in history to study the fascinating practices of skin care and the use of cosmetics by early cultures.

People have always endeavored to make themselves more attractive, and men and women have used an endless variety of materials and substances as cosmetics for the skin and hair. As we follow the development of styles in beauty from ancient times to modern days, we may not view all the changes as attractive. What appears beautiful to one group of people may appear unattractive to another group. Most people enjoy change in clothing fashions, in hairstyling, and in the use of cosmetics. This brief history will acquaint you with some of the ways men and women have tried to improve upon nature by changing and enhancing their appearance. You will also learn about some of the materials that have been used for body, skin, and hair care.

Color and Ancient Cosmetics

Ancient records show that coloring matter was used for the hair, skin, and nails, and that tatooing is an ancient practice. Coloring matter was made from berries, bark of trees, minerals, insects, nuts, herbs, leaves, and many other materials, and many of these colors have been used from ancient times to modern days.

Kohl is powder of antimony, a silver white, hard, crystalline, metallic material related to arsenic and tin that is used largely in chemistry and medicine. Kohl was used by the ancient Egyptians as eye makeup. Kohl was often applied to the eyelids to make eyes look larger and brighter. Lamp black was used on the brows and lashes to darken them, and was also used as a form of eyeshadow.

Red oxide of iron was used in the preparation of face paint. Some of the ingredients used in ancient cosmetic preparations would be considered extremely dangerous by modern standards.

The History of Grooming and Cosmetology

EGYPTIANS   The earliest uses of cosmetics have been traced to the ancient Egyptians who used cosmetic preparations generously for their personal use, for religious ceremonies, and for preparing the deceased for burial. The Egyptians used fragrances in their religious ceremonies, and incense was one of their most highly prized forms of fragrance.

The Egyptians believed in cleanliness and built a system for bathing that was later adopted by the Greeks and Romans. After bathing, the Egyptians kept their skin lubricated by applying fragrant oils, lotions, or ointments.

Combs and mirrors were often elaborate toilet articles. Cleopatra, Queen of Egypt (51 B.C.), is said to have used cosmetics and fragrances lavishly on her body, face, hair, and nails. Hairdressing was a fine art and elaborate wigs and headdresses were worn (Fig. 2.1).

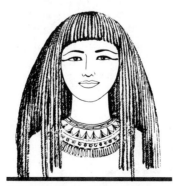

2.1—The ancient Egyptians wore elaborate wigs and headdresses.

HEBREWS   The early Hebrews were also known to be concerned with health and cleanliness. They brought cosmetics and fragrances to Judea from Egypt and manufactured many preparations for the care of the skin, hair, teeth, and nails. Hebrew people were considered to have beautiful, healthy skin and hair. Some of the early books of the Bible speak of fragrances and anointing the heads of guests of honor (Fig. 2.2).

GREEKS   From the Greek word "kŏsmêtikōs" (kos-**MET**-i-kos), meaning skilled in decorating, comes our word "cosmetics."

The cultural advance of the Greeks reached its peak in the years from 460 to about 146 B.C. They made lavish use of perfumes and cosmetics and used them in religious rites, for personal use, and for medicinal purposes.

Greek women used a facial preparation of white lead, applied kohl to their eyes, and used vermillion on their cheeks and lips. Vermillion is a brilliant red pigment consisting of mercuric sulfide, made by grinding cinnabar (the chief ore of mercury) to a fine powder. This product then was mixed with ointment or dusted on the skin in the same way modern cosmetics are applied.

The Greeks believed in cleanliness and built elaborate baths. They also developed excellent methods of dressing the hair and caring for the skin and nails (Fig. 2.3).

ROMANS   The ancient Romans assumed many of the customs of the Greeks and used fragrances and cosmetics lavishly. In about 454 B.C., Roman men began shaving off their facial hair, and a clean shaven face became popular. Women used facials made of milk and bread and sometimes fine wine. A mixture of chalk and white lead was used as a cosmetic for the face. Cheeks and lips were reddened by preparations made from vegetable

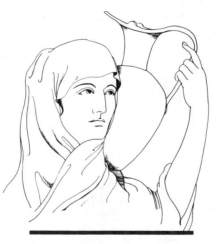

2.2—The early Hebrews were concerned with health and cleanliness.

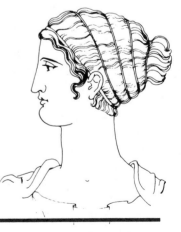

2.3—The Greeks developed excellent methods of dressing the hair.

dyes, and colored makeup was used on the eyelids and eyebrows. Some facials were made of corn, flour and milk, and flour mixed with fresh butter. The Romans formulated various formulas for bleaching and dyeing the hair.

Roman baths were magnificent public buildings with separate sections for men and women. Following the bath, rich oils and other preparations were used to keep the skin healthy and attractive. The Romans had a great variety of fragrances made from flowers, saffron, almonds, and other ingredients. They used many different grooming aids and cosmetics to maintain the health and attractiveness of their skin, hair, and nails.

A number of books were written on the composition of cosmetic preparations, and Roman poets wrote about the virtues of cleanliness and body, hair, and skin care (Fig. 2.4).

ORIENTALS   Orientals have a long and illustrious history of health practices. Grooming was an art among the people who could afford elaborate clothing. Perfumes and other products were formulated for self-care. In China, among the wealthy class, well cared for nails were desirable. In Japan, the makeup of the Geisha is still an intricate and highly stylized art. Orientals are known for their beautiful costumes, arts and crafts, high standards of cleanliness, and adherence to good health habits (Fig. 2.5).

AFRICANS   Africans have, since ancient times, developed many medicines and grooming materials from the substances found in their natural environment. They fashioned intricate and artistic hairstyles and sometimes used various colors of face paint to adorn their faces and bodies. Some of their costumes and hairstyles are seen today in modern versions (Fig. 2.6).

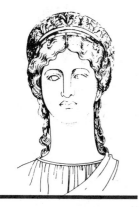

2.4—The ancient Romans used fragrances and cosmetics lavishly.

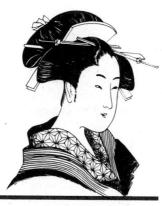

2.5—Orientals have a long and illustrious history of grooming as an art form.

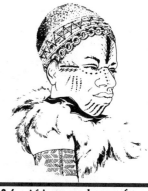

2.6—Africans are known for developing intricate hairstyles and using various color to adorn their faces and bodies.

If we traveled around the world we would find that people everywhere have contributed something to our present day knowledge of medicine, foods, cosmetics, and grooming practices (Fig. 2.7).

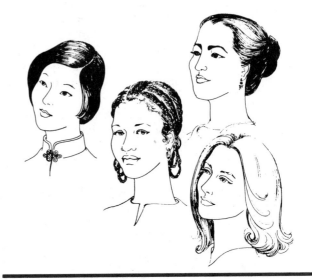

2.7 — We can draw on a variety of styles from studying different cultures.

Periods in History and Cosmetic Practices

THE MIDDLE AGES

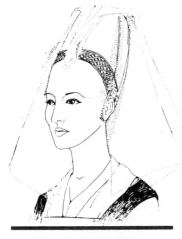

2.8 — The Middle Ages

The Middle Ages is the period in European history between classical antiquity and the Renaissance, usually regarded as extending from the downfall of Rome, 476, to about 1450. This was a time when religion played a prominent role in the lives and customs of the people. Beauty culture was also practiced. Tapestries, sculptures, and artifacts from this period in history show towering headdresses, intricate hairstyles, and the use of cosmetics for the care of the skin and hair. During the Middle Ages, bathing was not a daily ritual, but fragrant oils were used by those who could afford them. Women wore colored makeup on cheeks and lips but not on the eyes. During medieval times cosmetology and medicine were taught as combined subjects in English universities. Cosmetology and medicine were not officially separated until late in the 16th century (Fig. 2.8).

THE RENAISSANCE　The Renaissance is known as the period during which western civilization made the transition from medieval to modern history. It is known as the revival of arts and letters that spread from Italy, in the 14th century, to other countries. During the Renaissance many classical paintings and written records were produced that tell us a great deal about the grooming practices of the time. One of the most unusual practices of the period was the shaving off of the eyebrows and the hairline to show a greater expanse of forehead. The bare brow was thought to give women a look of greater intelligence.

Fragrances and cosmetics were used, but highly colored preparations for lips, cheeks, and eyes were discouraged. Paintings from this period show well-groomed brows, no eye makeup, and faintly colored lips and cheeks. During the Renaissance, there was great pride in physical appearance, and artists created elaborate costumes, combining line and color to produce elegance and harmony. The hair was carefully dressed and ornaments or headdresses worn (Fig. 2.9).

THE ELIZABETHAN ERA　During the reign of Elizabeth I (1558–1603), facial masks were in vogue. Formulas for lotions and packs were made from such ingredients as powdered eggshell, alum, borax and ground almond and poppy seeds. Milk, wine, butter, fruits, and vegetables were also used in cosmetics, and fragrances were used lavishly. Cosmetics were also used to color the cheeks and lips, but eye makeup was not in fashion. Elaborate hairstyles and wigs were popular (Fig. 2.10).

THE AGE OF EXTRAVAGANCE　Marie Antoinette was Queen of France from 1755 to 1793. This era was called the Age of Extravagance. During this time, women of status often bathed in strawberries and milk and used a number of extravagant cosmetic preparations. They used scented powder made from pulverized starch as face powder. Lips and cheeks were often highly colored in pink to orange shades. Small silk patches were used to decorate the face and

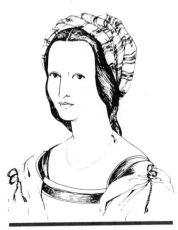

2.9—The Renaissance

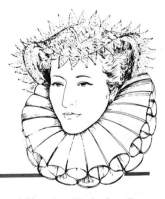

2.10—The Elizabethan Era

conceal blemishes. Eyebrows were shaped and a glossy substance applied to the eyelids, but intensive color was not used on or around the eyes. Men and women who could afford to do so wore enormous powdered wigs and extremely elaborate clothes (Fig. 2.11).

THE VICTORIAN AGE

The Victorian Age relates to the reign of Queen Victoria of England (1837–1901). Fashions in dress, hairstyles, and makeup were drastically influenced by the social mores of the Victorian Age, known as one of the most austere and restrictive periods in history. Makeup and elaborate clothing were discouraged except for use in the theater. In America, people tended to copy the fashions that were in vogue in Europe. Early photographs and paintings show that women used very little facial makeup. However, records show that both men and women had concern for cleanliness and personal care. To preserve the health and beauty of the skin, beauty masks and packs were made from honey, eggs, milk, oatmeal, fruits, vegetables, and other ingredients. Victorian women are said to have pinched their cheeks and bitten their lips to induce natural color, rather than use colored cosmetics, such as lipstick and rouge (Fig. 2.12).

THE 20'S

By the 1920's, industrialization had brought a new prosperity to America. Women were influenced by the clothes, makeup, and hairstyles of the stars of silent films. Women began to bob and Marcel wave their hair, and use eye makeup, lipstick, and rouge. Fashion features from the period were the brightly colored Cupid's bow mouth, and eyeshadow used beneath the lower eyelids. A wide variety of creams, oils, and lotions were manufactured for skin, hair, and body care (Fig. 2.13).

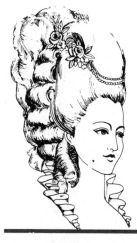

2.11—The Age of Extravagance

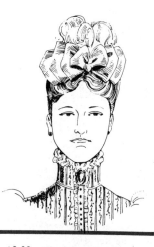

2.12—The Victorian Age

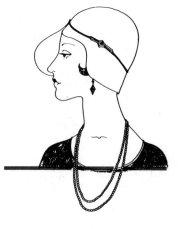

2.13—The 20's

THE 30'S   During the 1930's, men and women in America were strongly influenced by the media. Newspapers, magazines, radio, and motion pictures with sound kept people informed on fashions in the United States as well as in other countries. The permanent wave made it possible for women to have more varied hairstyles. A much admired female star was said to have started the popular trend of platinum blonde hair, pencil thin, highly arched eyebrows, and bright color on lips and cheeks. Sleek hair and a trim, neat mustache were popular for men (Fig. 2.14).

THE 40'S   World War II involved most of the civilized world, and most young men were in uniform in some branch of military service. A clean shaven face, closely cropped hair, and neatly pressed uniforms were required of servicemen. Motion pictures served as guidelines for women's fashions in clothing, hairstyles, and makeup. The attractive female stars of the 40's were dressed by leading designers. Their hair and makeup were done by professional stylists and artists. When styles were seen on the screen, millions of women copied them. For example, the natural, softly curved eyebrow, subtle eyeshadow, and mascara were favored to go along with the popular well-scrubbed look. Lip contours were also allowed to remain natural and colors for lips and cheeks were subdued. In spite of wartime shortages of goods and materials, sales of cosmetics and grooming aids continued to grow (Fig. 2.15).

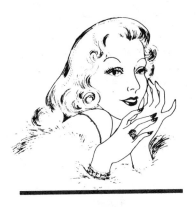

2.14—The 30's   2.15—The 40's

THE 50'S AND 60'S   Post-war prosperity accounted for a renewed interest in fashions, clothes, hairstyles, and makeup. European designers exerted a strong influence on clothing and hairstyles. Full service salons flourished and skin care and body massage clinics came onto the scene. Most families used a wider selection of grooming aids and cosmetics than ever before. Though many salons in the United States offered skin care and massage, hairstyling was the main source of income. Cosmetics manufacturers offered the consumer a wider choice in cosmetic formulas and colors. Colored foundations or makeup bases, cleansers, creams, lotions, moisturizers, and an array of lip, cheek, and eye colors flooded the market. Many popular motion picture stars of the period influenced makeup and hairstyles. Full eyebrows and full lips were fashionable. Heavy eyeliner and false eyelashes became popular and were applied to emphasize the eyes. Lip and cheek colors were mostly light tints. During the late 1960's, facial contouring with cosmetics became popular, and thin eyebrows came back into fashion (Figs. 2.16 and 2.17).

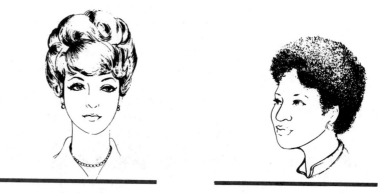

2.16—The 50's   2.17—The 60's

THE 70'S AND 80'S   The 1970's and 1980's brought exciting changes as manufacturers introduced a variety of new products for the care and beautification of the skin and hair. The new trend was to look your individual best, rather than to emulate any particular hair or makeup style. Makeup became more colorful for both day and evening wear. There was a new surge of interest on the part of both men and women in scientific skin care. Many more salons became full service salons, offering not only hair care and styling but a full range of grooming and beauty services (Figs. 2.18 and 2.19).

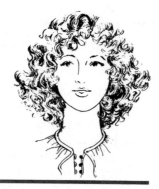

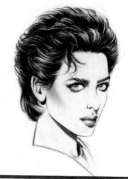

2.18—The 70's   2.19—The 80's

THE FUTURE   During the 1990's and on into the future, there is no doubt that new and interesting concepts of fashions in apparel, makeup, and hairstyles will continue to be created. Men and women of today are better informed about the scientific care of the skin and the use of cosmetics for improved health and attractiveness of the skin. As long as people are interested in the preservation of their health and appearance, the professional services of estheticians and other specialists in the field of cosmetology will continue to be in demand (Fig. 2.20).

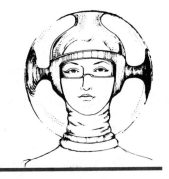

2.20—The Future

QUESTIONS   DISCUSSION AND REVIEW

A HISTORY OF SKIN CARE AND THE USE OF COSMETICS

1. Discuss the various materials that have been used for coloring matter in cosmetics.
2. What is kohl? How did Egyptians use kohl as a cosmetic?
3. How did Egyptians keep their skin lubricated?
4. The word "cosmetics" comes from what Greek word? What does it mean?
5. What products did the Roman women use in their facials?
6. When were cosmetology and medicine taught as combined subjects, and when were they officially separated?
7. Why did the women shave off their eyebrows during the Renaissance period?
8. Describe the ingredients used in facial masks during the reign of Elizabeth I (1558– 1603).
9. During what time in history were makeup and elaborate clothing discouraged?
10. How were the fashions of men and women influenced in the 1930's?

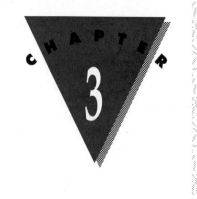

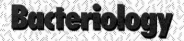

Bacteriology

LEARNING OBJECTIVES

After completing this chapter, you should be able to:

❶ List and explain the different types of bacteria and their classifications.
❷ Describe how bacteria can grow and reproduce.
❸ Explain how we can help to prevent the spread of bacteria in the salon.

INTRODUCTION

Ancient peoples had no knowledge of science and regarded disease as supernatural in origin. They believed that their Gods sent disease, pestilence, and harmful or unnatural occurrences (phenomena) as punishment. To appease the Gods, these ancient peoples developed rituals and sacrifices they hoped would prevent disease and injuries. As civilizations progressed people came to believe that certain diseases were contagious and could be transmitted by clothing and other objects. Although a number of theories existed regarding the existence of bacteria, a Dutch naturalist, Anton Van Leeuwenhock (1632–1723), is credited with discovering bacteria. He invented a microscope and ground lenses with magnifications of up to 300 diameters. This microscope, along with others he invented, enabled him to study bacteria, molds, protozoans, red blood corpuscles, plants, and animals.

Understanding Bacteriology

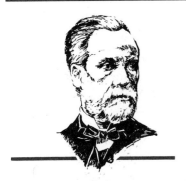

3.1—Louis Pasteur (1822–1895)

Bacteriology is the science that deals with the study of *micro-organisms* (meye-kroh-**OR**-gah-niz-ems) called bacteria.

Louis Pasteur (1822–1895), a French bacteriologist and chemist, proved that the activity of microbes caused fermentations and decompositions of substances (Fig. 3.1). Joseph Lister (1827–1912), an English physician, discovered a method for performing aseptic surgery which helped to prevent and control micro-organisms that caused infection. Great achievements have been made in the control and prevention of disease and many of the most dreaded diseases have been brought under control or eliminated. Every state has laws that make the practice of sterilization and sanitation mandatory for the protection of the public.

As an esthetician, you should understand how the spread of disease can be prevented and what precautions you must take to protect your health and your clients' health. Once you have an understanding of the relationship between bacteria and disease, you will understand the need for school and salon cleanliness and sanitation.

State boards of cosmetology and health departments require that a business that serves the public must follow certain sanitary precautions. Contagious diseases, skin infections, and blood poisoning are caused either by infectious bacteria being transmitted from one individual to another, or by the use of unsanitary implements (such as brushing machine brushes, spatulas, ionto rollers, high-frequency electrodes, suction cups, makeup brushes, tweezers, etc.). Dirty hands and fingernails are other sources of infectious bacteria.

Bacteria

Bacteria are minute, one-celled vegetable micro-organisms found nearly everywhere. They are especially numerous in dust, dirt, refuse, and diseased tissues. Bacteria are also known as *germs* (**JURMS**) or *microbes* (**MEYE**-krohbs). Bacteria can exist almost anywhere: on the skin of the body, in water, air, decayed matter, secretions of body openings, on clothing, and beneath the nails.

Bacteria can be seen only with the aid of a *microscope* (**MEYE**-kroh-skohp). Fifteen hundred rod-shaped bacteria would barely cover the head of a pin.

TYPES OF BACTERIA There are hundreds of different kinds of bacteria. However, bacteria are classified into two types, depending on whether they are beneficial or harmful.

1. Most bacteria are *nonpathogenic* (non-path-o-**JEN**-ik) organisms (helpful or harmless microbes or germs), which perform many useful functions, such as decomposing refuse and improving soil fertility. *Saprophytes* (sap-**RO**-fyts), nonpathogenic bacteria, live on dead matter and do not produce disease.
2. *Pathogenic* (path-o-**JEN**-ik) organisms are harmful and, although in the minority, produce disease when they invade plant or animal tissue. To this group belong the *parasites* (**PAR**-ah-syts), which require living matter for their growth.

It is because of pathogenic bacteria that beauty schools and salons must maintain certain sanitary and cleanliness standards.

CLASSIFICATION OF PATHOGENIC BACTERIA   Bacteria have distinct shapes that help to identify them. Pathogenic bacteria are classified as follows (Fig. 3.2):

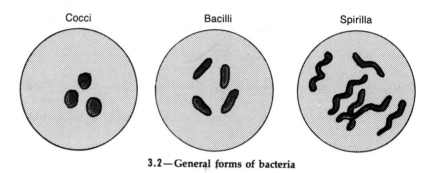

3.2—General forms of bacteria

1. *Cocci* are round-shaped organisms that appear singly or in the following groups (Fig. 3.3):
   a) *Staphylococci:* Pus-forming organisms that grow in bunches or clusters. They cause abscesses, pustules, and boils.
   b) *Streptococci:* Pus-forming organisms that grow in chains. They cause infections such as strep throat.
   c) *Diplococci:* They grow in pairs and cause, for example, pneumonia.

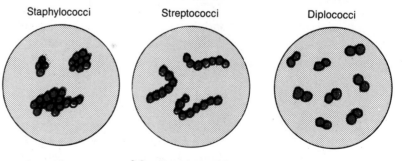

3.3—Groupings of bacteria

2. *Bacilli* are short rod-shaped organisms. They are the most common bacteria and produce diseases such as tetanus (lockjaw), influenza, typhoid fever, tuberculosis, and diphtheria (Fig. 3.4).

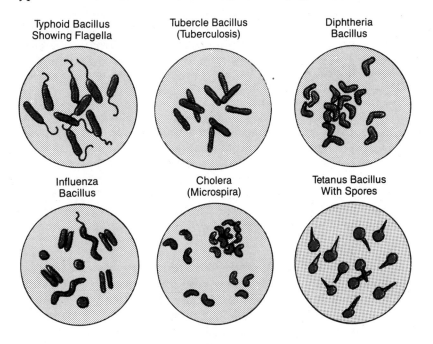

3.4—Disease-producing bacteria

3. *Spirilla* are curved or corkscrew-shaped organisms. They are subdivided into several groups. Of chief importance to us is the *treponema pallida* (trep-o-**NE**-mah **PAL**-i-dah), which causes *syphilis* (**SIF**-i-lis).

PRONUNCIATION OF TERMS RELATING TO PATHOGENIC BACTERIA	**SINGULAR**	**PLURAL**
	coccus (**KOK**-us)	cocci (**KOK**-si)
	bacillus (bah-**SIL**-us)	bacilli (ba-**SIL**-i)
	spirillum (speye-**RIL**-um)	spirilla (spi-**RIL**-a)
	staphylococcus (staf-i-lo-**KOK**-us)	staphylococci (staf-i-lo-**KOK**-si)
	streptococcus (strep-to-**KOK**-us)	streptococci (strep-to-**KOK**-si)
	diplococcus (deye-ploh-**KOK**-us)	diplococci (dip-lo-**KOK**-si)

Bacterial Growth and Reproduction

Bacteria generally consist of an outer cell wall and internal *protoplasm* (**PROH**-toh-plaz-em), material needed to sustain life. They manufacture their own food from the surrounding environment, give off waste products, and grow and reproduce. Bacteria have two distinct phases in their life cycle: the *active* or *vegetative stage*, and the *inactive* or *spore-forming stage*.

ACTIVE OR VEGETATIVE BACTERIA   During the active stage, bacteria grow and reproduce. These microorganisms multiply best in warm, dark, damp, or dirty places where sufficient food is available.

When conditions are favorable, bacteria grow and reproduce. When they reach their largest size, they divide into two new cells. This division is called *mitosis*. The cells formed are called *daughter cells*. When conditions are unfavorable, bacteria die or become inactive. (See chapter on cells, anatomy, and physiology.)

INACTIVE OR SPORE-FORMING BACTERIA   Certain bacteria, such as the anthrax and tetanus bacilli, form *spherical spores* with tough outer coverings during their inactive stage. The purpose is to be able to withstand periods of famine, dryness, and unsuitable temperatures. In this stage, spores can be blown about and are not harmed by disinfectants, heat, or cold.

When favorable conditions are restored, the spores change into the active or vegetative form, then grow and reproduce.

MOVEMENT OF BACTERIA   Cocci rarely show active *motility* (self-movement). They are transmitted on the air, in dust, or in the substance in which they settle. Bacilli and spirilla are both motile and use hairlike projections, known as *flagella* (flah-**JEL**-ah) or *cilia* (**SIL**-ee-a), to move about. A whiplike motion of these hairs propels bacteria about in liquid.

Bacterial Infections

There can be no infection without the presence of pathogenic bacteria. An infection occurs when the body is unable to cope with the bacteria and their harmful toxins. A *local infection* is indicated by a boil or pimple that contains pus.

A *general infection* results when the bloodstream carries the bacteria and their toxins to all parts of the body, as in syphilis.

PUS   The presence of pus is a sign of infection. Bacteria, waste matter, decayed tissue, body cells, and living and dead blood cells are all found in pus. Staphylococci are the most common pus-forming bacteria.

CONTAGIOUS DISEASE   A disease becomes *contagious* (kon-**TAY**-jus) or *communicable* (ko-**MU**-ni-kah-bil) when it spreads from one person to another by contact. Some of the more common contagious diseases that prevent a cosmetologist from working are tuberculosis, common colds, ringworm, scabies, head lice, and viral infections.

SOURCE OF INFECTION   The chief sources of contagion are unclean hands and implements, open sores, pus, mouth and nose discharges, and the common use of drinking cups and towels. Uncovered coughing or sneezing and spitting in public also spread germs.

BACTERIA ENTER BODY   Pathogenic bacteria can enter the body through:

1. A break in the skin, such as a cut, pimple, or scratch
2. The mouth (breathing air, or swallowing water or food)
3. The nose (air)
4. The eyes or ears (dirt)

BODY FIGHTS INFECTION   The body fights infection by means of:

1. Unbroken skin, which is the body's first line of defense
2. Bodily secretions, such as perspiration and digestive juices
3. White cells within the blood that destroy bacteria
4. Antitoxins that counteract the toxins produced by bacteria

Infections can be prevented and controlled through personal hygiene and public sanitation.

OTHER INFECTIOUS AGENTS   *Filterable viruses* (**FIL**-ter-a-bil **VI**-rus-es) are living organisms so small that they can pass through the pores of a porcelain filter. They cause the common cold and other *respiratory* (**RES**-pi-rah-torh-ee) and *gastro-intestinal* (digestive tract) (**GAS**-troh-in-**TES**-ti-nal) infections.

Parasites are organisms that live on other living organisms without giving anything in return.

Plant parasites or *fungi* (**FUN**-ji), such as molds, mildews, and yeasts, can produce contagious diseases, such as ringworm and *favus* (**FA**-vus), a skin disease of the scalp.

Animal parasites are responsible for contagious diseases. For example, the itch mite burrows under the skin, causing *scabies* (**SKAY**-beez), and infection of the scalp by lice is called *pediculosis* (pe-dik-yoo-**LOH**-sis).

Contagious diseases caused by parasites should never be treated in a beauty school or salon. Clients should be referred to a physician.

Immunity

Immunity (i-**MYOO**-ni-tee) is the ability of the body to destroy bacteria that have gained entrance, and thus to resist infection. Immunity against disease can be natural or acquired and is a sign of good health. *Natural immunity* is inherent resistance to disease. It is partly inherited and partly developed through hygienic living. *Acquired immunity* is something the body develops after it has overcome a disease, or receives through inoculation.

Human Disease Carrier

A human disease carrier is a person who is personally immune to a disease yet can transmit germs to other people. *Typhoid* (**TI**-foid) *fever* and *diphtheria* (dif-**THEER**-i-a) can be transmitted in this manner.

Destruction of Bacteria

Bacteria can be destroyed by disinfectants and by intense heat achieved by boiling, steaming, baking, or burning, and with ultra-violet rays. (This subject is covered in the chapter on sterilization and sanitation.)

VACCINATIONS Vaccinations involve the administering of an inoculation in order to produce immunity to a disease.

Vaccinations are effective against such diseases as polio, typhoid fever, smallpox, whooping cough, measles, and tetanus.

ANTIBIOTICS Antibiotics (an-tee-bye-**OT**-icks) are substances produced by various micro-organisms and fungi, that have the power to arrest the growth and to destroy other micro-organisms. An example is the antibiotic, penicillin. Penicillin is a powerful antibiotic found in the mold fungus penicillium and is produced in several forms for the treatment of a wide variety of bacterial infections.

The Body Defenses

The body is constantly defending itself against invasion by disease. Its defenses are called first-, second-, and third-line defenses.

FIRST-LINE DEFENSES Bacteria can enter the body through any orifice, such as the mouth or nose. Bacteria are taken into the body in food and liquids, and can enter by way of injuries that break, cut, or puncture the skin.

A healthy skin is one of the body's most important defenses against disease. It acts as a barrier by resisting the penetration of harmful bacteria.

The nose has mucus and fine hairs that serve as protection against bacteria. When a person sneezes or coughs, the body is reacting to protect itself against bacteria. Other barriers are created by the mucus membranes within the mouth, the gastric juices in the stomach, and the organisms within the intestines and other areas of the body.

Tears in the eyes also serve to flush out harmful bacteria and foreign objects.

SECOND-LINE DEFENSES The body also defends itself from harmful bacteria by producing inflammation. Redness and swelling reveal an increase in temperature and metabolic activity. The inflamed area will be sensitive to the touch. The white corpuscles go into action to destroy harmful micro-organisms in the bloodstream and tissues so that healing can take place.

THIRD-LINE DEFENSES The body can produce substances which can inhibit or destroy harmful bacteria. These protective substances are the antibodies.

Plants and Bacteria

Bacteria from some plants can produce diseases by forming substances that are injurious to health. Ringworm and athlete's foot are examples of diseases produced by fungi.

Insects (Parasites)

Many insects carry harmful micro-organisms, and lice, mites, bugs, and mosquitoes can inject them into the bloodstream. Malaria is an example of a disease caused by a certain kind of mosquito.

Prevention of Disease

To avoid the spread of disease, keep yourself and your surroundings clean. See that everything you use is clean before use, and sanitized after use. You must be aware of the importance of personal hygiene and public sanitation. You must refuse to perform a service for a person who obviously has a contagious disease or infection, and you should suggest, tactfully, that the client see a physician.

QUESTIONS DISCUSSION AND REVIEW

BACTERIOLOGY
1. Define bacteriology.
2. Why should the student and esthetician practice strict sanitary rules?
3. What are bacteria?
4. By what other terms are bacteria known?
5. Why are bacteria not visible to the naked eye?
6. Name and briefly describe two types of bacteria.
7. What are: a) parasites; b) saprophytes?
8. Name three general forms of bacteria and the shape of each.
9. Which bacteria grow in: a) clusters; b) chains?
10. How do bacteria multiply?
11. What is the difference between local infection and general infection?
12. What causes an infection?
13. Name two common pus-forming bacteria.
14. Name four common contagious diseases that prevent an esthetician from working.
15. What is a contagious or communicable disease?
16. How can infection be prevented in the salon?
17. Name four principal routes through which bacteria may enter the body.
18. In which four ways does the body resist infection?
19. What is immunity?
20. Differentiate between natural and acquired immunity.
21. What is a human disease carrier? Give two examples.
22. What will destroy bacteria?

C H A P T E R

4

Sterilization and Sanitation

LEARNING OBJECTIVES

After completing this chapter, you should be able to:

❶ List the differences between sterilization and sanitation.
❷ Discuss the different methods of sterilization and sanitation and the chemical agents used for each.
❸ Identify the methods of sanitation employed in the salon.
❹ Discuss why safety precautions and sanitary rules in the salon are necessary.
❺ Describe how the spread of disease can be prevented.

INTRODUCTION

Sterilization (ster-i-li-**ZAY**-shun) is the process of making an object germ-free by destroying all micro-organisms (bacteria, fungi, and viruses), both pathogenic (infectious) and nonpathogenic (not harmful).

Sanitation (san-i-**TAY**-shun) is the process of making objects clean and safe for use, to prevent the growth of germs and to reduce the risk of infectious disease.

Sterilization and sanitation are of practical importance to the esthetician because they deal with methods used either to prevent the growth of germs or to destroy them entirely. It is especially important to destroy those micro-organisms that are responsible for infectious and communicable diseases.

In the salon or school environment, it is impossible to sterilize implements and equipment as completely as is done in a hospital. It is vital, however, that you follow strict sanitation procedures in the school and salon. All work areas, all implements and equipment, and the dispensary must be kept in clean and sanitary condition at all times.

Note: A full service salon or school must have equipment to sanitize implements, such as combs, brushes, hair clips, rollers, etc. The esthetician requires only the equipment needed to sanitize implements, machines, and other items used for facials and makeup application.

Definitions Pertaining to Sanitation

1. *Sterilize* (**STERR**-i-lize)—To render sterile; to make free from all bacteria (harmful or beneficial)
2. *Sterile* (**STERR**-il)—Free from all germs
3. *Antiseptic* (an-ti-**SEP**-tick)—A chemical agent that kills or retards the growth of bacteria
4. *Disinfectant* (dis-in-**FECK**-tant)—A chemical agent that kills bacteria (stronger than an antiseptic)
5. *Disinfect* (dis-in-**FEKT**)—To destroy micro-organisms on any object
6. *Bactericide* (back-**TEER**-i-side)—A chemical agent that destroys micro-organisms
7. *Germicide* (**JUR**-mi-side)—A chemical agent that destroys micro-organisms; a bactericide
8. *Asepsis* (a-**SEP**-sis)—Freedom from disease causing germs
9. *Sepsis* (**SEP**-sis)—Contamination due to pathogenic germs
10. *Fumigant* (**FYOO**-mi-gant)—Germicidal vapor used to maintain clean equipment in a sanitary condition
11. *Sanitize* (**SAN**-i-tiz)—To render objects clean and sanitary

Methods of Sterilization and Sanitation

There are five widely used methods of sterilization and sanitation. These are grouped under three main headings: heat, chemical agents, and radiation.

HEAT *Boiling* is a method of sterilizing with moist heat. The process sterilizes objects by boiling them in water at 212°F (100°C) for 20 minutes. Schools and salons rarely use this method because it is time consuming and may damage certain objects, especially those made of plastic.

Steaming is another method for sterilizing objects with moist heat. It requires a steam pressure sterilizer, such as an autoclave. An autoclave is a strong, airtight metal vessel in which chemical reactions may be effected under pressure. This method is used in the medical field for various sterilization purposes. The equipment is too expensive and unwieldly for use in salons.

Baking is a method of sterilizing objects with dry heat. This process is often used in hospitals to sterilize bedding and similar materials.

CHEMICAL AGENTS There are various types of chemical agents that are used for sanitizing purposes. These include antiseptics, fumigants, and disinfectants (germicides).

Antiseptics and disinfectants are substances, usually in liquid form, that kill or retard the growth of germs. Antiseptics are generally milder and less powerful than disinfectants and are safer to use on the skin. Disinfectants are stronger than antiseptics and must be used with caution. They should not be used on skin. Fumigants are a form of disinfectant that kills germs through exposure to fumes. These must generally be used in closed areas.

Some soaps and detergents have antiseptic properties when used to wash the hands and implements; however, soap and water alone are not enough for thorough sanitizing, and must be used in conjunction with general antiseptics.

General antiseptics include alcohol, boric acid, tincture of iodine, hydrogen peroxide, chloramine, and sodium hypochlorite. Disinfectants include quaternary ammonium compounds (quats), formalin, formaldehyde, and alcohol. Although formaldehyde is no longer suspected to be a carcinogen and its use (as formalin) has been allowed by most State Boards of Cosmetology, it still should be used with caution. All of these substances should be diluted and used as recommended by the manufacturer. Refer to the chart included in this chapter for names, forms, strengths, and uses of various antiseptics and disinfectants. In addition to the products described herein, consult the State Board of Cosmetology or the Health Department in your state for further recommendations.

A good chemical agent should be easy to use, act quickly, be odorless, noncorrosive, economical, and safe to use.

RADIATION *Ultra-violet radiation*, especially in the shorter wavelengths, destroys most bacteria. Ultra-violet rays in an electrical sanitizer are used in schools and salons to keep implements sanitary once they have been sterilized. Ultra-violet radiation in this amount can be harmful to the eyes, so this kind of equipment must be used carefully.

Gamma ray radiation destroys micro-organisms through the action of ionized particles. This type of sterilization is used to sterilize medical instruments and devices in hospitals and is not suited for salon use.

> **Note:** Though several methods of sterilization are listed here, the most commonly used method by the esthetician is to wash the implements in soap and water, immerse or wipe them in alcohol, then place them in a dry sterilizer.

PRECAUTIONS FOR USING ANTISEPTICS AND DISINFECTANTS

1. Before performing any service in the salon, wash and sanitize your hands.
2. Be sure the work area and everything used for the service are clean and sanitary.
3. Keep all products and equipment organized to prevent accidental spills and breakage.
4. After completing the service, thoroughly clean and sanitize all reusable objects and the work area. Discard all disposable objects immediately.
5. To avoid contamination, use a spatula to remove a product from its container (Fig. 4.1). Never use the fingers. Never return a product to its container once it has been removed.
6. Always keep antiseptics and disinfectants sealed and in a safe place. They should be labeled clearly and never transferred to unlabeled containers, where they might be mistaken for some other product.
7. When using disinfectants, wear rubber gloves and make sure there is adequate ventilation.

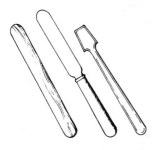

4.1—Spatulas

Sanitizers

Dry or cabinet sanitizers are airtight cabinets containing either an active fumigant or a source of ultraviolet radiation. The sanitized implements are kept clean by placing them in the cabinet until they are used (Fig. 4.2).

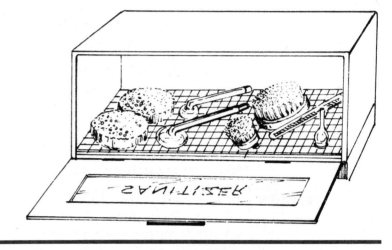

4.2—Dry/cabinet sanitizer

ULTRA-VIOLET RADIATION SANITIZERS   *Ultra-violet ray electrical sanitizers* are effective for keeping facial and makeup brushes or implements sanitized until ready for use. These materials must be washed before they are placed in the sanitizer. Follow the manufacturer's directions for proper use.

FUMIGANT SANITIZERS   *Fumigant sanitizers* are used by placing a tablespoon of borax and a teaspoon of formalin or another active fumigant on a small tray on the bottom of the cabinet. The fumes generated have a germicidal action and keep the implements placed in the cabinet sanitized. The implements must be washed before they are placed in the sanitizer. Follow the manufacturer's directions for proper use.

Chemical Sanitizing Agents

FORMALIN   *Formalin* (**FOHR**-mah-lin) is a relatively safe and effective sanitizing agent that can be used either as an antiseptic or disinfectant, depending on its strength. As usually purchased, formalin is composed of approximately 37 to 40 percent formaldehyde (for-**MAL**-de-heyed) gas in water. It is also available in powder and tablet forms. Formalin should be used with great care. Inhalation can cause damage to mucous membranes of the nose, and contact with the skin can cause irritation.

Formalin is used in various strengths. As a 25 percent or a 10 percent solution, it acts as a disinfectant. As a 5 percent solution, it is an antiseptic.

25 percent solution—(equivalent to 10 percent formaldehyde gas)—Use to sanitize implements. Immerse them in the solution for at least 10 minutes. Prepare by mixing two parts of formalin with five parts water. For anti-rusting action, add one part glycerine.

10 percent solution—(equivalent to 4 percent formaldehyde gas)—Use to sanitize combs and brushes. Immerse them in the solution for at least 20 minutes. Prepare by mixing one part formalin with nine parts water.

5 percent solution—(equivalent to 2 percent formaldehyde gas)—Use to cleanse the hands after they have been in contact with wounds, skin eruptions, and other sources of bacterial infection. Also use to sanitize bowls, countertops, chairs, etc. Prepare by mixing one part formalin with nineteen parts water.

QUATERNARY AMMONIUM COMPOUNDS

Quaternary Ammonium Compounds—*quats* (**KWAH**-ter-nah-ree ah-**MON**-nee-um **KOM**-pounds—**KWATS**) are effective disinfectants and are relatively safe to use. They are available under different trade and chemical names and come in liquid and tablet form. They are quick acting, odorless and colorless, nontoxic, and stable. Generally, they are diluted for use. A 1:1,000 solution is commonly used to sanitize implements.

▶ | **Caution:** Before using any quat, read and follow manufacturer's directions on the label and be familiar with any accompanying literature. Find out if the product should be diluted with tap water or distilled water. Find out if it contains a rust inhibitor. If it does not, add 0.5 percent *sodium nitrite* (**SOH**-di-um **NIGH**-trite) to the solution to keep metallic instruments from rusting.

To prepare 1:1,000 strength solution, if the product contains:

- 10% active ingredient—Add 1¼ oz. (37.5ml) quat solution to 1 gallon (3.8 liters) of water.
- 12% active ingredient—Add 1 oz. (30ml) quat solution to 1 gallon of water.
- 15% active ingredient—Add ¾ oz. (22.5ml) quat solution to 1 gallon of water.

ALCOHOL

Alcohols are organic chemicals and are especially important to estheticians. The most common forms are ethyl alcohol (ethanol or grain alcohol), which is the chief component of alcoholic beverages, methyl alcohol (wood alcohol), and isopropyl alcohol (rubbing alcohol). Phenol, a powerful disinfectant, is also an alcohol. Only ethyl alcohol can be ingested. Methyl and isopropyl alcohols have been denatured, that is, chemicals have been added to them to make them unfit to drink. They are still safe for external use, however, and they are all effective and safe sanitizers. Alcohols are flammable, and care should be taken when they are used near heat or open flame.

SODIUM HYPOCHLORITE *Sodium hypochlorite* (**SOH**-di-um **HY**-po-chlor-it), or common household bleach, provides the sanitizing ability of chlorine. One of the key advantages of bleach is its ability to destroy viruses. A 10 percent solution is normally used. Implements should be immersed for 10 minutes. Follow the manufacturer's directions for mixing and for use.

Antiseptics Used in Salons

NAME	FORM	STRENGTH	USES
Boric Acid	White crystals	2.5% solution	Cleanse the eyes.
Tincture of Iodine	Liquid	2% solution	Cleanse cuts and wounds.
Hydrogen Peroxide	Liquid	3% solution	Cleanse skin and minor cuts.
Alcohol	Liquid	60%–90% solution	Cleanse hands, skin, and minor cuts. Not to be used if irritation is present.
Formalin	Liquid	5% solution	Cleanse hands and implements.
Chloramine-T (Chlorazene; Chlorozol)	White crystals	½% solution	Cleanse skin and hands, and for general use.
Sodium Hypochlorite	Liquid; white crystals	½% solution	Rinse the hands.

Disinfectants Used in Salons

NAME	FORM	STRENGTH	IMMERSION TIME
Sodium Hypochlorite (household bleach)	Liquid	10% solution	10 minutes or more.
Quaternary Ammonium Compounds (quats)	Liquid; tablet	1:1,000 solution	20 minutes or more.
Formalin	Liquid	25% solution	10 minutes or more.
Formalin	Liquid	10% solution	20 minutes or more.
Alcohol	Liquid	70% solution	10 minutes or more.

Sanitizing Procedures

1. Wash implements thoroughly with soap and hot water.
2. Use plain water rinse to remove all traces of soap.
3. Immerse implements in a wet sanitizer containing approved disinfectant (bleach, quat, formalin, or alcohol) for the recommended time.
4. Remove implements from wet sanitizer, rinse in water, and wipe dry with a clean towel.
5. Store sanitized implements in individually wrapped plastic envelopes in a fumigant or ultra-violet cabinet sanitizer until ready to be used.

Sanitize electrodes and similar implements by gently rubbing the exposed surface with a cotton pad dampened with alcohol. Then place the articles in a dry sanitizer until ready for use.

To disinfect floors, sinks, and toilet bowls in the salon, use commercial household or industrial strength products such as Lysol, Pine Sol, or a similar disinfectant. Deodorizers are also useful to offset offensive smells and to impart a refreshing fragrance.

Whatever disinfectant product is used, follow the manufacturer's directions on the labels.

Safety Precautions

The Occupational Safety and Health Act (OSHA), enacted by the Federal government, and state and local "Right to Know" laws, require owners and managers of many businesses to inform workers and clients of the potential hazards of the materials they may come in contact with. OSHA regulations also require businesses to comply with safety standards and to maintain a safe work environment.

1. Purchase chemicals in small quantities and store them in a cool, dry place to avoid deterioration from contact with air, light, or heat.
2. Weigh and measure chemicals carefully when mixing.
3. Make sure there is adequate ventilation when mixing chemicals. Wear rubber gloves and safety glasses.
4. Keep all containers properly labeled.
5. Read all labels and follow directions carefully.
6. Do not breathe fumes from chemicals or solutions.
7. Avoid spills when mixing chemicals.

Sanitation

Sanitation is the application of measures to promote public health and to prevent the spread of infectious diseases. The importance of sanitation cannot be overemphasized. Cosmetic services bring the esthetician into direct contact with the client's skin. Understanding sanitary measures contributes to the protection of the client's health.

Various governmental agencies protect community health by providing for a wholesome food and water supply, quick disposal of refuse, and regular inspections of public facilities. These steps are only a few of the ways in which the public health is safeguarded.

DRINKING WATER Water for drinking purposes should be odorless, colorless, and free from any foreign contamination. Crystal clear water may still be unsanitary because of microscopic bacteria that cannot be seen by the naked eye. Most municipalities clean and filter the water used in the community.

AIR Air within a salon should be neither dry nor stagnant, nor should it have a stale or musty odor. Room temperatures should be maintained around 70°F. The salon may also be ventilated with the aid of exhaust fans or air conditioning units. Air conditioning has the advantage of permitting changes in the quality and quantity of air brought into the salon. Filters should be changed regularly. The temperature and moisture content of the air can also be regulated with air conditioning.

TRANSMISSION OF COMMUNICABLE DISEASES A person with an infectious disease is a source of contagion to others; hence, estheticians who have colds or any communicable diseases must not work on clients. Likewise, clients obviously suffering from an infectious disease must not be accommodated in a salon. In this way, the best interests of other clients will be served.

One of the most pressing concerns in public health today is the spread of AIDS (Acquired Immune Deficiency Syndrome), which is transmitted through sexual contact or contact with infected bodily fluids, such as blood. In some procedures in the salon, for example during manual extraction, the esthetician may be exposed to minute quantities of the client's blood. For maximum safety, the esthetician should wear surgical rubber or latex gloves during these procedures.

Sanitary Procedures

1. Change chemical solutions in sanitizers frequently.
2. Keep implements in a disinfectant solution or in a dry cabinet sanitizer until ready for use.
3. Sanitize all reuseable implements after each client.
4. Place all implements on a sanitary surface or in sanitary containers while in use.
5. Sanitize all bowls, trays, and other items before and after working on each client.
6. Sanitize all appliances after each client by washing and wiping with a cotton pad dampened with alcohol or another recommended solution.
7. All sanitary practices followed should conform to the regulations issued by the State Board of Cosmetology.
8. Every salon must be well-lighted, heated or cooled, and properly ventilated, and must be kept in a clean, sanitary condition.
9. The walls, curtains, and floor, or floor coverings, in a salon must be washable and kept clean.

10. All establishments must be supplied with hot and cold running water. Drinking facilities, such as a water cooler or drinking fountain (with disposable cups) should be provided.
11. All plumbing fixtures should be properly installed and maintained.
12. The premises should be kept free of rodents, flies, and other vermin.
13. The salon may not be used for cooking, for sleeping, or as living quarters.
14. Any waste material dropped on the floor must be picked up without delay and deposited in closed containers. Trash containers must be removed from the premises at frequent intervals.
15. Rest rooms must be kept in a sanitary condition and be provided with hot and cold running water, liquid soap, paper towels, and toilet tissues, as well as closed refuse containers.
16. The esthetician must wash and sanitize his or her hands thoroughly before and after serving each client and after using the rest room.
17. Freshly laundered towels or paper towels must be used for each client. Towels that are ready for use must be stored in clean, closed cabinets.
18. A clean towel should be placed on the headrest for each client.
19. When using a plastic item, such as a makeup cape, it must not come in contact with the client's skin.
20. The common use of powder puffs, lipcolor containers, cheekcolor applicators, eye makeup swabs, mascara brushes, lip brushes, eyebrow pencils and brushes, or any similar item is strictly prohibited.
21. Lotions, creams, powders, and similar cosmetics must be kept in clean, closed containers. Spatulas, not fingers, must be used to remove the products from jars. Sterile cotton pledgets or cosmetic sponges may be used to apply lotions and powders. Jars and bottles should be capped when not in use. Once a product is removed from its container, it must not be returned to the container.
22. All soiled and used items must be removed from the work area immediately after use. Never mix used items with sanitized, unused items.
23. Once a client has worn a salon gown or headband it may not be worn by another client until it has been washed and sanitized.
24. All implements and articles used when giving a face treatment or a facial makeup must be washed, sanitized, and placed in an airtight container or a cabinet sanitizer.
25. The esthetician must refrain from touching his or her own face or hair while performing a service. If it is necessary to do so, the hands must be sanitized again before touching the client or before handling any of the implements or articles being used for the service.
26. Pets of any type cannot be permitted in a salon or school.

> **Note:** The responsibility for sanitation rests with each student in the school and with each esthetician in the salon. The school owner or salon manager must provide the necessities for sanitation.
>
> The esthetician must obey all rules of sanitation issued by the Health Department and by the State Board of Cosmetology.

QUESTIONS DISCUSSION AND REVIEW

STERILIZATION AND SANITATION

1. What is sterilization?
2. What is sanitation?
3. Why are sterilization and sanitation important to the esthetician?
4. What does an antiseptic do?
5. What is asepsis?
6. What is sepsis?
7. Give three forms of heat sterilizing.
8. Which is stronger—disinfectant or antiseptic?
9. Give two forms of radiation.
10. What percent of formalin is used to sanitize implements?

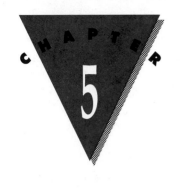

Cells, Anatomy, and Physiology

CHAPTER 5

LEARNING OBJECTIVES   *After completing this chapter, you should be able to:*

❶ Discuss cells, tissues, and organs, and how they work together to form the body's systems.

❷ Describe muscular structures and functions, and the various nerves that are affected during facial treatments.

❸ Explain the functions of the circulatory system and the importance of blood and lymph circulation.

❹ Discuss the effect on the various organs and systems when giving a massage and performing other steps during treatments.

INTRODUCTION   It is important for the esthetician to know how to care for the skin, to have a thorough understanding of its health, growth, and repair, and to understand how it functions. While the esthetician is not expected to be an anatomist, it is desirable to possess a working knowledge of the structure of those areas upon which treatments are given. This knowledge is helpful in understanding the reasons for certain steps required in giving facial treatments.

The human body is composed of cells, which reproduce by dividing. When grouped together, they form tissues, which in turn comprise organs, which, in combination, form systems. The skin, the membranous tissue which covers the body, is the largest organ of the body.

Cells

Cells are the basic units of all living things, from the simple, single-celled protozoa to the complex, multicellular human beings. The human body is composed of trillions of individual cells, which differ from each other in size, shape, structure, and function.

A cell is a minute portion of living substance consisting of *proto-plasm* (**PRO**-tuh-plazm), which is living matter surrounded by a membrane, containing a nucleus, cytoplasm, and various organelles or parts of the cell having special functions (Fig. 5.1).

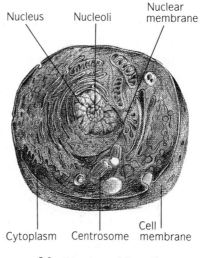

Nucleus   Nucleoli   Nuclear membrane

Cytoplasm   Centrosome   Cell membrane

5.1—Structure of the cell

STRUCTURE OF THE CELL

The cell contains the following structures:

Cell membrane (**MEM**-brayn)—encloses the protoplasm and holds the cell together. It is a filter that lets substances enter and leave the cell.

Nucleus (**NOO**-klee-us)—dense protoplasm found in the center, which plays an important part in the reproduction of the cell and in cell metabolism. It is surrounded by the nuclear membrane.

Cytoplasm (**SEYE**-toh-plaz-em)—less dense protoplasm that holds other organelles and contains food materials necessary for the growth, reproduction, and self-repair of the cell.

Centrosome (**SEN**-tro-sohm)—a small, round body in the cytoplasm, which also affects the reproduction of the cell. The centrosome plays an important role in maintaining the characteristics of the original cell.

CELL GROWTH AND PRODUCTION

As long as cells receive an adequate supply of food, oxygen and water, eliminate waste products and maintain proper temperature, they will continue to grow and thrive. Most body cells are capable of growth and self-repair during their life cycle.

In the human body, when a cell reaches maturity it reproduces by *mitosis* or indirect division (Fig. 5.2). This is a process in which a series of changes occur in the nucleus before the entire cell divides in half. This method of reproduction occurs in all human tissues, including hair and skin.

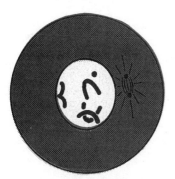

First Phase

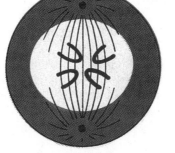

Second Phase

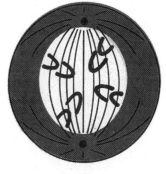

Third Phase

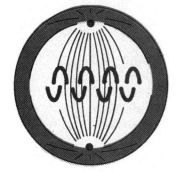

Fourth Phase

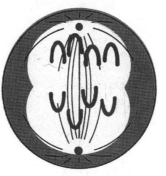

Fifth Phase

One cell has divided to create two cells.

5.2—Indirect division of the human cell

METABOLISM   *Metabolism* (meh-**TAB**-o-lis-em) is a complex chemical process in which cells are nourished and supplied with the energy needed to carry on their many activities. There are two phases to metabolism:

1. *Anabolism* (ah-**NAB**-o-lizm) builds up cellular tissues. During anabolism, the cells absorb water, food, and oxygen for growth, reproduction, and repair.
2. *Catabolism* (kah-**TAB**-o-liz-em) breaks down cellular tissues. During catabolism, the cells consume what they have absorbed to perform specialized functions, such as muscular effort, secretion, or digestion.

Tissues

Tissues are specialized groups of cells of like kind. Each type of tissue has a specific function and can be recognized by its characteristic appearance. Body tissues are classified in five groups:

1. *Connective tissue* supports, protects, and binds together other tissues of the body. Bone, cartilage, ligaments, tendons, and fat tissues are examples.
2. *Muscular tissue* contracts and allows movement in various parts of the body.
3. *Nerve tissue* transmits messages to and from the brain and controls and coordinates all body functions.
4. *Epithelial* (ep-i-**THEEL**-ee-ul) *tissue* is the protective covering on body surfaces. It includes the skin, mucous membranes, linings of the heart, digestive and respiratory organs and glands.
5. *Liquid tissue* carries food, waste products, and hormones. This type includes the blood and lymph.

Organs

Organs are structures consisting of two or more different tissues, which are combined to accomplish a specific function. The most important organs of the body are:

1. The brain (which controls the nervous system)
2. The heart (which circulates the blood)
3. The lungs (which supply oxygen to the blood)
4. The liver (which removes toxic products of digestion)
5. The kidneys (which excrete excess water and waste products)
6. The stomach and intestines (which process food)
7. The skin (which covers and protects the body). The skin is both a tissue and an organ.

Systems

Systems are groups of organs that cooperate for a common purpose, namely the welfare of the entire body. The human body is composed of the following systems:

1. *Skeletal* (**SKEL**-e-tahl) *System*—Bones
2. *Muscular* (**MUS**-kyoo-lahr) *System*—Muscles
3. *Nervous* (**NUR**-vus) *System*—Nerves
4. *Circulatory* (**SUR**-kyoo-lahr-tohr-ee) *System*—Blood and Lymph Supply
5. *Endocrine* (**EN**-doh-krin) *System*—Ductless Glands
6. *Excretory* (**EK**-skre-tohr-ee) *System*—Organs of Elimination
7. *Respiratory* (**RES**-pi-rah-tohr-ee) *System*—Lungs
8. *Digestive* (deye-**GES**-tiv) *System*—Stomach and Intestines
9. *Reproductive* (ree-proh-**DUK**-tiv) *System*—Organs of Reproduction

All of these systems are closely interrelated and dependent upon each other. While each forms a unit specially designed to perform a specific function, that function cannot be performed without the complete cooperation of some other system or systems. Many organs act as part of more than one system.

Skeletal System

The *skeletal system* is the physical foundation or framework of the body. (*See Color Plate 4.*) It is composed of differently shaped bones united by both movable and immovable joints. It serves as a means of protection, support and locomotion. The system consists of the bones, cartilage, and ligaments.

Besides the teeth, bone is the hardest structure of the body. It is composed of fibrous tissues firmly bound together, consisting of about one-third organic matter and two-thirds mineral matter. There are 206 bones in the human skeleton.

Bones have a number of functions:

1. They give shape and strength to the body.
2. They protect organs from injury.
3. They serve as attachments for muscles.
4. They act as levers for all bodily movements.

BONES OF THE SKULL　The *skull* is the skeleton of the head. (*See Color Plates 2 and 3.*) It is an oval, bony case that shapes the head and protects the brain. The skull is divided into two parts: the 8 bones of the cranium and the 14 facial bones. They are involved with scalp and facial manipulations. (*The bones listed below are numbered to correspond with the bones shown on Fig. 5.3.*)

1. The *occipital* (ok-**SIP**-i-tal) bone forms the lower back part of the cranium.
2. The two *parietal* (pa-**REYE**-e-tal) bones form the sides and top (crown) of the cranium.
3. The *frontal* (**FRUNT**-al) bone forms the forehead.
4. The two *temporal* (**TEM**-po-rahl) bones form the sides of the head in the ear region (below the parietal bones).
5. The *ethmoid* (**ETH**-moid) bone is a light spongy bone between the eyesockets and forms part of the nasal cavities.
6. The *sphenoid* (**SFEEN**-oid) bone joins all of the bones of the cranium together.
7. The two *nasal* (**NAY**-zal) bones form the bridge of the nose.
8. The two *lacrimal* (**LAK**-ri-mahl) bones are small fragile bones located at the front part of the inner wall of the eyesockets.
9. The two *zygomatic* (zeye-goh-**MAT**-ik), or *malar* (**MAY**-lur) bones, form the prominence of the cheeks.
10. The two *maxillae* (mak-**SIL**-ee) are the upper jawbones, which join to form the whole upper jaw.
11. The *mandible* (**MAN**-di-bel) is the lower jawbone and is the largest and strongest bone of the face. It forms the lower jaw.

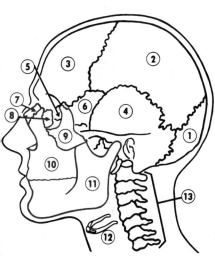

5.3—Diagram of the cranium, face, and neck bones

The following bones do not appear on Fig. 5.3: Two *turbinal* (**TUR**-bi-nahl) bones are thin layers of spongy bone situated on either of the outer walls of the nasal depression. The *vomer* (**VOH**-mer) is a single bone that forms part of the dividing wall of the nose. The two *palatine* (**PAL**-i-teyen) bones form the floor and outer wall of the nose, roof of the mouth, and floor of the orbits.

BONES OF THE NECK

12. The *hyoid* (**HEYE**-oid) bone, a U-shaped bone, is located in the front part of the throat and is commonly called the "Adam's apple."
13. The *cervical vertebrae* (**SUR**-vi-kal **VER**-te-bray) form the top part of the spinal column located in the region of the neck.

BONES OF THE CHEST (THORAX)

The *thorax* (**THO**-racks), or chest, is an elastic bony cage made up of the breastbone, the spine, the ribs, and connective cartilage. It serves as a protective covering for the heart, lungs, and other delicate internal organs. This framework is held in place by 24 ribs, 12 on each side.

BONES OF THE SHOULDER, ARM, AND HAND

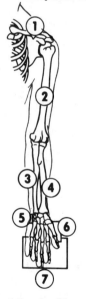

These descriptions correspond to the numbers on Fig. 5.4.

1. Each *shoulder* consists of one clavicle and one scapula, which forms the back of the shoulder.
2. The *humerus* (**HYOO**-mo-rus) is the largest bone of the upper arm.
3. The *ulna* (**UL**-nah) is the large bone on the little finger-side of the forearm.
4. The *radius* (**RAY**-dee-us) is the small bone on the thumb side of the forearm.
5. The *wrist*, or *carpus* (**KAHR**-pus), is a flexible joint composed of 8 small, irregular bones, held together by ligaments.

The hand is divided into two regions:

6. The *palm*, or *metacarpus* (met-a-**KAHR**-pus), consists of five long, slender bones, called *metacarpal* bones.
7. The *fingers*, or *digits* (**DIJ**-its), consist of 3 *phalanges* (fa-**LAN**-jeez) in each finger and 2 in the thumb, totalling 14 bones.

5.4—Bones of the shoulder, arm, and hand

The Muscular System

The *muscular* (**MUS**-kyoo-lahr) *system* covers, shapes, and supports the skeleton. (*See Color Plates 5 and 6.*) Its function is to produce all the movements of the body. The study of the structure, functions, and diseases of the muscles is called *myology*.

Muscles are contractile fibrous tissues upon which the various movements of the body depend for their variety and action. The muscular system relies upon the skeletal and nervous systems for its control. The system consists of more than 500 muscles, large and small, comprising 40 to 50 percent of the weight of the human body.

There are three kinds of muscle tissue: *striated*, striped or voluntary (Fig. 5.5), which are controlled by will, such as those of the face, arms, and legs; *nonstriated*, smooth or involuntary (Fig. 5.6), which function automatically, such as those of the stomach and intestines; and the *cardiac*, or the heart muscle (Fig. 5.7).

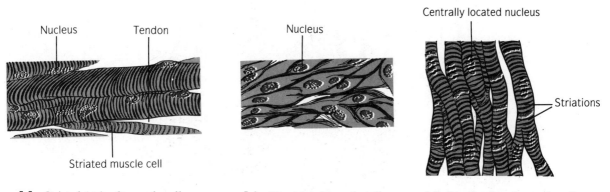

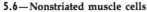
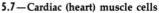

5.5—Striated (striped) muscle cells　　**5.6—Nonstriated muscle cells**　　**5.7—Cardiac (heart) muscle cells**

When a muscle contracts and shortens, one of its attachments usually remains fixed and the other one moves. The *origin* of a muscle is the term applied to the more fixed attachment, such as muscles attached to bones or to some other muscle. Muscles attached to bones are usually referred to as *skeletal muscles*.

The *insertion* of a muscle is the term applied to the more movable attachment, such as muscles attached to a movable muscle, to a movable bone, or to the skin.

Muscle tissue can be stimulated by any of the following:

1. *Chemicals*—Certain acids and salts
2. *Massage*—Hand massage and machines such as vibrators
3. *Electric current*—High-frequency
4. *Dry heat*—Heat lamps and heating masks
5. *Moist heat*—Steamers or moderately warm steam towels

MUSCLES AFFECTED BY MASSAGE　The esthetician is concerned with the muscles of the head, face, neck, arms, and hands. It is essential to know where these muscles are located and what they control. The direction of pressure in massage is usually performed from the insertion to the origin.

MUSCLES OF THE SCALP The muscles are numbered to correspond with the muscles shown on Fig. 5.8.

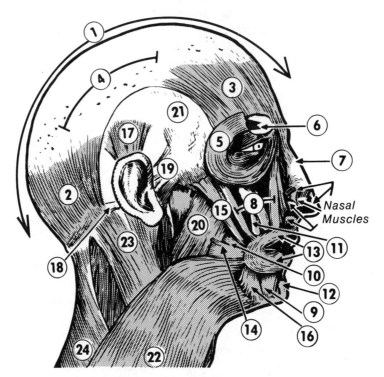

5.8—Diagram of the muscles of the head, face, and neck

1. The *epicranius* (ep-i-**KRAY**-ne-us), or *occipito-frontalis* (ok-**SIP**-i-toh fron-**TAY**-lis), is a broad muscle that covers the top of the skull. It consists of two parts:
2. The *occipitalis* (ok-**SIP**-i-ta-lis), or back part
3. The *frontalis* (fron-**TAY**-lis), or front part

The frontalis raises the eyebrows, draws the scalp forward, and causes wrinkles across the forehead. Both the occipitalis and the frontalis are connected by a tendon called:

4. The *aponeurosis* (ap-o-noo-**ROH**-sis)

MUSCLES OF THE EYEBROWS

5. The *orbicularis oculi* (or-bik-yoo-**LAY**-ris **OK**-yoo-leye) completely surrounds the margin of the eyesocket and closes the eyelid.
6. The *corrugator* (**KOR**-oo-gay-tohr) muscle is beneath the frontalis and orbicularis oculi and draws the eyebrows down and in. It produces vertical lines and causes frowning.

MUSCLES OF THE NOSE   7. The *procerus* (proh-**SEE**-rus) covers the top of the nose, depresses the eyebrow, and causes wrinkles across the bridge of the nose.

The other nasal muscles are small muscles around the nasal openings, which contract and expand the opening of the nostrils.

MUSCLES OF THE MOUTH   8. The *quadratus labii superioris* (kwah-**DRAY**-tus **LAY**-bee-eye suu-**PEER**-ee-or-ihs) consists of three parts. It surrounds the upper part of the lip, raises and draws back the upper lip, and elevates the nostrils, as in expressing distaste.

9. The *quadratus labii inferioris* (in-**FEER**-ee-or-ihs) surrounds the lower part of the lip. It depresses the lower lip and draws it a little to one side, as in expressing sarcasm.

10. The *buccinator* (**BUK**-si-nay-tor) is the muscle between the upper and lower jaws. It compresses the cheeks and expels air between the lips, as in blowing.

11. The *caninus* (kay-**NIGH**-nus) lies under the quadratus labii superioris. It raises the angle of the mouth, as in snarling.

12. The *mentalis* (men-**TAL**-is) is situated at the tip of the chin. It raises and pushes up the lower lip, causing wrinkling of the chin, as in doubt or displeasure.

13. The *orbicularis oris* (or-bik-yoo-**LAY**-ris **OH**-ris) forms a flat band around the upper and lower lips. It compresses, contracts, puckers, and wrinkles the lips, as in kissing or whistling.

14. The *risorius* (ri-**ZOHR**-ee-us) extends from the masseter muscle to the angle of the mouth. It draws the corner of the mouth out and back, as in grinning.

15. The *zygomaticus* (zeye-goh-**MAT**-i-kus) extends from the zygomatic bone to the angle of the mouth. It elevates the lip as in laughing.

16. The *triangularis* (treye-an-gyoo-**LAY**-ris) extends along the side of the chin. It draws down the corner of the mouth.

MUSCLES OF THE EAR   The three muscles of the ear are practically functionless.

17. The *auricularis* (aw-rik-yoo-**LAHR**-is) *superior* is above the ear.
18. The *auricularis posterior* is behind the ear.
19. The *auricularis anterior* is in front of the ear.

MUSCLES OF MASTICATION   20. The *masseter* (ma-**SEE**-tur) and

21. The *temporalis* (tem-po-**RAY**-lis) are muscles that coordinate in opening and closing the mouth, and are referred to as chewing muscles.

MUSCLES OF THE NECK   22. The *platysma* (pla-**TIZ**-mah) is a broad muscle that extends from the chest and shoulder muscles to the side of the chin. It depresses the lower jaw and lip, as in expressing sadness.

23. The *sterno-cleido-mastoid* (**STUR**-noh-**KLE**-i-doh-**MAS**-toid) extends from the collar and chest bones to the temporal bone in back of the ear. It rotates the head and also bends the head, as in nodding.

MUSCLES THAT ATTACH THE ARM TO THE BODY

The principal muscles that attach the arms to the body and permit movements of the shoulders and arms are as follows (Fig. 5.9):

24. The *trapezius* (tra-**PEE**-zee-us) and
25. The *latissimus dorsi* (la-**TIS**-i-mus **DOR**-see) cover the back of the neck and the upper and middle regions of the back. They rotate the shoulder blades and control swinging movements of the arm.
26. The *pectoralis* (pek-tohr-**AL**-is) *major* and *pectoralis minor* cover the front of the chest. They also assist in swinging movements of the arm.
27. The *serratus anterior* (ser-**RAT**-us an-**TEER**-ee-or) assists in breathing and in raising the arm.

MUSCLES OF THE SHOULDER, ARM, AND HAND

The following are the principal muscles of the shoulder and upper arm (Fig. 5.10):

1. The *deltoid* (**DEL**-toid) is the large, thick, triangular-shaped muscle that covers the shoulder, lifts and turns the arm.
2. The *biceps* (**BEYE**-seps) is the two-headed and principal muscle on the front of the upper arm. It lifts the forearm, flexes the elbow, and turns the palm downward.
3. The *triceps* (**TREYE**-seps) is the three-headed muscle of the arm, which covers the entire back of the upper arm and extends the forearm forward.

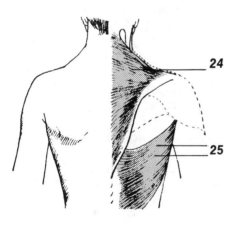

5.9—Muscles that attach the arms to the body

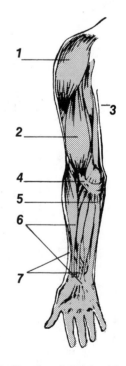

5.10—Muscles of the shoulder, arm, and hand

The forearm is made up of a series of muscles and strong tendons (Fig. 5.10). The esthetician is concerned with the following:

4. The *pronators* (pro-**NAY**-tors), the most important of the group, turn the hand inward, so that the palm faces downward.
5. The *supinators* (**SUE**-pi-nay-tors) turn the hand outward and the palm upward.
6. The *flexors* (**FLEKS**-ors) bend the wrist, draw the hand up, and close the fingers toward the forearm.
7. The *extensors* (eck-**STEN**-surs) straighten the wrist, hand, and fingers to form a straight line.

The hand has many small muscles overlapping from joint to joint, imparting flexibility and strength. When the hands are properly cared for, these muscles will remain supple and graceful.

The Nervous System

Neurology (nuu-**ROL**-o-jee) is the branch of anatomy that deals with the nervous system and its disorders.

The *nervous* (**NUR**-vus) *system* controls and coordinates the functions of all the other systems and makes them work harmoniously and efficiently. Every square inch of the human body is supplied with fine fibers, known as *nerves*.

The main purpose in studying the nervous system is to understand the effects various facial services have on the nerves, skin and face, and on the body as a whole.

The principal parts of the nervous system are the brain, the spinal cord, and the network of nerves. Generally, the nervous system is composed of three main divisions:

1. The *cerebro-spinal* (ser-**EE**-broh **SPEYE**-nahl) or *central* nervous system (CNS)
2. The *peripheral* (pe-**RIF**-er-al) nervous system
3. The *autonomic* (aw-toh-**NAHM**-ik) nervous system (ANS), which includes the *sympathetic* (sim-pah-**THET**-ik) and *parasympathetic* (**PA**-rah-sim-pah-**THET**-ik) systems

The *cerebro-spinal nervous system* consists of the brain and spinal cord. This system:

1. Controls consciousness and all mental activities.
2. Controls voluntary functions of the five senses: seeing, smelling, tasting, feeling, and hearing.
3. Controls voluntary muscle actions, such as body movements and facial expressions.

The *peripheral nervous system* is made up of the sensory and motor nerve fibers that extend from the brain and spinal cord and are distributed to all parts of the body. Its function is to carry messages to and from the central nervous system.

The *autonomic nervous system* is the portion of the nervous system that functions without conscious effort and regulates the activities of the smooth muscles, glands, blood vessels, and heart. This system has two divisions: the *sympathetic* and *parasympathetic systems*, which act in direct opposition to each other to regulate such things as heart rate, blood pressure, breathing rate, and body temperature, to aid the body in the maintenance of *homeostasis* (balance). The sympathetic division is primarily activated during stressful, energy-demanding, or emergency situations; the parasympathetic division is most active in ordinary restful situations.

TYPES OF NERVES

A *neuron* (**NOOR**-on), or *nerve cell*, is the primary structural unit of the nervous system (Fig. 5.11). It is composed of a cell body and long and short fibers called cell processes. The cell body stores energy and food for the cell processes, which convey the nerve impulses throughout the body. Practically all the nerve cells are contained in the brain and spinal cord.

Nerves are long, white cords made up of fibers (cell processes) that carry messages to and from various parts of the body. Nerves have their origin in the brain and spinal cord, and distribute branches to all parts of the body, which furnish impulses for both sensation and motion. Nerves are nourished through blood vessels, lymph spaces, and lymphatics found in the connective tissue surrounding them.

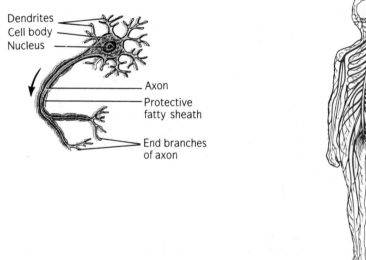

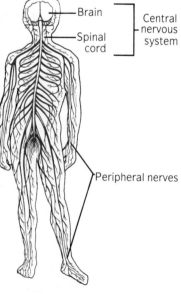

5.12—Spinal cord

Sensory or *afferent* (**AF**-fer-ent) *nerves,* carry impulses or messages from sense organs to the brain, where sensations of touch, cold, heat, sight, hearing, taste, smell, and pain are experienced.

Motor or *efferent* (**EF**-e-rent) *nerves,* carry impulses from the brain to the muscles. The transmitted impulses produce movement.

Sensory nerve endings, called receptors, are located near the surface of the skin. As impulses pass from the sensory nerves to the brain and back over the motor nerves to the muscles, a complete circuit is established and movement of the muscles results.

A *reflex* is an automatic response to a stimulus that involves the movement of an impulse from a sensory receptor along an afferent nerve to the spinal cord, and a responsive impulse along an efferent neuron to a muscle, causing a reaction. (Example: the quick removal of the hand from a hot object.) A reflex action does not have to be learned.

THE BRAIN
The *brain* is the largest mass of nerve tissue in the body and is contained in the cranium. The weight of the average brain is 44 to 48 ounces (approximately 1,418 grams). It is the central power station of the body, sending and receiving messages. Twelve pairs of cranial nerves originate in the brain and reach various parts of the head, face, and neck.

THE SPINAL CORD
The *spinal cord* consists of masses of nerve cells with fibers running upward and downward. It originates in the brain and extends down to the lower extremity of the trunk, and is enclosed and protected by the spinal column.

Thirty-one pairs of spinal nerves, extending from the spinal cord, are distributed to the muscles and skin of the trunk and limbs. Some of the spinal nerves serve the internal organs controlled by the sympathetic nervous system (Fig. 5.12).

NERVE FATIGUE
Nerve fatigue can be caused by excessive mental or muscular work, resulting in an accumulation of waste products. Weariness, irritability, poor complexion, and dull eyes may be signs of nerve exhaustion.

The supply of nerve energy is dependent upon proper intake of food and oxygen, and exercise. Rest and relaxation are absolutely necessary to renew nerve energy.

Appropriate massage manipulations help relieve nerve fatigue. When giving manipulations, the esthetician should always pause over nerve centers.

NERVE STIMULATION
Stimulation to the nerves causes muscles to contract or to expand. Heat on the skin causes relaxation; cold causes contraction.

Nerve stimulation may be accomplished by any of the following:

1. Chemicals—certain acids or salts
2. Massage—hand massage or vibrator
3. Electrical current—high frequency
4. Dry heat—heat lamps and heating masks
5. Moist heat—steamers or moderately warm steam towels

CRANIAL NERVES

There are 12 pairs of cranial nerves: All are connected to a part of the brain surface. They emerge through openings on the sides and base of the cranium and reach various parts of the head, face, and neck. They are classified as motor, sensory, and mixed nerves, and contain both motor and sensory fibers.

The cranial nerves are numbered according to the order in which they emerge from the brain, and are named by description of their nature or function.

First: Olfactory (ol-**FACK**-tur-ee)—A sensory nerve that controls the sense of smell.

Second: Optic (**OP**-tick)—A sensory nerve that controls the sense of sight.

Third: Oculomotor (ock-yoo-lo-**MO**-tur)—A motor nerve that controls the motion of the eye.

Fourth: Trochlear (**TROCK**-lee-ur)—A motor nerve that controls the motion of the eye.

Fifth: Trigeminal (trye-**JEM**-i-nul) or *trifacial* (trye-**FAY**-shul)—A sensory-motor nerve that controls the sensations of the face, tongue, and teeth.

Sixth: Abducent (ab-**DEW**-sunt)—A motor nerve that controls the motion of the eye.

Seventh: Facial (**FAY**-shul)—A sensory-motor nerve that controls the motion of the face, scalp, neck, ear, and sections of the palate and tongue.

Eighth: Acoustic (uh-**KOOS**-tick) or *auditory* (**AW**-di-tor-ee)—A sensory nerve that controls the sense of hearing.

Ninth: Glossopharyngeal (glos-o-fa-**RIN**-jee-ul)—A sensory-motor nerve that controls the sense of taste.

Tenth: Vagus (**VAY**-gus) or *pneumogastric* (new-mo-**GAS**-trick)—A sensory-motor nerve that controls motion and sensations of the ear, pharynx, larynx, heart, lungs, and esophagus.

Eleventh: Accessory (ack-**SES**-uh-ree)—A motor nerve that controls the motion of the neck muscles.

Twelfth: Hypoglossal (high-po-**GLOS**-ul)—A motor nerve that controls the motion of the tongue.

The cranial nerves of most interest to the esthetician in giving facial treatments are: fifth, trigeminal or trifacial; seventh, facial; and eleventh, accessory. The esthetician will also be interested in the spinal (*cervical*) (**SUR**-vi-kal) nerve, which originates in the spinal cord and is involved in scalp and neck massage.

FIFTH CRANIAL NERVE

The *fifth cranial* (*trifacial* or *trigeminal*) nerve is the largest of the cranial nerves. It is the chief sensory nerve of the face, and the motor nerve of the muscles that controls chewing. It consists of three branches: *ophthalmic*, *mandibular*, and *maxillary*.

The following important branches of the fifth cranial nerve are affected by massage. They are numbered according to their appearance on Fig. 5.13.

1. The *supra-orbital* (soo-prah-**OHR**-bi-tahl) *nerve* affects the skin of the forehead, scalp, eyebrows, and upper eyelids.
2. The *supra-trochlear* (soo-prah-**TROK**-lee-ahr) *nerve* affects the skin between the eyes and upper sides of the nose.
3. The *infra-trochlear* (in-frah-**TROK**-lee-ar) *nerve* affects the membrane and skin of the nose.
4. The *nasal* (**NAY**-zal) *nerve* affects the point and lower sides of the nose.
5. The *zygomatic* (zeye-goh-**MAT**-ik) *nerve* affects the skin of the temples, sides of the forehead, and upper part of the cheeks.
6. The *infra-orbital* (in-frah-**OR**-bi-tal) *nerve* affects the skin of the lower eyelids, sides of the nose, upper lip, and mouth.
7. The *auriculo-temporal* (o-**RIK**-yoo-loh **TEM**-po-rahl) *nerve* affects the external ear and the skin from above the temples to the top of the skull.
8. The *mental* (**MEN**-tahl) *nerve* affects the skin of the lower lip and chin.

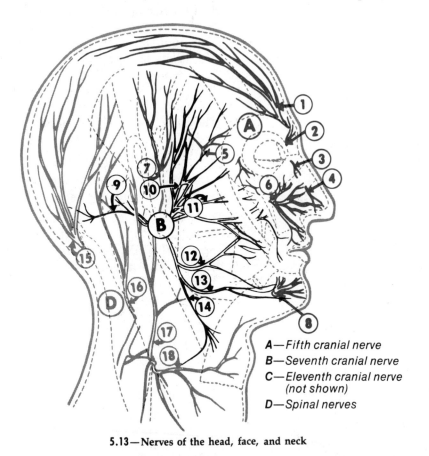

A—*Fifth cranial nerve*
B—*Seventh cranial nerve*
C—*Eleventh cranial nerve (not shown)*
D—*Spinal nerves*

5.13—Nerves of the head, face, and neck

SEVENTH CRANIAL NERVE

The *seventh cranial (facial) nerve* is the chief motor nerve of the face. It emerges near the lower part of the ear. Its divisions and their branches control all the muscles used for facial expression and extend to the muscles of the neck. Of all the branches of the facial nerve, the following are the most important:

9. The *posterior auricular* (po-**STEER**-i-ohr aw-**RIK**-yoo-lahr) *nerve* affects the muscles behind the ears at the base of the skull.
10. The *temporal* (**TEM**-po-rahl) *nerve* affects the muscles of the temples, sides of the forehead, eyebrows, eyelids, and upper part of the cheeks.
11. The *zygomatic* (zeye-goh-**MAT**-ik) *nerve (upper and lower)* affects the muscles of the upper part of the cheeks.
12. The *buccal* (**BUK**-ahl) *nerve* affects the muscles of the mouth.
13. The *mandibular* (man-**DIB**-yoo-lahr) *nerve* affects the muscles of the chin and lower lip.
14. The *cervical* (**SUR**-vi-kal) *nerve* affects the sides of the neck.

ELEVENTH CRANIAL NERVE

The *eleventh cranial (accessory) nerve*—spinal branch—affects the muscles of the neck and back. The branches are not shown on the illustration.

SPINAL (CERVICAL) NERVES

The *spinal (cervical) nerves* originate at the spinal cord. Their branches serve the muscles and scalp at the back of the head and neck, as follows:

15. The *greater occipital* (ok-**SIP**-i-tal) *nerve*, located in the back of the head, affects the scalp as far up as the top of the head.
16. The *smaller (lesser) occipital nerve*, located at the base of the skull, affects the scalp and muscles of this region.
17. The *greater auricular* (aw-**RIK**-yoo-lahr) *nerve*, located at the side of the neck, affects the external ears and the areas in front and back of the ears.
18. The *cutaneous colli* (kyoo-**TAY**-nee-us **CO**-li) *nerve*, located at the side of the neck, affects the front and sides of the neck, as far down as the breastbone.

NERVES OF THE ARM AND HAND

The principal nerves that, with their branches, supply the superficial parts of the arm and hand are (Fig. 5.14):

1. The *ulnar* (**UL**-nar) *nerve*—A sensory-motor nerve that serves the little-finger side of the arm and the palm of the hand.
2. The *radial* (**RAY**-dee-al) *nerve*—A sensory-motor nerve that serves the thumb side of the arm and the back of the hand.
3. The *median* (**MEE**-di-an) *nerve*—A sensory-motor nerve that serves the arm and hand.
4. The *digital* (**DIJ**-it-al) *nerve*—A sensory-motor nerve that serves all the fingers of the hand.

Ulnar
Radial
Median
Digital

5.14—Nerves of the arm and hand

The Circulatory System

The *circulatory* (**SUR**-kyoo-lah-tohr-ee) or *vascular* (**VAS**-kyoo-lahr) *system* consists of a closed system of vessels, including arteries, veins, and capillaries, which carry blood from the heart to all parts of the body, and then back to the heart. This system supplies body cells with food materials, and also carries away waste products. The circulatory system is vitally related to the maintenance of good health. Proper circulation is also a beauty aid to the entire body, as well as to the skin, hair, and nails.

The *blood vascular* (**BLUD VAS**-kyoo-lahr) *system* controls the circulation of the blood through the body in a steady stream, by means of the heart and the blood vessels, the arteries, veins, and capillaries.

THE HEART
The heart is the efficient pump that keeps the blood moving within the circulatory system. It is a muscular, cone-shaped organ, about the size of a fist. It is located in the chest cavity and is enclosed in a membrane called the *pericardium* (per-i-*KAHR*-dee-um). The vagus nerve and other nerves from the sympathetic nervous system regulate the heartbeat. In a normal adult, the heart beats about 72 to 80 times per minute.

The interior of the heart contains four chambers and four valves. The upper thin-walled chambers are the *right atrium* (**AY**-tree-um) and *left atrium*. The lower thick-walled chambers are the *right ventricle* (**VEN**-tri-kel) and *left ventricle*. *Valves* allow the blood to flow in only one direction. With each contraction and relaxation of the heart, the blood flows in, travels from the atria to the ventricles, and is then driven out, to be distributed all over the body. The atrium is also called the *auricle* (**OR**-ik-kel) (Fig. 5.15).

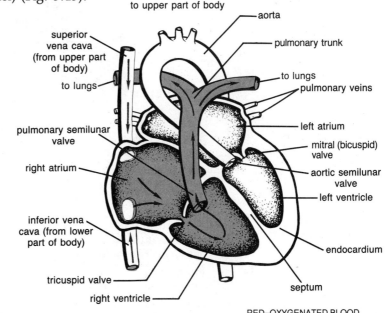

5.15—Diagram of the Heart

RED=OXYGENATED BLOOD
GRAY=UNOXYGENATED BLOOD

BLOOD VESSELS The arteries, veins, and capillaries are tubes that transport blood to and from the heart and to various tissues of the body.

Arteries are thick-walled muscular and elastic tubes that carry *pure* blood from the heart to the tissues.

Veins are thin-walled blood vessels that are less elastic than arteries. They contain cup-like valves to prevent back-flow, and they carry *impure* blood from the tissues back to the heart. Veins are located closer to the outer surface of the body than are the arteries (Fig. 5.16).

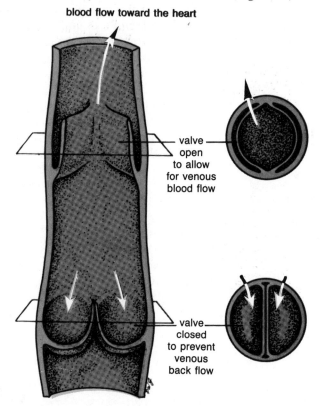

blood flow toward the heart

valve open to allow for venous blood flow

valve closed to prevent venous back flow

5.16—Cross sections of veins

Capillaries are minute, thin-walled blood vessels that connect the smaller arteries with the veins. The tissues receive nourishment and eliminate waste products through the capillary walls.

The blood is in constant circulation, from the moment it leaves the heart until it returns. Two systems take care of this circulation:

1. *Pulmonary* (**PUUL**-mo-ner-ee) *circulation* is the blood circulation that goes from the heart to the lungs to be purified, and then returns to the heart.
2. *General circulation* is the blood circulation from the heart throughout the body and back again to the heart.

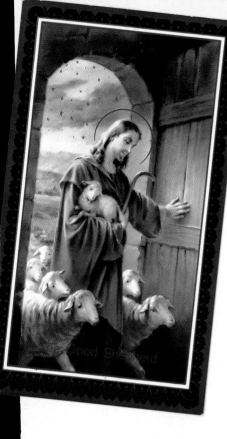

Blood is the nutritive fluid circulating through the blood circulatory system. It is a sticky, salty fluid, with a normal temperature that remains at 98.6°F (37°C). The 8 to 10 pints that fill the blood vessels of an adult make up about one-twentieth of the weight of the body.

Blood changes color as it gains or loses oxygen while passing through the lungs. Blood is bright red in color in the arteries (except in the pulmonary artery) and dark red in the veins (except in the pulmonary vein).

Blood is composed of *plasma*, the liquid portion that contains *red* and *white corpuscles*, and *platelets*. The red corpuscles carry oxygen to the cells. The white corpuscles, or *leucocytes* (**LOO**-ko-seyets), destroy disease-causing germs. Platelets are much smaller than the red blood cells. They play an important part in the clotting of the blood over a wound (Figs. 5.17–5.19).

Plasma is straw-like in color. About nine-tenths of the plasma is water. It carries food and secretions to the cells, and carbon dioxide from the cells.

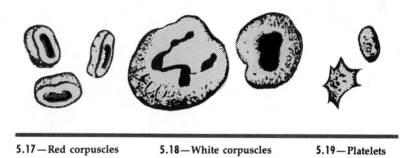

| 5.17—Red corpuscles | 5.18—White corpuscles | 5.19—Platelets |

FUNCTIONS OF THE BLOOD

The primary functions of blood are:

1. To carry water, oxygen, food, and secretions to all cells of the body
2. To carry away carbon dioxide and other waste products to be eliminated through the lungs, skin, kidneys, and large intestine
3. To help equalize the body temperature, thus protecting the body from extreme heat and cold
4. To help protect the body from harmful bacteria and infections, through the action of the white blood cells
5. To form clots, thereby closing injured blood vessels and preventing the loss of blood

ARTERIES OF THE HEAD, FACE, AND NECK

The *common carotid* (kah-**ROT**-id) *arteries* are the main sources of the blood supply to the head, face, and neck. They are located on either side of the neck and divide into internal and external carotid arteries. The *internal division* of the common carotid artery supplies the brain, eye sockets, eyelids, and forehead. The *external division* supplies the superficial parts of the head, face, and neck (Fig. 5.20).

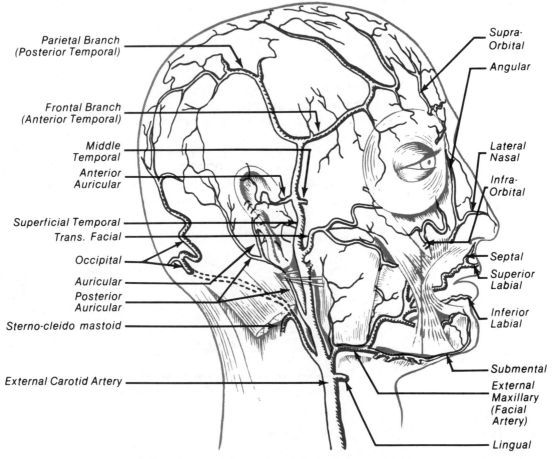

5.20—Diagram of the arteries of the head, face, and neck

THE EXTERNAL MAXILLARY ARTERY   The *external maxillary*, or *facial artery*, supplies the lower region of the face, mouth, and nose. These are some of its branches.

1. The *submental* (sub-**MEN**-tahl) *artery* supplies the chin and lower lip.
2. The *inferior labial* (**LAY**-bi-al) *artery* supplies the lower lip.
3. The *angular* (**ANG**-gew-lur) *artery* supplies the side of the nose.
4. The *superior labial artery* supplies the upper lip, *septum* (dividing wall) of the nose, and the wings of the nose.

SUPERFICIAL TEMPORAL ARTERY   The *superficial temporal* (**TEM**-po-rahl) *artery* is a continuation of the external carotid artery, and supplies the muscles, skin, and scalp on the front, side, and top of the head. The following are important branches.

1. The *frontal* (**FRUNT**-al) *artery* supplies the forehead.
2. The *parietal* (pa-**REYE**-e-tal) *artery* supplies the crown and sides of the head.

3. The *transverse* (trans-**VURS**) *facial artery* supplies the masseter.
4. The *middle temporal artery* supplies the temples and eyelids.
5. The *anterior auricular* (aw-**RIK**-yoo-lahr) *artery* supplies the anterior part of the ear.

THE OCCIPITAL ARTERY

The *occipital* (ok-**SIP**-i-tal) *artery* supplies the scalp and back of the head up to the crown. Its most important branch is the *sterno-cleido-mastoid artery*, which supplies the muscle of the same name.

THE POSTERIOR AURICULAR ARTERY

The *posterior auricular artery* supplies the scalp, behind and above the ear. Its most important branch is the *auricular artery*, which supplies the skin in back of the ear.

VEINS OF THE HEAD, FACE, AND NECK

The blood returning to the heart from the head, face, and neck flows on each side of the neck in two principal veins: the *internal jugular* and the *external jugular*. The most important veins are parallel to the arteries and take the same names as the arteries.

BLOOD SUPPLY FOR THE ARM AND HAND

The *ulnar* and *radial arteries* are the main blood suppliers for the arm and hand. The ulnar artery and its numerous branches supply the little-finger side of the arm and the palm. The radial artery and its branches supply the thumb side of the arm and the back of the hand. The important veins are located almost parallel with the arteries and take the same names as the arteries. While the arteries are found deep in the tissues, the veins lie closer to the surface of the arms and hands (Fig. 5.21).

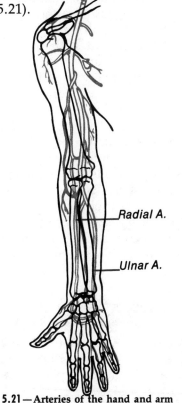

Radial A.

Ulnar A.

5.21 —Arteries of the hand and arm

The *lymph-vascular* (**LIMF-VAS**-kyoo-lahr) or *lymphatic system* is a separate circulatory system, consisting of the *lymph glands* and *lacteals* (**LAK**-teels). The lacteals are lymphatic capillaries that transfer *chyle* (**KILE**), which contains fats, absorbed from the intestine during digestion.

Lymph is a colorless, watery fluid that circulates through the lymphatic system and is similar in composition to the plasma of the blood.

The lymphatic system is the waste disposal and drainage system for the body tissues. Lymphatic capillaries serve as drains and join and form the larger lymphatic vessels. Some cellular products pass into the lymphatic capillaries. Before these substances reach the veins, they are filtered through the lymph nodes and then returned to the blood. The lymph carries nourishment from the blood to the cells and removes waste from the cells.

The main function of the lymphoid tissue is to remove bacteria and foreign materials, to manufacture lymphocytes, which make up some of the white blood cells, and to produce antibodies to combat infection. The tonsils are an example of lymphoid tissue.

The Endocrine System

The *endocrine* (**EN**-doh-krin) *system* is composed of a group of specialized *glands*, which regulate and control the growth, reproduction, and health of the body. Just as the nervous system is the body's electrical control system, the endocrine system is the body's chemical control system.

Glands are specialized organs that vary in size and function, and are intimately connected with the circulatory and nervous systems. The nervous system controls the functional activities of the endocrine glands, which have the ability to remove certain elements from the blood and to convert them into new compounds.

The endocrine, or ductless, glands are the major components of the endocrine system. They put their secretions directly into the blood stream, which in turn influence the welfare of the entire body. Because it produces vitamin D, the skin may also be considered part of the endocrine system.

The ducted glands, the sweat and sebaceous glands, are not part of the endocrine system. These glands possess canals that lead from the gland to a particular part of the body. These glands are discussed in the chapter titled, *Physiology and Histology of the Skin*.

The endocrine system is important to the esthetician because the hormones and other secretions produced may be affected by the skin care products used on the client.

The Excretory System

The *excretory* (**EK**-skre-tohr-ee) *system*, including the kidneys, liver, skin, intestines, and lungs, purifies the body by eliminating waste matter.

Each of the following plays a part in the excretory system:

1. The *kidneys* excrete urine.
2. The *liver* discharges bile.
3. The *skin* eliminates perspiration.
4. The *large intestine* evacuates decomposed and undigested food.
5. The *lungs* exhale carbon dioxide.

Metabolism of the cells of the body forms various toxic substances which, if retained, might poison the body.

The Respiratory System

The *respiratory* (**RES**-pi-rah-tohr-ee) *system*, whose most important organs are the *trachea* (**TRAY**-kee-uh), *bronchial* (**BRONK**-ee-ul) *tubes* and *lungs*, supplies the body with oxygen and removes carbon dioxide. The system is situated within the chest cavity and is protected on both sides by the ribs. The *diaphragm* (**DI**-a-fram), a muscular partition that controls breathing, separates the chest from the *abdominal* (ab-**DOM**-i-nal) *regions*.

The *nasal cavity* is the primary inlet for air. Air comes in through the nose, where it is warmed and filtered, then passed through the *pharynx* (**FAR**-inks), or throat, and then to the *larynx* (**LAR**-inks), or voice box. The *trachea*, or windpipe, connects the throat with the *bronchial tree*, which takes the air into the *lungs*.

The lungs are spongy tissues composed of microscopic cells into which oxygen from the inhaled air is absorbed. These tiny air cells are enclosed in a skin-like tissue. Behind this tissue are found the fine capillaries of the blood vascular system.

With each respiratory cycle, an exchange of gases takes place. During *inhalation* (in-ha-**LAY**-shun), oxygen is absorbed into the blood, while carbon dioxide is expelled during *exhalation* (eks-ha-**LAY**-shun). Oxygen is required to change food into energy.

Oxygen is more essential than either food or water. Although a person may live more than 60 days without food, and a few days without water, death occurs if air is excluded for more than a few minutes.

Breathing is necessary to carry on the life functions. The rate of breathing depends on activity. Muscular activities and energy expenditures increase the body's demands for oxygen. As a result, the rate of breathing is increased. A person requires about three times as much oxygen when walking than when standing.

Abdominal breathing is of value in building health. Costal breathing involves light, or shallow, breathing of the lungs, without action of the diaphragm. Abdominal breathing means deep breathing, which brings the diaphragm into action, and accomplishes the greatest exchange of gases.

The Digestive System

The *digestive* (deye-**GES**-tiv) *system* changes food into a soluble form, suitable for use by the cells of the body. It distributes the nutrients throughout the body. The digestive system consists of the *alimentary* (al-i-**MEN**-tuh-ree) *canal* and the *accessory glands* that produce the enzymes that digest and process the food. It is important to the esthetician because of the effects nutrition and elimination have on keeping the skin healthy.

The *alimentary canal* is a 27-foot long tube that begins at the mouth and ends at the *anus*. The *accessory glands* include the *salivary glands*, the *liver*, the *gallbladder* and the *pancreas*.

Food is ingested through the mouth, where it is broken into smaller particles. Saliva from the salivary glands moistens the particles and begins the digestive process. The food particles move through the *esophagus* (i-**SOF**-a-gus), or food pipe, into the stomach, where they mix with digestive juices to form a thick mass, called *chyme* (**KIM**).

Little by little, the chyme passes into the small intestine, a 21-foot long section of the alimentary canal, where most of the digestive process is carried out. Here, bile from the liver and enzymes from the pancreas release the nutrients from the food particles.

The nutrients are absorbed into the blood stream through the walls of the small intestine. Undigested food and wastes pass into the large intestine, where they are processed and made ready for removal from the body, with the aid of the excretory system.

The Reproductive System

The *reproductive system* performs the function of reproducing and perpetuating the human race. Although important to the perpetuation of the species, it is not of major importance to the esthetician, except as the sex hormones, testosterone (tes-**TOS**-tur-ohn) in males and estrogen (**ES**-tro-jin) in females, affect some skin functions.

QUESTIONS DISCUSSION AND REVIEW

CELLS, ANATOMY,
AND PHYSIOLOGY

1. What is the largest organ of the body?
2. What is a cell?
3. What is found in the structure of a cell?
4. How does a cell reproduce?
5. How is a cell nourished and what are the two phases of metabolism?
6. What are the five classified groups of tissues?
7. Is the skin a tissue or an organ?
8. What are the nine systems of the body?
9. What are the hardest structures of the body?
10. How many bones are in the body?
11. Name the eight cranium bones.
12. Name the fourteen facial bones.
13. What is the thorax made up of?
14. Where would you find the clavicle and scapula?
15. What is the largest bone of the upper arm?
16. The carpus is composed of how many bones?
17. What are the long slender bones of the palm called?
18. What is the function of the muscular system?
19. What is myology?
20. What is the muscle of the heart called?
21. Name five ways in which muscles can be stimulated.
22. Describe how the direction of pressure in the massage is usually performed.
23. Name the muscles of the scalp.
24. Name the muscles of the eyebrows.
25. Name the muscle of the nose.
26. Name the muscles of the mouth.
27. What is neurology?
28. What is the main purpose for studying the nervous system?
29. What are the three main divisions of the nervous system?
30. What are the two types of nerves?
31. What is the largest mass of nerve tissue?
32. Give the signs of nerve fatigue.
33. Give two other names for the fifth nerve.
34. Name the parts of the blood vascular system.
35. What carries the pure blood?
36. Which of the corpuscles destroy disease causing germs?
37. Which system is the waste disposal system for the body tissues?
38. Which system controls the chemicals in the body?
39. Why is the skin considered part of the endocrine system?
40. Kidneys, liver, skin, intestines, and lungs are all part of what system?
41. What is required to change food into energy?
42. Why is nose breathing healthier than mouth breathing?
43. Why is the digestive system important to the esthetician?

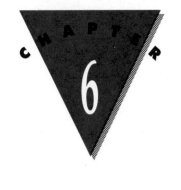

Physiology and Histology of the Skin

LEARNING OBJECTIVES *After completing this chapter, you should be able to:*

❶ Describe the structure and composition of the skin (histology).
❷ Explain how the skin is nourished.
❸ Explain how important the skin is to bodily health and how it reacts to the sensations of pressure, touch, temperature, and pain.
❹ List and explain the functions of the skin.

INTRODUCTION

The health and appearance of the skin (*integumentary system*) are of concern to everyone, but the scientific study of the skin is of particular importance to the esthetician. (*See Color Plate 1.*)

The skin is the largest and one of the most important organs of the body. A healthy skin is slightly moist, soft, flexible; possesses a slightly acid reaction; and is free from any disease or disorder. The skin also has immunity responses to organisms that touch or try to enter it. Its *texture* (feel and appearance) ideally is smooth and fine grained.

The skin varies in thickness from a twelfth to a fifth of an inch (.212 centimeters to .508 centimeters). The skin is thinnest on the eyelids and thickest on the palms of the hands and the soles of the feet. Continued pressure over any part of the skin will cause it to thicken (as in a callous) to provide more protection.

The skin of an adult covers about 18.2 square feet (1.69 square meters) and weighs approximately 6 pounds (2.73 kilograms). The skin is elastic, resistant, and under normal conditions renews itself. It functions as a protective covering for the body, preventing the entry of micro-organisms and other harmful substances. Sensory nerve fibers in the skin react to five separate and basic sensations: pressure, touch, temperature, (such as heat and cold), and pain.

Every inch of skin contains millions of cells, an intricate network of blood vessels, and nerves. In addition, the skin contains pores that are the openings for hair follicles, sebaceous glands, and sweat glands. The

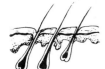

65 hairs

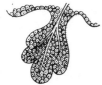

95–100 sebaceous glands

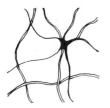

78 yards (70 meters) of nerves

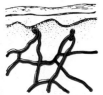

19 yards (17 meters) of blood vessels

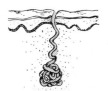

650 sweat glands

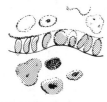

9,500,000 cells

sebaceous glands produce the sebum (oil) that lubricates the skin. Most skin problems are seen on the epidermis, the surface layer of the skin, but trouble can start in the dermis, the layer that lies just below the epidermis. The dermis is made of *collagen* (**KOL**-uh-jin) (a form of protein) fibers. This substance gives the skin strength, form, and flexibility. The blood vessels, fat cells, and oil and sweat glands are held together by collagen fibers. Wrinkles and sagging occur when the collagen fibers lose their flexibility.

The skin's unbelievable complexity is partially indicated when we consider the fact that each square inch contains (Fig. 6.1):

- 65 hairs
- 95–100 sebaceous glands
- 78 yards of nerves (70 meters)
- 19 yards (17 meters) of blood vessels
- 650 sweat glands
- 9,500,000 cells
- 1,300 nerve endings to record pain
- 19,500 sensory cells at the ends of nerve fibers
- 78 sensory apparatuses for heat
- 13 sensory apparatuses for cold
- 160–165 pressure apparatuses for the perception of tactile stimuli

The epidermis of the skin protects the delicate tissues of the body from injury. This protective ability of the skin is due to the fact that it is made of a substance called *keratin* (**KER**-a-tin).

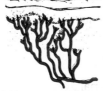

1,300 nerve endings to record pain

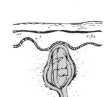

78 sensory apparatuses for heat

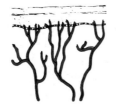

19,500 sensory cells at the ends of nerve fibers

13 sensory apparatuses for cold

160–165 pressure apparatuses for the perception of tactile stimuli

6.1—The structure of the skin contained within one square inch (6.452 square centimeters)

Keratin Composition

Keratin comes in two forms: hard, as in the hair, and soft, as in the skin. Being a protein, it contains the following elements: carbon, nitrogen, hydrogen, phosphorus, oxygen, and sulfur.

Soft Keratin—Soft keratin contains about 2 percent sulfur, 50 percent to 75 percent moisture and a small percentage of fats. Keratin is found in the skin, especially in the layer of the epidermis, where it occurs in the form of flattened cells or as dry scales.

FORMS OF KERATIN   *Hard Keratin*—Hard keratin, as found in hair, has a sulfur content of 4 to 8 percent, a lower moisture and fat content, and is particularly tough, elastic material. It forms continuous sheets (fingernails) or long endless fibers (hair). Hard keratin does not normally break off or flake away. It remains a continuous structure.

No other tissue of the body contains as much sulfur as is found in keratin.

Collagen

Collagen makes up a large part of the dermis—about 70 percent. It forms a network of microscopic interwoven fibers that gives the skin structural support for cells and blood vessels. Collagen allows for stretching and contraction of the skin, provides strength, and aids in the healing of wounds. The space between collagen fibers contains a protein called *elastin* (e-**LAS**-tin), which gives the skin its elasticity. Moisture is important to keeping the collagen network supple. It is the condition of the skin's collagen, not the facial muscles, that causes lines and wrinkles. With age, the collagen network tends to weaken, to lose moisture and resiliency, thus causing the skin to lose its tone and suppleness.

Hair and the Skin

Hair is an appendage of the skin, a slender, threadlike outgrowth of the skin and scalp (Fig. 6.2). There is no sense of feeling in hair, due to the absence of nerves.

Hair grows over the entire body, with the exception of the soles of the feet, the palms of the hands, some areas of the genitalia, the mucous membranes of the lips, the nipples, the navel, and the eyelids. Much of the hair on the body is invisible to the naked eye. The heavier concentration of hair is on the head, under the armpits, on and around the genitals, and on the arms and legs. Due to hormonal influence, males grow facial hair and hair on the chest. The genes that are inherited strongly influence the distribution of an individual's hair, its thickness, quality, color, rate of growth, and whether the hair is curly or straight.

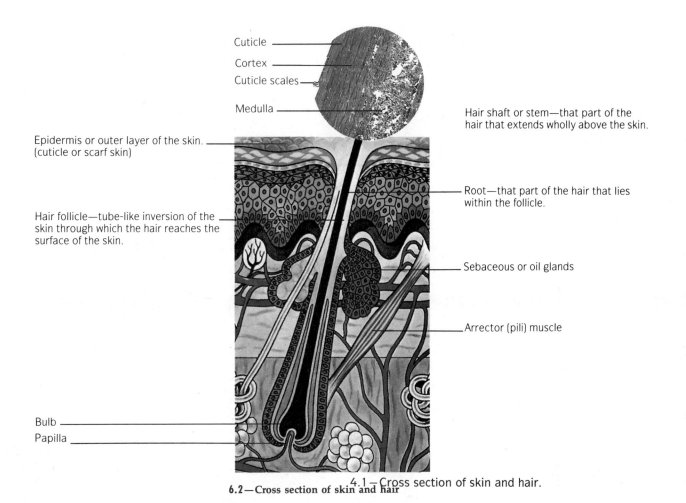

Cuticle

Cortex

Cuticle scales

Medulla

Hair shaft or stem—that part of the hair that extends wholly above the skin.

Epidermis or outer layer of the skin. (cuticle or scarf skin)

Root—that part of the hair that lies within the follicle.

Hair follicle—tube-like inversion of the skin through which the hair reaches the surface of the skin.

Sebaceous or oil glands

Arrector (pili) muscle

Bulb

Papilla

6.2—Cross section of skin and hair 4.1—Cross section of skin and hair.

Nails and the Skin

The nail, an appendage of the skin, is a hard translucent plate that protects the tips of the fingers and toes (Fig. 6.3). *Onyx* (**ON**-iks) is the technical term for the nail. The nail is composed of hard keratin. The hard, or horny, nail plate contains no nerves or blood vessels.

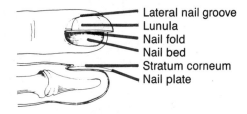

Lateral nail groove
Lunula
Nail fold
Nail bed
Stratum corneum
Nail plate

6.3—Fingernail

Histology of the Skin

The skin contains two clearly defined divisions: the epidermis and the dermis (Fig. 6.4).

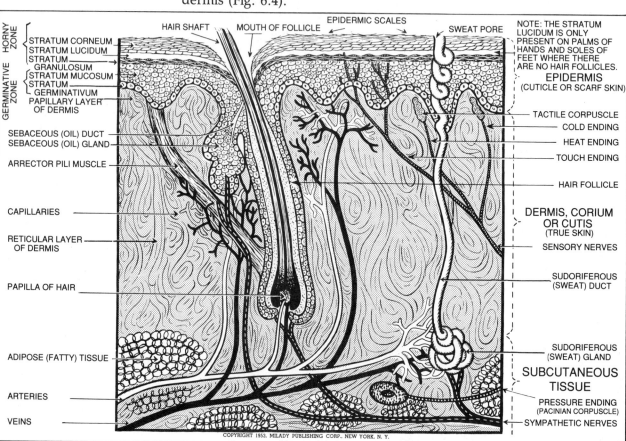

6.4—Histology of the skin, hair, and glands

EPIDERMIS

The *epidermis* (ep-i-**DUR**-mis) is the outermost layer of the skin. This layer is commonly called *cuticle* (**KYOO**-ti-kel) or *scarf skin*. The epidermis forms the protective covering of the skin of the body. It contains no blood vessels, but has many small nerve endings. The epidermis contains the following layers:

1. The ***stratum corneum*** (**STRAT**-um **KOHR**-nee-um), or horny layer, consists of tightly packed, scale-like cells, which are continually being shed and replaced.
2. The ***stratum lucidum*** (**LOO**-si-dum), or clear layer, consists of small, transparent cells through which light can pass. The stratum lucidum is only present on the palms of the hands and soles of the feet. It is not present where there are hair follicles.

3. The *stratum granulosum* (gran-yoo-**LOH**-sum), or granular layer, consists of cells that look like distinct granules. These cells are dying and undergo a change into a hard substance.

4. *Stratum spinosum* (spye-**NO**-sum), or prickle cell layer, is often classified with the stratum germinativum, to form the basal layer. Prickle-like threads join the cells.

5. The *stratum germinativum* (jur-mi-nah-**TIV**-um), formerly known as the *stratum mucosum* (myoo-**KOH**-sum), is composed of a single layer of cells. The stratum germinativum is responsible for the growth of the epidermis. It also contains a dark pigment called *melanin* (**MEL**-uh-nin), which protects the sensitive cells below from the destructive effects of excessive ultra-violet rays of the sun or ultra-violet rays from a lamp.

> **Note:** Stratum germinativum is also referred to as basal (**BAY**-sal) or Malpighian (mal-**PIG**-ee-un) layer.

DERMIS The *dermis* (**DUR**-mis) is the underlying, or inner layer, of the skin. It is also called *derma*, *corium* (**KOH**-ree-um), *cutis* (**KYOO**-tis), or *true skin*.

It is a highly sensitive and vascular layer of connective tissue. Within its structure are found numerous blood vessels, lymph vessels, nerves, sweat glands, oil glands, hair follicles, arrector pili muscles, and papillae. The dermis consists of two layers: the papillary or superficial layer, and the reticular or deeper layer.

1. The *papillary* (pa-**PIL**-ah-ry) layer lies directly beneath the epidermis. It contains small cone-shaped projections of *elastic* tissue that point upward into the epidermis. These projections are called *papillae* (pah-**PIL**-e). Some of these papillae contain looped capillaries, others contain nerve fiber endings called *tactile corpuscles* (**TAK**-til **KOR**-pus-lz).

2. The *reticular* (re-**TIK**-u-lar) layer contains the following structures within its network:

   a) Fat cells
   b) Blood vessels
   c) Lymph vessels
   d) Oil glands
   e) Sweat glands
   f) Hair follicles
   g) Arrector pili muscles

SUBCUTANEOUS TISSUE *Subcutaneous* (sub-kyoo-**TAY**-nee-us) *tissue* is a fatty layer found below the dermis. Some histologists consider this tissue as a continuation of the dermis. This tissue is also called *adipose* (**AD**-i-pohs), or *subcutis* (sub-**KYOO**-tis) *tissue* and varies in thickness according to the age, sex, and general health of the individual. It gives smoothness and contour to the body, contains fats for use as energy, and also acts as a protective cushion for the outer skin. Circulation is maintained by a network of arteries and lymphatics.

How the Skin is Nourished

Blood and lymph supply nourishment to the skin. As they circulate through the skin, the blood and lymph contribute essential materials for growth, nourishment, and repair of the skin, hair, and nails. In the subcutaneous tissue are found networks of arteries and lymphatics that send their smaller branches to hair papillae, hair follicles, and skin glands.

Nerves of the Skin

The skin contains the surface endings of many nerve fibers. They are:

1. *Motor nerve fibers*, which are distributed to the arrector pili muscles attached to the hair follicles. This muscle causes "gooseflesh" when you are frightened or cold.
2. *Sensory nerve fibers*, which react to heat, cold, touch, pressure, and pain. These sensory receptors send mesages to the brain (Fig. 6.5).
3. *Secretory nerve fibers*, which are distributed to the sweat and oil glands of the skin. These nerves regulate the excretion of perspiration from the sweat glands and control the flow of sebum to the surface of the skin.

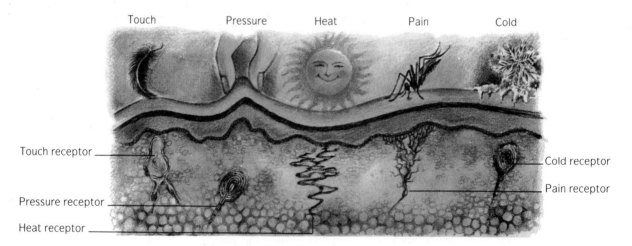

6.5—Sensory nerves of the skin

SENSE OF TOUCH   The papillary layer of the dermis houses the nerve endings that provide the body with the sense of touch. These nerve endings register basic sensations: touch, pain, heat, cold, pressure, or touch. Nerve endings are most abundant in the fingertips. Complex sensations, such as vibrations, seem to depend on the sensitivity of a combination of these nerve endings.

Skin Elasticity

The pliability of the skin depends on the elasticity of the dermis. For example, healthy skin regains its former shape almost immediately after being expanded.

Absorption of the Skin

NATURAL OPENINGS IN SKIN Although the skin is an intact outer layer of the body, it is in fact indented by hair follicles with their sebaceous (oil) glands and by the pores of the sudoriferous (sue-dur-**IF**-ur-us) (sweat) glands. These pockets, although normally resistant to bacterial attack (except in certain cases where they show as pimples, boils, blackheads or acne), will allow the entry of special drugs and chemicals into the body. These chemicals may be absorbed in order to combat infections of the skin (antiseptic creams and ointments) or they may be used as skin conditioners to help overcome dryness or damage (vitamin and hormone creams).

SKIN BREATHING The skin is said to "breathe" because it takes in oxygen and discharges carbon dioxide. The amount of carbon dioxide released by the skin in one hour is about one percent of the carbon dioxide released by the lungs at the same time. Therefore, it is dangerous to coat the skin entirely with a substance which interferes with this breathing process. There are cases where the use of gold paint to coat the body has resulted in death by asphyxiation.

SHRINKING PORES It is possible to make pore (follicle) openings smaller. Dirt, dead cells, makeup, and other substances can form a plug in the pore. This plug (commonly called a blackhead) stretches the opening of the follicle. When the plug is removed, the follicle becomes smaller. During a series of deep pore cleansing facial treatments, hundreds of enlarged follicles are cleansed, and as a result, the pores close, giving the complexion a more refined appearance (Fig. 6.6).

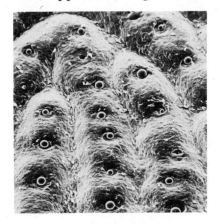

6.6—Sweat from pores on palm of hand

WATER Another problem to be considered is the effect of water on the skin. The skin, itself 50 to 75 percent moisture, is able to maintain this level only by the secretion of sebum which coats its surface (Fig. 6.7). This layer of oil slows down the evaporation of water in the skin and prevents excess moisture from penetrating into it. But if the natural oils are removed by any means whatsoever, especially from the hands, this protection is lost.

Let us examine the case where the hands are excessively exposed to cold, drying winds. As the oil barrier is lost, the skin cannot prevent its cells from becoming dry and scaly (chafed). If further exposed to drying winds, cracking and bleeding take place. This is more frequently noticed in winter than in summer, because the cold usually restricts the flow of blood to the dermis and the evaporation of the skin moisture cannot be balanced by a greater flow of blood and lymph (Fig. 6.8).

AGING SKIN The aging process of the skin is a subject of vital importance to everyone. Perhaps the most outstanding characteristic of the aged skin is its loss of elasticity. One factor that contributes to the loss of elasticity is that as we age subcutaneous tissue shrinks and is not as effective a support system in preventing the skin from wrinkling. Aging skin will be discussed in detail in Chapter 20, *Enemies of the Skin, Aging Factors, and Cosmetic Surgery.*

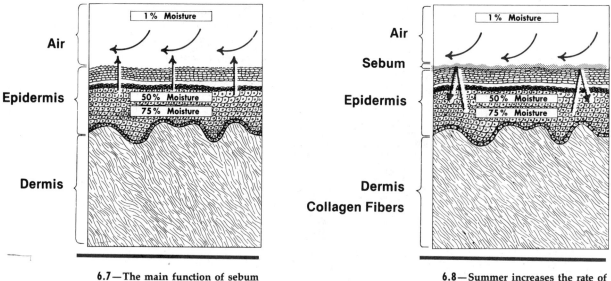

6.7—The main function of sebum is to act as a shield that prevents moisture from evaporating from the surface of the skin.

6.8—Summer increases the rate of sweating, and this enables the skin to be kept naturally moist, preventing drying and chafing.

Skin Color

The color of the skin, whether fair or dark, depends primarily on the melanin, or coloring matter, that is deposited in the stratum germinativum. To a limited extent, it depends on the blood supply in the skin. The pigment varies in different people. In various races and nationalities, the distinctive color of the skin is a hereditary trait.

Melanocytes

Special cells called melanocytes produce pigment granules which are scattered throughout the basal layer of the epidermis. Melanocytes are derived from nerve tissue and produce the pigment granules which are passed on to keratinocytes (epidermal cells that synthesize keratin) to give the skin most of its color. These granules are called melanosomes and produce a complex protein called melanin, a brownish, black pigment which serves as the skin's protective screen (Fig. 6.9).

People of different race have approximately the same number of melanocytes but they are more active in dark-skinned people. The lighter the skin, the fewer the melanocyte pigment cells. The darker the skin the more protection the melanin provides from the ultra-violet rays of the sun and from premature aging of the skin. Dark-skinned people also have fewer incidences of skin cancer.

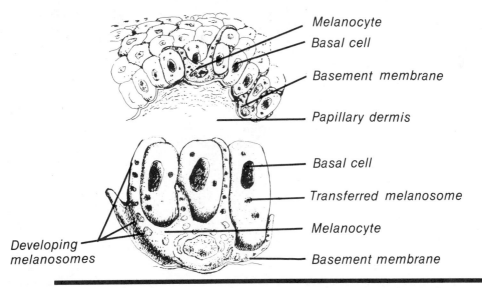

Melanocyte
Basal cell
Basement membrane
Papillary dermis

Basal cell
Transferred melanosome
Melanocyte
Basement membrane

Developing melanosomes

6.9—Melanocytes transfer pigment to the keratinocytes, the epidermal cells that synthesize keratin, to give the skin most of its color.

The Glands of the Skin

The skin contains two types of duct glands that extract materials from the blood to form different substances.

1. The *sudoriferous* (sue-dur-**IF**-ur-us) or *sweat glands* excrete sweat.
2. The *sebaceous* (si-**BAY**-shus) or *oil glands*, secrete sebum.

The *sweat glands* (tubular type) consist of a coiled base, or *fundus* (**FUN**-dus), and a tube-like duct which terminates at the skin surface to form the *sweat pore* (Fig. 6.10). Practically all parts of the body are supplied with sweat glands, which are more numerous on the palms, soles, forehead, and under the armpits. The sweat glands regulate body temperature and help to eliminate waste products from the body. Their activity is greatly increased by heat, exercise, emotions, and certain drugs. The excretion of sweat is under the control of the nervous system. Normally, one or two pints of liquids containing salts are eliminated daily through the sweat pores in the skin.

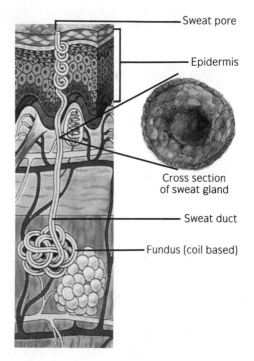

Sweat pore

Epidermis

Cross section
of sweat gland

Sweat duct

Fundus (coil based)

6.10—Sweat gland

SWEAT GLANDS   There are two kinds of sweat glands, the *apocrine* (**AP**-o-krin) and the *eccrine* (**ECK**-rin). The apocrine glands are tiny coiled structures attached to the hair follicles. Their secretions are released through the pores of the sebaceous (oil) glands.

The apocrine glands are found under the arms, in the genital area, and in the nipples of both males and females. The apocrine glands are more active during emotional changes, such as tension, fear or during sexual arousal. The secretion is odorless when released, but in a short period of time produces an offensive smell due to the bacteria on the skin's surface feeding on the fats of this secretion.

The eccrine (sweat) glands are found over the entire body, primarily on the forehead, the palms of the hands, and soles of the feet. Unlike the apocrine glands, the eccrine glands are not connected to a hair follicle and have a duct and pore through which secretions are brought to the skin's surface. The eccrine glands are more active when the body is subjected to physical activity and high temperatures. Eccrine sweat does not produce an offensive odor.

OIL GLANDS The *oil glands* (saccular type) consist of little sacs, whose ducts open into the hair follicle (Fig. 6.11). They secrete *sebum* (**SEE**-bum), which lubricates the skin and helps to prevent the evaporation of moisture from the skin. With the exception of the palms and soles, these glands are found in all parts of the body, particularly the face.

Sebum is a semi-fluid, oily substance produced by the oil glands. Ordinarily, it flows through the oil ducts leading to the mouths of the hair follicles. However, when the sebum becomes hardened and the follicle becomes blocked, a blackhead is formed. Deep cleansing of the follicles is of prime importance in keeping the skin free of blemishes.

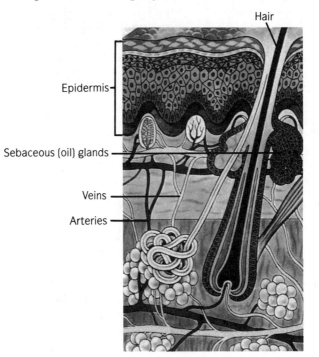

6.11 — Scalp hair, follicle, and oil glands

Functions of the Skin

The principal functions of the skin are: protection, sensation, heat regulation, excretion, secretion, and absorption.

1. *Protection*. The skin protects the body from injury and bacterial invasion. The outermost layer of the epidermis is covered with a thin layer of sebum, thus rendering it waterproof. It is resistant to different degrees of temperature, minor injuries, chemically active substances, and many microbes. If germs do invade, the skin becomes inflamed and in the process destroys them.
2. *Sensation*. Through its sensory nerve endings, the skin responds to heat, cold, touch, pressure, and pain. Extreme stimulation of a sensory nerve ending produces pain. A minor burn is very painful, but a deep burn that destroys the nerves may be painless.
3. *Heat regulation*. The healthy body maintains a constant internal temperature of about 98.6°F (37°C). As changes occur in the outside temperature, the blood and sweat glands of the skin make necessary adjustments in their functions. Heat regulation is a function of the skin, which is an organ that protects the body from the environment. Heat is lost by the evaporation of sweat.
4. *Excretion*. Perspiration from the sweat glands is excreted from the skin. Water lost by perspiration carries salt and other chemicals with it.
5. *Secretion*. Sebum is secreted by the sebaceous glands. Excessive flow of oil from the oil glands may produce *seborrhea* (seb-o-**REE**-ah). Emotional stress may increase the flow of sebum.
6. *Absorption* is limited, but it does occur. Only certain substances applied in a face cream can enter the body through the skin and influence the body to a minor degree.

The skin has an immunity responsiveness to many things that touch it or gain entry into it.

QUESTIONS DISCUSSION AND REVIEW

PHYSIOLOGY AND HISTOLOGY OF THE SKIN

1. Briefly describe the skin.
2. What is the appearance of a good complexion?
3. Name the two main divisions of the skin.
4. Locate the epidermis and give its main function.
5. Name the five layers of the epidermis.
6. Which epidermal layer is continually being shed and replaced?
7. Which epidermal layer consists of small, transparent cells?
8. Which epidermal layer starts to undergo a change into a horny (hard) substance?
9. Which layer of the epidermis is responsible for its reproduction and growth?

10. Describe the structure of the dermis.
11. Name the two layers of the dermis.
12. Which structures are found in the papillary layer?
13. Which structures are found in the reticular layer?
14. What is the function of the subcutaneous tissue?
15. About how much blood is found in the skin?
16. How is the skin nourished?
17. Name three types of nerve fibers found in the skin.
18. Which part of the body is abundantly supplied with nerve endings?
19. To which structures in the skin are the motor nerve fibers distributed?
20. What renders the skin flexible?
21. Where is the coloring matter (melanin) of the skin found?
22. To what five things will the sensory nerves of the skin react?
23. What are the functions of the nerve fibers distributed to sweat and oil glands?
24. What is meant by pliability of the skin?
25. What is the characteristic of aged skin?
26. What determines the color of the skin?
27. What are the six important functions of the skin?
28. What regulates the temperature of the body?
29. What is the normal temperature of the human body?
30. Name four appendages related to the skin.
31. Discuss two types of duct glands that are found in the skin.
32. Describe the structure of the sweat glands.
33. Where are the sweat glands found?
34. What is the function of the sweat glands?
35. Name four things capable of increasing the activity of the sweat glands.
36. Describe the structure of the oil glands.
37. Which substance is secreted by the oil glands?
38. What is the chief function of sebum?
39. Where are the oil glands found?
40. Discuss the principle functions of the skin and glands of the skin.

Disorders of the Skin, Dermatology, and Special Esthetic Procedures

LEARNING OBJECTIVES

After completing this chapter, you should be able to:

❶ Explain dermatology terms related to skin conditions and lesions.
❷ List and define skin conditions and lesions.
❸ Demonstrate the proper procedure for lifting blackheads and whiteheads.
❹ Explain the difference between disorders and diseases.

INTRODUCTION

The information in this chapter is designed to help you recognize and deal with skin disorders with which you may come in contact in the salon. You must be able to determine which skin disturbances can be treated and which require medical attention. Some skin disorders may be treated in cooperation with a dermatologist, but medical preparations prescribed by a dermatologist should not be applied by the esthetician without the written consent and instructions of the client's dermatologist.

Any skin disorder that you do not positively know to be a simple skin disorder, which can be rightfully handled in the salon, must be referred to a dermatologist. The client whose skin is inflamed, irritated, or appears to be in an abnormal condition, must be informed tactfully that you will need the permission of the client's physician before facial treatments can be given.

It is your duty to safeguard the health of the people who work in the salon as well as those who patronize the salon. It is to the client's benefit that she or he see a dermatologist before a poor skin condition worsens. If the client refuses to accept the estheticians advice, it is better to lose his or her patronage rather than risk contributing to the development of more serious problems.

Cosmetology and Dermatology Complement One Another

In recent years, many dermatologists have added the services of an esthetician to their staff. The dermatologist who is treating a patient for a skin disorder will prescribe the recommended treatment to be given by the esthetician. One of the more frequent treatments performed by the esthetician under the supervision of a dermatologist is the removal of blackheads and other debris from the follicles in an acned skin. Is is a known fact that acne pimples form in the follicles that are blocked by blackheads and other debris. This deep pore cleansing treatment is usually too time consuming for the dermatologist. The following is from *Dr. Zizmor's Skin Care Book,* by Jonathan Zizmor, M.D. and John Foreman, published by Holt, Rinehart and Winston Publishers. (Permission to reprint granted by the publisher.)

> Cosmetology and dermatology are services that ideally complement one another. Many of the treatments you'll receive at a skin salon or at the office of an individual cosmetologist are excellent for acne problems. Cosmetologists often spend two or three times as much time with you, for one-half to one-third of the fee charged by a dermatologist. They clean out pores, squeeze out blackheads and pimples, deep-moisturize the skin with special steam mist machines, apply wonderful-feeling facial masks, and lavish you with personal attention.
>
> If I have a patient undergoing treatment for acne, I often recommend supplementary visits to a cosmetologist. Many dermatologists don't have time to clean out pores and blackheads, nor do they all offer advice on artistic application of makeup. Cosmetologists do and can teach you all sorts of clever tricks.
>
> In addition to thorough skin cleansings, makeup lessons, and luxurious surroundings, cosmetologists will often be able to make great (if temporary) improvements on aged skin. They have machines and techniques to deep-moisturize the face and plump up the skin cells. Many establishments will also give a massage and remove unwanted hair.

Dermatology Defined

The following are terms the esthetician should know.

1. *Dermatology* (dur-mah-**TOL**-o-jee) is the study of the skin, its nature, structure, functions, diseases, and treatment.
2. A *dermatologist* (dur-mah-**TOL**-o-jist) is a skin specialist.
3. *Pathology* (pa-**THOL**-o-jee) is the study of disease.
4. *Trichology* (treye-**KOL**-o-jee) is the study of the hair and its diseases.
5. *Etiology* (ee-ti-**OL**-o-jee) is the study of the causes of disease.
6. A *diagnosis* (deye-ag-**NOH**-sis) is the recognition of a disease from its symptoms.
7. A *prognosis* (prog-**NOH**-sis) is the foretelling of the probable course of a disease.

Dermatology is the branch of medical science that relates to the skin and its diseases. In order for you to recognize skin conditions that may require the attention of a dermatologist, it is important to understand some of the basic terms and concepts of dermatology. For example, we refer to a normal skin as a skin that has no abnormalities. An abnormality that occurs in or on the skin in the form of blisters, pimples, or red spots is commonly referred to as "breaking out." They are called eruptions or rashes.

Symptoms are signs of disease. The symptoms in diseases of the skin are divided into two groups.

1. *Subjective* refers to symptoms that can be felt as itching, burning, or pains.
2. *Objective* refers to symptoms that can be seen as pimples, pustules, or inflammation.

Skin Conditions

The epidermis of the skin is composed of living cells, melanin (color factor) and keratin. The term *keratosis* (kerr-uh-**TO**-sis) refers to a condition of the skin involving keratin. *Hyperkeratosis* (**HIGH**-pur-kerr-uh-**TO**-sis) refers to an abnormal increase of the horny layer of the skin. An example of this condition is a callus, which usually appears on the palms of the hands or soles of the feet.

The following are terms that also apply to conditions of the skin:

1. *Parakeratosis* (par-uh-kerr-uh-**TO**-sis) refers to nuclei in the cells of the horny layer of the skin.
2. *Acanthosis* (ack-an-**THO**-sis) is a condition that is the result of an increased number of prickle cells.
3. *Dyskeratosis* (dis-kerr-uh-**TO**-sis) refers to imperfect keratinization of individual epidermal cells.
4. *Spongiosis* (spon-jee-**O**-sis) is a condition that produces a sponge-like appearance of the skin due to an increase of fluid in the cell layers.
5. *Pruritus* (proo-**RYE**-tus) is the medical term for a skin inflammation that causes itching.
6. *Erythema* (err-i-**THEEM**-uh) is the medical term for redness of the skin.
7. *Edema* (e-**DEE**-muh) is the medical term for swelling.
8. *Acute* (uh-**KUTE**) means severe.

Lesions of the Skin

A lesion is a structural change in the tissues caused by injury or disease. There are three types: primary, secondary, and tertiary. The esthetician is concerned with primary and secondary lesions only (Fig. 7.1).

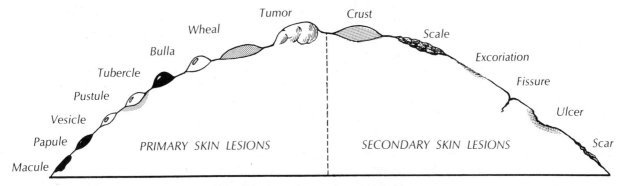

7.1 — Primary and secondary skin lesions

Knowing the principal skin lesions helps you to distinguish between conditions that may or may not be treated in a salon.

PRIMARY LESIONS

1. A *macule* (**MAK**-ul) is a small, discolored spot or patch on the surface of the skin, neither raised nor sunken, as freckles.
2. A *papule* (**PAP**-yool) is a small, elevated pimple in the skin, containing no fluid, but which may develop pus.
3. A *wheal* (**HWEEL**), is an itchy, swollen lesion that lasts only a few hours. (Example: hives or the bite of an insect, such as by a mosquito.)
4. A *tubercle* (**TOO**-ber-kel) is a solid lump larger than a papule. It projects above the surface or lies within or under the skin. It varies in size from a pea to a hickory nut.
5. A *tumor* (**TOO**-mohr) is an external swelling, varying in size, shape and color.
6. A *vesicle* (**VES**-i-kel) is a blister with clear fluid in it. Vesicles lie within or just beneath the epidermis. (example: poison ivy produces small vesicles.)
7. A *bulla* (**BYOO**-lah) is a blister containing a watery fluid, similar to a vesicle, but larger.
8. A *pustule* (**PUS**-chool) is an elevation of the skin having an inflamed base, containing pus.

SECONDARY LESIONS

The secondary lesions are those in the skin which develop in the later stages of disease. These are:

1. A *scale* is an accumulation of epidermal flakes, dry or greasy. (Example: abnormal or excessive dandruff.)
2. A *crust* (scab) is an accumulation of serum and pus, mixed perhaps with epidermal material. (Example: the scab on a sore.)
3. An *excoriation* (ek-skohr-i-**AY**-shun) is a skin sore or abrasion produced by scratching or scraping. (Example: a raw surface due to the loss of the superficial skin after an injury.)
4. A *fissure* (**FISH**-ur) is a crack in the skin penetrating into the derma, as in the case of chapped hands or lips.

5. An *ulcer* (**UL**-ser) is an open lesion on the skin or mucous membrane of the body, accompanied by pus and loss of skin depth.
6. A *scar* (*cicatrix*) (**SIK**-a-triks) is likely to form after the healing of an injury or skin condition that has penetrated the dermal layer.
7. A *stain* is abnormal discoloration remaining after the disappearance of moles, freckles, or liver spots, sometimes apparent after certain diseases.

Definitions Pertaining to Disease

Before describing the diseases of the skin and scalp so that they will be recognized by the esthetician, it is well to understand what is meant by disease.

1. A *disease* is any departure from a normal state of health.
2. A *skin disease* is an infection of the skin characterized by an objective lesion (one that can be seen), which may consist of scales, pimples, or pustules.
3. An *acute disease* is manifested by symptoms of a more or less violent character and of short duration.
4. A *chronic disease* is of long duration, usually mild but recurring.
5. An *infectious* (in-**FEK**-shus) *disease* is due to pathogenic germs taken into the body as a result of contact with a contaminated object or lesion.
6. A *contagious disease* is communicable by contact.

> **Note:** The terms "infectious disease," "communicable disease," and "contagious disease" are often used interchangeably.

7. A *congenital disease* is present in the infant at birth.
8. A *seasonal disease* is influenced by the weather, such as prickly heat in the summer, and forms of eczema, which are more prevalent in cold weather.
9. An *occupational disease*, such as dermatitis, is contracted while engaging in certain kinds of employment, and is caused by coming in contact with cosmetics, chemicals, or tints.
10. A *parasitic disease* is caused by vegetable or animal parasites, such as pediculosis or ringworm.
11. A *pathogenic disease* is caused by disease-producing bacteria, such as staphylococcus and streptococcus, pus-forming bacteria.
12. A *systemic disease* is due to under- or over-functioning of the internal glands. It may be caused by an inadequate diet.
13. A *venereal disease* is a contagious disease commonly acquired by contact with an infected person during sexual intercourse.

▶ **Caution:** Never try to diagnose a disease; always refer to a physician.

An *epidemic* is the manifestation of a disease that attacks simultaneously a large number of persons living in a particular locality. Infantile paralysis, influenza, or smallpox are examples of epidemic-causing diseases.

An *allergy* is a sensitivity which certain persons develop to normally harmless substances. Skin allergies are quite common. Contact with certain types of cosmetics, medicines, and tints, or eating certain foods, all may bring about an itching eruption, accompanied by redness, swelling, blisters, oozing, and/or scaling.

Inflammation is a sign of skin disorder characterized by redness, pain, swelling, and heat.

Disorders of the Sebaceous (Oil) Glands

There are several common disorders of the sebaceous (oil) glands which the esthetician should be able to identify and understand. (*See Color Plates 7 and 8.*)

COMEDONES

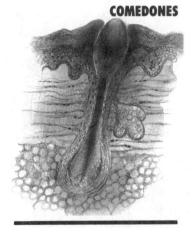

7.2—Blackhead (plug of sebaceous matter and dirt) forming around the mouth of hair follicle.

Comedones (**KOM**-e-donz), or blackheads, are a worm-like mass of keratinized cells and hardened sebum appearing most frequently on the face, chest, shoulders, and back. (*See Color Plate 9.*)

Blackheads accompanied by pimples often occur in youths between the ages of 13 and 20. During the adolescent period, the activity of the sebaceous glands is stimulated, thereby contributing to the formation of blackheads and pimples (Fig. 7.2).

When the hair follicle is filled with an excess of oil from the sebaceous glands and an accumulation of dead cells occurs, a blackhead forms and creates a blockage at the mouth of the follicle. Should this condition become severe, medical attention is necessary.

To treat blackheads, the skin's oiliness must be reduced by local applications of cleansers and the blackheads removed under sterile conditions. Thorough skin cleansing each night is a very important factor. Cleansing lotions often achieve better results than do common soap and water.

MILIA

Milia (**MIL**-ee-uh), or whiteheads, is a disorder of the sebaceous glands caused by the accumulation of dead, keratinized cells and sebaceous matter trapped beneath the skin. This may occur on any part of the face, and occasionally on the chest, shoulders, and back. Whiteheads look like small grains of sand under the skin.

ACNE

Acne (**AK**-nee) is a chronic inflammatory disorder of the skin, usually related to hormonal changes and overactive sebaceous glands during adolescence. Common acne is also known as *acne simplex* or *acne vulgaris*. (*See Color Plate 10.*)

Acne appears in a variety of different types, ranging from noncontagious pimples to deep-seated skin conditions. Though acne generally starts at the onset of puberty, it also afflicts adult men and women.

Modern studies show that acne is often due to heredity, but the condition can be aggravated by emotional stress and environmental factors. Adhering to a well-balanced diet, drinking plenty of water, and developing healthful personal hygiene habits are all recommended. Acne is not caused by any particular food, drink, or personal habit. Acne may also be present on the back, chest, and shoulders. Acne is accompanied by blackheads, pustules, and pimples that are red, swollen, and contain pus. The pus is seen as a yellowish or white-tinged center in some blemishes. In more advanced cases of acne, cysts appear, which are red, swollen lumps beneath the surface of the skin. (*See Color Plate 11.*)

Seborrhea (seb-o-**REE**-ah) is a skin condition caused by overactivity and excessive secretion of the sebaceous glands. An oily, or shiny, condition of the nose, forehead, or scalp indicates the presence of seborrhea. It is readily detected on the scalp by the unusual amount of oil on the hair. Seborrhea is often the basis of an acne condition.

Rosacea (ro-**ZA**-se-a), formerly called acne rosacea, is a chronic inflammatory congestion of the cheeks and nose. It is characterized by redness, dilation of the blood vessels, and the formation of papules and pustules. The cause of rosacea is unknown. Certain things are known to aggravate rosacea in some individuals. These include consumption of hot liquids, spicy foods or alcohol, being exposed to extremes of heat and cold, exposure to sunlight, and stress (Fig. 7.3).

A *steatoma* (stee-ah-**TOH**-mah), or sebaceous cyst, is a subcutaneous tumor of the sebaceous glands, ranging in size from a pea to an orange, the contents consisting of sebum. It usually occurs on the scalp, neck, and back. A steatoma is sometimes called a *wen* (Fig. 7.4).

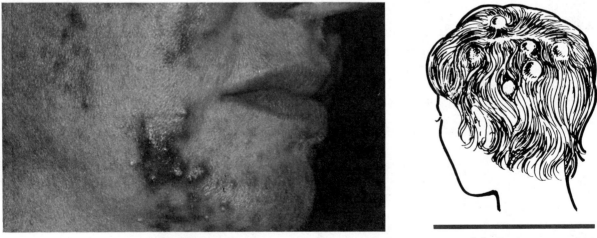

7.3—Rosacea   7.4—Steatoma

Asteatosis (as-tee-ah-**TOH**-sis) is a condition of dry, scaly skin, characterized by absolute or partial deficiency of sebum, usually due to aging or bodily disorders. In local conditions, it may be caused by alkalies, such as those found in soaps and washing powders.

A *furuncle* (fu-**RUN**-kel), also called a boil, is caused by bacteria that enter the skin through the hair follicles. It is a subcutaneous abscess that fills with pus. A boil can be painful and should be treated by a physician (Fig. 7.5).

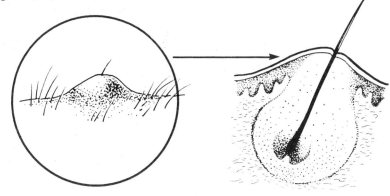

7.5—Furuncle (boil)

CYSTS When a follicle ruptures deep within the dermis, irritating oil and dead cells seep into the surrounding area and a *cyst* forms. The cyst appears as a large, hard, and painful lump underneath the surface of the skin. A cyst is a severe pimple that takes a longer time to reach the surface of the skin. (*See Color Plate 12.*) As the cyst works its way to the surface, it destroys many live cells and will often leave permanent scars. These scars are often referred to as *acne pits*. Quite often a wall (membrane) will form around the debris and medical treatment may be needed to clear the condition (Figs. 7.6a and 7.6b).

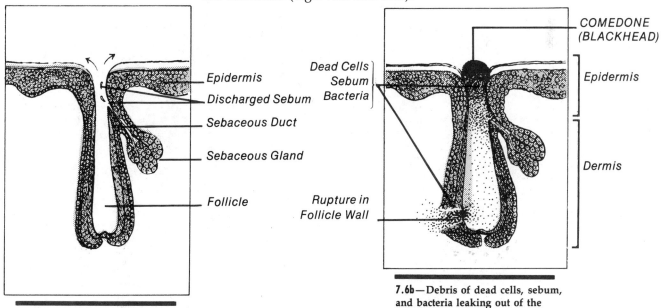

7.6a—Sebaceous gland functioning in a normal manner.

7.6b—Debris of dead cells, sebum, and bacteria leaking out of the follicle deep into the dermis. This can form into a painful cyst.

PIMPLES   When the follicle becomes filled with oil, dead cells, and bacteria, it often swells and ruptures causing the debris to escape into the dermis. The debris is irritating and causes an inflammation. White blood cells rush in to fight against the bacteria and create pus, a sticky, yellowish secretion. This is the beginning of a *pimple* and appears as an inflamed, red or blue-red lump.

When the overloaded follicle ruptures near the surface of the skin it is not so serious and will usually heal rapidly leaving no permanent mark. However, if the follicle breaks deeper underneath the skin, it will be more severe and may take longer to heal, leaving permanent scars.

When pimples are pinched or squeezed, the infectious material can spread to surrounding tissues, but common acne is not spread from one person to another. Unless proper treatment is given, permanent scarring can occur (Figs. 7.7a and 7.7b). (*See Color Plates 13 and 14.*)

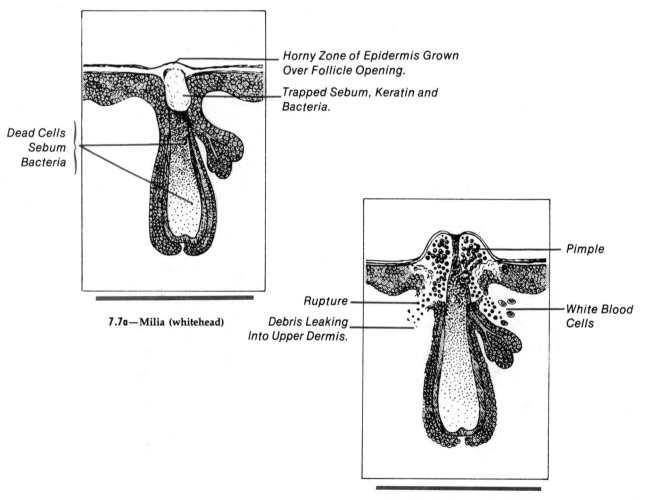

Horny Zone of Epidermis Grown Over Follicle Opening.

Trapped Sebum, Keratin and Bacteria.

Dead Cells
Sebum
Bacteria

7.7a—Milia (whitehead)

Pimple

Rupture

Debris Leaking Into Upper Dermis.

White Blood Cells

7.7b—Pimple in advanced stage

ACNE SCARS   There are three types of acne scars. These are called ice pick, acne pit, and raised scars. Proper treatment and care of the skin will help to prevent the conditions that produce scars.

Ice pick scars are large, visible, open pores that look as if the skin has been jabbed with an ice pick or other sharp, thin instrument. The follicle (pore) always looks open, as if a small hole has been made in the skin. This condition is caused by a deep pimple or cyst that has destroyed the follicle as the infection worked its way to the surface of the skin (Fig. 7.8).

Acne pit scars are indented and are due to pimples or cysts that have destroyed the skin and formed scar tissue. The scar has a slightly sunken or depressed appearance (Fig. 7.9).

When several large cysts have clumped together, and as scar tissue forms, a lumpy mass of raised tissue is created on the surface of the skin, known as *raised scars* (Fig. 7.10).

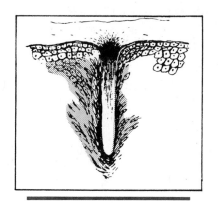

7.8—Ice pick pore scar

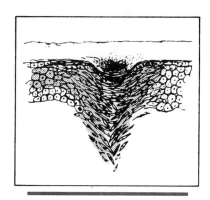

7.9—Acne pit scar

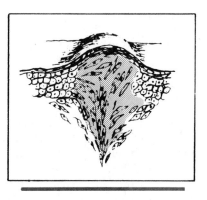

7.10—Raised scar

The Extraction of Blackheads and Other Blemishes

PREPARING FINGERS FOR THE EXTRACTION AND CLEANSING OUT OF BLACKHEADS, WHITEHEADS, AND PIMPLES

1. Prepare each forefinger with astringent-saturated cotton strips as follows: Squeeze out excess water from a clean wet cotton cleansing pad. (See Fig. 7.11.)
2. Unfold the pad and divide it in half. Place one half of the pad back in the bowl that holds the cleansing pads and/or sponges. (See Fig. 7.12.)

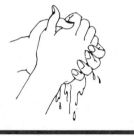

7.11—Squeeze out excess water from cleansing pad.

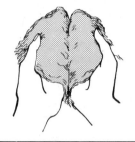

7.12—Divide pad in half.

3. Saturate the half of the pad you are holding with astringent. Squeeze out excess astringent.
4. Tear small strips from the astringent-saturated cotton. (See Fig. 7.13.)
5. Wrap the strips smoothly around the end of each forefinger. (See Fig. 7.14.)
6. Be sure the nails are well-padded. (See Fig. 7.15.)
7. Repeat this step as often as necessary. If more cotton strips are needed, use the second half of the pad that was set aside.

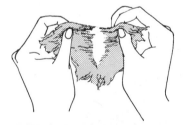

7.13—Tear strips from the pad.

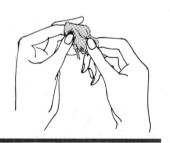

7.14—Wrap strip around forefinger.

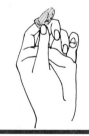

7.15—Secure strip around forefinger.

Note: Facial tissue is not recommended for use during the extraction of blackheads, whiteheads, and blemishes because it is too abrasive when applied with pressure to the skin. Tissue will not hold together when wet with water and astringent. Cotton is recommended, as it is much softer and less irritating to a sensitive skin, and will hold together when wet.

PROCEDURE FOR REMOVING BLACKHEADS

The skin must be prepared by using the vapor mist machine or warm, moistened towel applications. This is followed by the disincrustation (see page 255) and the suction apparatus, if available (see page 278), on greasy skins with open follicles and many blackheads. The Dr. Jacquet massage movements (see page 230) will follow the disincrustation. The blackheads can usually be coaxed from the follicle by a minimum amount of pressure.

Wrap fingertips with wet cotton strips that have been saturated with astringent. The fingertips and padded nails are used to exert firm pressure on the skin directly surrounding the blackhead, lifting the blackhead from the follicle. (See Fig. 7.16.) Concentrating on one blackhead at a time, the esthetician must work gently and carefully so as not to bruise the tissue.

When extracting blackheads and grease deposits from the nose, it is important not to press down on the cartilage which forms the semi-flexible part of the bridge of the nose. (See Fig. 7.17.) Apply pressure with the fingers in a vertical position on the nose, not in a horizontal position. (See Fig. 7.18.)

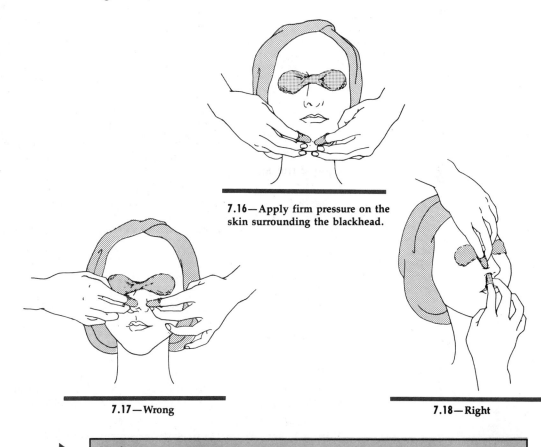

7.16—Apply firm pressure on the skin surrounding the blackhead.

7.17—Wrong

7.18—Right

▶ **Caution:** Never remove blackheads over broken blood vessels, doing so may cause more damage to the area.

The Extraction of Whiteheads and Other Blemishes

A *lancet* (**LAN**-sit) is a small, sharp, pointed surgical blade with a double edge. It is used to pierce or prick the skin. A lancet may be purchased at most surgical supply companies or ordered through a pharmacist. When purchasing this item it is called a "blood" lancet. Each lancet is sterilized and comes in a separately sealed envelope (Figs. 7.19 and 7.20). If the envelope is open, the lancet cannot be guaranteed to be sterile. A fresh lancet must be used for each client. Needles for pricking the dead cell layer of the skin also come presterilized and individually wrapped.

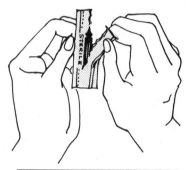

7.19—The lancet is sterilized and comes in a sealed envelope.

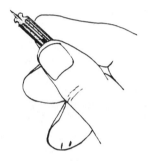

7.20—The lancet

Caution: The procedure of using a lancet needle to prick the surface layer of the skin is considered to be a medical procedure in some states, and may be illegal for either a cosmetologist, cosmetician, or esthetician to perform in a licensed cosmetology establishment. Please check with your state licensing agency to determine whether you may use this procedure in your state.

A metal comedone extractor is never used by the esthetician to aid in removal of blackheads, as this requires pressure that can cause the follicle walls to rupture, spilling sebum, keratin, and bacteria into the dermis. This debris causes irritation that can lead to the start of a pimple. The manual extraction of blackheads with cotton-wrapped fingers is the better and most professional method.

THE EXTRACTION OF WHITEHEADS

Whiteheads are removed in the same manner as blackheads except that an opening in the dead cell layer must first be made. This is done by placing a lancet or needle almost parallel to the surface of the skin and pricking the dead cell layer to make an opening for the debris to pass through. The whitehead is then removed by applying gentle pressure. (See Fig. 7.21.)

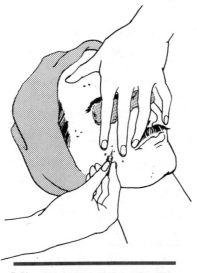

7.21—Removing whiteheads with a lancet

When treating an acned or problem-blemished skin, the most important step for the esthetician is the effective removal and cleansing out of blackheads, whiteheads, and other blemishes, such as pimples. Every pimple starts from a blackhead or clogged follicle. When the follicles are properly cleansed, the client's skin will begin to show marked improvement. It is important that the client understand that you cannot remove and clean out all blackheads, whiteheads, and pimples during one treatment. This would only cause needless irritation to the skin. The client must be told that you cannot undo in a one-hour treatment what it has taken months or years to accumulate.

> **Caution:** Proper cleansing when extracting blemishes is very important, so as not to spread infection elsewhere on the skin.

PROPER METHOD FOR CLEANSING PIMPLES FROM THE SKIN

Before extracting the debris from a pimple, it is important that the pimple has matured. (When the pimple is ready for cleansing, pus will be visible through the skin.) The surface of the pimple will have a yellowish, white head, often with a crust of dead cells forming a cap over the pimple. The esthetician must use his or her own judgment in determining if the pimple is ready to be drained. When in doubt, it is best to leave the pimple alone.

> **Caution:** If removal of a whitehead is difficult, refer client to a physician.

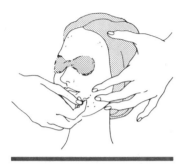

7.22—Prick the surface of the pimple very carefully with a sterilized lancet or needle.

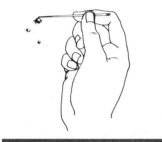

7.23—Debris will ooze from the area that was pricked.

It is of the utmost importance that the pimple break on the surface of the skin rather than underneath the skin where the pus and other debris can spread and cause more harm. To assure that a pimple breaks properly on the surface of the skin, a weak spot should be created on the head of the pimple, with the aid of a sterilized lancet or needle. This is done by placing the point of the lancet or needle almost parallel to the head of the pimple, and pricking the surface of the pimple very carefully. (See Fig. 7.22.) When the pimple is opened in this manner, you will be pricking only the surface of the epidermis. The area that is pricked will be the weak spot from which the debris will ooze. (See Fig. 7.23.)

Prepare the fingers with cotton strips that have been saturated with astringent. Apply gentle pressure to the sides of the pimple. If the debris does not ooze from the pimple, move the fingers to a new position around the pimple and try again. Do not use force. If, after applying pressure the second time, the debris still does not ooze from the pimple, prick the pimple again and repeat the gentle pressure. If the pimple still does not drain, it is not ready. (See Fig. 7.24.)

If the debris does begin to ooze out, apply pressure to several sides of the pimple and continue the pressure until clean blood begins to flow. It may be necessary to change the cotton strips on the fingers more than once when cleansing out a pimple. Discard the soiled cotton strips in a covered waste container to assure that they are out of sight of clients. Apply astringent to each pimple after it has been cleansed. Never attempt to open or lance a deep cyst, as to do so would only invite trouble. Remember you are an esthetician and not a physician.

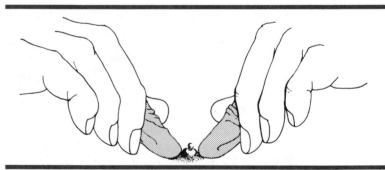

7.24—Apply gentle pressure to the sides of the pimple, with fingers wrapped in astringent-saturated cotton strips.

Caution: The cleansing of pimples must be done only under the most sanitary of conditions. Hands must be washed and sanitized. Because of the concern with the spread of such serious diseases as AIDS, disposable (rubber or plastic) gloves are preferred by many estheticians. If you use cotton, it must be clean and fresh from the container. Lancets and needles must be sterile, and, when used, they should be placed on a piece of cotton that has been saturated with alcohol or astringent.

DEEP CLEANING TREATMENT FOR BACK AND SHOULDERS

On occasion, a client being treated for acne on the face may ask if the esthetician will also treat blackheads and pimples on the back and shoulders (Fig. 7.25). This is a procedure that is left up to the discretion of the esthetician, and is dependent upon the policy of the school or salon. The back and shoulder treatment will add about one-half hour to the facial treatment and an additional charge should be made. The procedure is similar to the facial treatment.

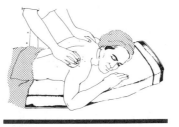

7.25—Back and shoulder treatment

Procedure

1. Cleanse the area by applying cleanser with upward and outward massage movements.
2. Remove the cleanser with wet cotton pads. (Only cotton is used for this treatment.)
3. Wipe the back and shoulders with a wet cotton pad that has been sprinkled with astringent.
4. Steam the back and shoulders with very warm towel compresses or a vaporizer.
5. Use the appropriate machines (galvanic disincrustation machine, high-frequency machine, etc.) to assist in the treatment. All of the machines may be used if available. The electric brushing machine may be used but not directly on acne or pimples.
6. Disincrustation may be done by applying cotton compresses that have been saturated with disincrustation lotion. The compresses are applied to the entire affected area. Please refer to page 255.
7. Complete the extraction of blackheads and cleansing of pimples.
8. The back is wiped or sprayed with astringent.
9. Treatment cream is massaged into the affected areas.
10. The mask is applied to the affected areas.
11. The mask is removed with wet cotton compresses.
12. The back is wiped or sprayed with astringent.
13. The back is blotted dry and a soothing, healing lotion is applied.

Disorders of Sudoriferous (Sweat) Glands

Bromidrosis (broh-mi-**DROH**-sis) or *osmidrosis* (ah-smi-**DROH**-sis), refers to foul-smelling perspiration, usually noticeable in the armpits or on the feet.

Anidrosis (an-i-**DROH**-sis), or lack of perspiration, is often a result of fever or certain skin diseases. It requires medical treatment.

Hyperidrosis (heye-per-heye-**DROH**-sis), or excessive perspiration, is caused by excessive heat, or general body weakness. The most commonly affected parts are the armpits, joints, and feet. It requires medical treatment.

Miliaria rubra (mil-ee-**AY**-ree-ah **ROOB**-rah), or prickly heat, is an acute, inflammatory disorder of sweat glands characterized by an eruption of small red vesicles, accompanied by burning and itching of the skin. It is caused by exposure to excessive heat.

Inflammations

Dermatitis (dur-mah-**TEYE**-tis) is a term used to denote an inflammatory condition of the skin. The lesions come in various forms, such as vesicles or papules.

Eczema (**EK**-se-mah) is an inflammation of the skin, acute or chronic in nature, presenting many forms of dry or moist lesions. It is frequently accompanied by itching, burning, and various other unpleasant sensations. All cases of eczema should be referred to a physician for treatment. Eczema may be the result of some type of allergy or internal disorder. The term "eczema" is applied to any number of surface lesions of the skin. It is usually a red, blistered, oozing area that itches painfully.

Psoriasis (so-**REYE**-a-sis) is a common, chronic, inflammatory skin disease whose cause is unknown. It is usually found on the scalp, elbows, knees, chest, and lower back, but rarely on the face. The lesions are round, dry patches covered with coarse, silvery scales. If irritated, bleeding points occur. While not contagious, it can be spread by irritating it.

Herpes simplex (**HUR**-peez **SIM**-pleks) is a viral infection of unknown origin, commonly called *fever blisters*. It is characterized by the eruption of a single group of vesicles on a red swollen base. The blisters usually appear on the lips, nostrils or other parts of the face, and rarely last more than a week. Indigestion may be one of the causes (Fig. 7.26).

Occupational disorders refer to abnormal conditions resulting from contact with chemicals or tints in the course of performing services in the salon. Some individuals may develop allergies to ingredients in cosmetics, antiseptics, cold waving lotions and aniline derivative tints, which may cause eruptive skin infections known as *dermatitis venenata* (**VEN**-e-na-tah). It is important that estheticians employ protective measures, such as the use of rubber gloves or protective creams whenever possible.

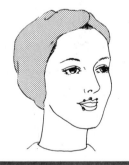

7.26—Herpes simplex

ANATOMY AND PHYSIOLOGY

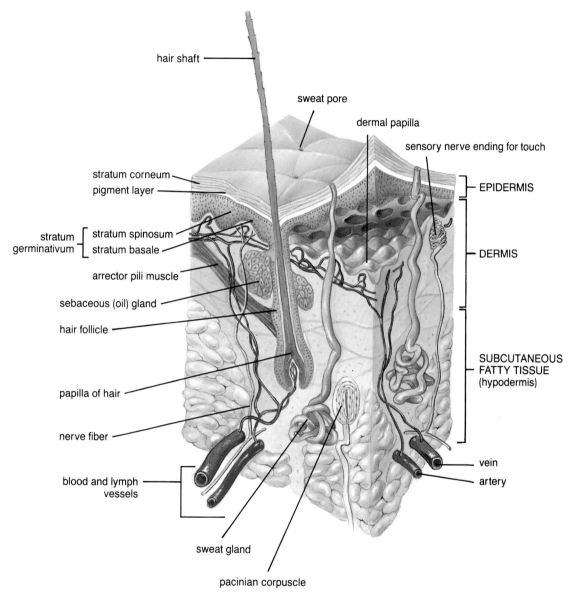

Plate 1 - Cross section of skin.

ANATOMY AND PHYSIOLOGY

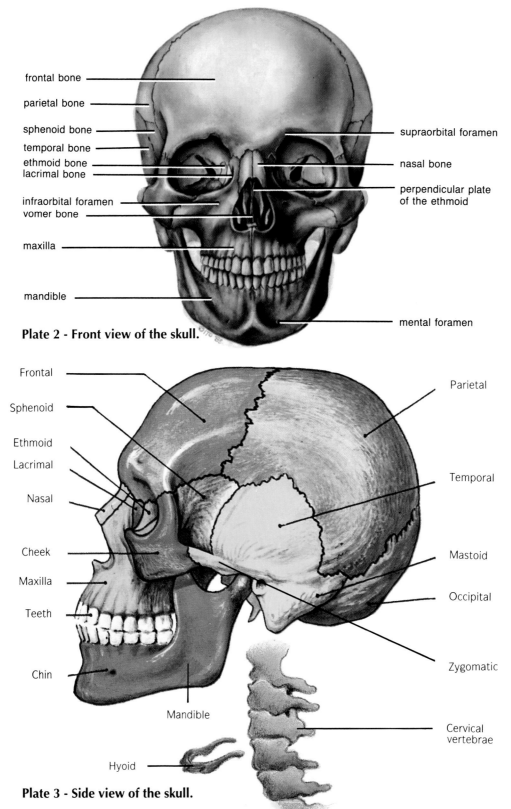

frontal bone

parietal bone

sphenoid bone

temporal bone

ethmoid bone

lacrimal bone

infraorbital foramen

vomer bone

maxilla

mandible

supraorbital foramen

nasal bone

perpendicular plate
of the ethmoid

mental foramen

Plate 2 - Front view of the skull.

Frontal

Sphenoid

Ethmoid

Lacrimal

Nasal

Cheek

Maxilla

Teeth

Chin

Mandible

Hyoid

Parietal

Temporal

Mastoid

Occipital

Zygomatic

Cervical
vertebrae

Plate 3 - Side view of the skull.

ANATOMY AND PHYSIOLOGY

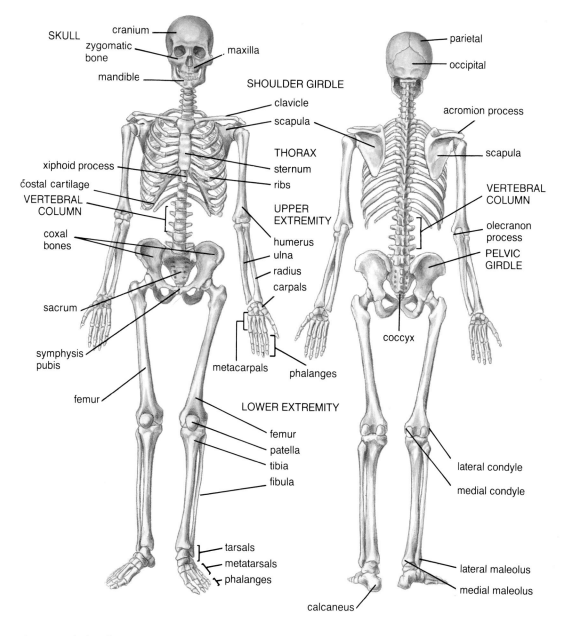

SKULL
cranium
zygomatic bone
maxilla
mandible

parietal
occipital

SHOULDER GIRDLE
clavicle
scapula

acromion process
scapula

THORAX
sternum
ribs

xiphoid process
costal cartilage
VERTEBRAL COLUMN

VERTEBRAL COLUMN
olecranon process

coxal bones

UPPER EXTREMITY
humerus
ulna
radius
carpals

PELVIC GIRDLE

sacrum

symphysis pubis

coccyx

femur

metacarpals
phalanges

LOWER EXTREMITY
femur
patella
tibia
fibula

lateral condyle
medial condyle

tarsals
metatarsals
phalanges

lateral maleolus
medial maleolus

calcaneus

Plate 4 - Skeletal system.

ANATOMY AND PHYSIOLOGY

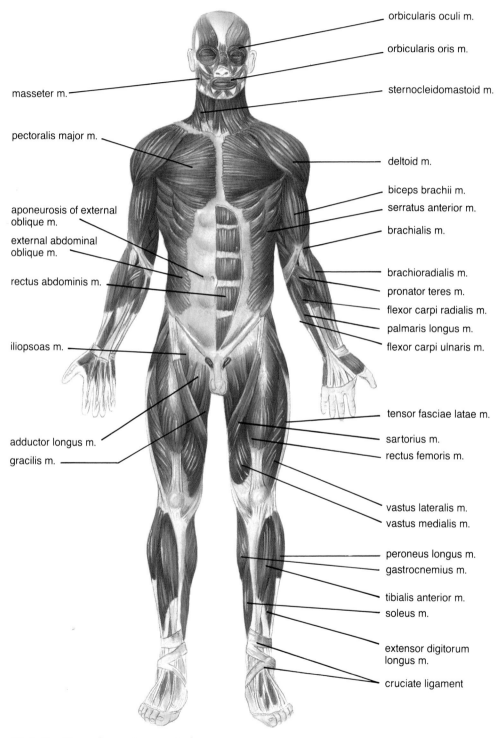

orbicularis oculi m.

orbicularis oris m.

sternocleidomastoid m.

masseter m.

pectoralis major m.

deltoid m.

biceps brachii m.

serratus anterior m.

aponeurosis of external oblique m.

brachialis m.

external abdominal oblique m.

rectus abdominis m.

brachioradialis m.

pronator teres m.

flexor carpi radialis m.

palmaris longus m.

flexor carpi ulnaris m.

iliopsoas m.

tensor fasciae latae m.

sartorius m.

rectus femoris m.

adductor longus m.

gracilis m.

vastus lateralis m.

vastus medialis m.

peroneus longus m.

gastrocnemius m.

tibialis anterior m.

soleus m.

extensor digitorum longus m.

cruciate ligament

Plate 5 - Muscular system, anterior.

ANATOMY AND PHYSIOLOGY

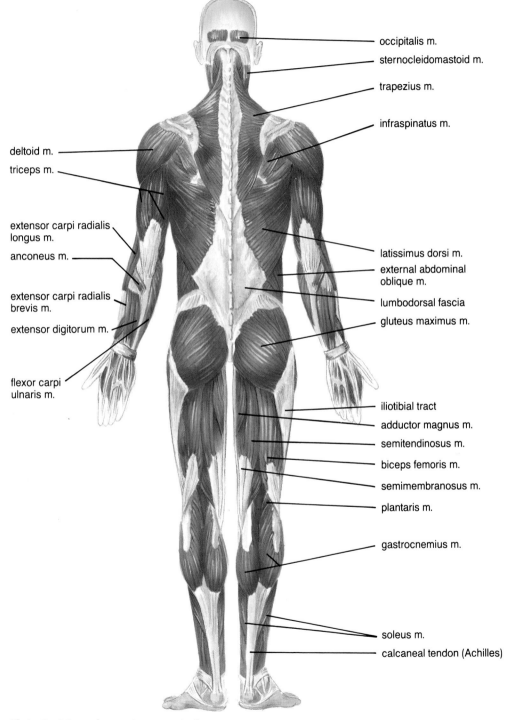

occipitalis m.

sternocleidomastoid m.

trapezius m.

infraspinatus m.

deltoid m.

triceps m.

extensor carpi radialis
longus m.

anconeus m.

extensor carpi radialis
brevis m.

extensor digitorum m.

flexor carpi
ulnaris m.

latissimus dorsi m.

external abdominal
oblique m.

lumbodorsal fascia

gluteus maximus m.

iliotibial tract

adductor magnus m.

semitendinosus m.

biceps femoris m.

semimembranosus m.

plantaris m.

gastrocnemius m.

soleus m.

calcaneal tendon (Achilles)

Plate 6 - Muscular system, posterior.

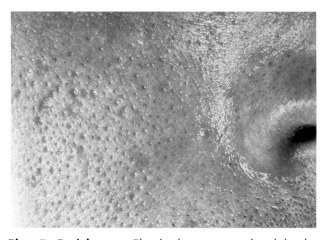

Plate 7 - Facial pores. Cheek of a young, male adult who had moderate acne. The pores are conspicuous. The larger, irregular depressions are small scars. The skin is obviously oily.

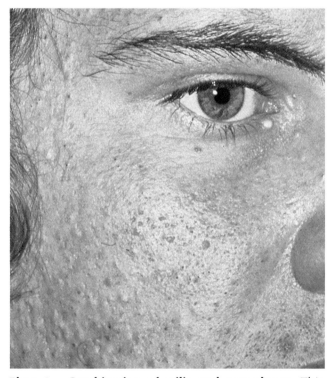

Plate 8 - Combination of milia and comedones. This teenage boy has a combination of many milia and comedones. With continued treatments from a well-trained esthetician, marked improvement can be achieved.

DISORDERS OF THE SKIN

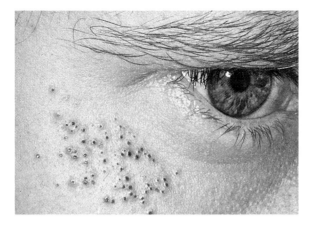

Plate 9 - Comedones in the eye area. This cluster of comedones around the eye area must be coaxed and extracted from the follicles with extreme care, and a minimum amount of pressure so as not to bruise the skin. Avoid using suction and the Dr. Jacquet massage movements when working in the eye area.

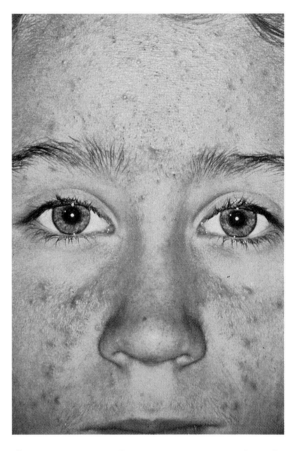

Plate 10 - Acne in the young. Acne started on the nose of this 12-year-old girl three years ago. Next, the forehead became involved. Recently, the acne descended onto the cheeks with more inflammatory lesions. This is a familiar sequence.

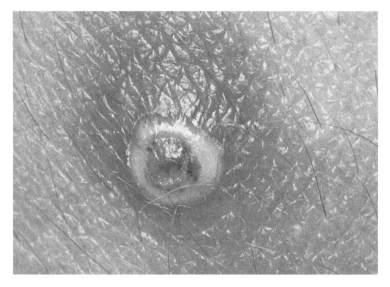

Plate 11 - The pustule. Pustules are very conspicuous lesions and are readily observable on all acne patients. A large, succulent pustule, acne pustules arise from comedones. Here, the brownish comedonal core floats on the yellow pus, surrounded by redness of the skin.

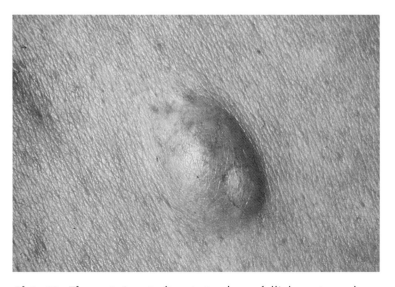

Plate 12 - The cyst. A cyst often starts when a follicle ruptures deep within the dermis causing irritating oil and dead cells to seep into the surrounding area. The esthetician should never attempt to open or lance a deep cyst, but should advise the client to seek medical treatment if the cyst does not seem to be working its way to the surface.

DISORDERS OF THE SKIN

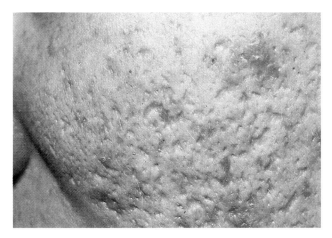

Plate 13 - Facial scarring. Variably shaped, crater-like depressions and pits are characteristic of facial scarring in severe acne. Retiform scars in a 17-year-old girl where very little clinical activity remains. Gouging with the fingernails probably contributed to her present appearance.

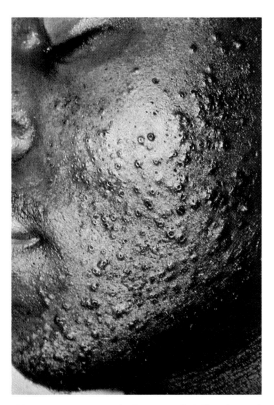

Plate 14 - Ingrown hairs. Pseudofolliculitis of the beard in persons with stiff, curved hairs (mainly adult blacks) is where the hair tips penetrate the skin just before they normally exit through the orifice. Each growing tip excites an inflammatory foreign-body reaction (ingrown hairs) creating perifollicular papules. These are not comedones. The condition persists as long as the victim shaves, eventually leaving crisscross scars.

(Plates 7 to 14 reprinted from ACNE MORPHOGENESIS AND TREATMENT by Gerd Plewig, MD and Albert M. Klingman, MD, Ph.D; permission of Publishers, Springer-Verlag, New York, U.S.A., Heidelberg, Berlin, Germany.)

CLEANSING AND MASSAGE

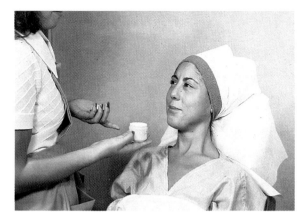

Plate 15 - Preparation of the client. When draping the head, applying cleanser, or performing a facial treatment or other movements, it is important to let the client know what is being done, what product will be used and why it will be beneficial.

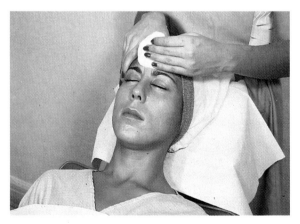

Plate 16 - Removing cleanser. A cotton pad is used to remove cleanser from the client's face.

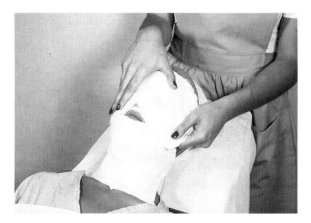

Plate 17 - Applying the cotton compress mask. This is the completed mask showing the face and neck covered with the exception of the nostrils and the mouth.

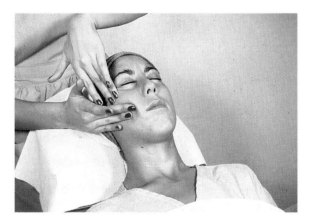

Plate 18 - Effleurage (stroking movement). Effleurage is a light, continuous movement applied to the skin with the fingers and palms in a slow and rhythmic manner.

Plate 19 - The skin scope. It is an elaborate magnifying lamp for analyzing the skin. It has a one-way magnifying mirror allowing the esthetician to scan the client's skin, while at the same time allowing the client to see his or her reflection in the magnifying mirror.

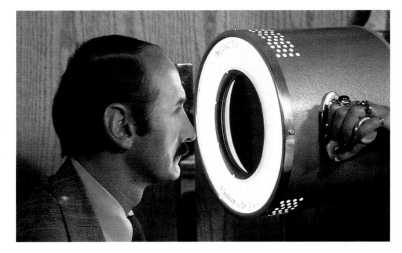

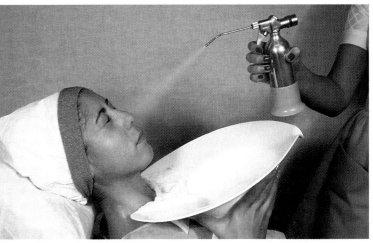

Plate 20 - The spray machine. The client is holding a cuvette (facial bowl) during the facial spray procedure.

Plate 21 - The brushing machine. This hand-held model is used to slough off the dead cells, and to remove any dirt and grime that clings to the surface of the skin.

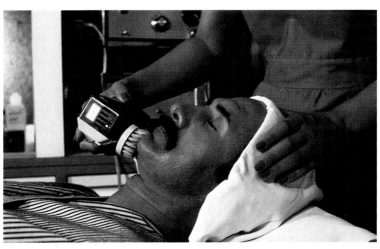

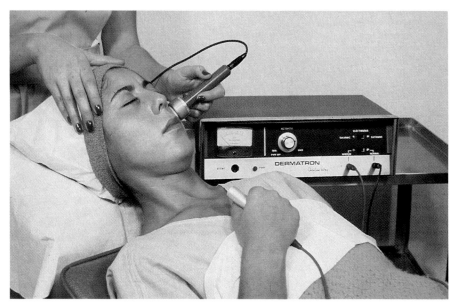

Plate 22 - The galvanic machine. The galvanic machine has important functions during a facial treatment. Its main function is to introduce water soluble products into the skin. This process is called iontophoresis. When using galvanic current there are two poles, a negative (-) and a positive (+).

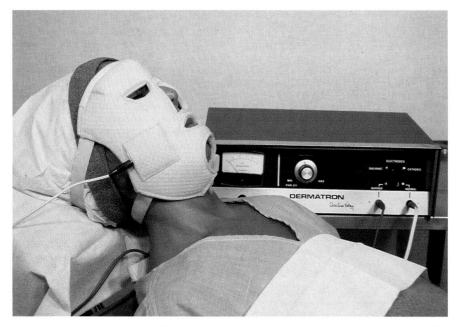

Plate 23 - The ionto mask. The ionto mask is used for ionization and/or disincrustation.

ADVANCED TOPICS IN ESTHETICS - CHEMICAL PEELING

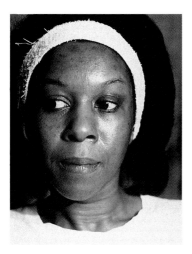

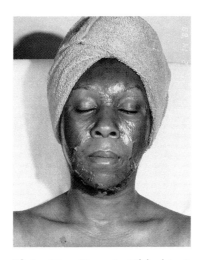

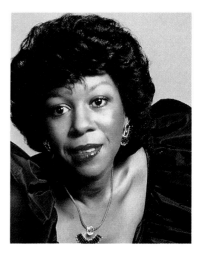

Plate 24 - Before. The skin is dull and has pigmentation marks.

Plate 25 - Day 4. Old skin is peeling back. Peeling starts at the mouth. Notice how tight and crispy the unpeeled areas are.

Plate 26 - After. Client is made up with light, translucent makeup. Her skin is clear and radiant.

(Plates 24 to 26 courtesy of Dr. Lee SaintMartin.)

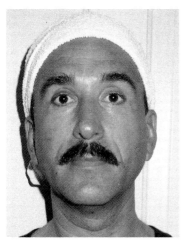

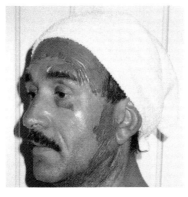

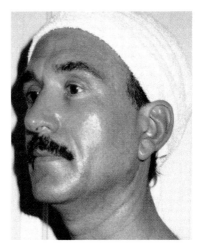

Plate 27 - Before. The skin looks dull.

Plate 28 - Day 5. About 60 percent of the old skin has peeled off. Notice how the unpeeled area on the forehead resembles parchment paper.

Plate 29 - After. Day 7 and the peeling is complete. Notice how clear and glowing the skin looks.

(Plates 27 to 29 courtesy of Mark Richard.)

Color Key 1

YOUR NATURAL EYE COLORS

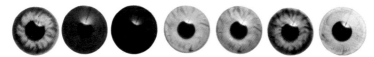

YOUR NATURAL HAIR COLORS AND MOST FLATTERING TINTS

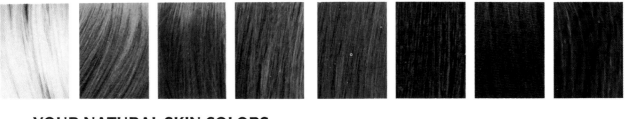

YOUR NATURAL SKIN COLORS

MAKEUP AND WARDROBE COLORS FOR PERSONS IN COLOR KEY 1

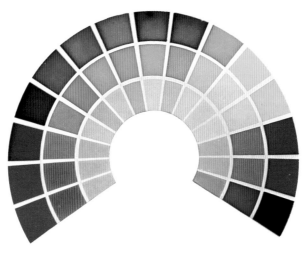

The purpose of this chart is to help you select your client's best colors for makeup, hair color and wardrobe; colors that will harmonize with their complexion tones. In Color Key 1, blue pigmentation predominates the undertones of the skin. When selecting a person's Color Key, the natural eye colors in the chart will be helpful in determining their correct Color Key. Light-skinned people who have a blue-pink undertone to their complexions, therefore, fall into Color Key 1. Some people in Color Key 1 have an olive undertone. Dark-skinned people in Color Key 1 may have a charcoal, or occasionally an ashen gray hue to their dark complexions. If you determine that a client's personal coloring is in Color Key 1, always choose colors from the Color Key 1 selection.

Color Key 2

YOUR NATURAL EYE COLORS

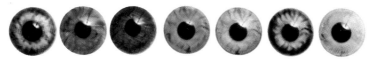

YOUR NATURAL HAIR COLORS AND MOST FLATTERING TINTS

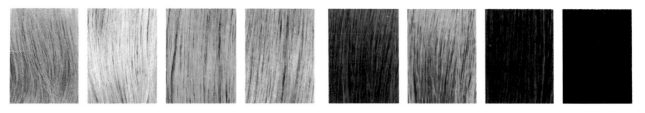

YOUR NATURAL SKIN COLORS

MAKEUP AND WARDROBE COLORS FOR PERSONS IN COLOR KEY 2

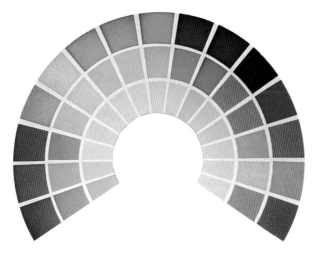

The purpose of this chart is to help you select your client's best colors for makeup, hair color and wardrobe; colors that will harmonize with their complexion tones. In Color Key 2, yellow pigmentation predominates. Light-skinned people with a peach-pink undertone to their complexion will, therefore, fall into Color Key 2. Dark-skinned people in Color Key 2 have a golden undertone. If you determine that a client's personal coloring is in Color Key 2, always choose colors from the Color Key 2 selection.

COLOR THEORY

Plate 31 - The laws of color.

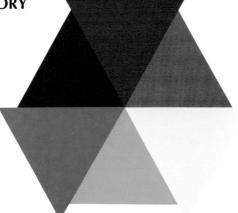

Primary

Red	Yellow	Blue

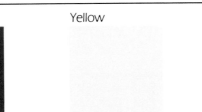

Secondary

Red

Yellow

Blue

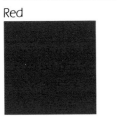 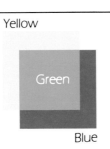 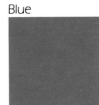

Orange

Green

Violet

Yellow

Blue

Red

Tertiary

Yellow

Blue

Blue

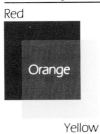 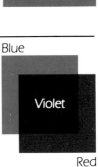

Yellow-Green

Blue-Green

Blue-Violet

Green

Green

Violet

Red

Red

Yellow

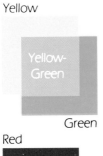 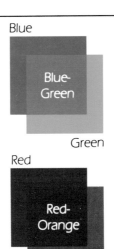

Red-Violet

Red-Orange

Yellow-Orange

Violet

Orange

Orange

Pigmentations of the Skin

In abnormal conditions, *pigment* can be affected from inside or outside the body. Abnormal colors accompany every skin disorder and many systemic disorders. A change in pigmentation is observed when certain drugs are taken internally.

Tanning is caused by excessive exposure to the sun.

Lentigines (len-ti-**JEE**-neez) (singular, lentigo), or freckles, are small yellow to brown colored spots on parts exposed to sunlight and air.

Stains are abnormal, brown, skin patches, having a circular and irregular shape. Their permanent color is due to the presence of blood pigment. They occur during aging, after certain diseases, and after the disappearance of moles, freckles, and liver spots. The cause of these stains is unknown.

Chloasma (kloh-**AZ**-mah) is characterized by increased deposits of pigment in the skin. It is found mainly on the forehead, nose, and cheeks. Chloasma is also called *moth patches* or *liver spots*.

Naevus (**NEE**-vus) is commonly known as a birthmark. It is a small or large malformation of the skin due to pigmentation or dilated capillaries. *Birthmarks* are present on the skin at birth. Special cosmetics have proven effective for some people with "portwine" or "strawberry" marks on the face. The portwine stain is usually found on the face and neck and may cover a large area of the face or a small patch of skin. It is pink to dark red in color. Strawberry birthmarks develop before or shortly after a child is born. Like the portwine stain, the bright reddish color can cover a large or small area of the face and neck. Treatment of such skin discolorations is limited, but makeup applied skillfully can conceal the stains. Some birthmarks are known to regress or disappear with time. In some cases, a specialist may advise plastic surgery or a tatoo method to conceal the birthmark.

Leucoderma (loo-ko-**DUR**-mah) refers to abnormal light patches of skin, due to congenital defective pigmentations. It is classified as follows:

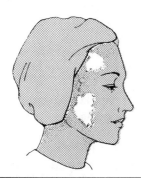

7.27—Vitiligo

1. *Vitiligo* (vit-i-**LEYE**-goh) is an acquired condition of leucoderma, affecting the skin or the hair. The only treatment is to apply a matching cosmetic color, making it less conspicuous (Fig. 7.27).
2. *Albinism* (**AL**-bi-niz-em) is a congenital absence of melanin pigment in the body, including the skin, hair, and eyes. The hair is silky and white. The skin is pinkish white and will not tan.

> **Note:** Color changes, a crack on the skin, a type of thickening, or any discoloration, ranging from shades of red to brown and purple to almost black, may be signs of danger and should be examined by a dermatologist.

Hypertrophies (New Growths)

Hypertrophy (high-**PUR**-truh-fee) is an abnormal increase in the size of a part or an organ; overgrowth; abnormal growth.

Keratoma (ker-a-**TOH**-ma), or callus, is a superficial, round, thickened patch of epidermis on the hands and feet caused by friction. If the thickening grows inward, it is called a corn. This condition is usually treated by a chiropodist.

A *mole* is a small, brown spot on the skin. Moles are believed to be inherited. They range in color from pale tan to brown or bluish black. Some moles are small and flat, resembling freckles, while others are more deeply seated and darker in color. Large, dark hairs often occur in moles. Any change in a mole requires medical attention.

▶ **Caution:** Do not treat or remove hair from moles.

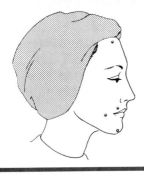

7.28—Verruca

Verruca (ve-**ROO**-kah) is the technical term for a wart. It is a viral infection of the epidermis. It can spread from one location to another, particularly along a scratch in the skin. Warts should be treated or removed by a physician. It is a growth that is benign. Children are more likely to have warts than are adults. Warts may appear on various parts of the body, but they appear most often on the hands and fingers. Warts can be destroyed by electrosurgery (electric current) or cryotherapy (freezing with dry ice or liquid nitrogen). Medication is also used in the treatment of warts. Warts sometimes disappear without treatment and self-applied medication is not advised (Fig. 7.28).

Skin Tags are made up of bead-like, fibrous tissue that stand away from the flat surface of the skin. They are often a dark color. Growths of this type can be removed by a surgeon.

Broken Capillaries—Dilated, split, or broken capillaries appear more prominently on the cheeks and nose. Broken blood vessels turn bluish in color and appear as fine lines. This condition may be caused by excessive friction, extremes of heat and cold, and poor circulation. The skillful use of cosmetics can help to conceal this condition.

Characteristics of Aging Skin

As a person ages, the deeper, or dermal, layers of the skin undergo changes. In most cases, the skin loses its elasticity, becomes thinner and dryer, showing deepening lines and wrinkles. The loss of elasticity of the skin and the loss of firmness of the underlying facial muscles contribute to deep folds and lines in the skin. A crepey appearance of the skin often follows illness, extreme loss of weight, improper lubrication of dry skin, or overexposure to sun or wind. Constant exposure to strong sunlight may also hasten the aging process.

Growths are more likely to appear on aging skin. Fine lines around the eyes, commonly known as crowsfeet, are usually caused by normal facial expressions, such as smiling or grimacing. Lines are also associated with swollen, puffy tissues (*edema*) around and under the eyes. Hormonal changes in the body (especially during menopause in women) may contribute to a diminished supply of natural oils and moisture needed to keep skin looking youthful. See pages 339–341.

Other Serious Disorders of the Skin

There are three kinds of skin cancer. The least malignant and most common is called *Basal Cell Carcinoma* (kahr-si-**NO**-muh). This type of cancer is characterized by light or pearly nodules and visible blood vessels.

Squamous (**SKWAY**-mus) *Cell Carcinoma* is different in appearance from the Basal type. It consists of scaly, red papules. Blood vessels are not visible. This cancer is more serious than the Basal Cell Carcinoma.

The most serious skin cancer is *Malignant Melanoma* (muh-**LIG**-nunt mel-uh-**NO**-muh). This cancer is characterized by dark brown, black, or discolored patches on the skin.

The esthetician should not attempt to diagnose bumps, lesions, ulcerations, or discolorations as skin cancer, but should be able to recognize serious skin disorders and suggest that the client seek medical attention without delay.

A *tumor* is an abnormal growth of swollen tissue that can be located on any part of the body. Some tumors are benign (mild in character and not likely to recur after removal), which means they are not harmful. Some tumors are malignant and are more serious, as they can recur after removal. Tumors are removed by surgery or X-ray treatment.

Venereal Diseases

Venereal diseases are those diseases associated with the sexual organs and are characterized by *chancre* (**SHANK**-ur) *sores* and rashes on the skin. *Syphilis* (**SIF**-i-lis) is a serious disease that is transmitted by contact with an infected person. When any sore, especially a sore that is hard and lacerated (with a hole in the center), first appears, a physician should be consulted. Without treatment, the sore may go away only to appear later in the form of a rash. This is called *secondary syphilis*. The condition may become latent. Secondary syphilis can cause degeneration of various parts of the body, ultimately causing death. *Gonorrhea* (gon-uh-**REE**-uh) is a more common disease than syphilis, characterized by a discharge and burning sensation when urinating. If left untreated, harmful bacteria can enter the bloodstream.

Allergies

Millions of people suffer from various forms of allergies. Some of the common allergies are as follows.

1. *Allergic dermatitis* (eczema) can be caused by a number of different factors: food, substances in the air, or materials the victim uses. Many objects contain metals that cause dermatitis. Necklaces, rings, hairpins and bracelets are a few of the objects that contain metal (such as nickel), which cause contact dermatitis. Some people are allergic to such substances as rubber, hair dyes, some types of makeup, and chemicals used in manufacturing or treating clothing and other items.

2. *Food allergies* are discussed in detail in Chapter 10.

3. *Hay fever* is considered an allergic condition that is caused by plant pollens in the air. Sneezing, coughing, and sinus congestion are a few of the symptoms of hay fever.

4. *Asthma* may be caused by a number of allergens to which an individual is sensitive. Asthma is characterized by symptoms that sometimes resemble those of a cold.

5. *Urticaria* (ur-ti-**KAR**-ee-uh) is the medical name for hives. It is an inflammation that is usually caused by an allergy to specific drugs or foods.

6. *Drug allergies* are allergic reactions to drugs and different kinds of medication. Whether a drug is bought with or without a prescription, any reaction should be reported to a physician.

7. *Dermatitis medicamentosa* (med-i-kuh-men-**TO**-sa) is the medical term applied to dermatitis that occurs after an injection of a substance, such as penicillin.

8. *Dermatitis venenata* is the medical term applied to dermatitis that occurs as the result of external contact with a substance, such as poison ivy, metal, or other allergens.

9. *Insect stings* can cause a reaction in some people. Many people have only a mild reaction to bee, wasp, or other insect stings, while others may experience a severe reaction.

ALLERGENS   The following is a list of common allergens:

Drugs	Fumes	Sprays
Laxatives	Tranquilizers	Insecticides
Sedatives	Cold remedies	Plastics
Sleeping pills	Antibiotics	Fabrics
Pollen	Diet pills	Plants
Mold spores	Dust	Flowers
Feathers	Animal hair	Metals

Substances in the environment

Substances that come in contact with the skin

Grooming products and cosmetics like hair spray

Leather dyes or polishes

Any person who has an allergy to any substance that is likely to cause a reaction should carry a medical identification card with information that would be helpful in case of emergency.

Regeneration and Repair of the Skin

The skin is capable of rapid regeneration and healing; however, rapid healing depends on a healthy and well-nourished body and a wound free of harmful bacteria and foreign matter. In a minor wound, such as a scratch, small cut, or scraped area, the epidermal cells start their regenerating process immediately and a new covering (epidermis) is formed. In case of severe injury, such as deep burns, cuts, and tears, the regeneration process is slower and skin transplantation may be required. The body responds to a wound by a temporary rise in body temperature and an increased pulse rate.

In addition to the recognition of primary and secondary lesions, which were explained at the beginning of this chapter, the esthetician should also be aware of any minor or major, large or small wounds or other imperfections on the skin. When the skin is injured, the client should see a physician and return for facial treatments when the injury has healed completely.

IMPERFECTIONS OF THE SKIN
An *abrasion* is rough and red where the skin has been scraped or worn away (Fig. 7.29).

A *laceration* is an uneven, jagged tear in the skin (Fig. 7.30).

A *cyst* is a sac-like, elevated (usually round) area that contains a liquid or clear semi-solid substance (Fig. 7.31).

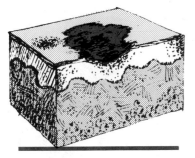

7.29 — Abrasion

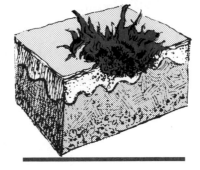

7.30 — Laceration

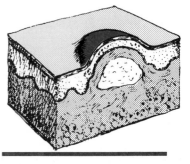

7.31 — Cyst

A *fissure* is a narrow opening or furrow in the skin (Fig. 7.32).

An *incision* is a cut or incised wound such as is made with a knife or other sharp instrument (Fig. 7.33).

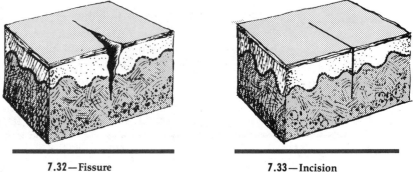

7.32 — Fissure   **7.33 — Incision**

A *scar* is a mark left on the skin after the healing of a wound or sore (Fig. 7.34).

A *nodule* is a small knot-like node beneath the surface of the skin (Fig. 7.35).

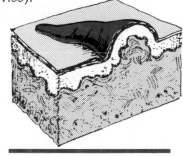

7.34 — Scar

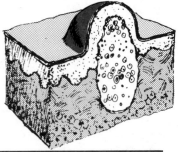

7.35 — Nodule

A *puncture* wound is a hole in the skin made by piercing the skin with a sharp, pointed object (Fig. 7.36).

A *polyp* is a growth that extends from the surface of the skin. Polyps may also grow within the body (Fig. 7.37).

An *ulcer* is an open sore on the external or internal surface of the skin, often accompanied by the formation of pus (Fig. 7.38).

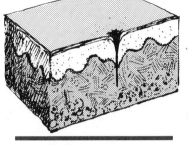

7.36—Puncture

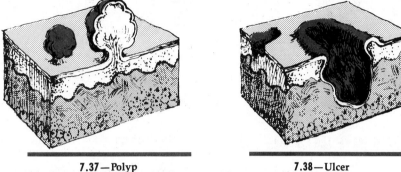

7.37—Polyp

7.38—Ulcer

QUESTIONS DISCUSSION AND REVIEW

DISORDERS OF THE SKIN, DERMATOLOGY, AND SPECIAL ESTHETIC PROCEDURES

1. Why should the esthetician be able to recognize common skin disorders?
2. What is the purpose of studying infectious diseases of the skin?
3. Why should the esthetician refuse to treat a client with an infectious or contagious disease?
4. Define dermatology.
5. What is a dermatologist?
6. What is a lesion?
7. What is the difference between objective and subjective lesions?
8. Discuss the primary lesions of the skin.
9. Discuss the seven secondary lesions of the skin.
10. Define disease.
11. What are the common terms for: a) comedones; b) milia?
12. What causes the formation of comedones?
13. Define acne.
14. Which of the following terms apply to disorders of the sebaceous (oil) glands? Milia, acne, bromidrosis, comedones, seborrhea?
15. Briefly describe: bromidrosis, anidrosis, hyperidrosis and miliaria rubra.
16. Define dermatitis.
17. Define eczema.
18. What is the characteristic appearance of psoriasis?
19. On which five parts of the body is psoriasis usually found?
20. Define herpes simplex. What is it commonly called?
21. Where do fever blisters usually occur?
22. What is albinism?
23. Discuss portwine and strawberry discolorations of the skin.
24. What are general causes of broken capillaries?

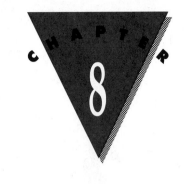

CHAPTER

8

Chemistry for Estheticians

LEARNING OBJECTIVES   *After completing this chapter, you should be able to:*

❶ Explain chemistry and its branches.
❷ Explain matter and its structure.
❸ Discuss how matter changes and its properties.
❹ Discuss why chemistry is important to estheticians.

INTRODUCTION

Chemistry is one of the physical sciences. Many people think chemistry only concerns chemists and persons involved in some scientific field. Actually, it concerns everyone in some way.

Every branch of medicine involves chemistry. The daily functioning of our bodies, both in health and in disease, is a matter of chemistry. Everything we eat is a chemical. Most of the clothing we wear is made of chemically combined substances, and practically everything else we use in our daily living depends on chemistry.

All material things are made up of atoms and molecules, arranged in various ways. The actions and reactions of these primary particles constitute the field of learning that we call chemistry. In one way or another, chemistry enters into practically everything with which we deal.

Skin, the basic structure that concerns the esthetician, is chemical in nature. So are all creams, lotions, masks, and makeup. While the esthetician is not expected to have the knowledge of a cosmetic chemist, he or she will find an understanding of the chemical characteristics of various materials invaluable.

Chemistry is the science that deals with the composition, structure, and properties of matter, and how matter changes under different conditions. The material covered here will pave the way for understanding the composition and functions of the materials and products used by the esthetician. These will be discussed fully in the next chapter, *Ingredient and Product Analysis*. A basic knowledge of modern chemistry is an essential requirement for an intelligent understanding of the various products used in facial treatments.

Through continuous study and research in chemistry, new products are constantly being developed for the benefit of both the esthetician and the client. It is important that the professional esthetician understand these products and learns how to use them so that the client will receive the maximum benefits.

Branches of Chemistry

There are two branches in the science of chemistry—*inorganic* and *organic*.

Inorganic chemistry is the study of all substances that do not contain carbon.

Inorganic substances are quick in their chemical reactions. Examples of inorganic substances are water, air, iron, lead, and iodine.

Organic chemistry is the study of all substances in which carbon atoms are present. Carbon can be found in all plants and animals, as well as in petroleum, coal, natural gas, and in many artificially prepared substances.

Most organic substances will burn. They are soluble in organic solvents, such as alcohol and benzene. They are not soluble in water.

Organic substances are slow in their chemical reactions. Examples of organic substances are grass, trees, gasoline, oil, soaps, detergents, plastics, and antibiotics.

Matter

Matter may be defined as anything that has mass and occupies space. It exists in three physical forms: solids, liquids, and gases.

Solids have shape and volume. Examples of solid objects are chairs, people, desks, etc.

Liquids are shapeless, but readily take the shape of their containers. Liquids cannot be compressed readily. Examples are water, lotions, and astringents.

Gases are also shapeless, but they expand easily and are compressible. An example is the air we breathe.

STRUCTURE OF MATTER   An *atom* is the smallest part of an element that possesses the characteristics of the element. All of the atoms in an element are identical. Therefore, an atom of hydrogen has the properties of hydrogen. If you took a piece of gold (an element) and divided it into smaller and smaller pieces, you would eventually come to a particle so small that it no longer showed the properties of the element.

Atoms consist of smaller particles—*protons*, *neutrons*, and *electrons*, which have a positive, neutral, or negative charge, respectively. The number of protons in an atom must equal the number of electrons.

A *molecule* is the smallest particle of an element or compound that possesses all the properties of the element or compound. If the molecule is of an element, it is an atom of the element. If it is of a compound, the atoms are different. For example, a molecule of hydrogen contains two or more atoms of hydrogen (H_2). A molecule of the compound water is composed of two atoms of hydrogen and one atom of oxygen (H_2O).

In general, when we talk about the chemical activity of an element, we refer to the tendency of its atoms to combine with other elements. Electrons are the most important factors for chemical reactions. For example, hydrogen is a very active element and readily combines with other elements, while neon is completely inactive and does not combine with other elements. Electrons of hydrogen atoms move readily. Electrons of neon atoms do not.

Matter exists in an almost infinite variety. This variety is made possible because atoms can join together with similar or dissimilar atoms to form an almost infinite variety of substances known as compounds. Matter exists in the form of elements, compounds, and mixtures.

ELEMENTS An *element* is the basic unit of all matter. It is a substance that cannot be made by the combination of simpler substances, and the element itself cannot be reduced to simpler substances. There are now 105 known elements, of which some of the more common are carbon, iron, sulfur, oxygen, zinc, silicon, and silver.

Each element is given a letter symbol, for example:

Carbon C

Iron . . . . Fe

Sulfur . . . . S

Oxygen . . . . O

Zinc . . . . Zn

Silicon . . . . Si

Silver . . . . Ag

COMPOUNDS When two or more elements unite chemically, they form a *compound*. Each element loses its individual properties and the new compound develops its own characteristic properties. For example, iron oxide (rust) has different properties from the two elements of which it is comprised— iron and oxygen. The new substance, which is a compound, cannot be altered by mechanical means, but only by chemical means.

There are many types of compounds. The four most important classes are as follows.

1. *Oxides* are compounds in which an element combines with oxygen. For example, one part carbon and two parts oxygen (CO_2) equal carbon dioxide, which, when frozen, is known as dry ice. One part carbon and one part oxygen (CO) equal carbon monoxide, better known as the poisonous exhaust from an automobile.
2. *Acids* are compounds consisting of hydrogen, a nonmetal such as nitrogen, and sometimes oxygen. For example, hydrogen + sulfur + oxygen = sulfuric acid (H_2SO_4). Acids turn testing paper, called blue litmus paper, red.
3. *Bases*, also known as alkalies, are compounds consisting of hydrogen, a metal, and oxygen. For example, sodium + oxygen + hydrogen = sodium hydroxide (NaOH), which is used in the manufacturing of soap. Bases turn red litmus paper blue, and have a slippery feel.
4. *Salts* are compounds formed by the reaction of an acid and a base. Water is also produced by the reaction. Two common salts and their formulas are sodium chloride, or table salt (NaCl), which contains sodium and chloride, and magnesium sulfate, or Epsom salts ($MgSO_4.7H_2O$), which contains magnesium, sulfur, hydrogen, and oxygen.

Elements and Compounds

TYPES AND DEFINITION	SMALLEST PARTICLE
Matter Solids Gases Liquids ELEMENTS: Simplest Form of Matter	ATOM: About 100 different kinds (cannot be broken down by simple chemical reactions).
COMPOUNDS: Formed by Combination of Elements	MOLECULE: Unlimited kinds possible (consists of 2 or more atoms chemically combined).

ELEMENTS FOUND IN SKIN OR HAIR	COMPOUNDS USED ON SKIN OR HAIR
CARBON NITROGEN OXYGEN SULFUR HYDROGEN PHOSPHORUS	WATER HYDROGEN PEROXIDE AMMONIUM THIOGLYCOLATE ALCOHOL ALKALIS

MIXTURES A *mixture* is a substance that is made up of two or more elements combined physically rather than chemically.

The ingredients in a mixture do not change their properties, as they do in a compound, but they retain their individual characteristics. For example, concrete is composed of sand, gravel, and cement. While concrete is a mixture having its own functions, its ingredients never lose their individual characteristics. Sand remains sand; gravel is still gravel; and cement is still cement.

CHANGES IN MATTER   Matter may be changed in two ways, either through physical or chemical means.

Physical change refers to an alteration in the form or the properties of a substance without changing the chemical nature of the substance or without forming any new substance. For example, ice (a solid) melts at a certain temperature and becomes a liquid (water), and water (a liquid) freezes at a certain temperature and becomes a solid. There is no change in the inherent nature of the water, but merely a change in its form.

A *chemical change* is one in which a new substance or substances are formed, with properties different from the original substance(s). For example, soap is formed from the chemical reaction between an alkaline substance (sodium hydroxide) and an oil or fat. The soap resembles neither the alkaline substance nor the oil from which it is formed. Chemical reaction between the two forms a new substance, having its own characteristic properties.

PROPERTIES OF MATTER   When we talk about the properties of matter, we are talking about how we distinguish one form of matter from another. The *physical properties* of matter are density, specific gravity, odor, color, and taste.

The *density* of a substance refers to its weight divided by its volume. For example, a volume of one cubic foot of water weighs 62.4 pounds (29 kilograms); therefore, its density is 62.4 pounds per cubic foot.

The *specific gravity* of a substance is also referred to as its *relative density*. This means that substances are referred to as either more or less dense than water. For example, copper is 8.9 times as dense as water; therefore, the specific gravity of copper is 8.9.

Every substance has a characteristic *odor* that helps identify it in many instances. For example, the characteristic odor of ammonium thioglycolate (a-**MOHN**-nee-um theye-oh-**GLEYE**-coh-layt), known as the "thio" odor, helps identify this compound.

Color also helps to identify many substances. For example, we recognize the color of gold, silver, copper, brass, and coal.

Taste helps identify many substances as well. For example, oil of wintergreen can be identified by its peppermint-type taste.

The *chemical properties* of a substance refer to the ability of the substance to react with other substances, and the conditions under which it reacts. Two of the more widely recognized chemical properties a substance possesses are *combustibility* and the ability to *support combustion*.

Phosphorus, for example, is a highly combustible substance. For that reason, it is used on the tips of matches. The heat produced by rubbing the match tip against a surface is enough to cause it to burst into flames. Wood has the ability to suport combustion; therefore, it is used in the manufacturing of matches. The phosphorus tip starts the fire; the wood supports the fire.

Properties of Common Elements, Compounds, and Mixtures

Knowledge of the properties of some of the most common elements, compounds, and mixtures can help the esthetician understand why certain cosmetic reactions occur.

Hydrogen (H) is a colorless, odorless, tasteless gas and is the lightest element known. It is found in chemical combination with oxygen in water, and with other elements in acids, bases, and most organic substances. It is flammable and explosive when mixed with air.

Oxygen (O) is the most abundant element found both free and in compounds. It composes about half of the earth's crust, half of the rock, one-fifth of the air, and 90 percent of the water. It is a colorless, odorless, tasteless gas. It combines with most other elements to form an infinite variety of compounds, called *oxides*. One of the chief chemical characteristics of this element is its ability to support combustion.

Nitrogen (N) is a colorless, gaseous element found free in the air. It constitutes part of the atmosphere, forming about four-fifths of the air. It is found chiefly in the form of ammonia and nitrates.

Air is the gaseous mixture that makes up the earth's atmosphere. It is an odorless, colorless solution and generally consists of about one part of oxygen and four parts of nitrogen by volume. It also contains a small amount of carbon dioxide, ammonia, and organic matter, which are all essential to plant and animal life.

Water (H_2O) is the most abundant of all substances, composing about 75 percent of the earth's surface and about 65 percent of the human body. Water is seldom pure. It usually contains dissolved minerals and bacteria. Water that contains certain mineral substances is an excellent conductor of electricity. Demineralized or distilled water is a nonconductor of electricity.

Hard water contains mineral substances, such as the salts of calcium and magnesium, which curdle, or precipitate, soap instead of permitting an even lather to form. Hard water may be softened by distillation, or by the use of borax, sodium carbonate, or sodium phosphate. To soften hard water effectively in salons, special equipment, such as a zeolite tank, is used.

Water serves many useful purposes in the salon. Only water of known purity is fit for drinking purposes. Suspended or dissolved impurities in water may render it unsatisfactory for cleaning objects and for use in facial treatments.

Impurities can be removed from water by filtration, passing water through a porous substance such as filter paper or charcoal; or by distillation, heating water in a closed vessel arranged so that the resulting vapor passes off through a tube and is cooled and condensed to a liquid. This process purifies water used in the manufacture of cosmetics.

In most cases, distilled or filtered water is used in the salon for machines that require water. Boiling water at a temperature of 212°F (100°C), will destroy most microbic life.

Hydrogen peroxide (H_2O_2) is a compound of hydrogen and oxygen. It is a colorless liquid with a characteristic odor and a slightly acid taste. Organic matter, such as silk, hair, feathers, and nails, are lightened by hydrogen peroxide. A 20 to 40 percent volume of hydrogen peroxide combined with a water solution is used as a lightening agent for the hair. A 10 percent volume solution possesses antiseptic properties.

Acidity and Alkalinity

The *pH* (potential of hydrogen) of a substance refers to its degree of acidity or alkalinity, and is measured on a scale of 0 to 14. Anything below 7 is acidic. The lower the pH number, the greater the degree of acidity. Anything from 7 to 14 is alkaline. The higher the pH number, the greater the degree of alkalinity. Although the precise neutral point on the scale is 7.0, the neutral range is considered to extend from pH 6.5 to 7.5 (Fig. 8.1).

The pH of a product can usually be tested by the use of indicator papers. Acids turn indicator papers pink or orange; alkalies turn them blue or green.

The pH is an important consideration for the esthetician. The pH of the skin's acid mantle ranges from 4.5 to 6 and is most often referred to as 5.5. It is generally believed that unless a cosmetic has a pH of 5.5, it is not compatible with the skin. Actually, many products would not be as effective if they had a reading of 5.5. For example, a cleanser formulated with a pH of 7, which is neutral, will cleanse the skin better than a cleanser with a pH of 5.5. A moisturizer that is slightly alkaline will have a softening effect on the skin. This makes it easier for the skin to absorb the beneficial ingredients in the moisturizer.

Products that are formulated for acne skins are more acidic to help fight germ penetration. The acid pH product will usually act as an anti-bacterial agent.

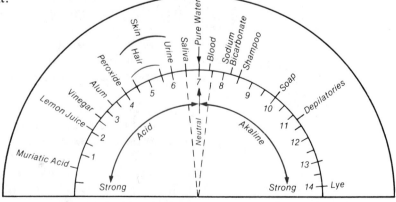

8.1—Average pH values

Chemical Reactions

Chemical reactions are the "balancing acts" of chemistry. When two or more chemicals are mixed together, they react in certain ways to form new chemicals. There are two types of chemical reactions of importance to estheticians, because they explain the working principles of many of the products used in skin care.

ACID-BASE REACTIONS

Acid-base reactions are also known as neutralizing reactions in which an acid reacts with a base, or alkali, to form a salt. For example, hydrochloric acid mixes with sodium hydroxide to form sodium chloride (salt) and water.

OXIDATION-REDUCTION REACTIONS

Oxidation-reduction reactions are among the most common types of chemical reactions, and are prevalent in all areas of chemistry. In oxidation, a substance loses electrons; in reduction, it gains electrons. Oxidation is always accompanied by reduction.

An *oxidizing agent* is a substance that takes electrons away from another substance. A *reducing agent*, on the other hand, gives electrons to another substance. These reactions are responsible for such phenomena as rusting, in which iron combines with oxygen to become iron oxide, or rust. The power from electric batteries is also a form of oxidation-reduction reaction.

Hydrogen peroxide is a typical oxidizing agent used by estheticians. It oxidizes the hair pigment, changing it to a colorless compound. During the action, the lightening agent is reduced and the pigment is oxidized.

Chemistry as Applied to Cosmetics

To better serve the public, estheticians should have an understanding of the chemical composition, preparation, and uses of cosmetics that are intended to cleanse and beautify the skin.

Cosmetics may be classified according to their use and function. Each type has a specific physical and chemical nature and the characteristics by which they can be recognized. The object in classifying cosmetics is to assist in their identification.

Any cosmetic may be a solution, a colloid, a suspension, or an emulsion. A *solution* is a homogeneous mixture of molecules. Solutions are preparations made by dissolving a solid, liquid, or gas into another substance. They are usually found in liquid form, but they may also be solid, as in some powders or gases, such as in air. Making a boric acid solution involves the dissolving of a solid into a liquid. Ammonia water is a mixture of a gas in water.

The substance dissolved in a solution is called the *solute*. The substance used to dissolve the solute is the *solvent*. Solutions are mixtures of solutes and solvents that do not separate on standing. Since a good solution is clear and transparent, filtration is often necessary, particularly if the solution is cloudy after mixing. The solute may be separated from the solvent by the application of heat, which evaporates the solvent.

Water is a universal solvent. It is capable of dissolving more substances than any other solvents. Water, glycerine, and alcohol readily mix with each other; therefore, they are *miscible*. On the other hand, water and oil do not mix with each other; hence, they are *immiscible*.

Solutions containing substances that evaporate, such as ammonia and alcohol, should be stored in a cool place.

A solution may be classed as dilute, concentrated, or saturated. A dilute solution contains a small quantity of solute in proportion to the quantity of solvent. A concentrated solution contains a large quantity of solute in proportion to the quantity of solvent. A saturated solution will not dissolve or take up more of the solute than it already holds at a given temperature.

Colloids and *suspensions* are liquid mixtures of immiscible materials, in which the molecules do not intermix, but stay separate. If the particles are large, the mixture is known as a suspension; if they are small, it is a colloid.

Since the particles have a tendency to separate on standing, a thorough shaking is required before using. Suspensions and colloids should not be filtered. Many skin lotions fall into either of these categories. Calamine lotion is one example.

Suspensions and colloids are made by first mixing the dry components, then adding a small amount of liquid to form a smooth paste, and finally adding the balance of the liquid.

Emulsions are permanent mixtures of two or more immiscible substances, such as oil and water, which are held in suspension with the aid of a binder, such as gum, or an emulsifier, such as soap. Emulsions are usually milky in appearance. If a suitable emulsifier and the proper mixing techniques are employed, the resultant emulsion will be stable. A stable emulsion can hold as much as 90 percent water. Depending on the ratio between the components, the emulsion may be either liquid or semi-solid in character. The amount of emulsifier used depends on its efficiency and the amount of water or oil to be emulsified.

Emulsions are prepared by hand or with the aid of a grinding and cutting machine, called a *colloidal mill*. In the process of preparing an emulsion, the emulsifier forms a protective film around the microscopic globules of either the oil or water. The smaller the globules, the thicker and more stable the emulsion will be.

Water is best for use in the emulsion type of skin cosmetic, since it helps carry chemicals more easily into the skin. If, however, these products are mixed in water alone, the small drops formed will, on standing, gradually separate into different layers. Therefore, water cannot be used with these insoluble substances, which, nevertheless, are still required for proper skin care.

Emulsions overcome the difficulties of applying water insoluble substances to the skin. For example, oils are required to condition the epidermis, either as special preparations, such as skin creams and conditioners, or in conjunction with other cosmetic treatments. But these oils are not soluble in water and would form a separate layer even after complete dispersion. If a mixture of oil and water is shaken vigorously, the oil will break into small droplets throughout the liquid. On standing, however, these dispersed oil droplets quickly rise to the surface, where they merge together as a separate layer.

If a special product, called an *emulsifier*, is present, it will coat the droplets of oil as they are formed. This stabilizes the oils and keeps them distributed throughout the water phase.

In commercial preparations, the droplets are often made by *homogenizers* or blenders. The main requirements are that the droplets be very small and uniformly dispersed in the product. They must be stable in this condition for at least the average shelf-life of the product.

There are two types of emulsions used in cosmetic preparations. They are oil-in-water (O/W) and water-in-oil (W/O) (Fig. 8.2).

Oil-in-water emulsions are made of oil droplets, dispersed in a water base. This base may, in addition, contain other dissolved substances required to carry out additional chemical reactions in the skin. The oil droplets may, in turn, contain water-insoluble chemicals.

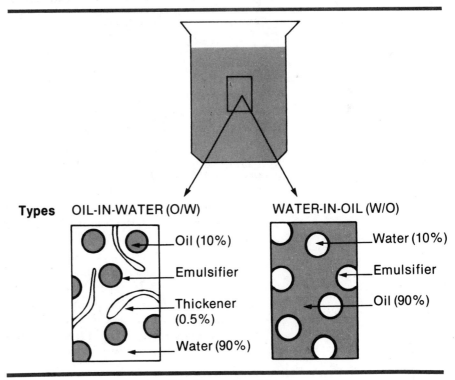

Types   OIL-IN-WATER (O/W)   WATER-IN-OIL (W/O)

Oil (10%) — Emulsifier — Thickener (0.5%) — Water (90%)

Water (10%) — Emulsifier — Oil (90%)

8.2—Types of emulsions

However, the purpose of an emulsion is to apply a suitably dispersed conditioner easily and evenly to the skin. Once contact is made with the skin, the finely dispersed oil is absorbed on the surface. (The released oils spread over the epidermis.)

The conditioning effect of the oil layer acts as an external lubricant to smooth and to help protect the surface of the epidermis.

The water molecules restore the natural moisture content of the epidermis. This makes the skin soft and smooth. Thus, the water content in the emulsion acts as an internal lubricant.

One advantage of O/W emulsions is that they may be easily rinsed away with water. A good example is an O/W cleansing lotion that can be removed easily with wet cotton pads or sponges.

Because they have a high water content, O/W emulsions are often milky, easy-flowing liquids. For special purposes, specific additives may be included as thickeners. These thickeners usually have extremely long, thread-like molecules that, by slowing down the movement of the emulsion molecules, make the emulsion thicker in both appearance and feel. Examples of O/W emulsions are moisturing lotions, cleansing lotions, sun tan lotions, and vanishing creams.

Typical Formula of an O/W Emulsion

IN AN EMULSION, THE FOLLOWING SUBSTANCES MAY BE FOUND:	
Oil type conditioner	A light mineral oil or lanolin
Emulsifier	A joining agent between the water and the conditioner, usually a form of soap
Thickener	To control the thickness of the emulsion or to make it look "richer"
Clouding agent	To give a pearly white, attractive appearance
Perfume and water	To disguise unpleasant odors and impart a pleasing odor to the skin

Water-in-oil emulsions are made of water droplets scattered within an oil base. As such, W/O emulsions are greasier than O/W emulsions. When formed with light mineral oils, they can be poured at normal temperature. Examples are cleansing creams, cold creams, night creams, massage creams, baby creams, and hair grooming creams.

W/O emulsions help to prevent moisture loss from the skin. They are also useful for removing grime from skin.

W/O emulsions do not mix with water and are usually thicker creams. O/W emulsions are easily diluted by water and, since they already consist of 65 to 90 percent water, can be free-flowing, milky, or creamy liquids.

However, when desired, O/W emulsions are thickened to form jellies or thick creams.

Because of the complicated chemical nature of emulsions, the water (the major part of the O/W emulsion) and the active ingredients will sometimes separate when standing. Once this occurs, the product is usually useless and should be discarded.

> **Note:** The percentage of water and oil in a product will vary, depending on the formulation of the product and the desired texture (such as cream or liquid).

Product Forms

Cosmetic products take a variety of forms, including powders, ointments, sticks, pastes, soaps, and creams. These forms will be discussed fully in the next chapter, *Ingredient and Product Analysis*.

QUESTIONS DISCUSSION AND REVIEW

CHEMISTRY FOR ESTHETICIANS

1. Define chemistry.
2. What are the two branches of chemistry?
3. What is the difference between organic and inorganic chemistry?
4. Define matter.
5. What is a liquid?
6. Define gases.
7. What is the smallest part of an element that possesses the characteristics of the element?
8. What are the smaller particles of an atom?
9. Define a molecule.
10. Describe an element.
11. What is a compound?
12. How many known elements are there?
13. What are the four most important classes of compounds?
14. How can matter be changed?
15. Give an example of a physical and a chemical change.
16. Give three characteristics that can help us to identify a substance.
17. What type of water is used in most salon machines?
18. What is the pH of the skin's acid mantle?
19. Why is the pH of a moisturizer slightly alkaline?
20. What is a universal solvent?
21. What are the differences between a dilute, a concentrated, and a saturated solution?
22. What are the two types of emulsions used in cosmetic preparations?

CHAPTER 9

Ingredient and Product Analysis

LEARNING OBJECTIVES   *After completing this chapter, you should be able to:*

❶ Discuss the products used in the practice of esthetics.
❷ Explain the product forms and ingredients.
❸ Discuss the different creams, lotions, and powders used in skin care.
❹ Define natural and organic cosmetics.
❺ Define the laws governing cosmetic manufacturing.
❻ Explain cosmetic labeling and cosmetic safety.
❼ Discuss how to deal with consumer complaints.

INTRODUCTION   The products the esthetician uses are the lifeblood of the facial treatment. The active ingredients in the product, regardless of its form, do the actual work of cleansing, normalizing, moisturizing, or otherwise treating the skin.

This doesn't minimize the importance of the work done by the esthetician. His or her skill in choosing the correct products, in applying them properly, and in performing the procedures correctly, lets the products do their work. Products and effort are equal partners in the facial process.

Products come in many forms and types. They may be available in the form of solids, liquids, or gases, or in combinations of these. They may be formulated as cleansers, moisturizers, deodorants, or as a host of other applications. Within each category, the products may be differentiated further by the skin type they are intended to treat. The esthetician must choose the correct formulation for the client's skin type as well as the correct product to perform the required function. Otherwise, the product may not work properly.

Regardless of its form or type, a product consists of ingredients, substances that work together to let the product achieve its purpose. Any given product will contain one or more ingredients that work together. Each ingredient in a product has a certain job.

Before using any product on a client, the esthetician should know what the product is supposed to do, how it works, and how it should be used. He or she should read the manufacturer's literature and follow the instructions.

The esthetician should be familiar with each ingredient in the product he or she uses and should know what that ingredient does. He or she should also be aware of potential side effects of particular ingredients.

Product Forms

Products come in many forms. They are available in dry or semi-dry form, such as powders and sticks; in liquid or semi-liquid form, such as liquids, creams, ointments, gels, and pastes; and in gas form, such as aerosols.

Powders are uniform mixtures of insoluble substances that have been blended to produce a product that has no coarse or gritty particles. They may be free-flowing, like talcum powder, or be pressed into cakes, like compact face powders. Mixing and sifting processes are used to make powders.

Sticks are a mixture of substances that are poured into a mold to solidify. No water is present. Lipstick is an example of a cosmetic stick product.

Liquids are free-flowing and have a watery consistency.

Creams are thicker and vary in consistency from pourable to spreadable. They are generally emulsions.

Ointments are semi-liquid mixtures of carriers and medicinal agents. No water is present. Ointments are prepared by melting the carriers and mixing the medicinal agent into the mixture. They are generally softer than sticks.

Pastes are soft, moist products, having a thick consistency. They are bound together with the aid of gum, starch, and water. If oils and fats are used, no water will be present.

Gels have a jelly-like consistency and are usually not emulsified.

Products in gaseous form are usually available as *aerosols*, which spray the product in a fine mist.

Ingredients

The ingredients in a product are either *active*, that is, they work directly on the skin, or *inactive*, that is, they don't work on the skin, but perform a function that helps the product, such as a preservative or a stabilizer.

Ingredients may come from plants, animals, vitamins, or minerals, or may be synthesized from chemicals. Plant materials include herbs, seaweed, fruits, sap from trees, etc. Animal products include lanolin, collagen, and albumin (al-**BEW**-min). Vitamins, such as vitamin A and vitamin E, are used widely in skin care products, as are minerals, such as kaolin (**KAY**-o-lin) and silica (**SIL**-i-kuh).

Chemically synthesized ingredients include alcohol and petroleum derivatives, such as mineral oil. The list of possible ingredients is almost endless.

Each ingredient has a specific part to play in any product formulation. Many ingredients can perform more than one function. Water, for example, is both a solvent and a vehicle. Some of the more important functions include:

Antioxidants—Substances, such as tocopherol (to-**KOF**-ur-ol) (vitamin E), that prevent damage due to oxidation.

Binders—Substances, such as glycerine (**GLIS**-ur-in), that hold products together.

Cleansers—Substances, such as soaps and detergents, that clean the skin. A *soap* is a compound formed in a chemical reaction between alkaline substances (potassium or sodium hydroxide) and the fatty acids in oil or fat. Besides soap, glycerine is also formed. Potassium hydroxide produces a soft soap; sodium hydroxide produces a hard soap. A good soap does not contain an excess of free alkali and is made from pure oils and fats. A *detergent* is a synthetic chemical preparation that differs from soap, but performs the same functions.

Colorants—Substances that give a product a characteristic color. These may be vegetable, animal, or mineral dyes or pigments. Colorants must be certified by the FDA before they may be used.

Emollients—Substances, such as aloe vera or acetylated lanolin alcohol, that soften and soothe skin.

Fragrances—Substances, such as essential oils, that give a product its characteristic odor.

Healing Agents—Substances, such as chamomile or zinc oxide, that heal the skin.

Humectants (hew-**MECK**-tunts)—Substances that have the ability to attract water. Humectants are found in moisturizing lotions and night creams that usually contain glycerine. Humectants in cosmetic products draw moisture to the surface of the skin, where it can soften and moisturize the dry cells on the surface of the skin. This not only makes the skin appear smoother, but also helps to diminish superficial lines caused by dryness.

Lubricants—Substances, such as mineral oil, that coat the skin and reduce friction.

Preservatives—Substances, such as methyl paraben, that kill bacteria and prevent products from spoiling.

Solvents—Substances, such as alcohol or water, that dissolve other ingredients.

Surfactants (sur-**FACK**-tunts)—Substances, such as sodium laureth sulfate, that let products spread more easily.

Vehicles—Substances, such as alcohol or water, that carry other ingredients. These usually make up the largest part of the product.

Some of the more commonly used ingredients include:

Alcohol—A colorless liquid or waxy solid obtained by the fermentation of certain sugars. It can be a powerful antiseptic and solvent. It is widely used in perfumes, lotions, and tonics.

Algae (**AL**-jee)—A sea product containing minerals and phytohormones (figh-to-**HOR**-mones). Algae products are used widely in facial masks and other products to remineralize and revitalize the skin.

Alum—A compound of aluminum, potassium, or ammonium sulfate, supplied in the form of crystals or powder. It has a strong astringent action. It is used in skin tonics and lotions and is also used in powder form as a styptic (**STIP**-tick), which is applied to stop bleeding in small cuts.

Ammonia Water—A colorless liquid with a pungent, penetrating odor. It is a by-product of the manufacturing of coal gas. As it readily dissolves grease, it is used as a cleansing agent, and is also used with hydrogen peroxide in lightening hair.

Boric Acid—A powder obtained from sodium borate, which is mined in the form of borax and crystallized with sulfuric acid. It is a mild healing and antiseptic agent. It is sometimes used as a dusting powder and in solution, as a cleansing lotion or eyewash.

Collagen—A fibrous substance, derived from the placenta (pluh-**SEN**-tuh) of cows, that is used as a super moisturizer. It is available in creams and lotions, or in sheets for use in facial masks.

Essential Oils—Oils derived from various herbs. These have the same properties as the herbs. They are used widely in skin care products and cosmetics. Essential oils are the basis for aromatherapy.

Herbs—Plant materials that contain phytohormones that have specific properties as healing agents, stimulating agents, soothing agents, emollients, and astringents. There are hundreds of different herbs used in skin care products and cosmetics.

Glycerine—A sweet, colorless, odorless, syrupy liquid, formed by the decomposition of oils, fats, or molasses. It is an excellent skin softener, and is an ingredient of cuticle oil, face creams, and lotions.

Potassium Hydroxide—A strong alkali used in making soaps and cosmetic creams.

Sodium Bicarbonate—Also known as baking soda, a precipitate made by passing carbon dioxide gas through a solution of sodium carbonate. It is a white powder used as a neutralizing agent.

Sodium Carbonate—Also known as washing soda, prepared by heating sodium bicarbonate. It is used widely in bath salts and as a water softener.

Sodium Hydroxide—A strong alkali used in making soaps.

Tincture of Iodine—A two percent solution of iodine in alcohol, used to treat minor cuts and bruises. *Mercurochrome* is a three to five percent peroxide solution of iodine, also used for cuts.

Witch Hazel—A commonly used herb in solution with alcohol and water, used as an astringent.

Zinc Oxide—A heavy white powder used as a dusting powder and in ointments for some skin conditions.

Cleansers

Cleansers are intended to clean the body by removing dirt, hair, or foreign odors from the skin. This classification includes soaps and detergents, bath accessories, deodorants, antiperspirants and depilatories.

Good toilet soaps should be made from purified fats that will not become rancid in the soap, and should not contain excessive free alkali. Soaps with a pH value above 9.5 dry and roughen the skin. A pH value of 8 is considered normal for skin. (See Table 1.)

Bath accessories include bath salts, bath oils, bath powders, and body oils. Bath salts and oils are used during the bath, while bath powders and body oils are used after the bath. (See Table 2.)

Few preparations can be classified separately as deodorant or antiperspirant products, since most combine the features of both. A *deodorant* is an agent that neutralizes or destroys disagreeable odors without suppressing the amount of perspiration. An *antiperspirant* checks perspiration by its astringent action. The skin surrounding the pores swells, thereby temporarily closing the pores.

Deodorants and antiperspirants are available in the form of aerosols, creams, sticks, solutions, and powders. (See Table 3.)

Depilatories are preparations used for the temporary removal of hair in the armpits and on the legs. They consist of various alkali sulfides, calcium thioglycolate compounds, or resins and waxes. They are available as liquids, soft creams, pastes, powders, or hard cakes.

Before applying a depilatory, conduct a test patch on the client's skin. If skin redness or blisters do not develop, it is safe to use the depilatory over a larger skin surface.

Chemical depilatories are made with hydrogen sulfide, which has the odor of spoiled eggs. They are generally used over the legs and arms. They soften and dissolve hair at the margin of the skin. To prevent irritation of the skin, use only as directed by the manufacturer.

Wax depilatories are odorless and are preferred for the face. After the melted wax with an embedded cloth hardens on the hairy surface, the patch is quickly removed, taking the embedded hairs with it.

Products for Skin Care and Cosmetics

All products designed to render the skin or face more attractive, to normalize, to moisturize or to treat specific conditions may be grouped under this heading. These include creams, lotions, powders, cosmetics, and other products.

Table 1—Kinds of Soaps

SOAPS	COMMON INGREDIENTS	USES
Castile soap (pure)	Olive oil and soda.	Best for the skin—produces little lather.
Green soap	Made from potash and olive or linseed oil and glycerine.	A medicinal liquid soap, used for oily skin.
Tincture of green soap	Mixture of green soap in about 35% alcohol and a small amount of perfume.	Used for correcting oily skin and scalp. Very drying, if used on normal or dry skin over a period of time.
Medicated soap	Contains a small percent of cresol, phenol, or other antiseptics.	Used for acne conditions.
Aerosol shaving cream	Contains alkalies, coconut oil, vegetable and animal fats, and a small amount of gum.	Used for shaving. The alkalinity softens the hair. The thick lather keeps the hair erect.
Shaving soap in pressure can	Shaving soap and gas under pressure.	Used the same as shaving soap.
Carbolic soap	A disinfectant soap containing 10% phenol.	Used for oily skin and acne infection.
Transparent soap	Contains glycerine, alcohol, and sugar, which render it transparent.	Used for normal skin.
Super-fatted soap	Contains a fatty substance, such as lanolin or cocoa butter.	Recommended for dry or sensitive skin. Keeps the skin soft after washing. Not suitable for hard water.
Naphtha soap	Contains naphtha, obtained from petroleum.	Do not use on face or scalp. Use mainly for laundry purposes.
Hard water soap	Contains coconut oil, varying amounts of washing soda or borax, sodium silicate and a phosphate.	Use only on oily skin. The alkaline substances will dry the skin.

Table 2—Bath Accessories

KIND	COMMON INGREDIENTS	USES
Bath salts	Carbonates or phosphates of sodium, color and perfume.	Soften and perfume the bath water.
Bath oils	Sulfonated oils (latherless) or sulfated fatty alcohols (produce lather), color, and perfume.	Sulfonated oils are drying to the skin. If the body skin is dry, do not use them.
Bath dusting powders	Perfumed talc and other absorbent substances.	Impart a mild fragrance to the skin, and aid in drying body moisture.
Body oils	Vegetable and animal oils.	Replace natural oils removed by bathing.
Foam-bath salts	Sulfated compound related to coconut oil.	Drying to the skin.

Table 3—Deodorants and Antiperspirants

KIND	COMMON INGREDIENTS	USES
Deodorant powders	Mixture of powder base, zinc compounds, boric acid, astringents, and antiseptics.	Destroy the odor of sweat without stopping perspiration.
Deodorant creams	Vanishing cream base, antiseptic, and astringent.	Destroy the odor of sweat without stopping perspiration.
Deodorant solutions	Solution containing an antiseptic, astringent, alcohol, glycerine and water.	Used to mask odor. The skin should be dry before wearing clothing. The acidity of the aluminum chloride will destroy clothing.
Deodorant sticks	Waxes and an astringent (zinc sulphocarbolate).	Easy to apply. Destroy odor without stopping perspiration.
Deodorant or antiperspirant creams or liquids	Strong astringents, such as aluminum compounds.	Contract the sweat gland at the place of application. Prevent excessive sweating under the arms.

CREAMS   Many types of *creams* are available for use on the face and body. These are either stable oil/water or water/oil emulsions. (See Table 4.)

LOTIONS   *Lotions* are popular products used to a considerable extent in various kinds of cosmetic treatments. They are available as clear solutions or as suspensions, which may have insoluble sediments that collect at the bottom of the container. (See Table 5.)

POWDERS   *Powders* are also widely used. Since each kind of powder serves a particular purpose, the esthetician should be acquainted with their advantages.

Face powder consists of a powder base, mixed with a coloring agent (pigment) and a suitable fragrance. A good face powder for normal skin should possess the following characteristics:

1. *Slip*—It has a smooth feel to the skin. This quality is imparted by talc or zinc stearate (**STEE**-uh-rate). French or Italian talc of 200-mesh size is the best for face powders.
2. *Covering power*—It has an easy and even spread to cover skin shine, skin defects, and enlarged pores. Zinc oxide, kaolin, or titanium dioxide may be used.
3. *Adherency*—It has the ability to remain on the skin. Zinc or magnesium stearate is used for this purpose.
4. *Absorbency*—It retains the fragrance, distributes the color, and absorbs perspiration and sebaceous secretions. Precipitated chalk and magnesium carbonate are used for this purpose.
5. *Bloom*—It imparts a velvet-like appearance to the skin. Chalk is used for this purpose.
6. *Color and odor*—It has a pleasant odor and a uniform shade.

Toilet powder or *bath powder* is used after bathing and shaving to relieve irritation. Talcum is the most satisfactory base for a toilet powder, as it is not absorbent and is not affected by moisture.

Cream powder is composed of a vanishing cream base mixed with a face powder. Cream powder combines the properties of both in one application.

Cake powder has a three percent gum tragacanth (**TRAG**-uh-kanth) solution mixed with a face powder. The gum binds the substances together in a compact form.

Liquid powder may contain oil, zinc oxide, stearates, talc, fragrance, and colorants. It spreads quickly and uniformly over the skin, producing a nondrying thin film, or foundation, over which facial cosmetics can be applied.

Table 4—Creams

KIND	COMMON INGREDIENTS	USES
Cold cream	Beeswax, vegetable or mineral oil, borax (1%), water, and perfume.	Suitable for cleansing dry or normal skin.
Liquefying cleansing cream	Mineral oil, petrolatum, mineral wax, perfume, small amount of water.	May be used on oily skin. Melts quickly, does not penetrate the skin. Long use will dry the skin.
Vanishing cream	75% water, stearic acid, combined with a small amount of an alkali. Cocoa butter, lanolin, glycerine, and alcohol are also used.	Used before makeup is applied and as a hand cream. Leaves a protective film on the skin. Skin may become very dry from its use.
Emollient cream (also called tissue cream and lubricating cream)	Waxes, lanolin, vegetable fats and oils, fatty acids, alcohols, and some mineral oil products.	Slightly penetrates and softens the skin. Used for the lubrication of the skin during massage.
Hormone cream	Emollient cream base containing sex hormones.	For women of middle age. Prevents dryness and age lines.
Moisturizing cream	Emollient cream base containing moisturizing agents.	For dryness in aging skin due to lack of moisture and natural oil.
Massage cream	Cold cream base, lanolin or casein (protein found in cheese).	Used for massage of normal or slightly dry skin.
Astringent cream	Mild ointment base containing zinc oxide and an astringent.	Recommended to correct excessive oiliness and to close pores.
Acne cream	Boric acid, sulfur, zinc oxide, cade oil, camphor, benzoin, and salicylic acids.	Helps clear the skin of simple acne and other minor lesions. Should be soft enough to spread easily without irritating the skin.
Foundation cream	Vanishing cream base is modified by increasing the glycerine content.	Applied to the face after cleansing, to provide a suitable base for makeup.
Eye cream and throat cream	Lanolin, vegetable oils, waxes, and astringent substances.	Lubricate and soften fine lines; make them less conspicuous.
Suntan cream	Contains a cream or ointment base and various color pigments.	Used to give the appearance of a darker skin color.

Table 5—Lotions

KIND	COMMON INGREDIENTS	USES
Aromatic water	Essential oil (oil of rose, geranium, lavender, etc.) dissolved in distilled water with the aid of talc.	Imparts a cooling and fragrant effect to skin tonics and lotions.
Cleansing lotions	Alcohol or a sulfonated compound.	For oily skin.
Astringent lotions	Zinc, alum, boric or salicylic acid, in solution of water, glycerine, and alcohol.	For oily skin and large pores.
Skin freshener lotions	Witch hazel, camphor, boric acid, mild organic acids, perfume, and coloring.	Slightly astringent solution for dry skin.
Acne lotions	Precipitated sulfur, glycerine, spirits of camphor, and distilled water.	Used to sponge the skin where simple acne exists.
Witch hazel	A solution of alcohol and water containing the astringent from witch hazel bark.	Used as an astringent and cooling lotion.
Eye lotions	Boric acid, bicarbonate of soda, zinc sulfate and glycerine, witch hazel, or other herbs.	Used to soothe, cleanse, and brighten the eyes.
Calamine lotion	Suspension of prepared calamine and zinc oxide in glycerine, bentonite and lime water.	Used as a soothing application to irritated surfaces of the skin and as a protective lotion.
Hardy's lotion	Corrosive sublimate, alcohol, zinc sulfate, lead acetate, and water.	Prescribed by a physician to remove freckles.
Medicated lotions	Antiseptics, sulfur compounds, or other medicinal agents.	Prescribed by a physician for acne or other skin eruptions.
Sunburn preventive lotion	Dilute solution of methyl salicylate in alcohol, glycerine, and water.	Filters out most of the ultra-violet rays of the sun and produces a uniform tan.
Sunburn remedial lotion	Dilute solution of astringent or cooling agent (camphor) in alcohol, glycerine, and water.	Helps to heal a first degree burn.

CHEEK AND LIP COLORS   The selection and application of proper makeup colors are the primary requisites for improving the complexion and beautifying the facial features. The introduction of a personalized makeup service in salons has increased the demand and sale of these cosmetics.

Cheekcolor, or *rouge*, is available in the form of sticks, compact powders, pastes, creams, and liquids. The three basic color bases are blue-red, yellow-red, and true red. *Powder rouge* resembles the composition of a face powder except that a suitable color is added and the entire mixture is moistened and molded with the aid of a binder. It is usually used with oily skin types.

Paste rouge is composed of fats and waxes and generally has a red or brownish-red color base. It is usually used with dry skin types. *Cream rouge* usually has a petroleum base and contains lanolin, fats, and waxes. It is also normally used with dry skin types.

Liquid rouge is composed of a dye dissolved in a solution of water, glycerine, alcohol, and wax. It is usually used with normal skin types.

The blood, as seen through the skin, reveals the natural coloring in the cheeks. The color of blood is bright red. Depending on its nature, the skin may acquire a bluish, purplish or orangy tone. The exact shade of rouge should match the natural skin color tone. Always select rouge to match the skin color tone rather than as a color scheme to match a garment.

Lipcolor contains high melting ingredients to which is added either an insoluble pigment or a soluble bromoacid dye. The color of the inner mucous membrane of the lower lip is a guide to color selection. If the lipstick blends with the color of this inner membrane, it will give the most natural effect.

Eye makeup comes in the form of liner pencils, mascara, and eye shadows. *Eyebrow pencils* consist of a wax base to which suitable coloring is added. Pencils come in various shades, although shades of brown and black are most common. They are used to darken eyebrows and lashes.

Mascara is also used to darken the brows and lashes. It is available in the form of cakes, liquids, and creams. *Cream mascara* contains a pigment in a vanishing cream base. *Liquid mascara* usually consists of an alcoholic solution of resin, colored with a dye. It is also available as a suspension of pigment in a gum binder. A brush, usually built into the container, is used for application to the lashes. (See Table 6.)

Eyeshadow is usually a suspension of pigments in a fatty base. It is available in a wide variety of colors, normally chosen to match current fashion trends. Color choice in eyeshadow should consider the color and tone of the skin, hair, and eyes, as well as the dress and the occasion.

There is also a wide range of miscellaneous cosmetic products. *Grease paint* is a mixture of fats, petrolatum, and coloring agents and is used mostly for theatrical purposes. *Cake* or *pancake makeup* is available in a compressed or compact form. It contains a dehydrated cream into which is blended a distinct color. It is removed from the container with a moist applicator pad and spread over the face. As the water evaporates, a thin film of cream and color adheres to the face. ***Beauty clay*** is composed of substances, such as kaolin, bentonite, Fuller's earth, or colloidal clay—honey, glycerine, zinc oxide, casein, oils, magnesium carbonate, starch, gum, tragacanth, astringents, water, or milk are added, depending on the nature of the pack. Beauty clays, or packs, are often used as facial masks to exert a cleansing, softening, astringent, refreshing, or stimulating action on the skin.

Table 6—Mascara

COLOR OF EYES AND EYELASHES	SHADE OF MASCARA
Black eyelashes with dark brown or black eyes	Black
Black eyelashes with blue or grey eyes	Blue or black
Brown, golden, or reddish eyelashes with brown eyes	Dark brown
Blonde, reddish, or light brown eyelashes with green, grey, or hazel eyes	Brown or green

Natural and Organic Cosmetics

The words ***natural*** and ***organic*** have been used in describing organically grown foods; that is, foods that have not been treated by chemical means. When the terms natural or organic appear on a cosmetic label they can become confusing. ***Natural*** means a substance is derived from or produced by nature; however, some materials that exist in nature can be synthesized in the laboratory. ***Organic*** materials are those which have been derived from something living, such as plants or animals. The two terms may be used interchangeably in describing cosmetic products, although some natural products may not be organic.

For example, a face pack may be composed of clay, which is a natural substance, but it doesn't come from living materials. Some natural animal oils used in cosmetics are mink oil, turtle oil, and lanolin (from the oil contained in sheep's wool). Oils derived from plants or seeds include almond oil, coconut oil, olive oil, and cocoa butter. Many other oils and substances can be added to this list. Vitamins and proteins as well as fruit and vegetable substances have also been added to modern day cosmetics.

While these additions to cosmetics may provide some therapeutic benefits, they may not live up to the advertising claims made by some manufacturers. It is not possible to include a complete study of cosmetic science here, but the interested esthetician will be able to find a number of excellent books that provide in-depth studies of cosmetics formulations.

Laws Governing Cosmetics Manufacture

There is a tremendous variety of cosmetics on the market today, and more are being introduced daily. The sales of these products have soared into the billions of dollars each year. Because of the growing use of cosmetic preparations, there has been an increase in efforts to protect the consumer from harmful and impure ingredients that might be used in the manufacturing of cosmetic preparations. Congress passed the first Food, Drug, and Cosmetic Act in 1938. This act made the manufacturer of products responsible to see that cosmetics were safe to use and not misbranded in any way. The Fair Packaging and Labeling Act, enacted by Congress in 1966, provided for the identification of a product by the listing on the label of the name of the product, the place of business of the manufacturer, the net quantity of the contents of the container, and other pertinent information. The label must also list all ingredients used in the product. Such rules and regulations protect the consumer who may be allergic to certain ingredients and provide information that help the consumer to make a responsible buying decision.

The Food and Drug Administration (FDA) is the federal regulatory agency that is responsible for enforcing rules and regulations regarding products (foods, drugs, and cosmetics) for public consumption and is a division of the U. S. Department of Health and Human Services.

The FDA can take legal action against a manufacturer if the product can be shown to be dangerous or has falsely claimed properties. Although the FDA does conduct some testing of products, it is the responsibility of the manufacturer to prove the quality and safety of their products and to supply substantiation of their claims.

Cosmetic Labeling

To become more familiar with the contents of various cosmetics products on the market, the esthetician should make it a practice to carefully read the labels on all products used in the salon.

By law, cosmetics are defined as any article or substance that is intended to be used in any manner on the body to cleanse, beautify, and alter appearance. Cosmetics are used topically, and have no ability to alter bodily functions. They are not drugs.

As of January 1976, the FDA has required that all of the ingredients contained in cosmetic preparations be listed in descending order, according to the amount of the ingredient the product contains. It is necessary for the esthetician to read the labels, to understand the functions of all the ingredients, and to follow directions for use of all products he or she uses, in order to avoid adverse reactions or misuse of products. For example, the eyes and areas around the eyes are very sensitive, and even a mild astringent may cause irritation if allowed to seep into the eyes.

There are many different kinds of reactions to cosmetics ingredients. Some products may cause irritation, while others may cause an allergic reaction. An irritation is easier to deal with than is an allergy, which may require extensive testing to find the substance that is causing the reaction. Fragrances and some types of preservatives are among the most common causes of allergic reactions.

Reactions to preparations may be detected immediately after they have been applied to the skin, or the reaction may occur several days after the application of the preparation. Symptoms of irritation or allergic reaction may include inflammation of the skin, burning or itching sensations, blisters, blotches, or rashes. When an irritant or allergen has been used near the eyes, the eyes may swell, puff, or produce tears. All cosmetics and grooming products should be kept out of the reach of children.

Making Products for Salon Use

A number of reference materials list formulas for making products for home or salon. Many of these cosmetics are made from ingredients that are commonly found in the family kitchen. While these products may be satisfactory for home use, they will rarely be suitable for professional use in the salon. It is more professional and is safer to use products from a reputable manufacturer. Commercially manufactured cosmetics have been formulated by experienced chemists. The formulations have been tested for safety and are manufactured under strict quality controls. Strict sanitary procedures must be observed to prevent contamination of the products. In addition to the potential legal liabilities involved in using homemade products in the salon, such products would be made in such small quantities that the cost of materials and the time involved in making the products would be prohibitive and would end up being far more expensive than commercial products.

▶ **Caution:** If a client is allergic to some ingredients in a product and has an adverse reaction that requires medical treatment, the manufacturer of the product is responsible, and is insured to cover possible claims. If a product made in the salon is used, the salon is responsible. Malpractice insurance does not cover cosmetic products formulated in the salon unless specified in the salon's insurance policy. These are some of the reasons it is not a good policy to make and package cosmetics for use or resale in the salon.

Manufacturers are not responsible for products that have been purchased in bulk, repackaged by the salon in smaller containers and resold. If a problem arises, the manufacturer can claim that the product was not used under sanitary and proper conditions, since it was not sold in its original package.

Cosmetics Safety

Many cosmetics are called hypoallergenic. This is not a guarantee that the product is harmless. It typically means that the product does not contain a fragrance.

Acne cosmetica, that is, acne caused by cosmetics, is not, in most cases, as severe as *acne vulgaris*, even though comedones are present. Certain preparations used on the hair and skin are thought to cause acne cosmetica. A dermatologist may recommend discontinuing the use of all cosmetic preparations.

The best way to guard against allergic reactions to cosmetics is to pretest a small quantity of the product with a test patch on the arm. If there is any reaction within 24 hours, the preparation should not be used. If a cosmetic causes a reaction that appears to be serious, the product should be taken to a physician who can determine what has caused the problem and can treat the condition. The manufacturer of the product should be notified immediately.

Consumer Complaints

Consumer complaints should be sent to the manufacturer and a copy sent to the Food and Drug Administration, Division of Cosmetics Technology, Washington, D.C. 20204.

Help clients avoid misuse of cosmetics: Maintain strict sanitary procedures in salon practices. All containers should be closed when not in use to prevent contamination. Hands should be clean before applying cosmetics and all makeup applicators (brushes, sponges, etc.) should be sanitized before use.

Cosmetics, such as lipcolors and eye makeup should not be passed around like community property. To use someone else's is to take a chance that harmful bacteria will spread from one person to another. Saliva should never be used to moisten eye makeup or other cosmetics. When water is needed to moisten cosmetics, use only fresh, clean water.

Some cosmetics deteriorate more rapidly than others. Storing cosmetics in the refrigerator or a cool place will help keep them fresh longer. Discard outdated, rancid, or stale cosmetics.

Cosmetics manufacturers maintain laboratories for extensive testing of products before releasing them for distribution and sale. The Food, Drug, and Cosmetics Act prohibits the use of unsanitary materials, unsanitary practices, and the packaging or storage of cosmetics that may cause contamination of the products. The act also prohibits the use of harmful colors or dyes in cosmetics, especially in products used on or near the eyes.

Cosmetics Advertising

The advertising of cosmetics is regulated by the Federal Trade Commission to prevent false and misleading advertising in any medium. The FDA regulates and requires proof of any claims made for a product. The FDA has the authority to fine manufacturers and force them to withdraw from sale, any product that does not meet these criteria.

The Cosmetics, Toiletry, and Fragrance Association (CTFA), an industry group, has a program that assists the FDA in its efforts on behalf of the consumer. Cosmetic firms and manufacturers belonging to CTFA voluntarily register with the FDA. They list all their products and their ingredients, except for flavors and fragrances, which have been declared exempt because of their proprietary nature. The manufacturers must also provide the FDA with information about new products and must report any consumer complaints they may receive.

QUESTIONS

DISCUSSION AND REVIEW

INGREDIENT AND PRODUCT ANALYSIS

1. Why should an esthetician be familiar with ingredients in products he or she uses?
2. What is the difference between *active* and *inactive* when referring to ingredients?
3. Name some of the sources for ingredients used in cosmetic products.
4. Give examples of chemically synthesized ingredients.
5. Give examples of healing agents.
6. What is a humectant?
7. Algae is an ingredient found in what cosmetic products?
8. Define collagen.
9. List the classifications of cleansers.
10. Explain the meaning of natural when used in cosmetics.
11. Define organic.
12. Why must manufacturers list all ingredients used in products?
13. How long does it take to detect reactions from cosmetic preparations?
14. What does hypoallergenic mean?
15. What is acne cosmetica?
16. Where do you send consumer complaints regarding cosmetics?

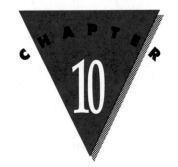

Nutrition and the Health of the Skin

LEARNING OBJECTIVES

After completing this chapter, you should be able to:

❶ Explain what nutrition is and why it is important to the health of the skin.

❷ List the three basic food groups and describe their importance.

❸ Explain calories and how diets can affect our skin.

❹ Explain why water is so important to the health of the skin.

❺ Discuss how hormones, medications and some of our habits can affect the skin.

❻ List different causes of some allergies.

❼ Discuss different vitamins used in cosmetics.

INTRODUCTION

Nutrition is the process by which food is assimilated and converted into tissue in living organisms. Nutritious foods promote the growth and repair of living organisms. Malnutrition is the state of being undernourished because of inadequate intake of essential nutrients. A person may be eating a lot of food, but if it is food that has been depleted of vitamins and other nutrients, the body will be poorly nourished. A well-balanced diet is the best insurance against vitamin and nutrient deficiency.

The skin is nourished by the blood and lymphatic systems of the body (the circulatory system). A major part of the circulatory system is devoted to the nourishment of the skin. Essential nutrients for growth, nourishment, and repair are circulated through the skin by the blood and lymph. Numerous networks of arteries, capillaries, and lymphatics throughout the subcutaneous skin layers supply nutrients to the glands and tissues of the skin. Good nutrition helps the skin to function in a normal way. A number of allergies, rashes, and other disorders of the skin are often the result of a poorly balanced diet.

Nutrition for Maintenance of Health

Metabolism is the name given to the sum total of all the body processes whereby the living body utilizes oxygen and food in building up and breaking down its tissues. Since the esthetician is dedicated to the maintenance and the enhancement of beauty and health, it is important that he or she knows that proper diet is reflected in the health of the skin, hair, and nails, and also contributes to a sense of well-being.

Numerous studies reveal that poor nutrition is directly responsible for slow development in many school children, and when they are given a nutritionally adequate diet, their personalities and abilities improve within a short time. A well-balanced diet is just as important for adults and is the best insurance against fatigue, listlessness, stress, anxiety, depression, poor disposition, and any number of diseases.

When the esthetician sees that the client's skin is obviously in poor condition due to inadequate nutrition, it may be helpful to discuss the benefits of a well-balanced diet to the health and appearance of the skin. Poor skin is often a symptom of a lack of vitamins. Excessively dry, oily, or blemished skin shows marked improvement when a healthful diet is combined with corrective facial treatments.

The Three Basic Food Groups

The three basic food groups are fats, carbohydrates, and proteins.

FATS Fats are important in the body because the sebaceous glands of the skin produce certain materials which help to lubricate the skin. The body also uses fat to help retain the heat it generates by depositing a layer of fat just under the skin over the greater part of the body. This layer of fat is generally thicker on females than on males of equal weight and becomes thicker as a person becomes overweight.

CARBOHYDRATES Carbohydrates include all the various types of sugars, starches, gums, pectins, and cellulose. The most important carbohydrate is glucose. It provides most of the body's energy. Glucose is stored in the muscles and liver as glycogen, which may be thought of as animal starch. Whenever the muscles are used, the glycogen stored in them is broken down to provide the energy needed for muscular work.

PROTEINS Proteins have been used in cosmetics since ancient times. Collagen (protein forming the chief constituent of connective tissue and bone) is one of the major sources of protein used in cosmetics. Proteins are the essential staff of life. No living thing exists without protein materials in its structure. The proteins are composed of various combinations of amino acids, which are the chief components of protein. Some of these amino acids are capable of being produced by the body from simpler materials, but others seem to be beyond the body's ability to manufacture. These are referred to as essential amino acids, which must be acquired from food.

It is not possible to do without essential amino acids, because the various proteins of the body require quantities of them. Without essential amino acids in the diet, the body would not be able to manufacture these proteins. Since the proteins are a part of our living processes, the body would not be able to exist without a supply of essential amino acids.

Protein Deficiency—When the body does not get the protein it requires, a child's growth can be retarded and an adult will lose weight. A few of the consequences of protein deficiency are: anemia, loss of resistance to infection, and impairment of internal and external organs.

Summary—Proteins are made from millions of small residues called amino acids (approximately 20 types). The amino acids are joined lengthwise by peptide or end bonds to form long chains of polypeptides (Fig. 10.1). Polypeptide chains may be:

1. Simple spiral or round chains. These are easily digested, releasing contained amino acids.
2. Complex chains bound together by cystine or sulfur-cross bonds.

Proteins may consist of:

1. Grade A type—(fish, meat, eggs, milk, etc.) that contain high levels of sulfur amino acids (cystine and cysteine).
2. Grade B type—(beans, peas, cereals, nuts, etc.) that contain low level of sulfur amino acids.

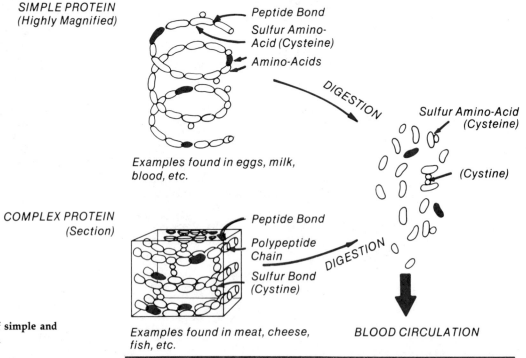

SIMPLE PROTEIN
(Highly Magnified)

— Peptide Bond
Sulfur Amino-Acid (Cysteine)
Amino-Acids

DIGESTION

Sulfur Amino-Acid
(Cysteine)

Examples found in eggs, milk, blood, etc.

(Cystine)

COMPLEX PROTEIN
(Section)

— Peptide Bond
Polypeptide Chain
Sulfur Bond (Cystine)

DIGESTION

10.1—The structure of simple and complex protein

Examples found in meat, cheese, fish, etc.

BLOOD CIRCULATION

Calories

It may seem somewhat removed from the study of skin care to go into the matter of calories and diet. However, health is part of the personal care picture, so a few simple facts about diet and health are important to understand the chemistry of the body.

From the dietary point of view, protein does not give as many calories of energy when it is burned as does an equal weight of fat. However, it is far more important to the body's efficiency than fat or carbohydrates. Proteins are the materials that the body uses to build tissue in the first place and to replace and repair tissue as it is "worn out" or injured.

It takes a certain amount of energy to keep us alive and healthy in our daily activities. The amount of energy required depends on the kind of work we do, our age, sex, height, and weight. This energy is measured in terms of calories, which are units of heat. A certain food is said to contain a given number of calories per ounce. This means that if an ounce of this food were burned in a special apparatus that could measure the heat energy released, it would be found to be so many calories.

We therefore use this term in describing the available energy from our various food materials. *All foods contribute calories to the total*. However, some foods contribute more than others per ounce. Butter, being almost all fat, is said to be very fattening, but it is no more fattening than an amount of carbohydrate or protein having the same caloric content. In reducing, it is not (scientifically at least) what you eat so much as it is *how much* you eat, figured on a caloric basis. It is the grand total of calories from all forms of food, measured against the grand total of energy the body uses up, that determines whether the dieter will gain, lose, or maintain normal weight.

DIETING AND ITS EFFECTS ON THE SKIN

When we cut our food intake for the purpose of losing weight, we also cut down on the intake of minerals and vitamins that are in foods. Since vitamins are essential to the process of burning up and getting rid of excess fat, it is obvious that enough must be taken in to be certain that we have a sufficient supply of energy on hand for the metabolic job of getting rid of the fat. At the same time, it is necessary to keep the protein content up, because, apart from trying to get rid of fat, the body must keep its muscles, blood, bones, and essential structures in good repair, and only protein can do this.

CRASH DIETS

When weight is reduced too fast, the skin will sag and wrinkle rather than gradually return to its former condition. Crash diets should not be undertaken without the supervision of a physician, as the entire body, and especially the skin, will suffer from lack of proper nourishment.

Enzymes, Vitamins, and Oxidation

Everyone has heard about vitamins, and most people have taken one or more at various times, but they know little about their place in body chemistry. Even fewer people have heard of or know about enzymes. Since their functions are essential to life and health and, therefore, to the underlying condition of the skin, we should consider their roles in keeping the skin, as well as the entire body, healthy.

When food is utilized in the body, the energy is extracted from it. This is accomplished by a breakdown of complex molecules into simpler ones, thus releasing the energy required to hold the large, complex molecules

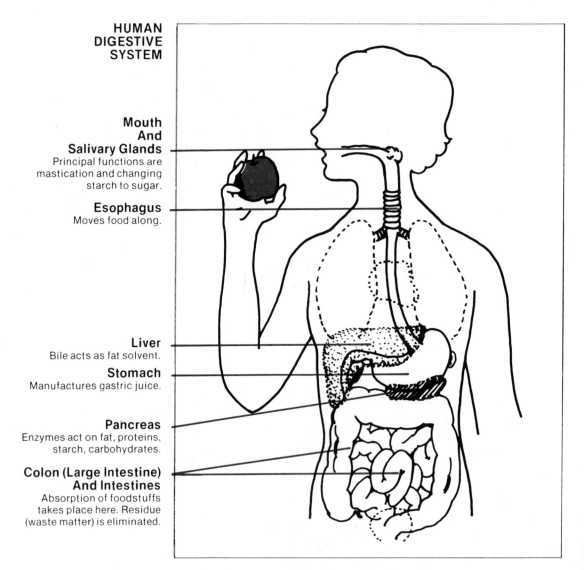

HUMAN DIGESTIVE SYSTEM

Mouth And Salivary Glands
Principal functions are mastication and changing starch to sugar.

Esophagus
Moves food along.

Liver
Bile acts as fat solvent.

Stomach
Manufactures gastric juice.

Pancreas
Enzymes act on fat, proteins, starch, carbohydrates.

Colon (Large Intestine) And Intestines
Absorption of foodstuffs takes place here. Residue (waste matter) is eliminated.

10.2—Human digestive system

together. How this is accomplished need not concern us here, as it is a very complicated process. However, it is sufficient for us to know that a great many substances present in our food finally end up as carbon dioxide and water, of which the body disposes. But, it is in this breaking up of larger molecules into smaller ones that vitamins and enzymes play their roles (Fig. 10.2).

ENZYMES Enzymes are substances that can bring about reactions that would not otherwise occur or that can speed up reactions that normally are very slow. They are sometimes called biological catalysts. They are all protein in nature; the protein being a special one for each different kind of enzyme. But most of them, or perhaps all of them, contain another substance, which is very small in size and weight. These additional materials are the ones that determine what kind of job the enzyme can do. Some enzymes will attack proteins and break them down into simpler compounds. Other enzymes will work on these broken down products and simplify them further, right down to the amino-acid stage. By means of this chopping up of materials bit by bit, they are finally reduced into carbon dioxide and water or into some other end product that the body no longer needs, which is then excreted.

The vitamins and some of the minerals that are important to our health are the small and relatively simple structures, which give the whole protein-vitamin complex its special importance. Since the breakdown of the foodstuffs can only be done by the hundreds of different enzymes, and since these enzymes are comprised, in part, of those relatively simple structures which we call vitamins, it should be clear why they are so essential to life and health.

Nourishment of the Skin

The skin is nourished by nutrients in the bloodstream. Therefore, a well-balanced diet is a form of health insurance for the skin. The skin must be kept healthy by proper cleansing, stimulation, moisturizing (when needed), and protection from the harmful effects of the environment. The skin also benefits from adequate, daily intake of water and other healthful liquids.

Nutrition Labeling and Information

Nutrition information has been added to food labels by many food producers. In addition to the name of the product, weight, and ingredients, the labels list the nutritional value of the food. The label tells the size of a serving, such as one cup, and how many servings are in the package or container. Calories are listed, as are the amounts in grams of protein, fat, and carbohydrates. Vitamins are listed in the same order on all labels to make it easier for the consumer to compare labels when shopping. Labels also show the percentage of the U.S. recommended daily allowances (U.S. RDA).

NUTRITION ESSENTIALS TO SKIN HEALTH

The nutritional needs of an individual depend on such factors as age, physical build, and amount of activity. There is such a great variety of foods on the market today that the main concern may be in knowing how to select the most nutritious foods that supply the daily requirements of individuals (Fig. 10.3). There are four broad food groups from which to select a balanced diet. These four groups are:

1. Milk and dairy products
2. Meat and alternatives, such as beans, peas, or nuts
3. Vegetables and fruit
4. Bread and grain

Dairy Group

Milk is good for everyone and should be included in the daily diet, unless a physician recommends the elimination of milk from the diet. The following are recommended daily amounts:

Children—2 to 3 cups
Teenagers—4 or more cups
Adults—2 or more cups

Other dairy products include yogurt, cheese, and butter.

Meat and Protein Alternatives Group

Good sources of protein are beef, veal, pork, lamb, organ meats, fish, poultry, and alternatives, such as nuts, peas, beans, and eggs. Two or more daily servings are recommended.

Vegetable-Fruit Group

Fruits and vegetables are important sources of Vitamins C and A. Four or more servings of fruits and vegetables, raw or cooked, should be eaten every day.

Bread-Cereal Group

Whole grain cereal is best. Size of serving may vary with the individual's age, activities, and body build. The main consideration is to provide the body with a well-balanced diet for maximum nutrition and maintenance of health. Four or more daily servings are recommended.

The nutrition chart on pages 152–155 shows the recommended daily allowance (RDA) of vitamins and minerals. Persons on a special diet must have a physician recommend foods to include and foods to avoid.

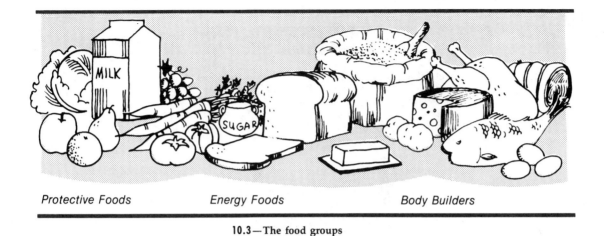

Protective Foods   Energy Foods   Body Builders

10.3—The food groups

Water—An Essential to Life

When studying the need for well-balanced meals, we should remember that water is essential to life. A person may go without food for a long period of time but only a few days without water or other fluids. Water makes up one-half to two-thirds of the human body. Water aids digestion, carries waste materials from the body, helps form body fluids, sustains the health of all cells, helps regulate the temperature of the body (perspiration) and much, much more. Although water or liquid is taken into the body in soups, juices, and beverages, these should not be totally substituted for water. Since water is essential to the healthful functioning of the body, it is easy to see why drinking enough water helps keep the skin healthy and attractive.

Nutrition and the Prevention of Disease

Scientists are constantly searching for ways to control and cure cardio-vascular disease, diabetes, cancer, and other diseases that may be diet related. Obesity (being overweight) is associated with some of these serious diseases. Good nutrition is also vital to mental health. The brain is a physical organ that controls our senses, thoughts, and emotions, and mental health depends on proper body chemistry for the brain to function properly. A chemical imbalance can lead to disturbed thoughts, extreme anxiety, delusions, and other symptoms of mental illness.

In many cases, persons exhibiting these symptoms have been found to be suffering from malnutrition. When nutritional therapy was applied, there was a noticeable improvement and in some cases a complete restoration of mental health.

Vitamin Information Chart—Courtesy of *Body Forum Magazine*

VITAMIN	NAME	NEED IN HUMAN NUTRITION	U.S. RDA	DEFICIENCY DISEASE
A	Retinol	Essential for growth and maintenance of body tissue, strong bones and teeth, and good eyesight. (Helps to form and maintain healthy function of eyes, skin, hair, teeth, gums, various glands, and mucous membranes. Also involved in fat metabolism.)	5,000 I.U., for adults and children four or more years of age, except pregnant and lactating women, for whom the RDA is 8,000 I.U.	Xerophthalmia; night blindness
B Complex	Thiamine (B$_1$)	Essential for utilization of carbohydrates in energy production. Promotes healthy central nervous system and mental attitude, and improvement of food assimilation and digestion.	1.5 mg	Beriberi
B Complex	Riboflavin (B$_2$)	Essential for good vision and healthy skin, nails, and hair. Functions with other substances to breakdown and utilize carbohydrates, fats, and proteins.	1.7 mg	Ariboflavinosis— lesions of the mouth, lips, skin, genitalia
B Complex	Niacin (Niacinamide or Nicotinic Acid)	Essential for healthy brain functions, nervous system, and skin. Important in tissue respiration. Essential for synthesis of sex hormones.	20 mg	Pellagra
B Complex	Cobalamin, Cyanocobalamin (B$_{12}$)	Essential for maintenance of healthy nervous system, and for utilization of carbohydrates, fats, and proteins.	6 mcg	Pernicious anemia; brain damage
B Complex	Para-Aminobenzoic Acid (PABA)	Helps to form folic acid and to utilize proteins.	Not established	Depression; headache; eczema
B Complex	Folacin or Folic Acid	Essential for division of body cells, for production of nucleic acids (RNA and DNA), and for utilization of sugar amino acids.	0.4 mg (400 mcg)	Anemia
B Complex	Inositol	Combines with choline to form lecithin, which in turn metabolizes fats and cholesterol. Important for healthy hair.	Not established	Eczema
B Complex	Choline	Combines with inositol to form lecithin, which in turn metabolizes fat and cholesterol. Essential for healthy liver and kidneys.	Not established	Kidney damage
B Complex	Pantothenic Acid; Panthenol; Calcium Pantothenate	Essential for conversion of fat and sugar to energy, for use of PABA and choline, and vital to proper function of adrenal glands.	10 mg	Hypoglycemia; other blood disorders; duodenal ulcers; skin disorders

SUBCLINICAL SYMPTOMS	NATURAL/FOOD SOURCES	ANTAGONISTS	TOXICITY LEVEL
Eyes—Inability to adjust to darkness; dry and inflamed eyeball; sties. Face and/or skin blemishes—rough, dry, prematurely aged skin. General—Loss of smell; loss of appetite; frequent fatigue; diarrhea.	Fish liver oil; carrots; green and yellow vegetables; liver; whole milk and dairy products; egg yolk; yellow fruits	Excessive consumption of alcoholic beverages; mineral oil; cortisone (and other drugs); polyunsaturated fatty acids with carotene (unless antioxidants are present)	More than 50,000 I.U. daily could produce some toxic effects.
Muscles—Cramps; general weakness; tenderness in calf. General—Loss of appetite; fatigue; loss of weight; burning sensation in soles of feet	Brewer's yeast; wheat germ; bran; liver	Cooking heat, air, water; caffeine; food processing techniques; sulfa drugs; sleeping pills; estrogen; alcohol	No known toxic effects
Eyes—Burning sensation; bloodshot	Milk; liver; enriched cereals; brewer's yeast; leafy green vegetables; fish; eggs	Water; cooking; sunlight; food processing techniques; sulfa drugs; sleeping pills; estrogen; alcohol	No known toxic effects
Nervous system—Hostility; suspicion; insomnia; loss of memory; irritability; anxiety. General—Abdominal pain; burning sensation in tongue; dry and scaly patches of skin	Liver; brewer's yeast; kidney; wheat germ; whole grains; fish eggs; lean meat; nuts	Water; food processing techniques; sulfa drugs; sleeping pills; estrogen; alcohol	Nontoxic, except some side effects may result from more than 100 mg daily.
Nervousness; heart palpitations; inflamed tongue	Liver; kidney; milk and dairy products; some types of meat	Water; sunlight; acids, alkalis; food processing techniques; sulfa drugs; sleeping pills; estrogen; alcohol	No known toxic effects
Fatigue; irritability; constipation; nervousness; graying hair	Liver; kidney; whole grains	Water; food processing techniques; sulfa drugs; sleeping pills; estrogen; alcohol	No known toxic effects
Gastrointestinal disorders	Liver; Tortula yeast; green vegetables	Water; food processing techniques; sulfa drugs; sleeping pills; estrogen; alcohol; sunlight	No known toxic effects
Loss of hair; constipation	Liver; brewer's yeast; whole grains; wheat germ; unrefined molasses; corn; citrus fruits	Water; food processing techniques; sulfa drugs; sleeping pills; estrogen; alcohol	No known toxic effects
Deteriorating kidneys; abnormally high blood pressure	Brewer's yeast; liver; kidney; wheat germ; egg yolk	Water; food processing techniques; sulfa drugs; sleeping pills; estrogen; alcohol	No known toxic effects
Restlessness; vomiting; abdominal pains; muscle cramps; burning sensation in feet	Whole grains; wheat germ; bran; kidney; liver; heart; green vegetables; brewer's yeast	Heat; cooking; canning; caffeine; food processing techniques; sulfa drugs; sleeping pills; estrogen; alcohol	No known toxic effects

Vitamin Information Chart—**Courtesy of** *Body Forum Magazine* (Continued)

VITAMIN	NAME	NEED IN HUMAN NUTRITION	U.S. RDA	DEFICIENCY DISEASE
B Complex	Pyridoxine (B₆)	Essential for metabolism of amino acids. Aids in blood building, utilization of fats, and normal functioning of brain, nervous system, and muscles.	2 mg	Anemia
B Complex	Biotin (also called Coenzyme R or Vitamin H)	Essential for utilization of proteins, carbohydrates, and fats, and for healthy hair and skin. Aids in the maintenance of the thyroid and adrenal glands, reproductive tract, and the nervous system.	0.3 mg (300 mcg)	Dermatitis; depression; anemia; anorexia
C	Ascorbic Acid	Principal function is to maintain collagen, which is necessary for the connective tissue that holds body cells together. It is involved in wound healing, the formation of red blood cells, and believed to be involved in disease resistance.	60 mg	Scurvy
D	Calciferol	Essential for utilization of calcium and phosphorus. Necessary for strong teeth and bones.	400 I.U.	Rickets; osteomalacia; senile osteoporosis
E	Tocopherol	Helps to protect oxidation of Vitamin A, selenium, two sulphur amino acids, polyunsaturated fatty acids, and some Vitamin C.	30 I.U.	Kidney and liver damage; anemia
K	Menadione	Essential for formation of prothrombin, a blood clotting chemical. Important to proper liver function and longevity.	Not established	Celiac disease; sprue; colitis; hemorrhage
P	Bioflavonoids	Essential for proper use of Vitamin C.	Not established	With Vitamin C: rheumatism; rheumatic fever

SUBCLINICAL SYMPTOMS	NATURAL/FOOD SOURCES	ANTAGONISTS	TOXICITY LEVEL
Loss of hair; water retention during pregnancy; nervous system disorder; cracks around mouth and eyes; increase in urination	Brewer's yeast; wheat bran; rice bran; wheat germ; liver; kidney; heart; blackstrap molasses; milk; eggs; cabbage; beef	Canning; long storage; roasting or stewing (meat); water; food processing techniques; sulfa drugs; sleeping pills; estrogen; alcohol	No known toxic effects
Mental depression; dry, peeling skin; muscular pains; poor appetite; lack of energy	Brewer's yeast; egg yolk; liver; milk; kidney	Water; food processing techniques; sulfa drugs; sleeping pills; estrogen; alcohol	No known toxic effects
Slow wound healing; loss of appetite; bleeding gums; muscular weakness; shortness of breath	Fresh fruits and vegetables	Heat; light; oxygen; water. Much Vitamin C is destroyed when vegetables are overwashed or cooked, and when fruit is overwashed.	No known toxic effect. Although not proven, excessive use of Vitamin C has been associated with kidney stones in some persons, and has a diuretic and/or laxative effect on some people.
Weakening bones, including teeth; weakening muscles	Fish liver oils; milk and dairy products; sunlight	Mineral oil	25,000 I.U. daily over a long period of time could produce a toxic effect in adults.
Muscle degeneration; enlarged prostate; red blood cell damage	Vegetable oils; whole raw seeds and nuts; soybeans	Food processing techniques; heat; freezing temperatures; oxygen; iron; mineral oil.	Nontoxic, except for persons with high blood pressure or chronic rheumatic heart disease
Diarrhea; bleeding nose	Yogurt; egg yolk; safflower oil; fish liver oils; kelp; alfalfa; leafy green vegetables	Aspirin; x-rays and radiation; frozen foods; industrial air pollution	Natural Vitamin K is considered nontoxic but more than 500 mcg per day of synthetic Vitamin K is not recommended.
High tendency to bleed easily	White pigments of citrus fruits; rutin	Same as for Vitamin C	No known toxic effects

Sources for the chart were: Raj Chopra, Private Formulations, Hempstead, N.Y.; *Dictionary of Nutrition,* by Richard Ashley and Heidi Duggal; *Remington's Pharmaceutical Sciences,* Managing Editor John E. Hoover; *Nutrition Almanac,* Nutrition Search, Inc.

SKIN — AN INDICATOR OF HEALTH

The professional skin care specialist is interested in the client's total health, but the main concern in the study of nutrition is its effect on the skin.

We know that the skin derives its nourishment from the bloodstream and that a well-balanced diet provides the nutrients that are essential to keeping the skin healthy and attractive. The skin reveals a lot about what the body may be lacking in essential nutrients. For example, a lack of Vitamin C over a period of time can cause *scurvy* (**SKUR**-vee), a disease that produces ugly skin lesions. *Pellagra* (pe-**LAG**-ruh) is the result of a severe Vitamin B deficiency that shows in a characteristic skin rash that can cause scarring. Other deficiencies that have a nutritional origin are such skin disorders as acne, eczema, psoriasis, and dermatitis (a skin inflammation).

Changes in the color of the skin can also be an indication of the body's nutritional state. This is due to the change in the color of the blood beneath the surface of the skin. A pale, dry skin may indicate anemia. Severe protein and calorie deficiency in children causes characteristic changes in skin and hair color. *Jaundice* (**JAWN**-dis) is characterized by a yellowish cast to the skin.

The skin is an indicator of any number of serious and minor internal problems. Liver disease will cause the skin to have a yellowish cast and the palms of the hands may be red. Yellow or white fatty papules around the eyes may indicate an elevated cholesterol level. High cholesterol levels can indicate heart trouble. Any persistent itching, change in color of the skin, or any type of growth that appears on the skin should be checked by a dermatologist without delay.

The Use of Sex Hormones on the Skin

A hormone secretion is produced in and by any one of the endocrine glands, such as the pituitary, adrenals, thyroid, etc. Hormones are carried by the bloodstream and body fluids to other parts of the body where they have specific functions.

Hormone creams may contain estrogen (female sex hormones) and/or progesterone (a female hormone active in preparing the uterus to receive a fertilized ovum). Cosmetic manufacturers usually advertise these creams as being especially beneficial to aging skin.

Hormones added to cosmetics may be beneficial, but they do not miraculously erase wrinkles, restore an aging skin to youthful bloom, or prevent youthful skin from going through the natural processes of aging as the body matures. Sex hormones in cosmetics may not be added in excessive amounts, and the amounts must appear on the label of the cosmetic container.

Habits That May Be Harmful to the Skin

Studies have shown that excessive use of tobacco, alcohol, or drugs can contribute to premature aging of the skin. Nicotine in tobacco affects the blood vessels and slows circulation. Alcohol dilates the blood vessels, but light intake of alcoholic beverages, especially wine, may not be harmful to the skin. It is the heavy, regular intake of alcohol that may cause blood vessels to dilate until tiny vessels burst in the white of the eyeball and beneath the skin. Excessive alcohol intake can cause the eyes to become puffy and can contribute to dehydrated, sagging skin.

Medication That May Affect the Skin

Allergies may be caused by substances other than food. Some people have a reaction to cosmetics, grooming products (such as hair spray and mouthwash), and various medications.

Anxiety, stress, emotional problems, hypertension, and nervousness are often the underlying causes of some types of skin reactions. Drugs given to alleviate these conditions may have side effects. Reddish eruptions may appear on the skin when a person has taken enough of a particular medication to become sensitized. Hives and rashes may be produced in some persons by the following medications: aspirin, penicillin, birth control pills, codeine, diet pills, barbiturates, and laxatives.

There are many other drugs and preparations that may cause skin reactions.

EFFECTS OF DRUGS ON SKIN   Tranquilizers, barbiturates, amphetamines, marijuana, heroin, or drugs of this type all affect the skin. The health of the individual and the amount or frequency of the ingestion of the substance will be factors in the extent of damage done to the skin. Drugs can interfere with the normal functioning of the body's internal organs and the brain. Allergies and rashes are not uncommon. The client who obviously smokes too much, drinks too much alcohol, or uses drugs should be made aware that facial treatments or makeup will not erase the damage these habits may do to the health and appearance of the skin.

Nutrition Is Important to Mothers and Infants

Women who have been accustomed to having facials and other beauty services will usually continue these throughout pregnancy. Modern women tend to remain active during pregnancy, and diet is especially important in maintaining the health of the mother and the unborn infant.

The mother-to-be can expect to gain some weight and her diet should therefore be supervised by a physician. Malnourished mothers may produce children with birth defects or deficiency-related diseases. Any changes in the skin during pregnancy should be brought to the attention of the client who, in turn, should have the condition checked by a physician.

Food Allergies

Persons who are allergic to certain foods exhibit such symptoms as tearing eyes, nausea, headaches, hives, diarrhea, constipation, or upset stomach, etc. Because allergy symptoms vary, it is difficult to determine the exact cause of the reaction. When an allergy is suspected, it is best to see an allergist (a specialist in the diagnosis and treatment of allergies).

An allergy is defined as a condition of sensitivity in an individual to a substance that, in similar amounts, is harmless to the great majority of people. Foods that most frequently cause allergy symptoms are milk, eggs, nuts, grains (such as wheat and corn), chocolate, fish, shellfish, and some fruits and vegetables.

Vitamins in Cosmetics

There is a great deal of controversy regarding the claims that the use of vitamins in cosmetic preparations has beneficial effects. Various vitamins are included in skin creams and lotions and the vitamins in these preparations may be absorbed to some extent by the skin. Most authorities agree that vitamins taken into the body by way of food is the best way to nourish the skin. However, vitamins in preparations applied to the skin may have a healing and softening effect.

Vitamin A is used in lubricating creams and lotions and is said to aid in softening the skin.

Vitamin E is used in deodorants, hair preparations, and in skin creams and lotions. Vitamin E is claimed to have healing and softening properties.

Vitamin D is also alleged to have skin healing properties.

Vitamin C (ascorbic acid) is used as a preservative and is used in cosmetic preparations.

Other vitamins are said to have special properties that are beneficial when applied to the surface of the skin.

Foods known for certain high vitamin content are often applied to the face in the form of packs and masks.

Metrics and Nutrition Information

Nutrition labeling is a program that has been developed by the Food and Drug Administration to provide consumers with information that may be helpful in the following ways:

1. To plan more nutritious and well-balanced meals
2. To get more nutrition for your food dollar by comparing the nutrition values of different brands
3. To select foods needed for special diets as recommended by physicians
4. To help you compare the calorie content in foods
5. To compare new foods to those already on the market

Nutrition labels show amounts in grams rather than ounces, because grams are a smaller unit of measurement. Many food components are in such small amounts that the use of grams (g), milligrams (mg), and micrograms (mcg) help to simplify the reading of labels. For example:

1 pound—454 g

1 ounce—28 g

1 gram—1,000 mg

1 milligram—1,000 mcg

Metrics and Cosmetics

Many manufacturers of drugs, cosmetics, food products, and other consumer goods are using metric terms on product labels. The metric system is used internationally. In the United States, legislation and school board regulations may make it mandatory for all school children to learn the metric system of weights and measures. *SI* is the symbol for The International System of Units.

Learning the metric system is valuable to the esthetician, because today many products are imported that have instructions written in metrics. The following charts will help you to understand and use the metric system. There are other more extensive charts and booklets available to serve as guides to learning the metric system.

There are only seven basic units for different types of measurement:

1. The unit of length is *meter*.
2. The unit of mass is *kilogram*.
3. The unit of temperature is *kelvin*.
4. The unit of time is *second*.
5. The unit of electric current is *ampere*.
6. The unit of light intensity is *candela*.
7. The unit of amount of substance is *mole*.

All other SI (International System of Units) are derived from these seven units.

Metric Conversion Factors

Approximate Conversions to Metric Measures

	SYMBOL	WHEN YOU KNOW	MULTIPLY BY	TO FIND	SYMBOL
Length	in	inches	2.5	centimeters	cm
	ft	feet	30	centimeters	cm
	yd	yard	0.9	meters	m
	mi	miles	1.6	kilometers	km
Area	in²	square inches	6.5	square centimeters	cm²
	ft²	square feet	0.09	square meters	m²
	yd²	square yards	.08	square meters	m²
	mi²	square miles	2	square kilometers	km²
	a	acres	0.4	hectares	ha
Mass (Weight)	oz	ounces	28	grams	g
	lb	pounds	0.45	kilograms	kg
		short tons (2,000 lb)	0.9	metric tons	t
Volume	tsp	teaspoons	5	milliliters	mL
	Tbsp	tablespoons	15	milliliters	mL
	in³	cubic inches	16	milliliters	mL
	fl oz	fluid ounces	30	milliliters	mL
	c	cups	0.24	liters	L
	pt	pints	0.47	liters	L
	qt	quarts	0.95	liters	L
	gal	gallons	3.8	liters	L
	ft³	cubic feet	0.03	cubic meters	m³
	yd³	cubic yards	0.76	cubic meters	m³
Temperature (Exact)	°F	degrees Fahrenheit	5/9 (after subtracting 32)	degrees Celsius	°C

ADDITIONAL INFORMATION ABOUT TEASPOON AND TABLESPOON MEASUREMENTS

60 drops = 1 teaspoon (5 ml)
3 teaspoons = 1 tablespoon (15 ml)
2 tablespoons = 1 fluid ounce (30 ml)
8 fluid ounces = 1 cup = 16 tablespoons (0.24 l)
2 cups = 1 pint = 16 fluid ounces (0.47 l)
2 pints = 1 quart = 32 fluid ounces (0.95 l)

1/8 cup = 2 tablespoons = 1 fluid ounce = 6 teaspoons (30 ml)
1/4 cup = 4 tablespoons = 2 fluid ounces (60 ml)
3/8 cup = 6 tablespoons = 3 fluid ounces (90 ml)
1/2 cup = 8 tablespoons = 4 fluid ounces (120 ml)
3/5 cup = 10 tablespoons = 5 fluid ounces (150 ml)
3/4 cup = 12 tablespoons = 6 fluid ounces (180 ml)
7/8 cup = 14 tablespoons = 7 fluid ounces (210 ml)
1 cup = 16 tablespoons = 8 fluid ounces (0.24 l)

Approximate Conversions From Metric Measures

	SYMBOL	WHEN YOU KNOW	MULTIPLY BY	TO FIND	SYMBOL
Length	mm	millimeters	0.04	inches	in
	cm	centimeters	0.4	inches	in
	m	meters	3.3	feet	ft
	m	meters	1.1	yards	yd
	km	kilometers	0.6	miles	mi
Area	cm²	square centimeters	0.16	square inches	in²
	m²	square meters	1.2	square yards	yd²
	km²	square kilometers	0.4	square miles	mi²
	ha	hectares (10,000 m²)	2.5	acres	a
Mass (Weight)	g	grams	0.035	ounces	oz
	kg	kilograms	2.2	pounds	lb
	t	metric tons (1,000 kg)	1.1	short tons	
Volume	mL	milliliters	0.03	fluid ounces	fl oz
	mL	milliliters	0.06	cubic inches	in³
	L	liters	2.1	pints	pt
	L	liters	1.06	quarts	qt
	L	liters	0.26	gallons	gal
	m³	cubic meters	35	cubic feet	ft³
	m³	cubic meters	1.3	cubic yards	yd³
Temperature (Exact)	°C	degrees Celsius	9/5 (then add 32)	degrees Fahrenheit	°F

QUESTIONS   DISCUSSION AND REVIEW

NUTRITION AND THE HEALTH OF THE SKIN

1. What is nutrition?
2. What are the three basic food groups?
3. Which food group is the most important to the body and why?
4. Why are crash diets bad for the skin?
5. Define enzymes.
6. How is water important to our body?
7. Can a lack of vitamins show in the skin's condition and if so, how?
8. List some habits that may be harmful to the skin and tell why.
9. List some of the medications that can cause hives and rashes.
10. What are some symptoms that people can experience from food allergies?
11. Who would you recommend your client to if you suspected that their problem was due to an allergy?
12. List the foods that most frequently cause allergy symptoms.
13. Which vitamin is said to have healing and softening properties?

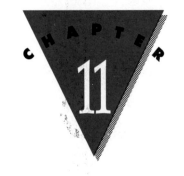

Client Consultation and Skin Analysis

LEARNING OBJECTIVES *After completing this chapter, you should be able to:*

❶ Explain the importance of the first impression of the professional and the salon.

❷ Discuss the importance of the consultation and some questions to ask during a consultation.

❸ Explain how to analyze the different skin types and which treatment is best for each.

❹ Discuss the importance of a skin care regimen for home care.

INTRODUCTION

There are many reasons why a person may seek treatment in a skin care salon. Usually the client has become conscious of the value of skin care treatments and feels it will be helpful in correcting his or her skin problems. Often a client will feel that facial treatments will be beneficial in maintaining the health and attractiveness of the skin. A growing number of people feel that a clear, healthy skin is an asset to their professional appearance and to their self esteem. In recent years, skin care has received a great deal of favorable press coverage and people are often influenced by this type of advertising. Often a potential client's interest is stimulated by a satisfied friend or acquaintance who is having skin treatments. In any case, good advertising of any kind means good business for the salon and a satisfied client is still the best means of advertising.

The Client's First Impression of the Salon

The initial impression the client has of the salon and of the people employed in the salon, may well determine if he or she will return for future services, or recommend the salon to others. Good impressions help you to build your clientele, and if you don't make a good first impression, you may not have another opportunity to do so.

The first contact with the client is often by way of the telephone. The person answering the telephone must have a pleasant voice and speak in a professional manner. He or she must also be knowledgeable about the salon's services, but it is vitally important that questions dealing with the actual skin treatment be answered only by the esthetician during the consultation. The receptionist who greets people as they enter the salon for information or by appointment must project professionalism in manner, voice, and appearance.

THE PROFESSIONAL ATMOSPHERE OF THE SALON

A professional atmosphere and an air of quiet efficiency, should be maintained in the salon at all times. Every detail should be in order before the arrival of the client. The person who receives the client should be immaculately groomed in the appropriate (career apparel) uniform or lab coat, and he or she should project a confident, friendly manner.

It is important to gain the client's trust and confidence from the moment he or she steps into the salon. The client should never be kept waiting beyond the appointed time and should always be properly introduced to the esthetician who will be performing the services for the client. Professional projection on the part of the receptionist and the esthetician enhances the status of, and builds the image of, the entire beauty culture industry.

THE PHYSICAL APPEARANCE OF THE SALON

Whether the salon is small or of modest appointments, or whether it reflects the utmost in luxury, it should be immaculately clean and uncluttered. The decor should be pleasant and furnished in good taste. A coordinated color scheme should be used throughout the salon.

It is desirable to have an office or consultation room or a combination of both that is separate from the room where the treatments are to be given. The consultation should not be given in the reception area where there is no privacy. An attractive display of products will create interest and help to promote sales. When the client's skin needs to be cleansed before the skin is analyzed, this step can be done in the consultation room or the esthetician may prefer to do this part of the consultation in the treatment room, then return to the consultation room to complete records and to select products for home use.

FREE CONSULTATIONS BUILD BUSINESS

The salon may offer free consultations on facial treatments and makeup to build interest, but profit for the salon and the esthetician's salary are made by the sale of services and products. It is important to use the consultation to build business when possible. The client may wish to have a treatment following the consultation, only to find that there are no openings available. Therefore, when the client calls for an appointment or comes in for the free consultation, it should be suggested, tactfully, that a time is also open for a facial treatment following the consultation. In this way, you will have an opportunity to give a treatment, possibly sell some products and gain the client on a regular basis. Once the client is interested enough to come to the salon for the consultation, he or she will usually be interested in having the treatments and also in purchasing products to help maintain his or her skin care regimen at home.

Discussing the Cost of Treatments and Products

As a professional person, the esthetician should not hesitate to recommend services and products that will be beneficial to the client. Since the client has taken the initiative to come into the salon, he or she will feel disappointed if not given an opportunity to discuss treatments and products as well as proper at-home care of the skin.

During the consultation, the client will usually inquire about the cost of facial treatments. For best results, the esthetician should suggest a series of treatments. One treatment is usually not enough to get the results the client is looking for. It should be explained to the client that a single one-hour treatment cannot undo a condition that has taken months and some-

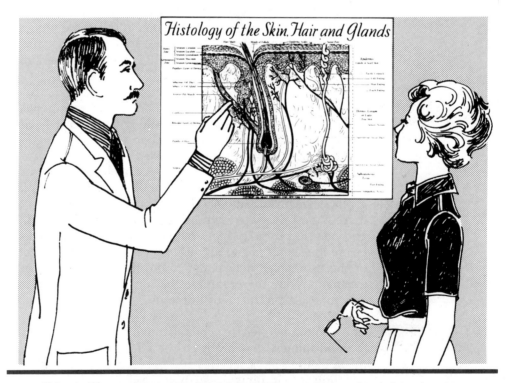

11.1—A skin care chart is often helpful during the consultation when it is necessary to explain the functioning of the skin to a client.

times years to acquire. With a series of treatments, more positive results can be achieved.

Many salons offer a special arrangement so that when the client is unsure about a series of treatments, the cost of the introductory treatment can be applied to the series. For example, your salon may offer a series of six treatments for a fixed amount that would be less than the same six treatments if given as single treatments. The client would recognize that with the series of treatments, there is a substantial savings. The advantage of this plan is not only to keep the client coming back for services and products, which means better business for the salon, but to give the client the full advantage of the treatments and products under the professional supervision of the esthetician.

Credentials

The esthetician's credentials, such as diplomas, certificates, or licenses should be displayed on a wall. This assures the client that he or she is receiving the services of a qualified esthetician. The consultation room should also have a skin care chart for reference purposes (Fig. 11.1).

The Client's Records

During the consultation it is necessary to keep record cards at hand and to write down the necessary information for the client's records (Fig. 11.2).

CONSULTATION CARD

Name ....

Address ....

City .... State .... Zip ....

Tel. (Home) .... (Business) ....

Ref. by: ....
(Person, advertising, etc.)

Date of Consultation ....

Age .... Sex ....

Known allergies ....

Medication ....

SKIN CLASSIFICATION

Facial Area		Facial Area	
Normal		Acne .... How many years	
Dry		Vulgaris .... Chronic	
Dehydrated		Cystic .... Rosacea	
Aging		Scars (acne, etc.)	
Thin, sensitive skin		Wrinkles	
Oily		Superficial lines	
Open pores		Deep lines	
Comedones (blackheads)		Relaxed elasticity	
Milium (whiteheads)		Good elasticity	
Asphyxiated .... (blocked pores and follicles)		Couperose (broken capillaries)	
		Discolorations	

REMARKS ....

....

....

Rec. Treatment ....

11.2—Consultation card

The salon record card should contain the following information:

1. The client's name, home address, and telephone number should be noted.
2. Any information that should be considered before treatments are given, such as the client's medical history and if the client is presently taking or using any kind of medication. It should also be noted if the client is or has been under the care of a physician or dermatologist. The client who is wearing a pacemaker must not have treatments that include galvanic current and high frequency.
3. Any abnormalities of the skin should be noted.
4. The record card should show whether the client is allergic to any substance of any kind. A test patch may be required and results noted.
5. In some cases where diet may be a factor in the condition of the skin, the client's general dietary habits may be recorded.
6. The client's age and weight should be noted, especially if he or she is dieting.
7. Separate cards may be kept to record the client's skin type, texture, and personal coloring. All procedures and products used during the consultation or treatments should be recorded for future reference. The reference cards are essential to record changes in treatments, when the changes were made, and to keep a record of progress or lack of progress of the treatments.
8. It is helpful to note on the consultation card, how the client was referred to the salon. This helps you to determine what source of advertising is drawing clients. If the salon has been recommended by another client, you may want to thank him or her.

The esthetician may use the back of the consultation card to record the date and the service/treatment performed at that time.

If makeup is applied following a skin care treatment, a list of cosmetics used and any special procedures should be recorded.

> **Note:** Records should be kept of products that the client has purchased for home use, as well as those used in the salon treatments. Quite often a client will want to purchase a product that he or she has used before, but has lost or thrown the container away and cannot remember the name of the product or color.

Procedure for the Analysis

After the client is seated in the consultation room and the appropriate information is obtained, this is a good time to ask the client how he or she learned about the salon. This information helps you to be aware of which type of advertising is reaching potential clients.

You may be able to determine at a glance the client's skin problem, but you should proceed with the complete skin analysis, using the magnifying lamp. This procedure will assure the client that you know what you are doing, and that he or she will receive the proper treatment for his or her particular skin condition.

Before examining the client's skin, the esthetician's hands should be sanitized with alcohol and dried with a towel or tissue. It is important to allow the client to see that sanitary practices are being observed.

If the client is a woman wearing heavy makeup, her face will need to be cleansed before using the magnifying lamp or the Wood's lamp. Sometimes only a small area will need to be cleansed in order to analyze the skin. The client may prefer not having her eye and lip makeup removed if she is not getting a facial treatment.

The purpose of the skin analysis is to determine the condition of the skin and select the proper treatments. The age and general health of the client should be observed, as these are important factors in the analysis of the skin. During the consultation and as the analysis proceeds, the esthetician should make the client aware of the benefits of professional skin care. For example, the esthetician might discuss the client's skin condition and how the treatment will be beneficial.

SKIN ANALYSIS IS DONE BEFORE EACH TREATMENT

When the skin is analyzed in the treatment room (the skin analysis done near the beginning of each treatment), the skin should be cleansed first, and eye pads used, to protect the eyes from the magnifying lamp.

The skin is analyzed before every treatment, because its general condition can be different due to seasonal changes. It is important to keep records of the progress of all treatments that are given.

The consultation is important to establish the client's needs and desires, but it is the analysis that helps the esthetician to determine the correct treatments for the client's skin care needs.

The esthetician must train his or her sight and touch in order to know what to look for during the skin analysis. At first glance the appearance of the skin may be misleading. Makeup used heavily by some women can be so cleverly applied that the skin's actual condition is hidden. This is why it is necessary to thoroughly cleanse the skin. Dryness and oiliness of the skin, blackheads, blemishes, and other problems will exist in varying degrees. The examination of the skin must be done with careful concentration.

PROCEDURE FOR SKIN ANALYSIS

1. Cleanse the skin thoroughly, following the step-by-step professional cleansing method.
2. Remove the cleanser and place eye pads on the client's eyes to protect them from the light of the magnifying lamp and/or Wood's lamp.
3. Let the client know what you are doing as you progress with the analysis. Study the skin of the entire face and neck under the magnifying lamp.
4. Using the middle finger of both hands, take a small (about one inch) section of skin between the fingers and stretch it slightly to reveal the texture of the skin and size of the openings of the follicles. The trained esthetician will be able to recognize the difference between large pores that are clear, and those that are clogged. Lines, flakiness and other problems will show clearly underneath the magnifying lamp.

IMPERFECTIONS AND DISEASED CONDITIONS OF THE SKIN

If the esthetician detects a skin disease that may require the attention of a dermatologist, the client should be told, tactfully, that the condition cannot be treated in the salon. The esthetician should not attempt to diagnose a skin disease, nor tell the client what the problem may be.

The esthetician must remember that he or she is not a physician and should never treat any skin condition that is outside of the realm of cosmetology. When unsure of any skin condition that is present, the client should be encouraged to consult a dermatologist. The dermatologist will then advise the client when the condition permits salon treatments.

The Classification of Skin Types

During the analysis of the skin, the esthetician must be able to determine the client's skin type and texture, and to discuss it with the client in a tactful manner. The skin is classified as one of the following types.

BRIEF DESCRIPTION OF SKIN TYPES

1. The *normal skin* is usually in good condition and has a sufficient supply of sebum and moisture. Normal skin is usually free of blemishes but can benefit from maintenance treatments to keep it healthy and attractive.
2. *Dry skin* is lacking in oil or moisture or both. Treatments can help to eliminate the drying conditions by stimulating the sebaceous glands to produce the natural oils and retain the moisture that is needed to keep the skin lubricated.
3. *Mature* or *aging skin* is usually loose, crepey, wrinkled, and/or lined. Treatments will help to slow down the aging process and help diminish surface lines.
4. *Oily skin* has an overabundance of sebum, and it may or may not be blemished. Treatments will help to normalize the production of sebum and clear blemishes.

5. If mild cases of blackheads, pimples and *acne skin* are not corrected, the condition can worsen. Treatments help to control blackheads, pimples, and acne by cleansing the impurities from the follicles and helping to normalize the production of sebum.

6. *Couperose skin* is identified by small broken capillaries beneath the surface. Treatments help to strengthen the walls of the capillaries and improve the health and appearance of the skin.

7. A *combination skin* may have dry and oily areas, or it may have a combination of conditions. Treatments help to normalize the functioning of the sebaceous glands and improve the health and appearance of the skin.

Professional terms should be explained to the client. For example, the esthetician may tell the client that his or her skin has overactive sebaceous glands or that the stratum corneum layer is dehydrated. The term "sebaceous" should be explained, and that the dead cells on the surface of the skin lack moisture.

A More Detailed Explanation of Skin Types

Clients will often have questions about their skin types and the causes of specific skin conditions. The following explanations can be given in the esthetician's own words. Additional information may be given according to the client's individual needs.

NORMAL SKIN   A normal skin is a skin that appears to be functioning normally and is neither too dry nor too oily. It is usually free of blemishes that require extensive treatments. The normal skin will benefit from maintenance treatments that help to keep it healthy and attractive.

When caring for a normal skin, the main objectives of the esthetician are to cleanse the skin so that dead cells are removed from the surface and impurities are removed from the follicles. The metabolism of the skin can be improved by stimulation and the client should be advised about products that can be used at home for everyday skin care. Regular care will assure that normal skin will continue to function in a normal way.

DRY SKIN   The skin may become dry due to too much sun, wind, harsh soaps, poor diet, aging, lack of enough fluid intake, excessive steaming of the face, the use of drying packs and masks, the use of drying cosmetics, medication taken internally or applied externally, or factors in the environment. The skin is often dry due to inactivity of the sebaceous glands that produce the sebum (oil) that lubricates the skin. Facial treatments and home maintenance will help stimulate the sebaceous glands and normalize the production of sebum.

Dry Skin that Is Lacking Natural Oil (Sebum)—A dry skin may be classified as "oil dry" when the sebaceous glands are sluggish and fail to produce sebum. The skin may have dry and oily areas that must be treated separately. When discussing the client's dry skin condition, the esthetician can explain that the application of heavy creams may in some cases interfere with the production of sebum and that the natural oil of the skin is far more beneficial than applying heavy oils or creams. The purpose of the treatment and special products is to try to stimulate the sebaceous glands into supplying the natural oil (sebum) the skin needs to keep it well-lubricated. The natural oils can be supplemented when necessary to relieve dryness.

Dry Skin that Lacks Moisture (Dehydrated)—A skin may have a sufficient amount of oil, but still feels dry and flaky due to lack of water in the skin. This is known as "dehydrated" skin. A dehydrated skin is prone to fine lines and wrinkles. Most often a dehydrated skin will appear to be thin, and in some cases small capillaries can be seen near the surface of the skin. Dry skin can appear to be fine in texture but coarse to the touch.

If the client's skin seems to be dehydrated from factors that require medical attention (such as diet, lack of fluids, or medication), the esthetician should recommend that the client seek the advice of his or her physician or dermatologist. In the meantime, facial treatments to improve the general health of the skin and to help it to retain moisture will be beneficial.

A dry skin may have a normal amount of sebaceous secretion (sebum) and may still be flaky and feel taut and dry. This condition is due to lack of surface moisture. Special treatment will help alleviate this condition. Dehydration of the skin may be a temporary condition varying from season to season and from various factors in the environment. There is a theory that using too heavy a cream or oil on dry skin may inhibit its production of natural oils by the sebaceous glands.

MATURE (AGING OR SENILE SKIN)

Dry skin is often due to the natural aging processes of the body. As a person advances in years, the body's processes slow down and cells are not replaced as rapidly as they were when the person was younger. It is not difficult to diagnose aging skin, but skin ages at different rates due to the following factors:

1. The skin ages due to neglect and the external treatment it has received.
2. Exposure to too much sun, wind, salt water, or polluted air will hasten the aging process.
3. Physiological disease, ill health, and psychological (emotional) problems can cause the skin to appear older.
4. Extreme weight loss can result in loss of muscle tone and lined and sagging skin, which in turn gives the skin an aged appearance.
5. Medications, lack of proper diet, and the misuse of alcoholic beverages and smoking may affect the appearance of the skin.

HELP FOR MATURE SKIN The mature client's skin can be improved but the natural aging process cannot be reversed, nor the skin restored to the same vital condition of youth. The client should be advised that treatments can make the skin look and feel better, but there are no miracle treatments that restore aging skin. Cosmetic (plastic) surgery or skin refining, along with proper salon treatments (and the enhancement of makeup) may help to achieve the desired results.

THE ELASTICITY OF THE SKIN Aging skin will often lack elasticity. The skin is tested for elasticity by taking a small section of the facial skin or neck between the thumb and forefinger and giving the skin a slight outward pull. When the skin is released, and if the elasticity is good, the skin will immediately return to its normal shape. If the skin is slow to resume its normal shape, it is lacking elasticity.

DISCOLORATION OF THE SKIN The client may be taking a certain type of medication that has caused uneven pigmentation of the skin, such as light and dark areas. The skin may also appear quite yellow or flushed. Some foods and liquids can cause a reaction that changes the color of the skin. Overexposure to sunlight, especially while taking some medications, can cause blotching and discoloration. The esthetician may be able to recommend a treatment that will help to diminish the blotched condition. In some cases, the use of makeup will conceal the discoloration.

OILY SKIN Oily skin is characterized by an over production of sebum (oil) and will feel thicker than dry or normal skins. The oily skin also has enlarged pores (follicles) that may be filled with dirt and grease. Oily skin is caused by a combination of factors. For example, during adolescence there may be an imbalance of hormones or a change in hormone levels that helps to increase the production of sebum. A diet rich in fats and oils may contribute to the oily condition of the skin. A hot, humid climate may also stimulate the sebaceous glands to produce more sebum.

Oily skin is more prone to pimples and blemishes, due to being well-lubricated by the excessive oil, but is less prone to wrinkles and fine lines than is dry skin. However, lines and wrinkles that do appear on an oily skin will be deeper and more pronounced. The oil helps to keep moisture in the skin from evaporating and forms the acid mantle, which protects the skin from germ penetration.

If oily skin is not cleansed properly, dirt, dead cells, and grease can clog follicles and become blackheads (also called comedones), which often lead to pimples on the surface of the skin giving it a sallow appearance. Whiteheads are accumulations of sebum underneath the surface of the skin.

Pimples are infected ducts that have become clogged with oil, dead cells, and dirt. Blackheads are breeding grounds for infectious bacteria and, if not given proper attention, can develop into pimples. An occasional pimple may develop into acne.

It is not uncommon for a person with an oily skin to wash the face too frequently. It is generally believed that excessive oil means that the skin is dirty and that washing away the excess oils will prevent blemishes. However, too much washing can actually aggravate a skin problem. Excessive washing or scrubbing the face removes only the surface oil and not the debris (oil, dirt, dead cells and bacteria) trapped beneath the surface of the skin.

Some believe that excessive drying of the surface of an oily skin stimulates the sebaceous glands to produce more oil. Actually, too much washing or cleansing, especially with harsh products, removes the skin's acid mantle and leaves it vulnerable to germ penetration. The acid mantle is the skin's natural defense against germ penetration, and when it is removed by too much cleansing, it may take up to a half hour or more for the skin to return to its normal acid balance.

ENLARGED PORES (FOLLICLES)   Clients will often ask if large pores (follicles) can be made smaller. Actually you can no more change the characteristics of the skin than you can change the color of your eyes. Enlarged pores (follicles) can be made to appear smaller, but it is impossible to shrink follicles to the degree that the skin will look like fine parchment-type skin that has small, almost invisible pores. Blackheads, grease deposits, dead cells, makeup, and other debris, fill and stretch the pores and prevent them from closing. Once this material is removed by deep cleansing, and the pores are kept cleaned out, they will close and tighten. Although the skin will still have enlarged pores, they will not seem as large or noticeable.

ACNE SKIN   *Acne skin* has the same characteristics as oily skin and is especially common during adolescence when it affects the face, shoulders, and back. The first signs of acne are usually seen during puberty, when there is an increase in hormone production, which stimulates the sebaceous glands. This leads to blackheads which in turn can develop into pimples and acne. Not everyone with blackheads, will develop acne, but everyone with acne has blackheads. It has not been determined why some people develop acne while others do not. Acne has a demoralizing effect on a person and, if neglected, can cause scars and pits that will not be outgrown.

Dr. Harold T. Hyman, a former teacher of medicine at the Columbia University College of Physicians and Surgeons and the author of a number of books for physicians states in *The Complete Home Medical Encyclopedia* that "Acne is not a skin disease; it is a skin manifestation of revolutionary changes that occur in the body at and throughout adolescence."

Women often experience a flare up of pimples and blemishes usually around the mouth and chin prior to the onset of the menstrual cycle. This is due to a high proportion of androgen (a male sex hormone) at the time of their periods, when the estrogen level tends to fall.

Acne skin can be treated to keep the condition under control. In the book, *The Complete Guide to Skin and Hair for Cosmetologists*, by Charles W.

Whitmore, M.D. and William H. Young, Ph.D., it is stated: "With today's knowledge of acne, all but the most severe cases can be kept under control. Control, however, takes more than good intentions. It involves time, patience, and adherence to certain procedures." The esthetician should advise the client as to the best home care procedure. The client with an acne skin should be told that every pimple starts with a blackhead or clogged pore. Deep cleansing treatments prevent the follicles from becoming clogged with the debris that causes the problem.

It is not uncommon for a dermatologist to refer patients to an esthetician for deep pore cleansing treatments. The esthetician should not hesitate to recommend that the client see a dermatologist for severe cystic acne. The female client should be advised not to use heavy makeup to conceal an acne condition, but to work diligently to clear the condition so that the skin is returned to its natural healthy state.

SEBORRHEA   *Seborrhea* is a functional disease of the sebaceous glands, characterized by an excessive secretion or disturbed quality of sebum, which collects upon the skin in the form of an oily coating or of crusts or scales. The skin will often have enlarged follicles and will appear coarse and shiny from the excess oil. An itching or burning sensation often accompanies seborrhea.

ROSACEA   *Rosacea*, like seborrhea, is characterized by excessive oiliness of the skin. The nose and cheeks are the most frequently affected. The face will have a flushed appearance and, if neglected, the skin can become lumpy where the papules and pustules are formed. Although sometimes referred to as "acne rosacea" this skin condition is not to be confused with acne. Rosacea is not the same type of skin condition that appears during adolescence, because it usually does not appear before the age of 35. Rosacea is more common in adult females than in males. However, when a male develops rosacea, it usually becomes quite severe. Rosacea can be aggravated by consumption of too much alcohol and heavily spiced foods. The client should be advised to avoid squeezing or picking lumps that appear on any area of the face. In ordinary cases, soothing treatments will be helpful. In recent years rosacea has been treated successfully by dermatologists. The client should be encouraged to consult a dermatologist for medication.

COUPEROSE SKIN   *Couperose skin* is characterized by broken capillaries that can be seen beneath the surface of the skin. These small red vessels are usually more prominent in a thin skin. A couperose condition can be combined with other problems and each area of the face must be treated for that specific condition. When the blood vessels are not elastic enough to handle the flow of blood that is forced through them, they stretch and break. Extremes of heat and cold on the face, strong alcoholic beverages, and some foods can affect the vessels.

Note: Blood cells pass through the tiny narrow capillaries single file and it is through the capillary walls that the cells receive oxygen, nutrients, hormones, and antibodies. It is also through the walls that cellular waste is returned to the bloodstream. Healthy cells are dependent upon healthy capillaries. Vitamin P (bioflavonoids and flavones) combined with Vitamin C is often helpful in strengthening the walls of the capillaries. Vitamin P is found in vegetables and is concentrated in the white pulp of the rinds of citrus fruits.

The esthetician should not promise that treatments will clear the couperose condition, but proper care can help to prevent further damage. The client may wish to consult a dermatologist about medically removing unsightly, broken, surface capillaries.

THE COMBINATION SKIN ("T" ZONE)

The combination skin is characterized by the existence of two or more different conditions. For example, the skin may be oily around the nose, forehead, and chin, but dry on the rest of the face. When treating a combination skin, each area is treated for its particular condition. For example, when applying a mask, a mask formulated for oily skin is applied to the oily areas of the face and a mask formulated for dry skin is applied to dry areas.

Differences in Light and Dark Skins

An esthetician is not expected to be an anthropologist but he or she should be able to recognize some of the important differences in the skins of persons from different ethnic origins. There are subtle undertones in skin color that must be considered when selecting makeup for women, and there are other physical characteristics of light and dark skins.

ETHNIC DIVISIONS BY COLOR

The peoples of the earth are classified into three major divisions of humankind. These are: The *Negroid* (black), *Caucasoid* (white), and the *Mongoloid* (yellow) races. Negroid refers to the major ethnic division of human species characterized by skin color that ranges from light brown to black or ebony. In modern day, dark-skinned people of the Negroid ethnic division, are referred to as "black" people, even though skin tones may range from very light to very dark and will have varied undertones. Caucasoid refers to the major ethnic division of human species characterized by skin that is very light (but may have varied undertones) to dark brown or olive. In modern society, light-skinned people are often referred to as "white" or caucasian. Mongoloid refers to the major ethnic division of the human species characterized by a yellowish cast to the skin. They are also called Asians. Their skin tones may range from light ivory to a deeper brown or golden brown. American Indians and Eskimos have a predominantly reddish undertone to the skin, while the people of India have predominantly brown skin.

People from various ethnic groups are also characterized by other physical features such as curly or straight hair and distinguishing facial and body structure. Skin color is a matter of pigmentation and is explained in more detail in the chapters on makeup and cosmetic color selection. Our concern here is to understand some differences in structure and function that exist between light and dark skin that the esthetician must take into consideration when giving a skin analysis.

ANALYSIS OF BLACK SKIN

All skins must be analyzed carefully before treatments are given. The esthetician must be particularly careful during the analysis of dark skin, because skin imperfections (blemishes, flaws, blackheads, etc.) that are readily visible on light skin may not be so easy to detect on dark skins due to the dark pigment of the skin. A magnifying lamp must always be used and the Wood's lamp should be used (when available) to analyze dark skin. In most cases, dark (black) skins will be healthy and even in color. The skin will most often have good texture and may only need maintenance treatments. On the other hand, the black client may need treatments for excessive oiliness or for other conditions that may be treated by an esthetician. The esthetician must be aware of products that are especially formulated for specific skin types.

CHARACTERISTICS OF BLACK SKIN

Black skin usually has more and larger sebaceous glands. Due to the shiny surface of black skin, it is often thought that all black skin is oily. Actually, light is reflected to a greater degree on dark skin and this often gives the impression that the skin is moist or oily when it may actually lack moisture and/or oil. It is true that the follicles of black skin most often have a greater abundance of sebum, but usually this is due to enlarged follicles. A great many black people have normal skin, but it is not uncommon for the skin to be dry, or extremely oily. The condition of dark skin, like any other skin, will be affected by climate and extremes of heat and cold.

MATURITY AND BLACK SKIN

Black skin does not usually show signs of maturity (aging) as early as light skin. This is due to the deeper pigment color of the skin filtering out the ultra-violet radiation of the sun, which is one of the leading causes of weakening of the skin's elasticity. Loss of the skin's elasticity results in lining and wrinkling of the skin. Black skin is also thicker and has more protection from environmental elements due to a heavier buildup of dead surface cells. Black skin is, in most cases, stronger and more durable and is therefore less prone to lines and wrinkles. Most black people show few signs of aging even at age 50 or 60. Hair may show signs of graying long before the skin begins to show age. Once black skin starts to age, however, wrinkles and depression lines appear to be deeper than those on lighter skins.

TREATMENTS FOR BLACK SKIN

Treatments for black skin are basically the same as for light skin, but because the darker skin is firmer, with a thicker buildup of dead surface cells, it is usually more resistant to electric current such as galvanic and high-frequency current. Electric brushing and epidermabrasion treatments (peeling) give excellent results for the black skin. The treatment rids the skin of the dead surface cells, which often give the skin an ashen appearance. It is important to remember that both epidermabrasion and brushing are not done on the skin during the same treatment.

Since black skin will often have a greater abundance of thick sebum in the follicles, disincrustation will prove to be helpful for deep pore (follicle) cleansing. When galvanic current is used for disincrustation, it may be necessary to use a stronger current due to the darker skin being resistant to electric current. Disincrustation is followed by the Dr. Jacquet massage movements, which help to move the excess sebum forward and out of the sebaceous ducts. Before doing the Dr. Jacquet movement, the skin should be dry and free of oil so the fingers can hold the skin firmly without slipping.

The suction machine (when available) follows the Dr. Jacquet movements. Whether or not the Dr. Jacquet movements are used in the facial treatment, the suction can be used on all types of skin to vacuum debris from the follicles and to stimulate the skin.

Interesting Facts About Light and Dark Skins

1. Perspiration acts as a cooling system for the body. Dark-skinned people tend to perspire more than light-skinned people, therefore they generally have better heat tolerance.
2. Body temperature in persons with dark skin remains lower when in strong sunlight or extreme heat than it does in persons with light skin. Persons with light skins are able to withstand extremes of cold better than dark-skinned people.
3. Sebaceous glands tend to be more numerous and larger in dark skin than in light skin.
4. Dark skin flakes, sheds, and casts off (exfoliates) dead cells more easily than light skin.
5. Dead cells that flake off of dark skin contain pigmentary granulations. Dead cells from a light skin will not contain pigmentary granulations unless the skin has been tanned.
6. Skin cancer is seen less frequently in dark skin due to the deeper pigmentation, which tends to filter out sun radiation.
7. The dead-cell layer of the epidermis is thicker on dark skin than on light skin.
8. Acne is rarely as severe in dark-skinned people as in light-skinned people, even though there are more sebaceous glands in dark skins.

9. Warts, which are more frequent in children than in adults, are practically nonexistent in persons with dark skin.

10. Allergies due to use of products are less frequent in persons with dark skin. This is believed to be due to dark skin being thicker and having a heavier surface cell layer.

11. Keloids are more common in dark skins than in light skins. A keloid is a rounded, thick scar that results from excessive growth of fibrous tissue during connective tissue repair. For example, acne scars on light skin can be more easily improved by dermabasion, while this treatment may be risky for dark skin due to keloid formation.

12. As a rule, neither dark nor lighter-skinned people have sebaceous glands on the palms of the hands or the soles of the feet.

Advising the Client About Skin Care at Home

The main purpose of the consultation is to provide a needed and wanted service that also gains clients for the salon. The client should never be made to feel that the sole purpose of the consultation is to sell products. Once the client trusts the integrity of the esthetician, it is not too difficult to sell the products needed to back up the salon treatments and the recommended home care regimen. It is not wise to discourage the client from using the products he or she now uses at home, but the esthetician should explain the importance of using products that are formulated for the client's particular skin type. It can be stressed that following a proven regimen of skin care is for the client's benefit if maximum results are to be achieved. Failure to follow salon treatments with proper at-home care would be a waste of the client's time and money.

Some salons employ a person who is trained to handle all sales of cosmetics. In this case the esthetician makes out the cosmetic list for the client and the order is filled by the salesperson. The salesperson can refill orders for clients as products are needed. It is estimated that over 90 percent of the clients who come for salon treatments purchase products following the first treatment, and will continue to use all or some of the products.

It is better not to sell the client large containers of products as he or she may not return to the salon for additional treatments until they are in need of refills. Small containers of cleansers, protective lotions, and treatment creams usually last about four to six weeks. No matter what products the client has been using, it is never courteous to make derogatory remarks about the products. It can be suggested that the client set aside any odds and ends of cosmetics for the time being in order to allow the professional treatments and products to take affect.

Cleansing the Face at Home

All types of skins are cleansed in the same manner because it is the best method and the least trouble. The home cleansing routine is similar to the cleansing that is done during the professional treatment given in the salon. This cleansing method involves no messy procedures, and leaves the skin feeling clean and refreshed.

PROCEDURE
1. Show the client how to make wet cotton pads for cleansing the face. This is the same method used when making pads for the professional salon treatment.
2. The pad is squeezed to remove excess water. About one level teaspoon of cleanser is placed on the pad.
3. The cleanser is applied to the neck and face by dabbing some of the cleanser lightly on the neck, cheeks, and forehead.
4. The client is instructed on how to cleanse the face, starting with the neck and moving to the jaw, cheeks, chin, area beneath the nose, the nose, forehead, and the eye areas. Pads are discarded after use.
5. Astringent or skin-freshening lotion is applied to the face with a clean, wet cotton pad. This is an important step as it removes all the residue of the cleanser and restores the skin's natural pH acid balance. If the client prefers to rinse the face with water, rinsing can be done following the use of the astringent or skin-freshening lotion. Some cosmetic companies manufacture a special wash or cream soap in place of the cleansing cream or lotion. If used, this product should be of the non-drying kind.
6. Directly after cleansing and the use of the astringent, and while the face is still moist, protection fluid or a night treatment cream may be applied. The protection fluid or cream will trap the moisture next to the skin, keeping the skin moist longer.

During the cleansing instruction, the client should be advised not to push on, or drag the facial skin and muscles. Gentle upward and outward motions are essential to keep from stretching delicate tissue.

Claims and Guarantees

During the first consultation and before a treatment, clients with acne will often ask if treatments can be guaranteed to clear up the acne condition. In most cases these clients have tried other treatments, medications, and products bought from the shelves of department and drugstores. Some advertising of the products may claim to clear acne and the client may have experienced disappointment when the expected results were not achieved.

The client may look upon salon treatments as a last resort. Some clients may be skeptical of any suggestions the esthetician may make, and feel that treatments may be a waste of time and money. When this happens, it is necessary to explain to the client that treatments for acne skin condition have proved to be successful for the majority of people who have received them over the years. Also, facial treatments are being given by licensed nurses and estheticians in dermatologists offices, and in salons throughout the country. Positive results are achieved and facial treatments are beneficial in almost all cases.

Many clients do not understand the causes of acne and may have developed some misconceptions about this type of skin problem. It is important to answer the client's questions and explain how cleaning the pores regularly brings about improvement in the skin. The client should expect improvement, but he or she should also be aware that a treatment that works wonders for one person may do little for another. An esthetician cannot guarantee a cure nor make exaggerated claims.

REFUNDS Sometimes a client will ask if his or her money will be refunded if the treatment fails to clear the skin. Just as a doctor cannot guarantee that a certain medication will cure an illness or the patient's money will be refunded, estheticians cannot promise refunds. It is better not to perform a service if the client does not have confidence in the sincerity and professionalism of the esthetician and the reputation of the salon.

Questions Frequently Asked During the Consultation

Question: I don't feel clean unless I use soap and water on my face. Some people have told me to use soap and water, and others that soap and water should never be used. What is the answer?

Answer: Most modern day soaps contain ingredients that do a good job of cleansing the surface of the skin. If we lived in an ideal environment that was free from dirt and pollutants in the air and that had a controlled atmosphere, then soap might be adequate for keeping the skin clean and healthy. Since we are subjected to extremes of temperature, pollutants, and other harsh effects of our environment, most skins benefit from specially formulated products and professional treatments. A skin cleansing cream or lotion will cleanse the surface of the skin without drying or irritating the skin. A great deal of modern research has been done and money spent over the years to find a more effective method for cleansing the skin. Modern science has been able to improve on basic soap and water for cleansing the skin. For people who like to use water when cleansing the face, after cleansing with cleanser and astringent or freshener, they may splash and rinse with water as much as they like.

Question: Why is it necessary to use a skin-freshening lotion or astringent after cleansing?

Answer: Astringents and mild skin fresheners actually further the cleansing of the skin. These products are effective in removing the residue of cleansers and help to restore the skin's natural pH acid level and temporarily tighten the pores.

Question: My skin is dry. Does this mean I need to apply oil to compensate for the oil my sebaceous glands are not producing?

Answer: When skin is dry, it can be oil dry and/or moisture dry. Oil will not replenish moisture in the skin but it can provide a protective film to keep moisture from evaporating from the skin. It is best to use an emulsion containing oil and moisture specially formulated for your type of skin.

Question: My skin is oily. Does this mean I don't need to use a moisturizer?

Answer: Oily skin can be dehydrated (lacking water) especially due to health or environmental conditions. Oily skin may have dry areas such as around the eyes. Under these conditions a moisturizer is as beneficial for an oily skin as for one that is dry. Oily skin needs moisture to help prevent wrinkles. It is best to use a product especially formulated for your skin type.

Question: My skin gets very dry, itchy, and flaky, not only on my face but also on the rest of my body, especially during the winter months. What is the best type of soap to use for bathing?

Answer: Because of the high alkalinity of bar soaps (average pH range from 9 to 10), it can cause irritating stress and aggravation to the skin. This is due to the mismatch of the skin's pH (approximately 5.5) and that of bar soap.

This problem has been overcome by the development of the synthetic detergent-based soap bar. To the average person, the word "detergent" sounds strong and harsh because we have seen and heard the word used so often for household cleansers. For this reason the manufacturer will often refrain from using the word detergent on the package. Actually the manufacturer can adjust the detergent cleansing bar to be less drying and irritating by formulating it to be completely alkali free, with a neutral pH of 7. This does not disturb the acid mantle of the skin. In addition the manufacturer can add emollients and/or cold cream to the formula to help prevent itching and flaking. Look for the words beauty bar or cleansing bar on the package. If you see the word soap, it is not what you are looking for.

Question: I have been told that cosmetics applied to the skin do not penetrate the skin.

Answer: In recent years, it has been substantiated that most chemicals applied to the skin will penetrate to some degree. Some ingredients have been known to accumulate in the body and cause serious and dangerous side effects. An example of this would be mercury, which was used in bleaching creams, and *hexachlorophene*, an antibacterial used in products such as soaps and antiperspirants. Both were removed from the market during the early 1970's by the Food and Drug Administration.

Question: My grandmother never used anything on her face but soap and water and she had a beautiful complexion. Why can't I get by with this kind of skin care today?

Answer: Your grandmother may have been one of those people who have a naturally healthy and attractive skin. However, she was not confronted with some of the enemies of the skin that have come about in recent times. Air pollution, chemicals in water, and preservatives in food are just a few of the things in our modern environment that may affect the skin. Today it is more important than ever to give the skin proper, daily care.

QUESTIONS — DISCUSSION AND REVIEW

CLIENT CONSULTATION AND SKIN ANALYSIS

1. Why is the first impression so important when dealing with a client?
2. Explain why it is important to speak in a pleasant and professional manner when answering the telephone.
3. Describe what the appearance of a professional salon should look like.
4. What is the reason for skin analysis?
5. Can the condition of your client's skin change from treatment to treatment?
6. List the different skin types.
7. Is it important for a client to practice a home care regimen at home? Explain your answer.
8. What guarantees can an esthetician make about skin treatments?

Client Preparation and Draping

CHAPTER 12

LEARNING OBJECTIVES

After completing this chapter, you should be able to:

❶ Explain how to set up a treatment room and prepare a client for treatment.
❷ Demonstrate the proper draping for the male and female clients.
❸ Demonstrate the different head drapings for your clients.
❹ Demonstrate how to make cleansing pads, eyepads, and compresses.

INTRODUCTION

Before a facial treatment can be given, the esthetician must be sure the treatment area is ready and that all implements and supplies are on-hand and ready for use. The professional esthetician must be efficient and well-organized at all times. During the preparation for the treatment, it is essential that the client feel at ease and comfortable. When draping the head, applying cleanser, or performing other movements, it is important to let the client know what is being done and why it will be beneficial. For example, when draping the client's head, the esthetician might say, "Mrs. Green, I'm going to drape this towel around your head to protect your hair. Would you lift your head just a little, please? Thank you. Are you comfortable?"

It is important to do all your preparation in a confident professional manner. You can move quickly without seeming hurried, and you can work in a relaxed manner without seeming too slow. Your sense of confidence will impress the client who will in turn have confidence in you as a professional esthetician. (*See Color Plate 15.*)

Procedure for Preparing the Treatment Area

The facial treatment area should be located in the most quiet area of the school or salon. All implements and supplies should be ready before the arrival of the client.

IMPLEMENTS AND SUPPLIES Everything that is to be used for the facial treatment should be set out and arranged in an orderly manner. This would include such items as:

1. Cleanser, astringent, treatment creams
2. Cotton pads, compresses and/or sponges
3. Towels, tissues, swabs, spatulas
4. Machines and other apparatus
5. Coverlet and other items of this type

▶ **Caution:** All creams and masks should be removed from the container with a spatula. Never, under any circumstances, should the fingers be dipped into any of the products to be used.

Preparation of the Client for the Facial Treatment

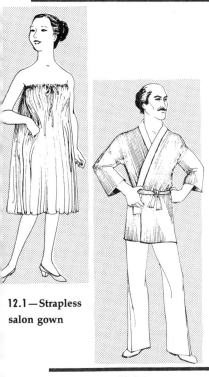

When greeting the client it is important to put him or her at ease immediately. To prevent the client from worrying about personal belongings being misplaced or stolen while in the treatment room, it is best to have a place to hang the client's coat and other garments in the treatment room. Hooks with several hangers are usually sufficient. If an outside cloakroom is used for coats, it should be in the reception room where it can be observed by someone on the staff. A woman should place any valuables in her handbag and keep the handbag with her at all times.

Female clients wear a strapless salon gown (Fig. 12.1). Undergarment straps can be removed from the shoulders and tucked into the top of the gown. A woman usually removes her dress or blouse. A male client changes into a kimono-type salon robe (Fig. 12.2). He removes his shirt, undershirt and tie. Salon gowns and robes should be made of attractive, washable, no-iron fabric. A clean gown or robe is given to each client. Beauty supply dealers offer a choice of gowns and robes, or some salons have special styles and colors of costumes custom made.

12.1—Strapless salon gown

12.2—Kimono-type salon robe

MAKING THE CLIENT COMFORTABLE

After the client is in the treatment chair, place a towel across the client's chest and a coverlet over the body. Fold the outer edge of the towel over the top of the coverlet. Remove the client's shoes and tuck the coverlet around the feet. (Fig. 12.3.)

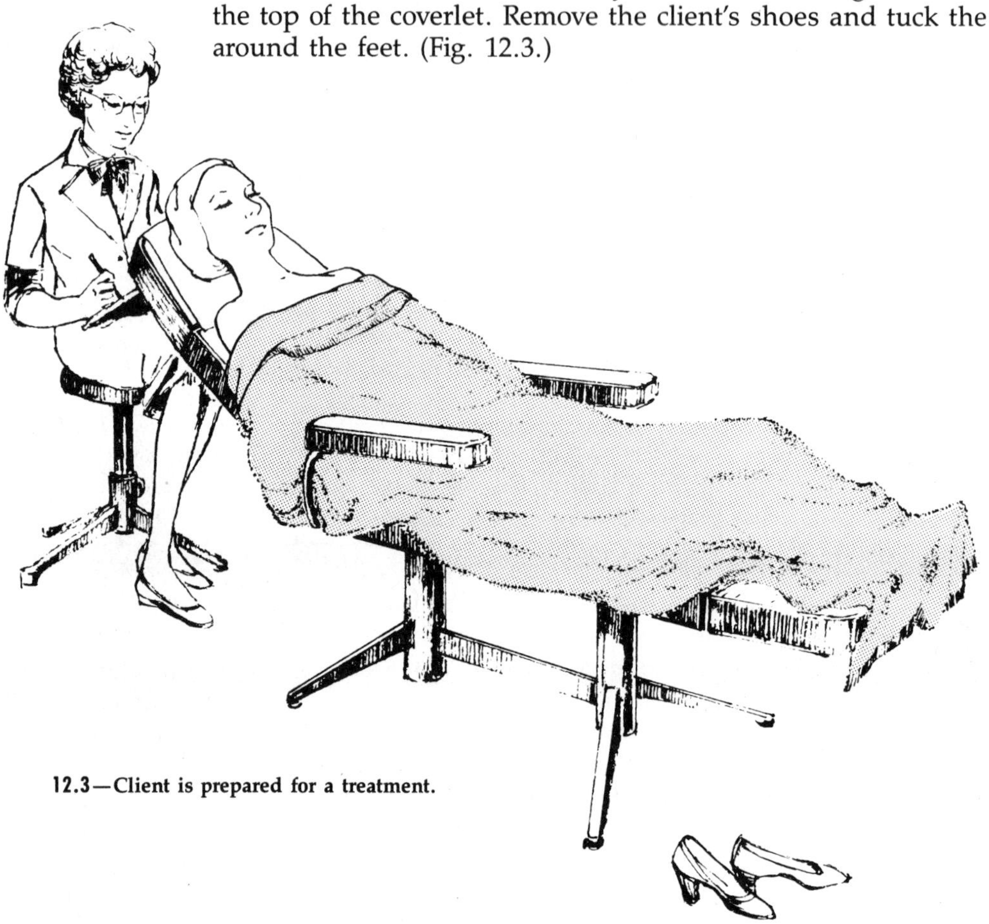

12.3—Client is prepared for a treatment.

Draping the Head

The purpose of the head drape is to cover and protect the client's hair during the facial treatment. There have been several types of commercial head coverings on the market over the past years. Some types are of a turban design, and others are designed with elastic similar to a shower cap. The most popular type of head covering used in facial and beauty salons is the cloth or paper towel. For years, most salons have rented cloth towels from a commercial laundry service. These towels, however, often have obvious and unsightly stains such as dye and nail polish that did not come out in the wash. Also, in some areas, the price of laundry service has risen drastically in recent years. To combat these problems, more salons are now installing electric washers and dryers to provide their own supply of clean towels. The washer and dryer pay for themselves within a short time because towels, smocks, and coverlets can be laundered.

Another alternative to the commercial laundry service is the use of paper towels. They are ideal for use in schools and salons that are operated on a tight budget.

DRAPING WITH THE CLOTH TOWEL

1. Fold the towel lengthwise from one of the top corners to the opposite lower corner and place it over the headrest with the fold facing down. Place the towel on the headrest before the patron enters the facial area. (See Fig. 12.4.)

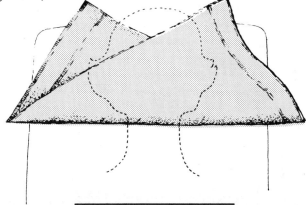

12.4—Place the folded towel on the headrest.

2. When the client is in a reclining position, the back of the head should rest on the towel so that one side of the towel can be brought up to the center of the forehead to cover the hair line. (See Fig. 12.5.)
3. With the other hand, bring the other side of the towel over to the center and cross it over. (See Fig. 12.6.)
4. Use a regular bobby pin to hold the towel in place. Check to be sure that all strands of hair are tucked under the towel, earlobes are not bent, and the towel is not wrapped too tightly. (See Fig. 12.7.)

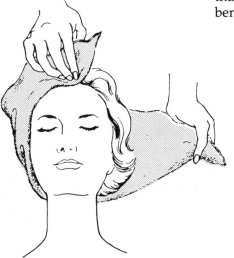

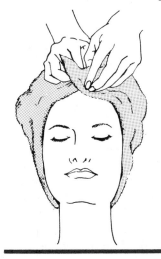

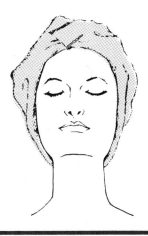

12.5—Place towel around client's head.

12.6—Join towel at center of client's head.

12.7—Secure towel with a bobby pin.

DRAPING WITH THE PAPER TOWEL

To keep the paper towel snug to the head and from tearing along the hairline when it becomes damp, line the paper towel with a 2-inch wide elastic band (the type used for wrapping a sprained wrist or ankle). These elastic bands can be purchased at any drugstore and can be cut crosswise to give three equal bands. They are easy to wash and sanitize.

1. Fold the paper towel over an elastic band lengthwise from one of the top corners to the opposite lower corner. (See Fig. 12.8.)

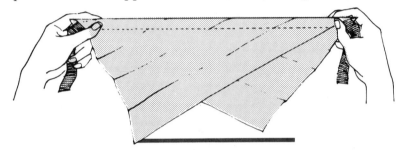

12.8—Fold the paper towel over an elastic band.

2. Place the straight edge of the towel across the client's forehead about 1 inch lower than the hairline. Have the client place his or her fingers in the center of the band to keep the towel from slipping while the band is tied at the nape of the neck. (See Fig. 12.9.)

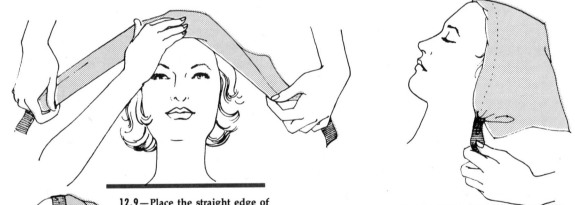

12.9—Place the straight edge of the towel across client's forehead.

12.10—Tie the band.

12.11—Apply a second elastic band, if necessary.

3. Have the client lift his or her head slightly off the headrest while you are tying the band. Slide the towel back so that the edge of the towel just covers the hairline. A spatula is used to tuck hair strands under the towel. Check to see that the client's earlobes are not bent and that the headband or towel is not wrapped too tightly. (See Fig. 12.10.)

4. For the beginning student, a second elastic band may be applied over the edge of the towel and tied in the back. When the student becomes experienced in giving facial treatments the second band may be eliminated. (See Fig. 12.11.)

Preparation of Cotton Pads and Compresses

Prepare all cotton cleansing pads, eyepads, and the cotton compress pads that are used in facial treatments before the treatment begins. In a busy salon that gives facial treatments, the esthetician should check the appointment book at the beginning of each work day to see how many appointments are booked for that day. Enough pads and compresses can then be made for the entire day. Store pads and compresses in a covered container. Remove enough pads from the container before each treatment and place them in a plastic or glass bowl that is within easy reach during the facial treatment. An inexpensive ice bucket may be kept in the facial area to store the prepared pads and compresses. For each client you will need one pair of eyepads, one cotton compress mask, and three cleansing pads. The pads and compresses that are not used on the day they are made can be stored safely in a covered container for the next workday (Fig. 12.12).

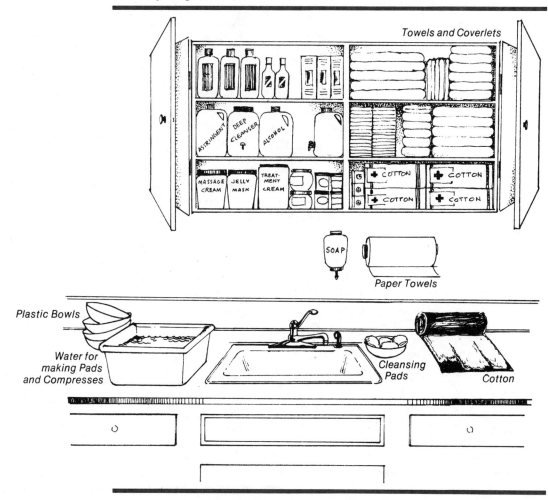

12.12—A neat, well-organized dispensary

HOW TO MAKE CLEANSING PADS, EYEPADS, AND COMPRESSES

Have all the cotton you need ready before you begin to submerge the pads or compresses in water. For sanitary reasons, keep the water used for making cleansing pads and cotton compresses in a metal, enamel, or plastic basin. Pads should never be made in a sink where hands or articles are washed. The following is the procedure for making cleansing pads and compresses:

1. Divide a roll of beautician's cotton into three equal strips, each approximately 4 inches wide. This is about the width of the average hand. Tear the cotton (do not cut) so that the edges are frayed and the cleansing pads are less lumpy when the edges are folded under. (See Fig. 12.13.)
2. To make cleansing pads, hold one of the cotton strips in one hand and pull downward with the other hand until the cotton tears, giving you a piece of cotton that is approximately 4 inches wide by 5 to 6 inches long. You need three of these pieces for each facial treatment. (See Fig. 12.14.)

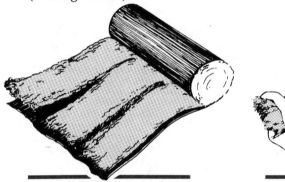

12.13—Divide a roll of cotton into three equal strips.

12.14—Tear a 4 inch by 4 inch piece of cotton.

3. Submerge the cotton under water as you support the pad with your fingers. Tuck the edges of the cotton under while turning it in your hand. (See Fig. 12.15.)
4. Form a round pad with the cotton. (See Fig. 12.16.)
5. Place it on the palm of one hand quickly, then place the other palm over the pad. Squeeze the excess water from the pad. (See Fig. 12.17.)

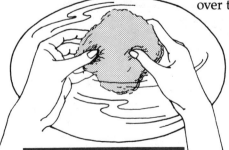

12.15—Submerge the piece of cotton in water.

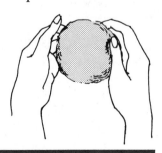

12.16—Form a round pad.

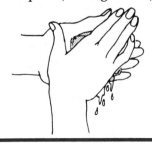

12.17—Squeeze excess water from pad.

EYEPADS Eyepads can be made from scrap pieces of cotton. There are two types of eyepads, *round* and *butterfly pads*. Both styles of eyepads are correct and the choice is up to the esthetician. The pads should be large enough to cover the entire eye area. If the round eyepads fall from the client's face, they are usually not wet enough. The advantage of the butterfly pad is that it will not fall from the eyes as easily as the round-type pad.

Round Eyepads The following are the two steps for making round eyepads (Fig. 12.18):

1. Dip a piece of cotton about 2½ inches by 2½ inches into water and tuck the edges under while forming a round-shaped pad.
2. Press the pad between your palms to squeeze out the excess water. (See Fig. 12.19.)

Butterfly Pads The following are the three steps for making butterfly eyepads (Fig. 12.20):

1. Dip a piece of cotton about 2 inches by 6 inches into water. (See Fig. 12.21.)
2. Twist the cotton in the center with a one-half turn. (See Fig. 12.22.)
3. Fold the pad in half and squeeze out the excess water. (See Fig. 12.23.)

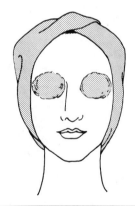

12.18—Round eyepads.

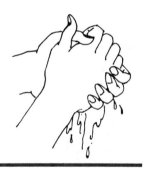

12.19—Squeeze excess water from pad.

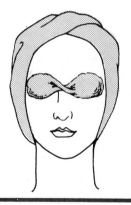

12.20—Butterfly pads

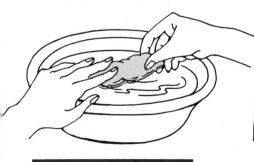

12.21—Dip cotton in water.

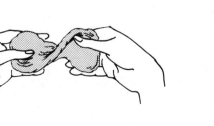

12.22—Twist cotton in the center.

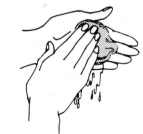

12.23—Fold cotton in half and squeeze out excess water.

**HOW TO MAKE THE
COTTON COMPRESS MASK**

1. To make the cotton compress mask, you need a piece of cotton 4 inches wide and 9 inches long. (See Fig. 12.24.)
2. Using both hands, push the cotton strips evenly under the water. Before the cotton has a chance to spread out, take one end of the strip and, with the right hand, lift the strip completely out of the water and quickly place the left hand under the opposite end of the strip. (See Fig. 12.25.)
3. Fold the wet cotton strip in half. (See Fig. 12.26.)
4. Fold the wet cotton strip in half again. (See Fig. 12.27.)
5. Squeeze out the excess water so that it remains fairly wet, but will not drip when applied. When the compress mask is being used to apply an herbal tea compress, the cotton is saturated with the tea. (See Fig. 12.28.)

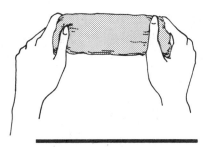

12.24—Start with a piece of cotton 4 inches wide by 9 inches long.

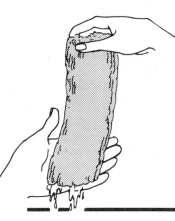

12.25—Saturate the cotton with water.

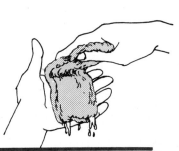

12.26—Fold the cotton in half.

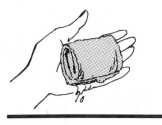

12.27—Fold the cotton in half a second time.

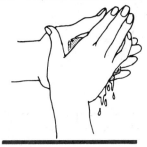

12.28—Squeeze out excess water.

QUESTIONS DISCUSSION AND REVIEW

**CLIENT PREPARATION
AND DRAPING**

1. Why is it necessary to have everything ready in the treatment room before the arrival of the client?
2. How should creams and masks be removed from containers?
3. What is the purpose of the head drape?
4. What are the most popular types of head covering?
5. What is used when making eyepads, cleansing pads, and compresses?

C H A P T E R

13

Cleansing the Skin

LEARNING OBJECTIVES   *After completing this chapter, you should be able to:*

❶ Explain how to properly apply and remove cleansing creams.
❷ Demonstrate how to apply a cotton compress and why it is used.

INTRODUCTION

In this chapter you will learn the basic application methods for applying cleanser, treatment creams, and protective fluids. You will learn how to prepare cotton pads and sponges and how to use them effectively in the application and removal of cosmetics. Using correct cleansing methods is important for maintaining the health of the facial skin.

Before every treatment, it is important to take a very close look at the skin before cleansing it. Many surface signs of the client's skin condition can be removed by the cleanser and wet cotton pads or sponges during the initial cleansing. For example, if the client's skin is oily, the skin will look shiny or greasy; if the client's skin is dry, the skin will often be flaky.

The cleansing procedure should be both a restful and a stimulating experience for the client. Help the client to relax by speaking in a quiet and professional manner. Explain the benefits of the products and services and answer any questions the client may have.

It is important that the client remain comfortable and relaxed throughout the facial treatment. Cold or iced pads, sponges, or compresses can feel shocking and unpleasant to the client. These items should be kept at a comfortable temperature. The excess water should be squeezed from a pre-prepared cotton pad so that water does not drip on the client during the cleansing procedure.

Product Application

The following method of application is used throughout the text when applying cleansers, massage creams, treatment creams, and protective fluids. Please refer to Face Area Chart (Fig. 13.1) for numbers in parenthesis.

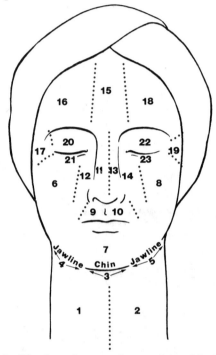

13.1—Face Area Chart. This chart has been designed to help the esthetician identify the exact areas of the face and neck during the explanation of various techniques and manipulations. When an explanation of a movement is followed by a number, or numbers in parenthesis (*1–2), refer to the chart for the exact location.

1. The hands must be sanitized before touching the client's face. While applying the product, don't lift your hands from the client's face until you are ready to apply the product to the eyelids. (See Fig. 13.2.)
2. Apply approximately one level teaspoon or less of the product to the fingers of either hand (not the palms). (Water soluble cleansing lotion is preferred when cleansing the face because it can be easily removed with moistened cotton pads or sponges.) (See Fig. 13.3.)

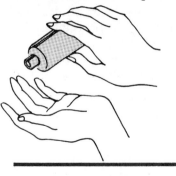

13.2—Apply product to fingers.

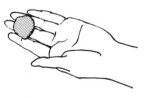

13.3—Use one teaspoon or less of the product.

3. With the other hand, use circular motions to distribute the product over both sides of the fingers. You are now ready to apply the product to the client's neck and face. (See Fig. 13.4.)

4. Start applying the product by placing both hands, palms down, on the neck (*1 and *2). Slide hands back toward ears until the pads of the fingers rest at a point directly beneath the earlobes. (See Fig. 13.5.)

5. Reverse the hand with the back of the fingers now resting on the skin and slide the fingers along the jawline to the chin (*7). (See Fig. 13.6.)

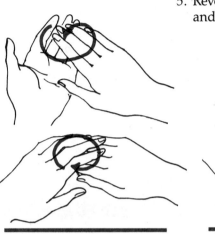

13.4—Distribute the product over both sides of the fingers.

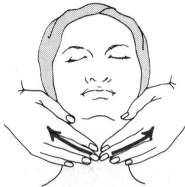

13.5—Start applying the product on the neck.

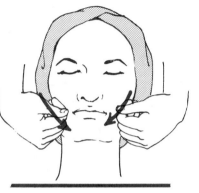

13.6—Slide the fingers along the jawline to the chin.

6. Reverse the hands again and slide the fingers back over the cheeks (*6 and *8), until the pads of the fingers come to rest directly in front of the ears. (See Fig. 13.7.)

7. Reverse the hands again and slide the fingers forward over the cheekbones to the nose. (See Fig. 13.8.)

8. With the pads of the middle fingers, make small circular motions on the flair of the nostrils on each side of the nose. (See Fig. 13.9.)

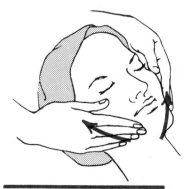

13.7—Slide the fingers back over the cheeks.

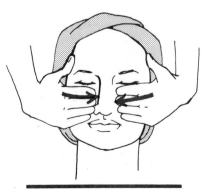

13.8—Slide the fingers forward over the cheekbones to the nose.

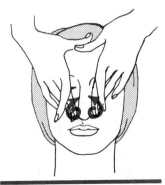

13.9—Use small circular motions on each side of the nose.

9. Slide the fingers up to the forehead (*15) and outward toward the temples (*17 and *19), pausing with a slight pressure on the temples. (See Fig. 13.10.)

10. Bring the left hand over and lift the right eyebrow with the middle and ring fingers. With the middle and ring fingers of the right hand, apply the product to the eyelid with downward strokes. (See Fig. 13.11.)

11. Move the middle and ring fingers of the right hand over to the left side of the face and lift the left eyebrow. With the middle fingers of the left hand, apply the product to the left lid with downward strokes. (See Fig. 13.12.)

12. Repeat steps 4 through 11, three to five times, or until the product is well applied to the face and neck.

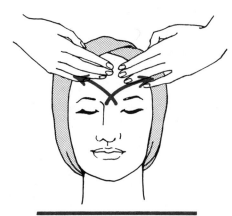

13.10—Slide the fingers up to the forehead.

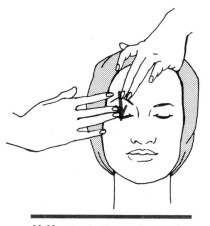

13.11—Apply the product to the right eyelid.

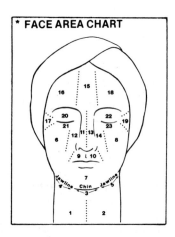

* FACE AREA CHART

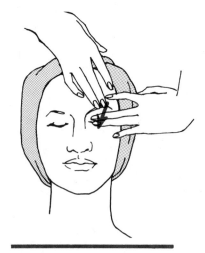

13.12—Apply the product to the left eyelid.

The Cleansing Procedure

Some estheticians prefer to use wet cotton pads when cleansing and working on the face. Others prefer to use facial sponges. Both methods are correct and equally professional. Many estheticians use both methods. For example, an esthetician that usually uses the sponges will use cotton pads when working on an acne skin. In some areas, the professional facial sponges are not readily available, whereas, cotton can be purchased at all drug and variety stores. Supply houses refer to cotton as "beautician's" cotton. Even when using sponges, an esthetician needs some cotton during the treatment for eyepads, extracting blackheads, and the cotton compress mask. (*See Color Plate 16.*)

PROCEDURE FOR REMOVING LIPCOLOR

Before starting the cleansing procedure, the client's lipcolor should be removed. To remove lipcolor, fold a tissue into about three folds and apply a small amount of cleansing lotion to the tissue. Avoid having too much cleanser as it can get into the client's mouth. Start cleansing the lips at the outside corner of the lips and slide the tissue to the center of the lips. Alternate the strokes on both sides of the mouth. Turn the tissue to the clean side and repeat the procedure until all the cleanser is removed and the lips are clean.

PROCEDURE FOR REMOVING CLEANSER WITH A COTTON PAD

1. Starting at the base of the neck, cleanse the neck using upward strokes. Refer to facial chart (*1 and *2). To keep the pad from slipping from the hand, pinch the edge of the pad between the thumb and upper part of the forefinger. It is important that most of the surface of the pad remains in contact with the skin. Do not exert pressure on the hyoid bone (Adam's apple). (See Fig. 13.13.)

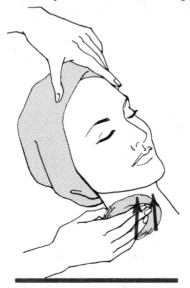

13.13—Cleanse the neck using upward strokes.

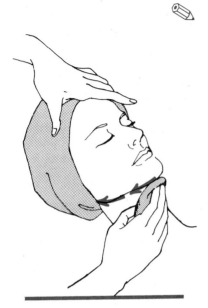

13.14—Cleanse along the jawline.

> **Note:** When cleansing the bearded area of a man's face, the cleansing movements should be done in the direction of the beard growth.

2. Place the pad directly under the chin (*3) and slide the pad along the jawline (*4), stopping directly under the ear. (See Fig. 13.14.)
3. Repeat the movement on the other side of the face (*5). Alternate back and forth three times on each side of the face. (See Fig. 13.15.)
4. Starting at the jawline, use upward movements to cleanse the cheek (*6). (See Fig. 13.16.)
5. Continuing the straight upward movement, cross over the chin (*7) to the left cheek (*8). (See Fig. 13.17.)
6. Continue the cleansing movement with approximately six strokes on each cheek. (See Fig. 13.18.)
7. Cleanse the area directly underneath the nose (*9 and *10). Start at the center and work outward toward the corners of the mouth. Alternate the movements back and forth three times on each side of the face. (See Fig. 13.19.)
8. Starting on the bridge of the nose, cleanse the right side of the nose and the area directly next to it. Use light outward movements (*11 and *12). Repeat the same step on the left side of the nose (*13 and *14). (See Fig. 13.20.)
9. Place the pad flat on the center of the forehead (*15) and slide to the right temple. Apply a slight pressure on the temple. Return the pad to the center of the forehead (*15) and repeat the same step on the left side (*18 and *19). Repeat the movement three times on each side of the forehead. (See Fig. 13.21.)

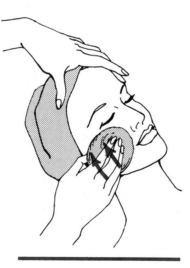

13.15—Repeat the cleansing movement back and forth three times on each side of the face.

13.16—Cleanse the cheek with upward movements.

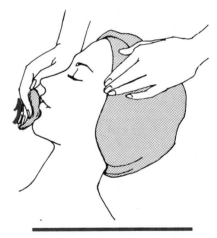

13.17—Cross over the chin to the left cheek and continue cleansing.

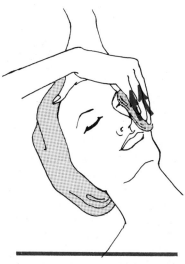

13.18—Continue cleansing, using six strokes on each cheek.

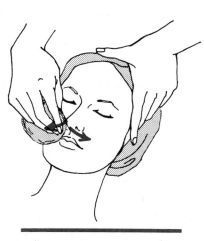

13.19—Cleanse the area directly underneath the nose.

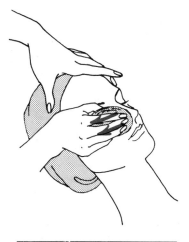

13.20—Cleanse the right and left side of the nose.

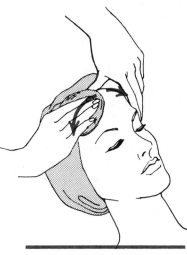

13.21—Cleanse the forehead area.

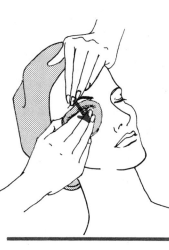

13.22—Cleanse the eyelids and lashes.

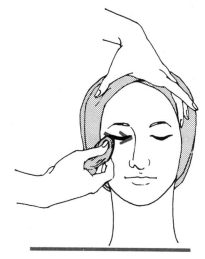

13.23—Cleanse under the lower lashes and eye area.

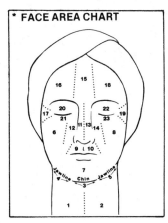

* FACE AREA CHART

10. With the middle and ring fingers of the left hand, lift the eyebrow. Use downward movements with the cleansing pad to cleanse the eyelid and lashes. Repeat this step as often as necessary to remove eye makeup. While cleansing the eyes, rotate the pad to provide a clean, unused surface. (See Fig. 13.22.)

11. Place the edge of the pad under the lower lashes at the outside corner of the eye, and slide the pad toward the inner corner of the eye. The mascara will gradually work loose and can be wiped clean. Be especially gentle when cleansing the eyes, since the skin around the eyes is very sensitive and can become irritated. Repeat steps 10 and 11 on the left eye. (See Fig. 13.23.)

CONVERTING THE COTTON PAD TO FORM CLEANSING MITTS

With the same cotton pad continue as follows:

1. Shake the pad vigorously until it opens to its original square shape. Divide the pad through the center. (See Fig. 13.24.)
2. With the palm of the left hand facing downward, grasp one of the pieces of cotton between the first and middle fingers. (See Fig. 13.25.)
3. Wrap the cotton underneath the first, middle, and ring fingers. Swing the end upward between the ring and little fingers. (See Fig. 13.26.)
4. Secure the end under the middle finger. Be sure the cotton extends beyond the tips of the fingers enough to cover the nails. (See Fig. 13.27.)
5. You should now have a mitt with the clean side of the cotton on the outside. Repeat the same steps with the second piece of cotton on the right hand. You will have two mitts ready for the cleansing procedure. (See Fig. 13.28.)

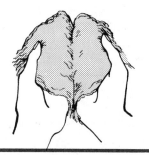

13.24—Divide the pad through the center.

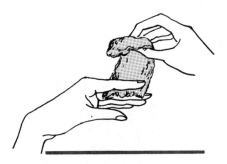

13.25—Grasp the cotton between the first and middle fingers.

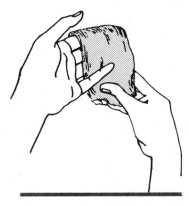

13.26—Wrap the cotton underneath the first, middle, and ring fingers.

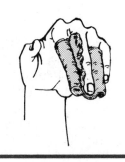

13.27—Secure the end under the middle finger.

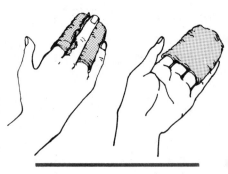

13.28—The finished cotton mitt

**CONTINUE THE
CLEANSING PROCEDURE**

1. Begin a rolling movement upward on the neck (*1 and *2) with one hand following the other. Cleanse one side of the neck then repeat on the other side. Stroke approximately six times on each side of the neck. (See Fig. 13.29.)
2. Position mitts directly underneath the chin (*3). Slide both mitts simultaneously along the underside of the jaw (*4 and *5), stopping at a point directly under the ears. Repeat the movement five times. (See Fig. 13.30.)
3. Start a rolling movement with both hands on the right cheek (*6). Work from a jawline up to the right temple (*17) and gradually move to the corner of the mouth. (See Fig. 13.31.)
4. Continue the rolling movement across the chin (*7) to the left cheek (*8), and repeat the same movement. (See Fig. 13.32.)
5. Cleanse the area directly underneath the nose, both hands working simultaneously, from the center outward, toward the corners of the mouth (*9 and *10). Repeat this movement approximately five times. (See Fig. 13.33.)

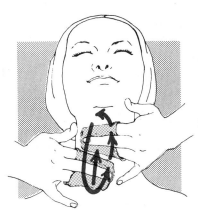

13.29—Rolling movement upward on the neck

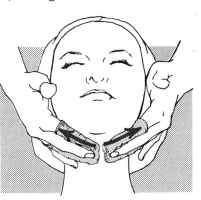

13.30—Movement along the underside of the jaw

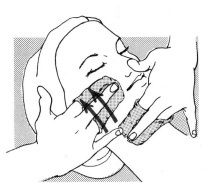

13.31—Rolling movement with both hands on the right cheek

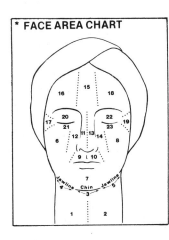

* FACE AREA CHART

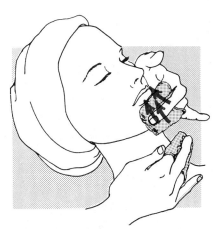

13.32—Rolling movement across the chin

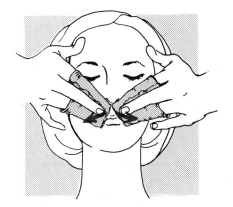

13.33—Cleanse the area directly underneath the nose.

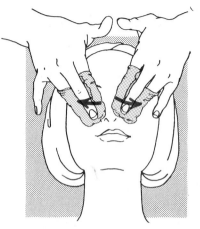

13.34—Cleanse the sides of the nose and the area directly alongside of the nose.

6. With both hands working in outward movements, cleanse the sides of the nose and the area directly alongside of the nose (*11, *12, *13, and *14). Repeat the movement five times. (See Fig. 13.34.)
7. Start a rolling motion, hand over hand, in the center of the forehead (*15). Gradually move over the forehead toward the right temple (*17). Continue the rolling movement back across the forehead to the left temple (*19), then continue back to the center of the forehead and stop. (See Fig. 13.35.)
8. Lift the right brow with the left mitt and cleanse the eyelid and lashes. Gently use downward movements, three to five times. (See Fig. 13.36.)
9. Cleanse underneath the eye (*21), working from the outside corner of the eye toward the nose. (See Figs. 13.37 and 13.38.) Either of the hand positions shown here are considered correct. Use the position that is most comfortable.
10. Repeat the above procedure on the left eye using the right mitt to lift the brow.
11. Discard cotton mitts.

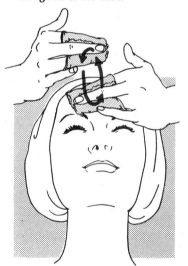

13.35—Rolling movement across the forehead

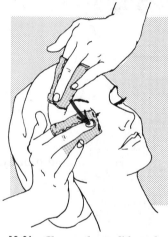

13.36—Cleanse the eyelids and lashes.

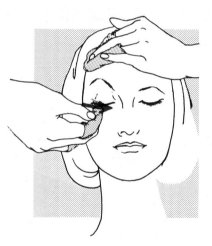

13.37—Cleanse underneath the eye.

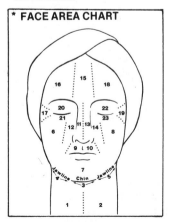

* FACE AREA CHART

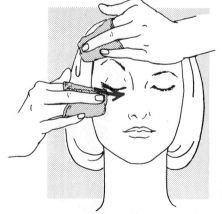

13.38—The movement starts from the outside corner of the eye moving toward the nose.

PROCEDURE FOR CLEANSING THE FACE WITH SPONGES

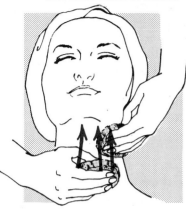

13.39—Rolling movement upward on the neck

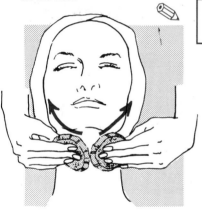

13.40—Position sponges under chin.

During the treatment, keep the sponges in a small basin of lukewarm water. The basin can be glass, metal, or plastic. It must be placed within reach of the esthetician, usually on a shelf, utility table, or cart where the treatment products are kept. Some utility tables have a swing-out basin, which is used to rinse the cleanser and other products from the sponges. Sometime during the facial treatment, when it will not interrupt the steady progress of the treatment, replace the water with fresh water. The best time to do this is while the client is having his or her face vaporized or while a warm moist towel is being applied. Another good time to change the water is while the mask is on. The following is the procedure for cleansing the face with sponges:

1. Begin with a rolling movement upward on the neck (*1 and *2) with one hand following the other. Cleanse one side of the neck, then repeat on the other side. Stroke approximately six times on each side of the neck. (See Fig. 13.39.)

> **Note:** When cleansing the bearded area of a man's face, the cleansing movements should be done in the direction of the beard growth.

2. Position sponges directly underneath the chin (*3). (See Fig. 13.40.) Slide both sponges (simultaneously) along the underside of the jaw (*4 and *5), stopping at a point directly under the ears. (See Fig. 13.41.) Repeat the movement five times.
3. Start a rolling movement with both hands on the right cheek (*6). Work from the jawline up to the right temple (*17), and gradually move to the corner of the mouth. (See Fig. 13.42.)
4. Continue the rolling movement across the chin (*7) and repeat the same movement on the left cheek (*8). (See Fig. 13.43.)

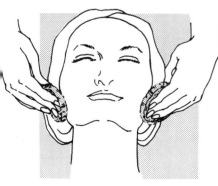

13.41—Slide sponges along the underside of the jaw.

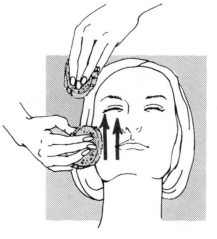

13.42—Rolling movement starting on the right cheek

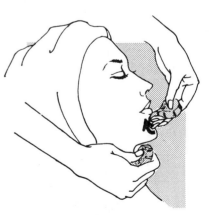

13.43—Rolling movement across the chin and moving to the left cheek

5. With both hands working simultaneously, cleanse the area directly underneath the nose, from the center outward, toward the corners of the mouth (*9 and *10). Repeat this movement approximately five times. (See Fig. 13.44.)

6. With both hands working in outward movements, cleanse the sides of the nose and the area directly alongside the nose (*11, *12, *13, and *14). Repeat the movement five times. (See Fig. 13.45.)

7. Start a rolling motion, hand over hand, in the center of the forehead (*15). Gradually move over the forehead toward the right temple (*17). Continue the rolling movement across the forehead to the left temple (*19), then continue back to the center of the forehead and stop. (See Fig. 13.46.)

8. Lift the right brow with the left sponge and cleanse the eyelid and lashes. Gently use downward movements, three to five times, or until all eye shadow and liner is removed. (See Fig. 13.47.)

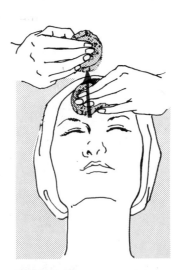

13.44—Cleanse the area directly underneath the nose.

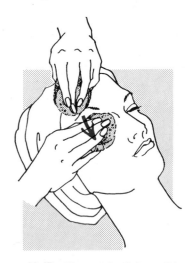

13.45—Cleanse the sides of the nose and the area directly alongside the nose.

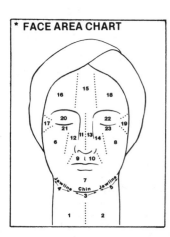

* FACE AREA CHART

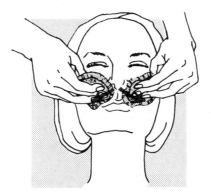

13.46—Rolling movement across the forehead

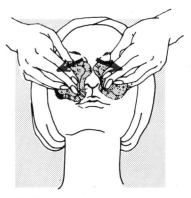

13.47—Cleanse the right eyelid and lashes.

9. Cleanse underneath the eye (*21), working from the outside corner toward the nose. (See Fig. 13.48.)
10. Repeat the above procedure on the left eye. (See Figs. 13.49 and 13.50.)

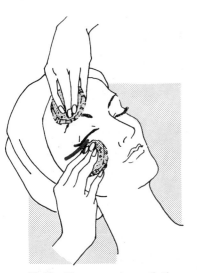

13.48—Cleanse underneath the right eye.

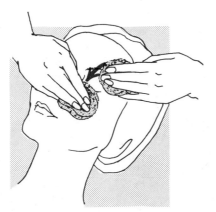

13.49—Cleanse the left eyelid and lashes.

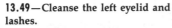

13.50—Cleanse underneath the left eye.

The Cotton Compress Mask

The cotton compress mask has been used for removing the treatment mask in facial treatments for many years. An article entitled, "A Scientific Facial for the Matron," from a 1938 *Modern Beauty Shop Magazine*, describes how a large piece of cotton is dipped in water, wrung out, divided into sections and placed over the treatment mask, completely covering the face with the exception of the nostrils and mouth. It also describes how squares of ice are used to massage the entire face with a quick rotary motion. Following the ice massage, the cotton compresses are used to remove the mask. (See Fig. 13.51.) In another part of the treatment, the article describes how wet cotton is folded to form a "patter" with which the face is patted or slapped lightly all over to relax any tight facial feelings. (See Fig. 13.52.)

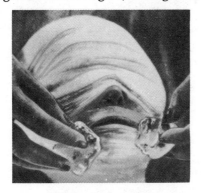

13.51—Ice massage

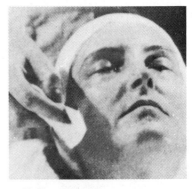

13.52—The "patter" movement

**HOW TO APPLY THE
COTTON COMPRESS MASK**

1. Unfold the folded cotton strip and carefully divide it lengthwise into three separate strips. Try to keep the thickness of each strip as even as possible. (See Fig. 13.53.)
2. Secure pads on the client's eyes. Take the strip that feels the thinnest and mold it to the client's neck. Be sure the strip does not overlap on the underside of the chin and jawline. (See Fig. 13.54.)

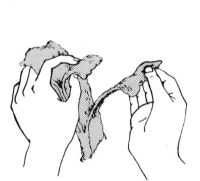

13.53—Separate cotton into three strips.

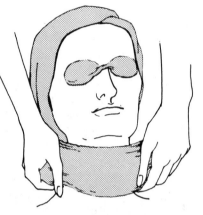

13.54—Mold the thinnest strip to the client's neck.

3. Take the second strip of cotton (save the thickest piece for last) and place the center of the cotton on the chin and under the lower lip. (See Fig. 13.55.)
4. Carefully, but firmly, mold the cotton under the jaw, chin, and lower part of the cheeks. (See Fig. 13.56.)

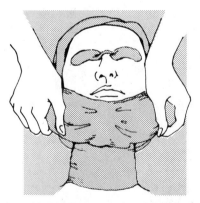

13.55—Place the second strip (not the thickest) on the chin.

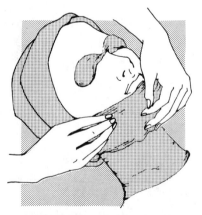

13.56—Mold the strip under the jaw, chin, and lower part of the cheeks.

5. Take the third and thickest cotton strip and place it over the upper portion of the face (eyepads remain in place) and carefully stretch the cotton. (See Fig. 13.57.)
6. Stretch the cotton carefully as you pull and mold it to fit the facial contours. (See Fig. 13.58.)
7. Take the cotton covering the tip of nose and pull it down until it tears, forming a thin strip to be placed over the area between the nose and upper lip. (See Fig. 13.59.)
8. This is the completed mask showing the face and neck covered, with the exception of the nostrils and the mouth. (See Fig. 13.60.) (*See Color Plate 17.*)

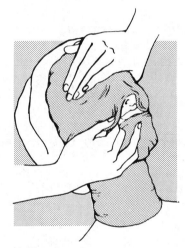

13.57—Place the thickest strip over the upper portion of the face.

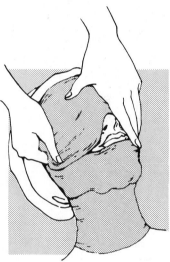

13.58—Mold the strip to fit the facial contours.

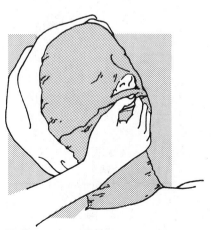

13.59—Create a thin strip between the nose and upper lip.

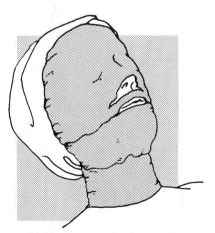

13.60—The completed mask

HOW THE COMPRESS IS USED TO REMOVE A TREATMENT MASK

1. Massage over the surface of the compress mask with an ice cube (if available), using rotary movements. The ice will feel cool and refreshing. It will also firm the skin and temporarily close the follicles. As the ice melts, the water will seep into the compress, helping to soften the treatment mask underneath. (See Fig. 13.61.)
2. Starting on the upper part of the face, place the hands, palms down, on each side of the face. Begin to slide both the left hand and the cotton compress strip slowly toward the right side of the face. Concentrate on picking up as much of the treatment mask as possible. The eyepads will come off at the same time and should be discarded. Fold the strip in half so that the side of the compress that has the treatment mask on it is inside, and the compress strip has two clean surfaces. Squeeze the cotton over a waste container to remove any excess water. (See Fig. 13.62.)
3. Tear this piece of cotton down the center. (See Fig. 13.63.)
4. Form cotton cleansing mitts over the fingers. (See procedure for making cotton mitts, on page 198.) (See Fig. 13.64.)
5. Use the cotton mitts to further remove the remaining traces of the mask. If necessary, clean cotton mitts can be made by reversing the same cotton mitt. (See Fig. 13.65.)
6. When all traces of the treatment mask have been removed, move down to the next cotton compress strip and repeat the same steps. (See Fig. 13.66.)
7. Repeat the same movements on the neck using the third cotton compress strip. (See Fig. 13.67.)

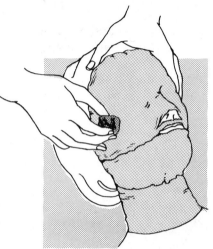

13.61—Massage the surface of the mask with an ice cube.

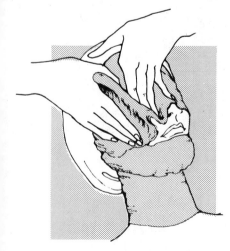

13.62—Start to remove the upper portion of the mask.

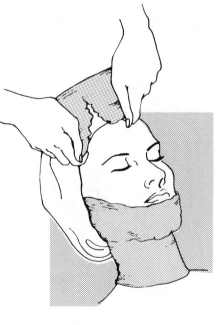

13.63—Tear the removed portion in half.

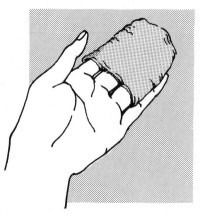

13.64—Form cleansing mitts with removed portions.

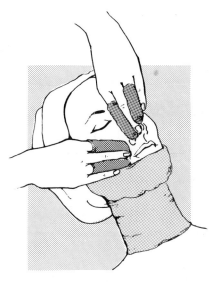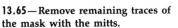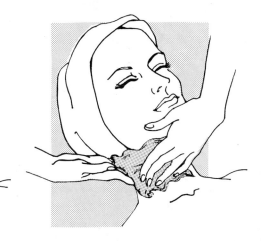

13.65—Remove remaining traces of the mask with the mitts.

13.66—Working downward, remove the next cotton compress.

13.67—Remove the remaining cotton compress.

QUESTIONS   DISCUSSION AND REVIEW

CLEANSING THE SKIN

1. What type of cleansing lotion is preferred for the cleansing procedure?
2. How does the facial chart for cleansing help the esthetician?
3. What are two of the preferred materials used when cleansing the face?
4. How would you remove lipcolor from your client?
5. Discuss the correct way to remove eye makeup.
6. Should you use cold water when removing cleansing products? Explain.
7. Should you change the water during the facial?
8. When is the cotton compress used?

Techniques for Professional Massage

LEARNING OBJECTIVES

After completing this chapter, you should be able to:

❶ Describe the benefits of massage.
❷ Explain the different types of massage.
❸ Describe and locate the different nerves and muscles of the face and neck.
❹ Demonstrate hand exercises for the esthetician.
❺ Define and demonstrate the different massage movements.
❻ Explain and demonstrate the purpose and procedure of massage #1, massage #2 and the Dr. Jacquet movements.

INTRODUCTION

The facial massage is one of the most beneficial and pleasing steps in facial treatments. The client enjoys the relaxation and stimulation that results from the massage and benefits from the soothing effects of the creams and lotions that are used to cleanse and refresh the skin.

Massage is essential to facial treatments because it benefits the client both physically and psychologically. Various techniques are used in salons. With practice, the professional esthetician will become proficient in giving the best massage for the client's individual needs. Massage should never be too prolonged, too deep, nor given when it is not beneficial to the client.

The following beneficial results may be obtained by proper facial massage:

1. Massage nourishes the skin and all its structures, by stimulating blood circulation. Blood brings oxygen, which is essential to cell growth, to the cells and carries away waste products and carbon dioxide, thereby helping to cleanse the skin of impurities.
2. Massage reduces fat cells in the subcutaneous tissue. This helps firm the skin and underlying tissue.
3. Massage promotes warmth by increasing the blood supply and circulation. It increases the secretion of sebum (oil) and perspiration,

which in turn open the pores. Waste products, dirt, grease, and other impurities are then easier to remove.

4. Massage makes the skin softer and more pliable. It tones muscles and retards aging of the skin.

5. Massage manipulations can help deplete excess fluids in the tissues and reduce puffy or sagging areas.

6. Massage strengthens, nourishes, and tones muscle fiber.

7. Massage soothes and rests the nerves. The client feels renewed, invigorated, and pleased with the physical results of the facial massage.

8. Massage improves the appearance of the skin. It increases the production of sebum, which helps to maintain the moisture content of the cells. The moisture helps the skin retain a dewy, youthful look and improves its texture.

9. Massage sometimes relieves pain by helping tense muscles relax.

10. Massage loosens and helps to clear away dead surface cells and other debris, revealing the healthier skin underneath.

To obtain proper results from a facial massage, the esthetician must have a thorough knowledge of all the structures involved: the muscles, nerves, and blood vessels. (Fig. 14.1)

A KNOWLEDGE OF NEURO-MUSCULAR ANATOMY IS NECESSARY IN ORDER TO LOCATE THE AREAS OVERLYING MUSCLE MOTOR POINTS AND THE REGIONS WHERE MOTOR NERVES ARE SUFFICIENTLY NEAR THE SURFACE OF THE SKIN TO BE STIMULATED.

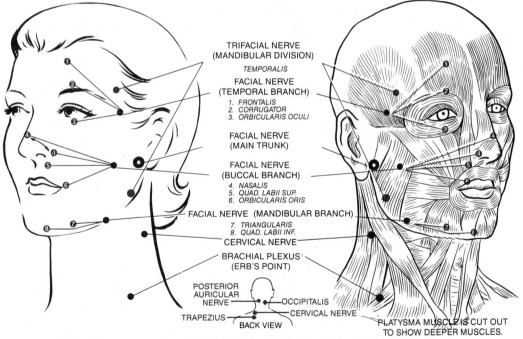

TRIFACIAL NERVE
(MANDIBULAR DIVISION)

TEMPORALIS

FACIAL NERVE
(TEMPORAL BRANCH)

1. FRONTALIS
2. CORRUGATOR
3. ORBICULARIS OCULI

FACIAL NERVE
(MAIN TRUNK)

FACIAL NERVE
(BUCCAL BRANCH)

4. NASALIS
5. QUAD. LABII SUP.
6. ORBICULARIS ORIS

FACIAL NERVE (MANDIBULAR BRANCH)

7. TRIANGULARIS
8. QUAD. LABII INF.

CERVICAL NERVE

BRACHIAL PLEXUS
(ERB'S POINT)

POSTERIOR
AURICULAR
NERVE

OCCIPITALIS

CERVICAL NERVE

TRAPEZIUS

BACK VIEW

PLATYSMA MUSCLE IS CUT OUT
TO SHOW DEEPER MUSCLES.

14.1—Motor nerve points of the face and neck. To obtain the maximum benefits from a facial massage, the esthetician must consider the motor nerve points that affect the underlying muscles of the face and neck.

Almost every muscle and nerve has a motor point. The position of motor points will vary in location on individuals due to differences in body structure. However, a few manipulations on the right motor points will readily induce relaxation at the beginning of the massage treatment.

Skillfully applied, massage influences the structures and functions of the body, either directly or indirectly. The immediate effects of massage are first noticed on the skin. The part being massaged responds by a more active circulation, secretion, nutrition, and excretion.

Types of Massage

There are many different types of massage, based on both body structure and body energy. *Swedish massage* manipulates deep muscle tissues by a series of massage movements. Most massage movements given during a facial massage are based on these techniques.

Accupressure massage works with accupressure points on the body. *Shiatsu* combines stretching of limbs with pressure on accupressure points. Many of the motor points on the face and neck are accupressure points and respond to manipulation by the esthetician. Some of these techniques are also used during a facial massage.

Reflexology is a form of therapeutic massage that manipulates areas on the hands and feet. Although not a part of a facial massage, this type of massage may be useful in the salon as an added service.

Aromatherapy massage uses essential oils, which penetrate the skin during massage movements. These oils may be used during facial massage.

Lymphatic drainage massage uses gentle pressure on the lymphatic system to move waste materials out of the body more quickly.

Most facial massages combine techniques from many of these types of massage to benefit the client.

 Note: Also see Chapter 23 for further discussion on some of these advanced topics.

Hand Exercises for the Esthetician

The esthetician's hands should be flexible and relaxed, yet strong, controlled, and supple. Hand mobility is important in maintaining a regular rhythm and regulating the pressure of hand movements. Hand exercises help the esthetician maintain control of the hands when doing fast or slow movements. Exercises for flexibility let the esthetician work on the contours of the face with gentle movements.

The following exercises should be done everyday to improve hand mobility:

1. Hold hands at chest level and shake vigorously for about twenty-five counts. This exercise limbers and warms the hands and increases circulation. (See Fig. 14.2.)

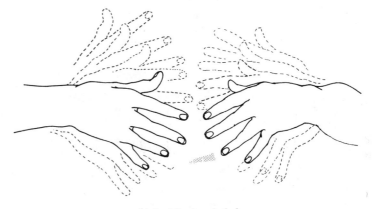

14.2—The hand shake

2. Hold hands at chest level with fists clinched. Pretend that you are holding a small ball in the palm of your hands. Make a fist, squeezing as hard as you can, while counting to five. Now throw the ball away, spreading the fingers wide as you count to five. Repeat the exercise 10 to 20 times. This exercise is excellent for strengthening the hands and wrists. (See Fig. 14.3.)

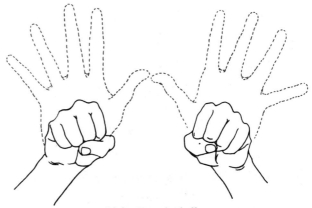

14.3—Toss the ball

3. Place both hands palms down on a flat surface. Start with the thumbs and count each finger from thumb to little finger, as it is tapped in rhythm. Count 1, 2, 3, 4, 5. Then starting with the little finger tap each finger to the count of 5, 4, 3, 2, 1. This exercise is similar to playing a piano and is especially good for building coordination and hand control. (See Fig. 14.4.)

4. Place palms together at chest level. Keep them together as you bend the left wrist as far back as it will go; then do the same with the right wrist. Keep bending the wrists in rhythm for 20 counts. This exercise strengthens the hands and wrists and makes them more flexible. (See Fig. 14.5.)

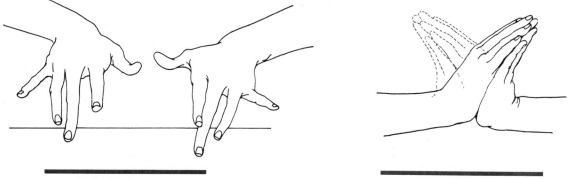

14.4—Playing piano

14.5—Palm press

5. Starting with the thumb of the left hand, massage all the fingers on that hand. The massage is done by rubbing each finger from the knuckles to the tip, one by one, until the fingers have been thoroughly massaged. Repeat exercise with the right hand. This exercise stimulates circulation, warms the hands, and keeps them supple. (See Fig. 14.6.)

6. Hold the clenched hands at chest level and rotate in circular movements at the wrists for 20 counts. Reverse the rotating movements for 20 counts. This exercise limbers and strengthens the wrists. (See Fig. 14.7.)

14.6—Massage the fingers.

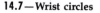

14.7—Wrist circles

POSTURE   It is important to maintain correct posture during hand movements so that the hands and arms can move freely. When standing, a basic stance with one foot placed slightly ahead of the other, knees slightly bent, will improve balance and prevent fatigue.

Practicing Facial Massage

There are a number of ways to practice facial massage when first learning the massage movements. When learning to give massages, it is necessary to practice until you acquire the right touch and finger dexterity. Although in the classroom students practice massage movements on one another, there are times when you may want to practice at home outside of class time. The following exercises will help you perfect your massage techniques.

1. Practice massage movements on a mannequin head that is anchored to a wig block clamp. This can be done in front of a mirror, such as at a comb-out or makeup station, so you can study the movements by looking at the reflection in the mirror. (See Fig. 14.8.)
2. Practice on a styrofoam wig block. It is important that the styrofoam block show facial features. Styrofoam blocks are inexpensive and may be found at most beauty supply or variety stores. Hold the head in your lap, as this type of wig block will break under the pressure of a wig block clamp. (See Fig. 14.9.)
3. Practice on your knee. Anytime you have a few minutes to practice massage movements, you can practice on your knee. Although the knee is smaller than a face, it is still possible to practice the movements effectively. (See Fig. 14.10.)
4. When practicing massage movements for the chest, shoulders, and back, stand behind a chair and use the back of the chair to practice the movements. When the routine gets to the neck, proceed with techniques 1, 2, or 3. (See Fig. 14.11.)

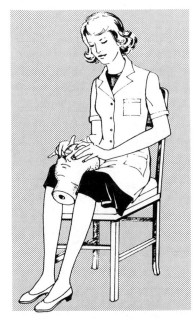

14.8—Practice on a mannequin head.

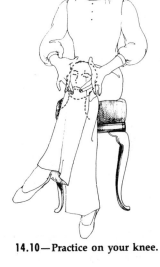

14.9—Practice on a wig block.

14.10—Practice on your knee.

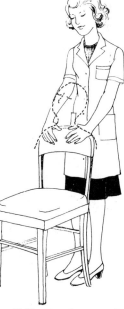

14.11—Practice on a chair.

> **Note:** Products such as cleansers, astringents, and massage creams are not used when practicing, but should be used when working on a client or student. Use cotton pads or sponges that have been moistened in water only.

Manipulative Movements of Massage

Every massage treatment utilizes one or more of the basic massage movements. Each manipulation is applied in a definite way, for a particular purpose, according to the condition of the skin and the desired results. The result of a massage treatment will depend on the amount of pressure, direction of movement, and the duration of each type of manipulation.

▶ > **Caution:** Do not give a massage when certain conditions exist, such as inflamed and swollen joints, glandular swelling, abrasions of the skin, or diseased skin.

There are five basic movements used in massage: *effleurage*, *petrissage*, *friction*, *tapotement*, and *vibration*.

EFFLEURAGE (STROKING MOVEMENT)

Effleurage (ef-loo-**RAHZH**) is a light, continuous movement applied to the skin with the fingers (digital) and palms (palmar) in a slow and rhythmic manner. Over large surfaces, use the palm. Over small surfaces, use the cushions of the fingertips. Effleurage is frequently applied to the forehead, face, scalp, back, shoulders, neck, chest, arms, and hands for its soothing and relaxing effects. Massage movements are usually directed toward the origin of muscles to avoid damage to muscular tissues. (*See Color Plate 18.*)

For the correct position for stroking, slightly curve the fingers with just the cushions of the fingertips touching the skin. Do not use the end of the fingertips for massage movements: Fingertips cannot control the degree of pressure. Also, the free edges of the fingernails are likely to scratch the skin (Figs. 14.12 and 14.13).

For the correct position of the palms for stroking, hold the whole hand loosely. Keep the wrist and fingers flexible and curve the fingers to conform to the shape of the area being massaged (Fig. 14.14).

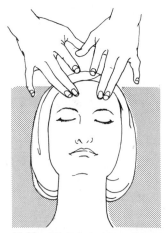

14.12—Digital stroking of face

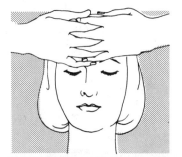

14.13—Digital stroking of forehead

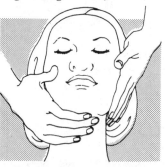

14.14—Palmar stroking of face

PETRISSAGE (KNEADING MOVEMENT)

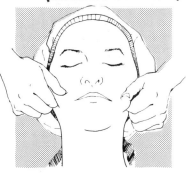

14.15—Digital kneading of cheeks

Petrissage (pay-tri-**SAHZH**) is a kneading movement in which the skin and flesh are grasped between the thumb and forefinger. As the tissues are lifted from their underlying structures, they are squeezed, rolled, or pinched with a light, firm pressure. This is the primary manipulation in the Dr. Jacquet movement.

The pressure should be light but firm. When grasping and releasing the fleshy parts of the face, maintain a smooth, rhythmic movement (Fig. 14.15). Kneading movements give deeper stimulation, improve circulation, and invigorate the part being treated. They also help empty the oil ducts.

Fulling is a form of petrissage, used mainly in massage of the arms. With the fingers of both hands grasping the arm, apply a kneading movement over the flesh. The kneading movement must be used with light pressure on the underside of the client's forearm and on the upper arm.

FRICTION (DEEP RUBBING MOVEMENT)

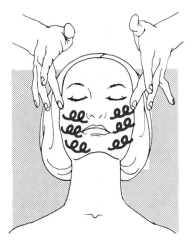

14.16—Circular friction of face

Friction maintains pressure on the skin, while the fingers or palms are moved over the underlying structures. Friction has a marked influence on the circulation and glandular activity of the skin. Circular friction movements are usually employed on the scalp, arms, and hands (Fig. 14.16). Lighter circular friction movements are generally used on the face and neck.

Chucking, *rolling*, and *wringing* are variations of friction movements, employed principally to massage the arms. The chucking movement is accomplished by grasping the flesh firmly in one hand and moving the hand up and down along the bone, while the other hand keeps the arm in a steady position.

The rolling movement requires that the tissues be compressed firmly against the bone and twisted around the arm. Both hands of the esthetician are active as the flesh is twisted down the arm in the same direction.

Wringing is a vigorous movement in which the esthetician's hands are placed a little distance apart on both sides of the arm. While the hands are working downward, the flesh is twisted against the bones in opposite directions (Fig. 14.17).

14.17—Wringing movement of arm

TAPOTEMENT (PERCUSSION MOVEMENT)

Tapotement (tah-**POT**-ment) or *percussion* (per-**KUSH**-un) consists of tapping, slapping, and hacking movements. This form of massage is the most stimulating. It should be applied with care and discretion.

In facial massage, only light digital *tapping* is used. The fingertips are brought down against the skin in rapid succession. The fingers must be flexible to create an even force over the area being treated (Fig. 14.18).

Slapping and *hacking* movements are used to massage the back, shoulders, and arms. In slapping movements, keep the wrists flexible so the palms come in contact with the skin in light, firm, and rapid slapping movements. One hand follows the other. With each slapping stroke (which must be nothing more than a firm, light, and quick contact with the skin), lift the flesh slightly (Fig. 14.19).

Hacking movements use the wrists and outer edges of the hands. Both the wrists and fingers must move in fast, light, firm, flexible motions against the skin in alternate succession.

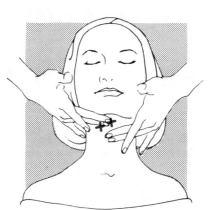

14.18—Tapping under chin

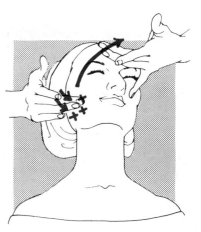

14.19—Light slapping and lifting on cheek

VIBRATION (SHAKING MOVEMENT)

Vibration is accomplished by rapid muscular contractions in the arms of the esthetician, while the balls of the fingertips are pressed firmly on the point of application. It is a highly stimulating movement. Use it sparingly and never for more than a few seconds duration on any one spot. Muscular contractions can also be produced with a mechanical vibrator (Fig. 14.20).

JOINT MOVEMENTS

Joint movements are restricted to the massage of the arm and hand. These movements are applied either with or without resistance (Fig. 14.21).

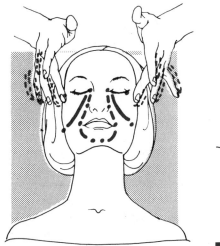

14.20—Vibratory movement of face

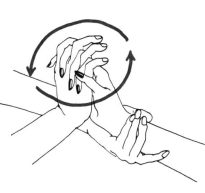

14.21—Joint movements

Massage Techniques

There are several acceptable methods of facial massage. These include the procedures that are shown in this textbook; the manipulations that appear in *Milady's Standard Textbook of Cosmetology* and *Milady's Van Dean Manual*; and procedures developed by your instructor.

The specific manipulations used and the number of times that each massage movement is repeated may depend on several factors, such as the condition of the skin and the amount of time the esthetician would like the massage to last. The massage routine is usually longer in treatments given without the aid of machines.

Rest and relaxation are brought about by giving light but firm, slow, rhythmic movements, or very slow, light hand vibrations over the motor points for a very short time. Another technique is to pause briefly and use light pressure over the motor points.

Stimulation of body tissues is brought about by movements of moderate pressure, speed, and time, or by light hand vibrations of moderate speed and time.

Reduction of body contours or fatty tissues are brought about by firm kneading or fast, firm, but light slapping movements over a fairly long period of time. Moderately fast hand vibrations with firm pressure will also accomplish this reduction.

In giving facial manipulations, remember that an even tempo, or rhythm, induces relaxation. Do not stop or interrupt the massage once the manipulations have been started. Should it become necessary to remove the hands from the client, feather them off the face and then very gently replace them with feather-like movements.

The frequency of facial massage depends on the condition of the skin, the age of the client, and the condition to be treated. As a general rule, normal skin can be kept in excellent condition with a facial treatment with massage once or twice a month, accompanied by the proper home care.

Therapeutic lamps, high-frequency current, and vaporizers may be used in conjunction with massage. See Chapter 18 for a discussion of machines used in skin care.

MASSAGE TIPS
1. Help the client relax.
2. Provide a quiet, comfortable atmosphere. Speak in a well-modulated and soft tone of voice.
3. Maintain a clean, orderly arrangement of supplies.
4. Follow a systematic procedure.
5. Be sure your fingernails are kept well cared for with no rough edges to scratch the client's face during the treatment.
6. If your hands are cold, warm them before touching the client's face.
7. Project professionalism in everything you do and say in the presence of the client.
8. Make every client feel that you are giving the best massage for his or her individual needs, and answer all questions in a friendly, professional manner (Fig. 14.22).

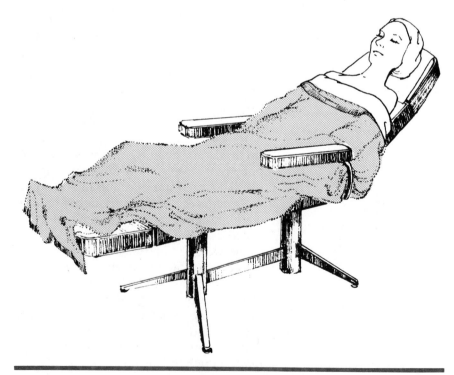

14.22—Client prepared for facial massage

Develop the following qualities:

1. A firm, sure touch that inspires confidence in the client
2. Strong, flexible hands for application of the various massage movements
3. Self-discipline and time organization
4. An understanding of human psychology

Keep the hands soft by using creams, oils, and lotions. Bevel nails until smooth to prevent scratching of the client's skin. Keep the wrists flexible and the palms warm and dry.

Use a spatula to apply one teaspoon of massage cream to your fingertips. Place your palms together and rotate your hands in a circular movement to distribute the cream over the entire surface of the hands. Place your hands palms down on the center upper part of the client's chest. Slide the hands outward toward the shoulders, then around the shoulders to the upper back and up to the neck. Repeat this movement three or four times until the treatment cream is applied evenly. Distribute ½ teaspoon of the cream to the fingers and apply it to the front of the neck and face, using the basic product application method.

The Standard Massage*

1. Linear movement over forehead: Slide fingers to temples. Rotate with pressure on upward stroke. Slide to left eyebrow, then stroke up to hairline gradually moving hands across forehead to right eyebrow. (See Fig. 14.23.)
2. Circular movement over forehead: Starting at eyebrow line, work across middle of forehead, and then toward the hairline. (See Fig. 14.24.)
3. Criss-cross movement: Start at one side of forehead and work back. (See Fig. 14.25.)

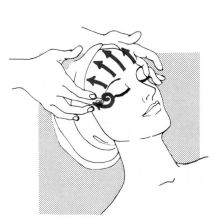

14.23—Linear movement over forehead

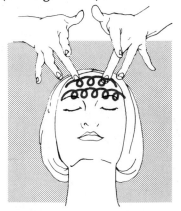

14.24—Circular movement over forehead

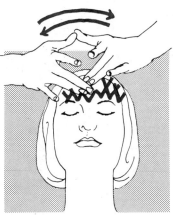

14.25—Criss-cross movement

* The STANDARD MASSAGE has been reprinted from the STANDARD TEXTBOOK OF COSMETOLOGY and the VAN DEAN manual. Those instructors and students who have previously mastered the routine may wish to continue its use.

4. Chin movement: Lift chin, using a slight pressure. (See Fig. 14.26.)
5. Lower cheek movement: Use circular movement from chin to ear and rotate. (See Fig. 14.27.)
6. Mouth, nose, and cheek movements. (See Fig. 14.28.)
7. Stroking (headache) movement: Slide fingers to center of forehead, then draw fingers, with slight pressure, toward temples, and rotate. (See Fig. 14.29.)
8. Brow and eye movement: Place middle fingers at inner corners of eyes and index fingers over brows. Slide to outer corners of eyes, under eyes, and back to inner corners. (See Fig. 14.30.)
9. Nose and upper cheek movement: Slide fingers down nose. Apply rotary movement across cheeks to temples, and rotate gently. Slide fingers under eyes and back to bridge of nose. (See Fig. 14.31.)
10. Mouth and nose movement: Apply circular movement from corners of mouth up sides of nose. Slide fingers over brows and down to corners of mouth. (See Fig. 14.32.)

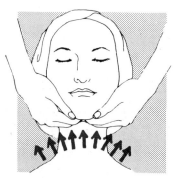

14.26—Chin movement

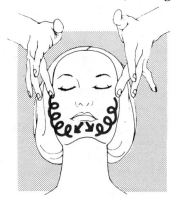

14.27—Lower cheek movement

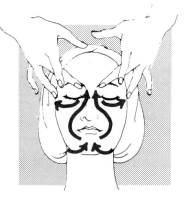

14.28—Mouth, nose, and cheek movements

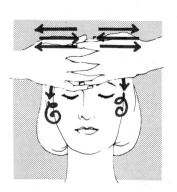

14.29—Stroking (headache) movement

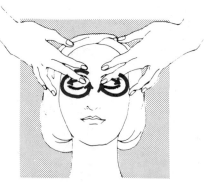

14.30—Brow and eye movement

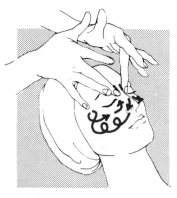

14.31—Nose and upper cheek movement

11. Lip and chin movement: Draw fingers from center of upper lip, around mouth, going under lower lip and chin. (See Fig. 14.33.)
12. Optional movement: Hold head with left hand; draw fingers of right hand from under the lower lip, around mouth, to center of upper lip. (See Fig. 14.34.)
13. Lifting movement of cheeks: Proceed from the mouth to ears, and then from nose to top part of ears. (See Fig. 14.35.)
14. Rotary movement of cheeks: Massage from chin to ear lobes, from mouth to middle of ears, and from nose to top of ears. (See Fig. 14.36.)
15. Light tapping movement: Work from chin to earlobe, mouth to ear, nose to top of ear, and then across forehead. Repeat on other side. (See Fig. 14.37.)

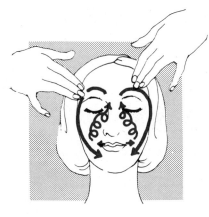

14.32—Mouth and nose movement

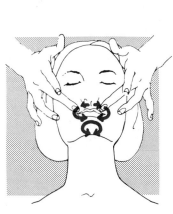

14.33—Lip and chin movement

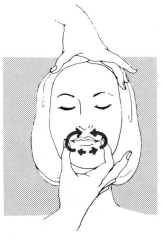

14.34—Optional movement

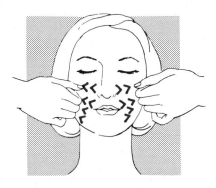

14.35—Lifting movement of cheeks

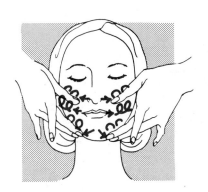

14.36—Rotary movement of cheeks

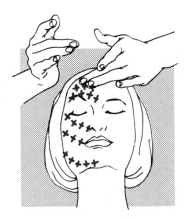

14.37—Light tapping movement

16. Stroking movement of neck: Apply light upward strokes over front of neck. Use heavier pressure on sides of neck in downward strokes. (See Fig. 14.38.)

17. Circular movement over neck and chest: Starting at back of ears, apply circular movement down side of neck, over shoulders, and across chest. (See Fig. 14.39.)

18. Infra-red lamp (optional): Protect eyes with eye pads. Adjust lamp over client's face, leave on for about five minutes. (See Fig. 14.40.)

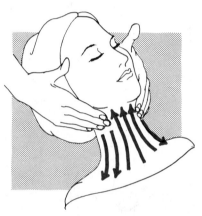

14.38—Stroking movement of neck

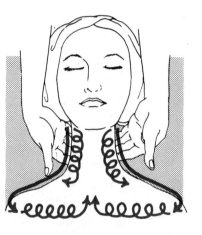

14.39—Circular movement over neck and chest

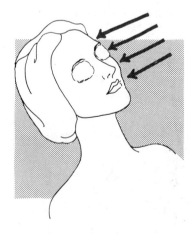

14.40—Infra-red lamp (optional)

CHEST, BACK, AND NECK MANIPULATIONS (OPTIONAL)

Some instructors prefer to treat these areas first before starting the regular facial. A suggested procedure is as follows:

1. Apply and remove cleansing cream.
2. Apply massage cream.
3. Give manipulations as outlined below.
4. Chest and back movement: Use rotary movement across chest and shoulders, then to spine. Slide fingers to base of neck. Rotate three times. (See Fig. 14.41.)
5. Shoulders and back movement: Rotate shoulders three times. Glide fingers to spine, then to base of neck. Apply circular movement up to back of ear, and then slide fingers to front of earlobe. Rotate three times. (See Fig. 14.42.)
6. Back massage (optional): To stimulate and relax client, use thumbs and bent index fingers to grasp the tissue at the back of the neck. Rotate six times. Repeat over shoulders and back to the spine. (See Fig. 14.43.)
7. Remove cream with tissues or warm, moist towel.
8. Dust the back lightly with talcum powder and smooth.

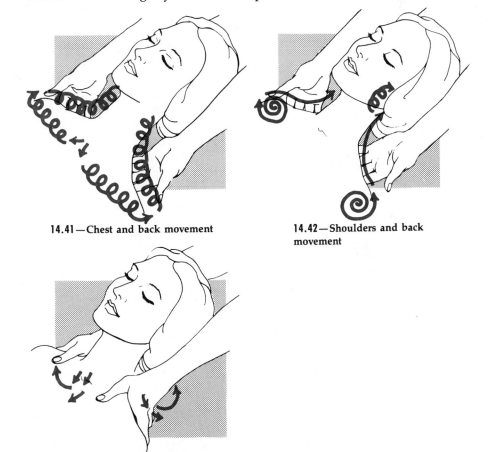

14.41—Chest and back movement

14.42—Shoulders and back movement

14.43—Back massage (optional)

Massage Number 1

Massage #1 was developed for use by estheticians and has been thoroughly salon-tested. The sequence of movements in this massage permits a smooth and graceful flow of one movement into another.

The main purpose of Massage #1 is to continue the cleansing process, help remove dead surface cells, and increase blood circulation. Massage cream that is not formulated to penetrate the skin is used for this massage. (Cold cream may be used when massage cream is not available.) Deep penetrating creams should not be used in this massage procedure because they would act as vehicles to carry dirt and makeup deeper into the pores. Massage #1 is done after the skin has been vaporized or towel steamed, as the steam will not penetrate through the massage cream. Apply the massage cream to the face, but not to the eyelids.

PROCEDURE FOR MASSAGE #1

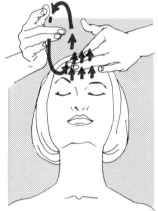

14.44—Linear movement over forehead

1. With the middle and ring fingers of each hand, start upward strokes in the middle of the forehead at the browline. Working upward toward the hairline, one hand follows the other as the hands move toward the right temple. This same movement is continued, moving back across the forehead to the left temple, then back to the center of the forehead. Repeat the movements three to five times. (See Fig. 14.44.)

2. With the middle finger of each hand, start a circular movement in the middle of the forehead along the browline. Continue this circular movement while working toward the temples. Bring the fingers back quickly to the center of the forehead at a point between the browline and the hairline. Repeat the circular movements to the temple. Return the fingers to the middle of the forehead at the hairline, then repeat the circular movements to the temple. Each time the fingers reach the temple, pause for a moment and apply slight pressure to the temple. Repeat three to five times. (See Fig. 14.45.)

3. With the middle and ring fingers of each hand, start a criss-cross stroking movement at the middle of the forehead, starting at the browline, moving upward toward the hairline. Move toward the right

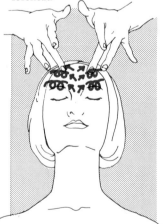

14.45—Circular movement over forehead

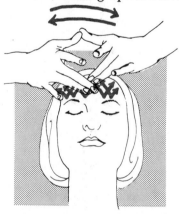

14.46—Criss-cross movement

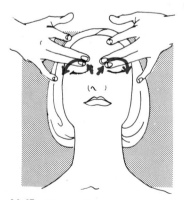

14.47—Brow and eye movement

temple, and back to the center of the forehead. Now move toward the left temple, and back to the center of the forehead. Repeat three to five times. (See Fig. 14.46.)

4. Place the ring fingers under the inside corners of the eyebrows and the middle finger over the brows. Slide the fingers to the outer corner of the eye, lifting the brow at the same time. (See Fig. 14.47.)

5. Start a circular movement with the middle finger at the outside corner of the eye. Continue the circular movement on the cheekbone to a point under the center of the eye, then slide the fingers back to the starting point. Repeat six to eight times. (See Fig. 14.48.)

6. Start a light tapping movement with the pads of the fingers. Tap lightly around the eyes as if playing a piano. Continue tapping, moving from the temple, under the eye, toward the nose, up and over the brow, and outward to the temple. Do not tap the eyelids directly over the eyeball. Repeat six times. (See Fig. 14.49.)

7. With the middle finger of each hand, start a circular movement down the nose and continuing across the cheeks to the temples. Slide the fingers under the eyes and back to the bridge of the nose. Repeat the movements six times. (See Fig. 14.50.)

8. With the middle and ring finger of each hand, slide the fingers from the bridge of the nose, over the brow (lifting the brow), and down to the chin. Start a firm circular movement on the chin with the thumbs. Change to the middle fingers at the corner of the mouth. Rotate the fingers five times and slide the fingers up the sides of the nose, over the brow, then stop for a moment at the temple. Apply slight pressure on the temple. Slide the fingers down to the chin and repeat the movements six times. (See Fig. 14.51.)

Note: The downward movement on the side of the face should have a very light touch to avoid dragging the skin downward.

9. With the pads of the fingertips, start a light tapping movement (piano playing) on the cheeks, working in a circle around the cheeks. Repeat the movements six to eight times. (See Fig. 14.52.)

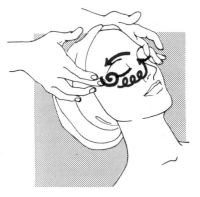

14.48—Circular movement around eye and cheekbone

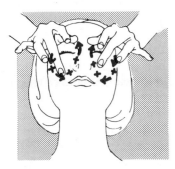

14.49—Light tapping movement around eyes

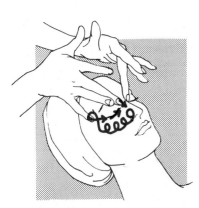

14.50—Circular movement down nose and across cheeks

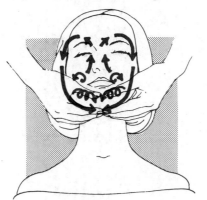

14.51—Nose, brow, and chin movement

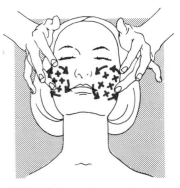

14.52—Light tapping movement on the cheeks

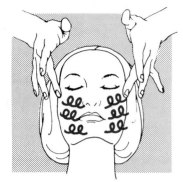

14.53—Rotary movement of cheeks

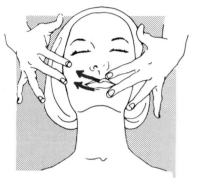

14.54—Scissor movement from center of the mouth to cheekbone

10. With the middle finger of each hand, start a circular movement at the center of the chin and move up to the earlobes. Return the middle fingers to the corner of the mouth, then continue the circular movements to the middle of the ears. Return the middle fingers to the nose and continue the circular movements to the top of the ear. Repeat three to five times. (See Fig. 14.53.)

11. With the index and middle fingers of each hand, start the "scissor" movement, moving from the center of the mouth, upward over the cheekbone, stopping at the top of the cheekbone. Alternate the movement from one side of the face to the other using the right hand on the right side of the face and the left hand on the left side of the face. Repeat eight to ten times. (See Fig. 14.54.)

12. With the middle finger of both hands, draw the fingers from the center of the upper lip, around the mouth, under the lower lip, and continue under the chin. Repeat six to eight times. (See Fig. 14.55.)

13. With the index finger above the chin and jawline (the middle, ring, and little fingers should be under the chin and jaw), start a "scissor" movement from the center of the chin, then slide the fingers to the earlobe. Alternate one hand after the other, using the right hand on the right side of the face and the left hand on the left side of the face. Repeat eight to ten times on each side of the face. (See Fig. 14.56.)

14. Apply light upward strokes over the front of the neck. Use firmer downward pressure on the sides of the neck. Repeat ten times. (See Fig. 14.57.)

> **Note:** Blood returning to the heart from the head, face, and neck flows down the jugular veins on each side of the neck. All massage movements on the side of the neck are done with a downward (never upward) motion.

15. With the middle and ring fingers of the right hand, give two quick taps under the chin, followed with one quick tap with the middle and ring fingers of the left hand. The taps should be done in a continuous

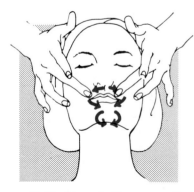

14.55—Lip and chin movement

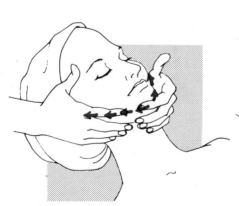

14.56—Scissor movement from the center of chin to the earlobe

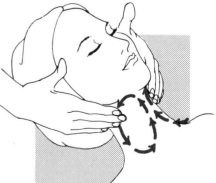

14.57—Stroking movement of neck

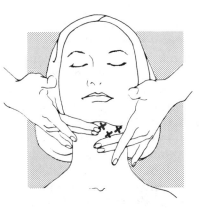

14.58—Tapping movement under the chin

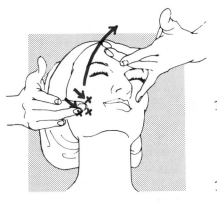

14.59—Tapping movement of cheeks

movement, keeping a steady rhythm. The taps should be done with a light touch, but with enough pressure so that a soft slapping sound can be heard. Continue the tapping movement while moving the hands slightly to the right and then left, so as to cover the complete underside of the chin. Without stopping or breaking the rhythm of the tapping, move to the right cheek. (See Fig. 14.58.)

16. Continue the tapping on the right cheek in the same manner as under the chin, except the tapping with the left hand will have a lifting movement. The rhythm will be: tap, tap, lift, tap, tap, lift, tap, tap, lift. Repeat this rhythmic movement 25 times. Without stopping the tapping movement, move the fingers back under the chin and over the left cheek, repeating the tapping and lifting movements. (See Fig. 14.59.)

17. Without stopping the tapping movement, move back under the chin and over to the right corner of the mouth. Break into a rolling movement with the first three fingers of each hand. One finger follows the other as each finger lifts the corner of the mouth. Repeat the movement 20 times. Continue the rolling movement as you quickly move under the chin to the left corner of the mouth. Repeat the rolling movement 20 times. (See Fig. 14.60.)

18. Without stopping the rolling movement, quickly move up to the outside corner of the left eye and continue the rolling movement 20 times. Continue the rolling movement across the forehead to the outside corner of the right eye. Continue this rolling movement 20 times. (See Fig. 14.61.)

19. Continue the rolling movement back and forth across the forehead, gradually slowing the movement. Let the movements grow slower and slower as the touch becomes lighter and lighter. Taper the movement off until the fingers are gradually lifted from the forehead. This slowing down of movement is often called "feathering." (See Fig. 14.62.)

Note: Avoid tapping directly on the jawbone, as this will feel unpleasant to the client.

This completes Massage #1.

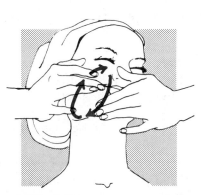

14.60—Rolling movement around mouth

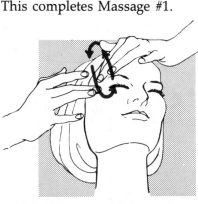

14.61—Rolling movement around eyes

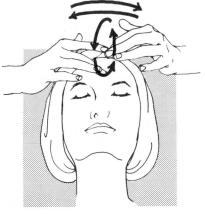

14.62—Rolling movement across forehead

Massage Number 2

Massage #2 is given with continuous and rhythmic movements, one hand following the other. It is done with slow, soothing, relaxing effleurage movements. The main purpose of Massage #2 is to aid the deep penetration of treatment creams and lotions and to induce relaxation. This is brought about by the heat that is built up from the stroking movements.

Massage #2 is given after the surface of the skin has been cleansed to prevent any dirt and makeup from being forced into the pores. It may be done when facial treatments are given with or without machines. Massage #2 is always given when deep penetration is required and other means of deep penetration of products such as iontophoresis (eye-on-to-fo-**REE**-sis), electric heating mask, or warm wax mask are not available. Massage #2 is given in almost all machineless treatments but is omitted in the treatment of acne skin.

Massage #2 is very relaxing. It is excellent for the client who seems to be tense. The massage promotes the feeling of calmness and tranquility; it is not unusual for the client to fall asleep during Massage #2. It is always followed by the treatment mask.

To encourage continuous relaxation, refrain from talking to the client during the massage and the mask treatment.

PROCEDURE FOR MASSAGE #2

Use a spatula to apply one teaspoon of treatment cream to your fingertips. Place your palms together and rotate your hands in a circular movement to distribute the cream over the entire surface of the hands. Place your hands palms down on the center upper part of the client's chest. Slide the hands outward toward the shoulders, then around the shoulders to the upper back and up to the neck. Repeat this movement three or four times until the treatment cream is applied evenly. Distribute ½ teaspoon of treatment cream to the fingers and apply the cream to the front of the neck and face, using the basic product application method.

1. With both hands (palms down) on the upper part of the chest, move the hands outward and around the shoulders to the center of the back and up on the neck using firm lifting movements. Let the hands follow the contours of the client's body. Repeat the movement six times. (See Fig. 14.63.)
2. With the surface of your hands, make circular movements from the center of the chest outward to the shoulders. When the hands reach the shoulders make several circular movements with the thumb, then slide the hands to the center of the back and up on the neck. Repeat six times. (See Fig. 14.64.)
3. Start upward movements at the base of the neck, rotating one hand after the other. Repeat 16 times. (See Fig. 14.65.)

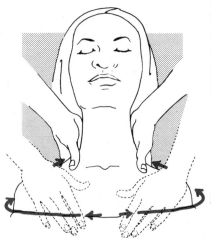

14.63—Lifting movements around chest, shoulders, back, and neck

Note: This movement is done on the neck only. The movements are not to be continued on the chin or jawline.

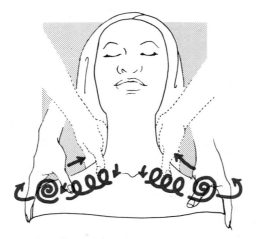

14.64—Circular movements around chest, shoulders, back, and neck

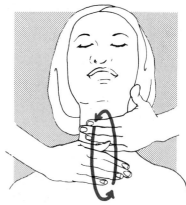

14.65—Rotating movement of the neck

4. With the hands alternating one after the other, start a firm, sliding movement from under the chin, ending when the fingers reach the upper cheekbone. Use the left hand on the left side of the face and the right hand on the right side of the face. Repeat 16 times. (See Fig. 14.66.)
5. Start with the hands flat on the cheeks, making firm, sliding upward movements, alternating one hand after the other. Do the movement 16 times on the right cheek, then repeat on the left cheek. (See Fig. 14.67.)
6. With the middle and ring fingers of each hand, start upward rolling movements at the corner of the right side of the mouth. Repeat 16 times on each side of the mouth. (See Fig. 14.68.)

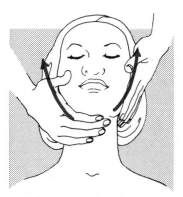

14.66—Sliding movement under chin

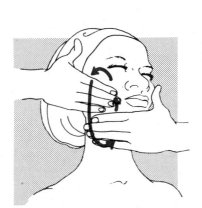

14.67—Sliding movement of the cheeks

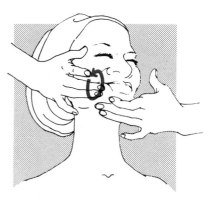

14.68—Rolling movement of the mouth

7. With the index and middle fingers of each hand, start a "scissor" movement from the center of the mouth upward, over the cheekbone, stopping at the top of the cheekbone. Use the left hand on the left side of the face and the right hand on the right side of the face. Repeat the movement 16 times on each side of the face. (See Fig. 14.69.)
8. With the middle and ring fingers of each hand, start a criss-cross movement at the outside corner of the right eye. Repeat the movement 16 times at the corner of the left eye. (See Fig. 14.70.)
9. With palms down, finish the massage with firm, alternating hand movements. Start at the browline and work upward to the hairline. Hand pressure should go from firm to very light until the hands are gradually feathered off the forehead. Repeat the movement 16 times. (See Fig. 14.71.)

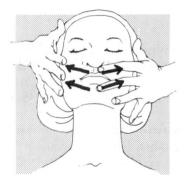
14.69—Scissor movement from the mouth to the cheekbone

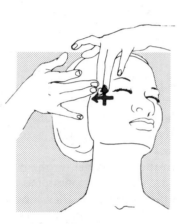
14.70—Criss-cross movement at the outside corner of the eye

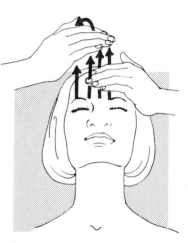
14.71—Alternating movement from browline to hairline

Dr. Jacquet Movements

Some years ago in Europe, the famous dermatologist, Dr. Jacquet, introduced a massage method that is especially effective in the treatment of oily skin and acne-blemished skin.

Gather a small section of the skin between the thumb and forefinger and squeeze gently. At the same time, give the skin a slight twisting or kneading movement. This helps to empty the oil ducts. The movement is somewhat similar to squeezing the peel of an orange until a fine spray of oil is expelled. The *Dr. Jacquet movement* keeps the sebum moving forward and out of the follicles. When the movement is done as part of a facial treatment, it should follow the disincrustation step.

The following movements combine the Dr. Jacquet method with variations on the original technique, so that the client will receive the maximum benefits.

The Dr. Jacquet movement must be done with care because the pressure of the movement can cause pain and too much kneading can stretch the skin. Do not use the movement in the eye area. If used close to the eye area, keep pressure to a minimum.

It may be necessary to forego the Dr. Jacquet movements over large areas of the skin that are strongly infected.

PROCEDURE FOR THE DR. JACQUET METHOD

1. Start with a slight twisting or kneading movement on the chin. (See Fig. 14.72.)
2. Continue with a kneading movement on the cheeks. (See Fig. 14.73.)
3. When the skin on the forehead is too tight to twist between the thumb and forefinger, place the tips of the fingers parallel to one another approximately ¾ inch apart on the forehead. Push the fingertips toward one another so that the skin is pinched gently between the fingers. Continue this movement across the entire forehead. (See Fig. 14.74.)

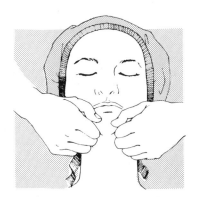

14.72—Chin movement   14.73—Cheek movement   14.74—Forehead movement

QUESTIONS   DISCUSSION AND REVIEW

TECHNIQUES FOR PROFESSIONAL MASSAGE

1. Briefly list the benefits of massage.
2. Explain the different types of massage.
3. Define reflexology.
4. Explain aromatherapy massage.
5. Describe lymphatic drainage massage.
6. Why is hand exercise important to the esthetician?
7. How often should you do hand exercises?
8. What are the five basic movements used in massage?
9. How often should normal skin have a facial treatment?
10. What is the main purpose of massage #1?
11. Give an example of a cream used in massage #1.
12. Why don't we use a penetrating cream with massage #1?
13. What is the main purpose of massage #2?
14. Which type of skin is benefited most by the Dr. Jacquet movements?

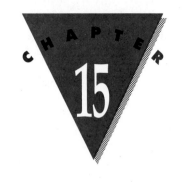

Mask Therapy in Facial Treatments

LEARNING OBJECTIVES *After completing this chapter, you should be able to:*

❶ Discuss how to use commercial masks and their applications.

❷ Explain how to prepare a custom mask for your client from fruit, vegetables, and herbs.

❸ Demonstrate the proper application of gauze and discuss why we use it in our facial treatment.

❹ Explain and demonstrate the purpose and procedure of the wax treatment.

INTRODUCTION The use of masks dates back to ancient times. It is believed that former civilizations discovered that some types of clay, mud, and earth had healing powers. When applied to the skin, these natural substances left it softer, smoother, and aided in the healing of blemishes and wounds. Natural, warm springs, containing minerals and sulphur, were also thought to be highly beneficial to health. Modern health resorts worldwide feature health treatments that consist of baths in these natural springs. Today, a great variety of natural and synthetic products are marketed as facial masks to improve the appearance of the skin. These preparations are usually in paste, gel, or dry powders, which are meant to be mixed with other ingredients. Masks are applied to the face while moist and allowed to dry, or set, thus producing a tightening and stimulating sensation. When removed from the face, dead cells and other impurities are removed with the mask. Some masks, such as the wax mask or the peel-off type mask, cause the skin to perspire. The perspiration is trapped beneath the mask so that it does not evaporate. Instead, the moisture is forced into the corneum layer of the skin where it plumps up fine lines. Masks are applied to the face after it has been cleansed.

Many commercial masks on today's market claim to remove oil, blackheads, dead surface cells, and other debris from the follicles and surface of the skin; however, some of these claims are exaggerated. The removal of blackheads, dead cells, and other debris from the skin is a job done more thoroughly by the esthetician. A mask should be used at the end of a facial treatment, for its beneficial ingredients and its calming, soothing, toning, and hydrating effects.

Classification and Benefits of Facial Masks

Masks are generally classified as warm or cold. A good mask will have the following qualities:

1. The mask must be safe to use and nontoxic.
2. The mask should be smooth and contain no gritty particles and it should be of a consistency that spreads over the face easily.
3. The mask should be removed easily with cotton compresses, sponges, and tepid water. If a peeling mask is used, it must peel off the face without causing discomfort to the client.
4. The mask should produce a toning and tightening sensation to the skin.
5. Following the removal of the mask, the skin should feel clean, stimulated, firm, smooth, and refreshed.
6. Some masks absorb and remove excess surface oils from the skin.

> **Note:** Any one or more of the above effects may be achieved depending on the type of mask that is being used.

INGREDIENTS USED IN MASKS

Glycerine is often added to masks for its moisturizing benefits.

Zinc oxide is added to some masks because it tends to neutralize excess alkali or acid on the skin. It has soothing properties, is mildly astringent and antiseptic, and encourages healing.

Calamine is a basic ingredient used in masks to produce a soothing action, especially on surface capillaries.

Magnesium, used in a mask, results in a stimulating astringent action that tones the skin.

Fuller's earth is a basic ingredient used in hardening masks. It also creates a stimulating effect and its drawing action absorbs oil and dead cells.

Sulfur is used in masks, since it produces a drying effect and has the ability to slow down oil gland activity; it also dissolves dead surface cells.

None of these ingredients are considered harmful, but the client's skin should be analyzed carefully and the skin condition determined beforehand, so that the appropriate mask can be selected.

SOLUTIONS AND OILS USED IN MASKS

Almond oil is added to basic mask ingredients and will give mild stimulation. Its nondrying effect is especially desirable for dehydrated skin.

Rose water and *orange flower water* are often used in basic masks for their mild, stimulating, and toning effects.

Witch hazel is used for its soothing qualities when the skin is irritated. It is mildly astringent.

CLAY AND GEL MASKS

Masks come in two basic forms—clay (kaolin and Fuller's earth) and gels. Clay type masks absorb oil and debris from the skin leaving it with a smoother, more even texture. Often mild bleaching agents are added to the clay mask. Clay produces a healing action that is beneficial in reducing inflammation. The length of time the mask is left on the face should be timed according to the manufacturer's directions.

The gel mask may be clear or tinted and should be spread on the face evenly. Most masks are applied with a spatula and can be easily smoothed on the face with the fingers. Some masks, however, are applied with a brush.

There are two types of gel masks. One is known as the "peel-off" type. This mask is allowed to dry on the face. The mask prevents evaporation of perspiration and forces the moisture into the corneum layer of the skin. The mask can usually be peeled off the face in one piece.

The second type of gel mask (also called the jelly mask) does not necessarily need to dry on the face since its active ingredients can be more beneficial to the skin before it dries out. This type of mask is usually very hydrating to the skin. Its active ingredients are often more beneficial to the skin than the peel-off type of mask. It will not absorb or remove oil, dead cells, or debris but is beneficial because of its calming, soothing, and refreshing effects on the skin.

BASIC MASK APPLICATION

Commercial masks used in the salon usually come in bulk form. Once the esthetician has determined the mask to be used for the client's particular skin condition, enough mask for one application is removed with a spatula from the bulk container and placed in a smaller container. Some masks, such as a yeast mask, come in dry powder or flake form and must be premixed. This type of mask is mixed directly prior to the application to prevent it from drying out during the facial treatment, and is often applied with a brush. Premixed masks may be applied with a spatula and smoothed with the fingers. When using either a brush or a spatula, the application of the mask starts on the client's neck. It is then applied on the jaws, cheeks, chin, the area between the nose and lip, the nose, and the forehead. Avoid applying mask to the lips and the area surrounding the eyes. Eye pads are placed on the client's eyes and the mask is left on the face for the required amount of time.

> **Note:** Masks such as the yeast mask or the herbal jelly mask are beneficial for most types of skin conditions and may be applied to the entire face and neck. Others, however, are formulated for a particular skin condition such as dry skin or oily skin. In the case of a combination skin, such as definite dry and oily areas, each area of the face must be treated separately for its particular condition: Masks formulated for dry skin are applied to the dry areas and mask formulated for oily skin are applied to the oily areas.

ADVANTAGES OF USING COMMERCIAL MASKS

Most estheticians use a commercially prepared mask because it is both faster and safer to use. If you compare the time and effort spent finding and collecting the ingredients needed for making the mask, and time spent preparing the mask, it is not worthwhile. Commercial masks are formulated by professional chemists and are manufactured by reliable companies, which have all products tested for safety and packaged under strict sanitary conditions.

For those estheticians who would still like to prepare some of their own masks, there are numerous books (found in health stores and bookstores) that contain interesting formulas for making facial masks.

> **Note:** See Chapter 13 for the proper method of removing a treatment mask with wet cotton compresses or sponges.

CUSTOM-DESIGNED MASKS

The esthetician will usually use prepared masks, but there are times when a custom-designed mask prepared from fresh fruits, vegetables, eggs, herbs, milk, vitamin oils, or extracts may be preferred. Custom-designed masks are generally left on the face for 10 to 15 minutes during a 1 hour treatment.

These masks are generally beneficial unless the client is allergic to a particular substance. The following list will acquaint you with some of the ingredients used in custom-designed masks and their benefits to the skin.

> ▶ **Caution:** Always ask clients if they have any allergies to the fruits or vegetables you are using before applying them.

1. There are several fresh fruit masks. Fresh strawberries may be crushed or sliced and applied to the face (usually over or between layers of gauze) for a mildly astringent and stimulating mask. Lemons and grapefruits are generally too acidic to use directly on the skin. Bananas may be sliced or crushed to make a mask for dry and sensitive skin, since they are rich in vitamins, potassium, calcium, and phosphorus and leave the skin soft and smooth.

2. Avocados may be crushed and applied to the face, as they are rich in vitamins, and essential oils, and produce a beneficial mask for dry or sensitive skin.

3. Other fruits and vegetables that are mildly astringent and have excellent soothing qualities are: papaya, tomatoes, apples, and cucumbers. These fruits or vegetables may be sliced very thinly or crushed, then applied to the face. Gauze helps to hold the mask in place.

4. Thinly sliced or grated raw white potatoes (applied over or between layers of gauze) are often used for oily or blemished skin. In addition, this mask will reduce puffiness in the eye area.

5. The white of an egg can be beaten until fluffy and applied to the face as a mask. Egg white has a tightening effect and is said to clear impurities from the skin. It is beneficial to all skin types.

6. Yogurt, buttermilk, and mayonnaise are mildly astringent and are used for masks on all skin types. Their cleansing action leaves the skin feeling refreshed.

7. Honey is used for its toning, tightening, and hydrating effect.

8. Oatmeal and yeast are also used as mildly stimulating facial masks.

9. In some cases, a mild bleaching mask may be desirable. Fresh lemon juice can be used as it has a slight bleaching action. However, lemon juice is acidic and may not be suitable for all types of skin.

10. When vitamins are applied to the skin in a facial mask, they may produce the following effects:

    Vitamin A—Softens and lubricates dry, rough skin
    Vitamin C—Used for its astringent effect
    Vitamin D—Considered to have exceptional healing qualities
    Vitamin E—Used to lubricate and soften dry, rough skin

11. Herbs are used in masks for their natural qualities. They are steeped in water to make a tea. The tea is then applied to the face with a saturated cotton compress mask. It may also be mixed with other ingredients, such as the herbal jelly mask. The mask is left on the face for approximately 10 minutes. Herbs commonly used in facial masks are: comfrey, camomile, thyme, and menthol (derived from mint and peppermint). These are just a few of the herbs used in masks, and it is advisable to use commercially prepared herbal masks unless you are familiar with the action of the various herbs when applied to different skin types. (For more on herbs, see Chapter 22.)

Herbal Teas for Masks and Compresses

Make a cup of herbal tea using an herb that will be beneficial for the type of skin that is being treated. For example, use camomile tea for its calming, soothing, and softening properties: It helps reduce swelling and relieves irritations, and is excellent for a dry, sensitive skin. Peppermint tea is cooling, soothing, and mildly antiseptic. Peppermint tea is also rich in Vitamins A and C and is especially good for an oily skin. Add one or two drops of green food coloring to the peppermint tea if desired, for esthetic effect. For acne, use comfrey-root tea for its healing, astringent, soothing, and softening qualities. Comfrey root is a source from which "allantoin" comes. Allantoin increases the speed of cell growth. Allantoin is used in many cosmetics, such as hand lotions, after shave lotions, and skin creams to help heal wounds and skin ulcers, and to soothe the skin. The herbal tea may be applied with a cotton compress or made into an herbal jelly mask.

HOW TO PREPARE AN HERBAL JELLY MASK

To make the herbal jelly mask you will need the following ingredients:

6 oz (170 g) herbal tea made with distilled water

6 oz (170 g) glycerine

1 oz (28 g) pectin (dry)

Pectin is a mildly acidic extract from the rinds of citrus fruits and from the skin and pulp of apples. It is used to thicken and set jellies. Pectin can be found in many supermarkets or in health food stores.

To prepare the mask, stir the glycerine as you slowly add the pectin powder. When the pectin is well-blended into the glycerine, slowly add the herbal tea, stirring all the while. Keep mixing until the pectin is well-blended; an electric mixer may be used. The mask should be allowed to stand overnight to allow it to thicken. This is enough for approximately 20 to 24 applications and the mask will stay fresh for several days. The formula may also be made in smaller amounts. For example:

3 oz (85 g) herbal tea

3 oz (85 g) glycerine

½ oz (14 g) pectin (dry)

Before using an herbal jelly mask, check with your client to see that she or he is not allergic to the herb you have chosen.

> **Note:** This herbal jelly mask was formulated especially for use by the professional esthetician.

The Use of Gauze for Mask Application

Gauze is a thin, transparent fabric of loosely woven cotton, that is often purchased for household uses. It is not the same quality gauze that is used for medical purposes and is commonly called "cheesecloth."

Certain ingredients used in facial masks do not cling or hold to the face. Such is the case with a yeast mask, which crumbles easily, and grated or pulverized fruit or vegetables, which tend to run. These ingredients are applied over a layer of gauze. The gauze holds the mask on the face, but allows the ingredients to seep through. In some cases, it is necessary to apply a second layer of gauze over the mask.

PROCEDURE
1. A piece of gauze is cut to cover the entire face and neck of the client. The piece of gauze is moistened with water, then applied and molded to the contours of the face. It is not necessary to cut a slit for the nostrils as the client can breathe easily through the gauze. However, on occasion a client may express a feeling of claustrophobia (claus-tro-**PHO**-bia), an abnormal fear of being closed or confined in space. In this case a slit or hole can be cut in the cloth for the eyes, nose, and mouth. (See Fig. 15.1.)
2. The mask ingredients are applied over the gauze, starting at the neck and ending on the forehead. Eye pads are applied over the gauze. (See Fig. 15.2.)
3. After the mask has been on the face for the desired amount of time, it is removed by carefully lifting and rolling the gauze from the face. Most of the mask will come off with the gauze. Any remaining mask may be removed from the face with wet cotton pads or sponges. (See Fig. 15.3.)

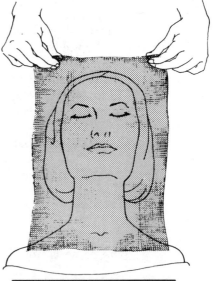

15.1—Cover entire face and neck with gauze.

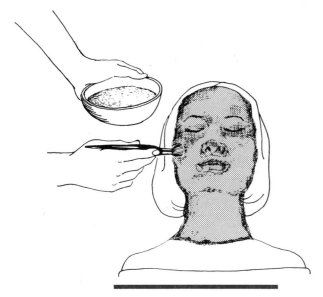

15.2—Apply the mask ingredients over the gauze.

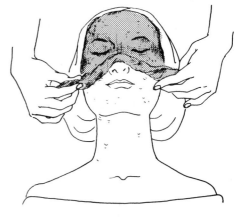

15.3—Lift and roll the gauze upward to remove.

The Wax Mask

The wax-mask treatment has been a favorite treatment of estheticians around the world for many years. Spectacular results can be seen immediately and the treatment can be given as an alternate treatment with deep-pore cleansing and epidermabrasion treatments. It is another treatment that can be given without the use of machines. The wax-mask treatment is beneficial and impressive to the client, because instant results can be seen. The treatment is most beneficial to skins that are dehydrated, dry, and/or aging. The wax mask is not recommended for acne skin conditions but it may be used on oily skins.

The purpose of the wax mask is to insure deep penetration of a product. The warmth of the mask relaxes the skin, allows the product to penetrate, and forms a vacuum that provokes the skin to perspire. The perspiration cannot escape and is forced into the stratum corneum layer. When the treatment is completed, the skin will appear moist and of good color, and superficial lines will be diminished.

FORMULA FOR THE WAX MASK The waxes and oils used for the treatment come in combinations of beeswax, paraffin (**PAR**-uh-fin), petroleum jelly, mineral oil, and other similar oils and waxes. If prepared wax is not available from a supplier, a simple formula can be prepared by melting 3½ ounces (98 grams) of paraffin wax with 4½ ounces (126 grams) of petroleum jelly. Both ingredients can usually be found in a grocery or drugstore.

PROCEDURE FOR THE WAX MASK TREATMENT

Before proceeding with the wax-mask treatment, the following steps should be completed:

1. The client's face is cleansed.
2. The skin is analyzed.
3. The vaporizer is used for approximately 10 minutes. (Warm, moist towel compresses may be applied to the face.)
4. The massage cream is applied. Massage #1 is done for approximately 7 minutes and the massage cream removed. If machines are available, brushing, suction, and spray will follow Massage #1.
5. The treatment cream is applied and the wax mask applied over the cream.

HOW TO PREPARE THE WAX MASK

1. The safest method for melting wax is the use of a thermostatically controlled heating pot. The heating pot warms the wax to approximately 130° F (54.4° C), keeping the wax at the right temperature throughout the treatment or throughout the day as needed. (See Fig. 15.4.)
2. Before applying the mask to the client's face, it must be tested for comfort on the inside of your own wrist to be sure it is not too hot. (See Fig. 15.5.)

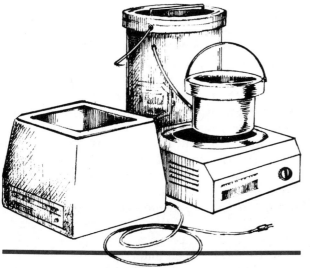

15.4—Heating pot

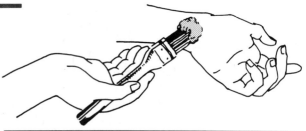

15.5—Test the temperature of the wax mask.

PROCEDURE FOR WAX MASK APPLICATION

1. The warm melted mask is applied to the face and neck with a brush. A natural bristle brush will be better than a nylon or plastic brush. The brush should be ½ to ¾ inch wide. The first step in the application of the wax is to apply the warm wax to the neck, starting at the hollow of the throat. (See Fig. 15.6.)
2. Brush the wax upward on the jaw and chin. (See Fig. 15.7.)

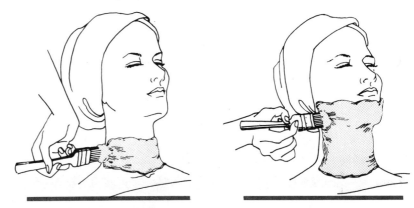

15.6—Start to apply the warm melted wax to the face and neck with a brush.

15.7—Continue upward on the jaw and chin.

3. Brush the wax under and around the nose. Avoid getting any of the wax in the nostrils. The wax is then brushed upward on the cheeks and around the eye. Avoid brushing the wax on the delicate tissue of the upper or lower eyelids. (See Fig. 15.8.)

 Caution: Never use hot wax over couperose skin areas.

4. Apply the wax to the forehead. The client's hair should be tucked under a headband or wrap to avoid getting wax on the hair. (See Fig. 15.9.)

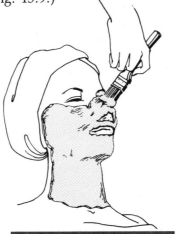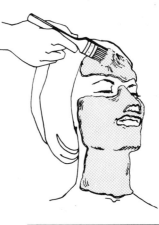

15.8—Apply the wax under and around the nose.

15.9—Apply the wax to the forehead.

5. A piece of gauze (cheesecloth) is placed over the first layer of wax. (See page 238.) Some estheticians prefer purchasing gauze with pre-cut spaces (cut out openings) for the eyes, nose, and mouth. (See Fig. 15.10.)

6. Continue to build the wax up until it is approximately ¼ inch thick. The application of wax will take several minutes. The wax-mask treatment should be completed in 1 to 1½ hours. After the wax is applied, pads are placed over the eyes and the client is allowed to relax. Approximately ½ hour should elapse from the beginning of the application of wax until it is ready to be removed. (See Fig. 15.11.)

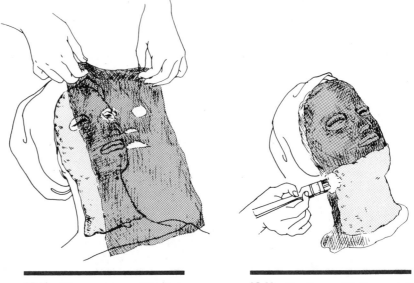

15.10—Place gauze over the first layer of wax.

15.11—Continue with the second layer of wax.

REMOVAL OF THE WAX MASK

1. When ready to remove the mask, use a wooden spatula to work the mask loose from the face and neck. (See Fig. 15.12.)
2. The mask is carefully lifted from the face in one piece. (See Fig. 15.13.)
3. It is impressive for the client to see the complete mask sculpture of his or her face. (See Fig. 15.14.)

Following the removal of the wax mask, the face is cleansed with a moist cotton pad or sponge that has been sprinkled with 10 to 15 drops of mild astringent or skin freshener.

If a spray machine is available, a light spray over the face is refreshing. The final step in the treatment is to apply a protective fluid. Following the completion of the treatment, the client should be allowed to inspect his or her face in a hand mirror in order to fully appreciate the results of the treatment.

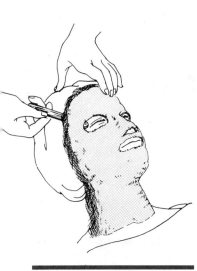

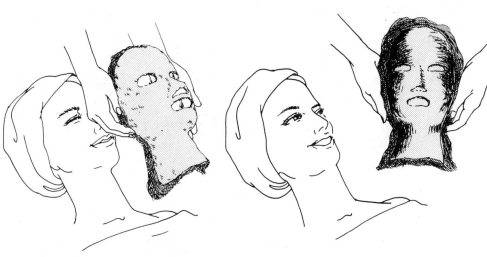

15.12—Use a wooden spatula to remove the mask.

15.13—Lift mask from face in one piece.

15.14—Show the client the mask sculpture.

Note: An added fee is sometimes charged for the wax mask treatment due to the added expense of the materials used.

QUESTIONS   DISCUSSION AND REVIEW

MASK THERAPY IN FACIAL TREATMENTS

1. What is the difference between facial masks and facial packs?
2. What is the primary purpose of a facial mask?
3. Discuss how the wax mask helps to moisturize the skin.
4. Name at least four benefits of facial masks.
5. What are some of the benefits of a clay mask?
6. What is a custom-designed mask?
7. Discuss the two types of gel masks and how they benefit the skin.
8. Why is gauze used when applying some masks?
9. Why do most estheticians prefer using preprepared commercial masks?
10. How are vitamins said to benefit the skin when used in facial masks?
11. What is allantoin and why is it often used in cosmetics?
12. What is the main purpose of the wax mask?

Facial Treatments without the Aid of Machines

LEARNING OBJECTIVES

After completing this chapter, you should be able to:

❶ Discuss the importance of a facial without the aid of a machine in the salon.

❷ Explain the procedures that can be done in the salon and the type of skin each is used for, also explaining the benefits of each.

INTRODUCTION

The treatments included in this chapter are all accomplished without the aid of machines. This knowledge is invaluable because you may work in a salon that has not yet invested in machines for scientific skin care. Although you will have the knowledge to give facial treatments with the aid of machines, it is advantageous that you be able to give a professional facial treatment without them. You may be called upon to give a treatment when machines are not available or when the client may request a treatment without the use of machines. There may be a time when a machine is not working properly and you will need to know how to continue the treatment without the aid of the machine. The facial treatments in this chapter may also be given with the use of one or more machines, when they are available.

Towel Steaming of the Face

Although it is not as convenient as the electric vaporizer, towel steaming of the face can bring about the following beneficial effects:

1. Opens follicles, allowing a deeper cleansing of dirt, grease, blackheads, and other debris from the follicles
2. Softens dead surface cells, which aids in their removal
3. Helps to stimulate the sebaceous glands
4. Aids the sweat glands to rid themselves of toxins and other impurities
5. Increases the circulation of the blood to the face so that the tissues are nourished
6. Leaves the skin feeling soft and glowing
7. Leaves the client feeling relaxed

The most important thing to remember when steaming the face is to use towels that are very warm but never hot. Terry cloth towels are best because they are thicker and hold heat longer. The size of the towel should be about 16 inches by 24 inches (40.64 centimeters by 60.96 centimeters) so that it can be wrapped around the face. Two towels will be needed for each treatment.

PROCEDURE
1. Fold the towel in half lengthwise. (See Fig. 16.1.)
2. Fold the towel in half once more. (See Fig. 16.2.)
3. Submerge the towel in very warm water. (See Fig. 16.3.)

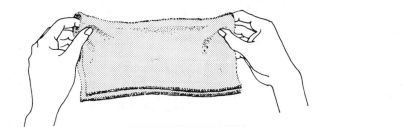

16.1—Fold the towel in half.

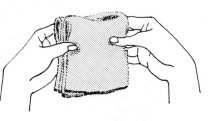

16.2—Fold the towel in half a second time.

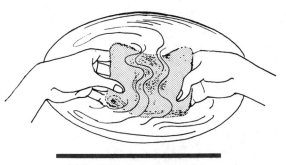

16.3—Submerge the towel in water.

4. An alternate method for wetting the towel is to form a cylinder and hold it directly under a tap of very warm running water. (See Fig. 16.4.)
5. Wring the towel out thoroughly. Step behind the client and unfold the towel, except for the first lengthwise fold. Place the center of the folded edge of the towel directly under the client's lower lip. (See Fig. 16.5.)
6. Drape the towel so that it covers the under part of the chin, jaw, and upper neck. Fold the ends of the towel over each other, covering the upper part of the face. The nostrils and mouth are not covered in order to permit the client to breathe easily. (See Fig. 16.6.)
7. With both hands, press the towel to the face. The towel should remain on the face approximately 2 minutes during which time the second towel is prepared. The first towel is lifted from the face and the second towel applied in the same manner as the first. The first towel is prepared again for application. This routine continues for 10 minutes. Be sure the towels are heated evenly, as a towel that is partially warm and partially cool can feel unpleasant to the client. (See Fig. 16.7.)

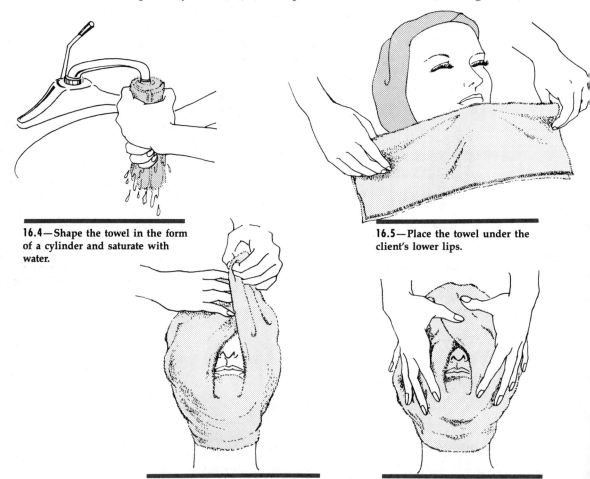

16.4—Shape the towel in the form of a cylinder and saturate with water.

16.5—Place the towel under the client's lower lips.

16.6—Drape the towel.

16.7—Secure the towel.

Normal Skin Facial

PROCEDURE
1. Prepare the client.
2. Sanitize your hands with alcohol or astringent.
3. Cleanse the client's face thoroughly with cleansing lotion, followed by a mild skin freshener.
4. Analyze the face. (Use eyepads and the magnifying lamp.)
5. Apply warm wet towels to the client's face to open pores for deep cleansing and to soften dead cells for easy removal.
6. Proceed with Massage #1.
7. Remove the massage cream with tissue and a wet cotton pad or sponges that have been sprinkled with a mild astringent.
8. Apply a treatment cream to the face and neck, and place the client under an infra-red heat lamp for 3 to 5 minutes.
9. Proceed with Massage #2. The infra-red lamp may be left on during the massage.
10. Apply the treatment mask for 10 minutes.
11. Remove the mask.
12. Wipe face and neck with a mild astringent.
13. Apply protective lotion.
14. Complete the treatment.
15. Complete the cleanup procedure.

Alternate treatments for normal skin can be the wax mask or the epidermabrasion treatment.

> **Note:** In Chapter 11 it is explained that, with regular maintenance treatments, a normal skin will continue to function in a healthy, normal way.

Dry Skin Facial

PROCEDURE
1. Prepare the client for the treatment.
2. Sanitize your hands with alcohol or astringent.
3. Cleanse the client's face thoroughly with cleansing lotion, followed by a mild skin freshener.
4. Place eyepads on the client's eyes and analyze the skin underneath the magnifying lamp.
5. Place a folded towel that has been thoroughly saturated with warm water on the client's face. (Refer to instructions.) The warm towel will soften dead surface cells so that they can be removed easily and the follicles opened for deeper cleansing.

6. Apply massage cream. Follow the basic steps for product application, except the cream is not applied to the eyelids. Proceed with Massage #1. The purpose of this massage is to continue the cleansing of the skin, to stimulate blood circulation, and to remove dead cells. *It is important that a massage cream and not a deep-penetrating cream be used for Massage #1.*

7. Remove the massage cream with a soft facial tissue, followed by a wet cotton pad or sponges that have been sprinkled with skin freshener. A rolling movement with cotton mitts (see Chapter 13), is used to assure the complete removal of the massage cream.

8. Apply the treatment cream to the face, including the eye area. Cover the client's eyes with moist cotton pads. Place the client under the infra-red lamp for 3 to 5 minutes and then do Massage #2. The infra-red lamp may be left on during Massage #2.

9. Apply the mask for dry skin. If the treatment cream that was used is of a texture that leaves an oily film on the surface of the skin, the excess should be removed with a wet cotton pad or sponges that have been sprinkled with skin freshener. If the cream that is being used is not of an oily texture and is water soluble, the mask may be applied directly over the cream. Leave the mask on for 10 minutes.

10. Apply the cotton compress mask over the treatment mask. Massage an ice cube over the mask with a rotary motion. The melting ice will seep through the cotton, helping to soften the treatment mask underneath and tone the skin. This procedure will feel cool and refreshing to the client and will help to close the pores. The mask is now removed.

11. Wipe the client's face and neck with a wet cotton pad or sponge that has been sprinkled with a mild skin lotion.

12. Apply moisturizer or protection fluid using the basic product application movements.

13. After finishing the treatment:
    a) Return the chair to an upright position.
    b) Remove the protective head covering from the client's head.
    c) Remove the protective towels and body covering.
    d) Assist the client with shoes and other belongings.

14. Cleanup procedure:
    a) Discard all disposable supplies and materials.
    b) Clean containers, close them tightly, and return them to their proper places.
    c) Tidy up the facial booth. Return used articles to be sanitized and unused articles to the dispensary.
    d) Wash and sanitize your hands.

Dehydrated Skin Facial

> **Note:** In Chapter 11, *Client Consultation and Skin Analysis,* a dehydrated skin is defined as a skin that is flaky, with superficial lines, due to a lack of water. A dehydrated skin can be a temporary condition brought on by several factors, such as heating of rooms during winter or the use of certain medications.

The treatment for dehydrated skin without the use of machines is given in the same way as the treatment for a dry skin, except for the following additional steps:

1. After the massage cream is removed, a hydrating lotion (moisturizer) is applied and the client is placed under the infra-red lamp for 5 minutes.
2. The treatment cream is applied over the hydrating lotion and Massage #2 is given.

The rest of the treatment is the same as for dry skin.

Alternate treatments for the dry and/or dehydrated skin can be (1) the wax mask or (2) the epidermabrasion treatment.

> **Note:** See Chapter 15 for wax-mask procedure.

Oil Dry Skin Facial

In Chapter 11, *Client Consultation and Skin Analysis,* an oil dry skin is defined as a skin that has sluggish sebaceous glands and fails to produce enough sebum. The facial treatment for oil dry skin without the use of machines is given in the same manner as the treatment for a dry skin. The treatment for oil dry skin will help to stimulate the sebaceous glands to produce sebum. The products that are used will help supplement natural oils and relieve dryness.

Alternate treatments for an oil dry skin can be (1) the wax mask or (2) the epidermabrasion treatment.

If the client has been using a cream that is too heavy for the oil dry condition, she or he should be advised that in some cases a heavy cream can interfere with the natural production of sebum, which the skin produces to combat dryness.

Facial Treatment for Mature (Aging) Skin

In Chapter 11, *Client Consultation and Skin Analysis*, it is explained that the natural aging process cannot be reversed nor can the aging skin be restored to the same vital condition of youth. However, salon treatments and proper home care can make the skin look and feel better.

The treatment for the mature (aging) skin without the use of machines is given in the same manner as the treatment for a dry skin and/or a dehydrated skin. Alternate treatments for the mature skin can be (1) the wax mask or (2) the epidermabrasion treatment. If time allows, it is recommended that the mature (aging) client receives Massage #2, which is usually omitted, when the wax mask is given.

> **Note:** See instructions for the wax mask in Chapter 15.

Oily Skin Facial

PROCEDURE
1. Prepare the client.
2. Sanitize your hands.
3. Cleanse the client's face.
4. Analyze the client's skin. Use eyepads and the magnifying lamp.
5. Apply warm wet towels to the face to open pores for deep cleansing and to soften the dead cells for easy removal.
6. Apply massage cream and proceed with Massage #1.
7. Remove the massage cream.
8. Do the disincrustation step with cotton compresses. (See page 255.) Use eyepads with the infra-red lamp.
9. Do the Dr. Jacquet massage.
10. Extract and expel blackheads and whiteheads. Use eyepads and the magnifying lamp.
11. Cleanse the face with astringent.
12. Massage #2 may be given for an oily skin, but is usually omitted.
13. Apply the mask formulated for oily skin. (Use eyepads.)
14. Remove the mask.
15. Wipe the client's face and neck with a wet cotton pad or sponges that have been sprinkled with astringent.
16. Apply protection fluid.
17. Complete the treatment.
18. Complete the cleanup procedure.

A Combination Skin Facial

PROCEDURE When treating a combination skin, each area of the face and neck is treated for the problem in that particular area. For example: If your client has an oily "T" zone (oily forehead, nose, and chin) and the rest of the face and neck are dry or normal, you would apply a mask for oily skin on the oily "T" zone and a mask for dry or normal skin in the areas that are dry or normal.

1. Prepare the client for the treatment.
2. Sanitize your hands.
3. Cleanse the client's face.
4. Analyze the face. (Use eyepads and the magnifying lamp.)
5. Apply warm wet towels to the face to open pores for deep cleansing and softening of dead cells for easy removal.
6. Proceed with Massage #1.
7. Remove the massage cream with tissue and a wet cotton pad or sponges that have been sprinkled with a mild astringent.
8. Apply cotton compresses that have been saturated with disincrustation lotion to the oily areas that have open pores and blackheads. Apply a hydrating fluid (moisturizer) to areas not covered with disincrustation compresses. Apply eyepads and place the client under the infra-red lamp for approximately 7 to 10 minutes. (The infra-red lamp is placed at a distance that will not dry the compresses, but will keep them warm.)
9. Do the Dr. Jacquet massage in the areas that are oily, with open pores and blackheads.
10. Expel blackheads and whiteheads.
11. Wipe the client's face with a wet cotton pad or sponge that has been sprinkled with a mild astringent.
12. Apply a treatment cream or lotion and place the client under the infra-red lamp for 3 to 5 minutes.
13. Proceed with Massage #2. The infra-red heat lamp may remain on during the massage.
14. Apply a treatment mask formulated for the skin condition for approximately 10 minutes. (Use eyepads.)
15. Remove mask with cotton compress mask or sponges.
16. Wipe the client's face and neck with a wet cotton pad or sponge that has been sprinkled with a mild astringent.
17. Apply protection lotion.
18. Complete the treatment.
19. Complete the cleanup procedure.

Acne Skin Facials (Problem Blemished)

> **Note:** When treating an acne skin, only cotton pads should be used for cleansing and mask removal. Since acne skin contains infectious matter, all pads and compresses must be disposed of after use. No massage or brushing is done on acne skin except the Dr. Jacquet massage.

1. Prepare all materials to be used for the treatment.
2. Prepare the client to receive the treatment.
3. Sanitize hands.
4. Cleanse the client's face with cotton pads.
5. Analyze the client's skin under the magnifying lamp. Use cotton pads over the eyes.
6. Apply warm wet towels to the face to open pores for deep cleansing and to soften the dead cells for easy removal.
7. Cotton compresses that have been saturated with disincrustation lotion are applied to the problem blemished areas, and to those areas where there are blackheads, open pores, and excessive oil. Eyepads are placed over the eyes and an infra-red lamp (if available) should be placed at a far enough distance to keep the compresses warm but not dry them out. This step takes 7 to 10 minutes.
8. Give the Dr. Jacquet massage.
9. Extract whiteheads and blackheads, and cleanse out pimples.
10. Cleanse the face with a wet cotton pad that has been sprinkled with 10 to 15 drops of astringent.
11. Apply the acne treatment cream. Eyepads are placed over the client's eyes and the infra-red lamp is used for approximately 7 minutes to aid in deep penetration.
12. Apply a treatment mask formulated for the skin condition for approximately 10 minutes. (Use eyepads.)
13. Remove the mask with the wet cotton compress mask.
14. Astringent is applied to the face with a wet cotton pad.
15. Special protective fluid for acne skin is applied to the face.
16. The treatment is completed.
17. The cleanup procedure is completed.

Special Acne Facial Treatment

When the client has a severe acne condition, it is important to start a series of treatments that will not cause undue irritation, but will be soothing to the skin. The client should be advised that it will take a number of treatments before the clogged pores (follicles) and blemishes can be cleansed and healed. Results will require the client's cooperation with home and salon treatments in order to soften the surface of the skin so the infection that is clogging the follicles, and being held down in the skin, can escape to the surface where it can be removed.

During the beginning of special acne treatments, the client may experience a "flare-up"; that is a sign that the infectious material is working its way to the surface. The special treatments will be more beneficial if the client can come to the salon twice a week as well as adhere to a strict home care regimen.

The esthetician's main objective is to soften the surface of the skin and clean out large, infectious pimples that have yellowish caps and are ready to be extracted. A sterilized needle or blood lancet is used to prick the blemish when it is necessary to open it. No facial massage or brushing is done when giving the special acne treatment.

PROCEDURE FOR THE SPECIAL ACNE TREATMENT

1. Everything that is to be used during the treatment must be ready before the treatment begins.
2. Prepare the client for treatment.
3. Sanitize hands.
4. Cleanse the skin with cleansing lotion followed by astringent. Use cotton pads only.
5. The skin is analyzed carefully.
6. Warm towel compresses are applied for approximately 10 minutes.
7. The disincrustation procedure is started. Cotton compresses that have been saturated with disincrustation lotion are applied. An infra-red lamp may be used. The lamp is placed at a distance that will keep the compresses warm but will not dry them. Disincrustation should take approximately 7 to 10 minutes. The Dr. Jacquet movements are not done for the first treatments on strong acne skin, as the skin may be too sensitive.
8. Blackheads are extracted and pimples are cleansed. Moist cotton pads that have been sprinkled with astringent are used to cleanse the face.
9. The treatment cream is applied. Eyepads are placed over the client's eyes and an infra-red lamp is used to aid deep penetration of the cream into the skin.
10. The acne treatment mask is applied. If the treatment cream is water soluble, the mask is applied directly over the treatment cream.
11. The mask is removed with a wet cotton compress mask.
12. The face is wiped with a wet cotton pad that has been sprinkled with astringent.
13. Special protective lotion for acne skin is applied to the face.
14. The treatment is completed.
15. The cleanup procedure is completed.

Home Care for Acne Skin

Acne is not considered a disease but rather a manifestation of changes that take place in the body, especially during adolescence. Proper care of the skin and good health habits will do much to prevent the onset of acne, but once acne gets a start, it must be kept under control to keep the condition from worsening. With today's knowledge of the skin and its functions, if proper treatments are followed, acne can be controlled and in most cases, cleared. The client should be told that it takes time, patience, and cooperation to achieve results. It is important that the client maintain a strict home care regimen in addition to salon treatments. The client must avoid picking and squeezing blemishes if the spread of infection is to be controlled.

The following guide for home treatment care of the skin will help the client to control acne and help the esthetician to clear the condition sooner.

PROCEDURE FOR HOME FACIAL TREATMENT

1. Every morning and evening, the face should be cleansed with moist cotton pads: First with cleansing lotion, then with astringent. After the morning cleansing, a protective lotion for acne is applied. In the evening after cleansing, a night treatment cream or fluid formulated for acne skin should be applied.
2. At least twice a week the following home facial is given.
   a) Prepare the disincrustation lotion by mixing 1 tablespoon (15.0 grams) of baking soda (bicarbonate of soda) in 1 pint of distilled warm water. Commercial disincrustation lotion should be purchased from the salon if available.
   b) Cleanse the face with cleansing lotion followed by astringent.
   c) Place cotton compresses that have been saturated in the disincrustation solution over the areas of the face that have enlarged follicles, blackheads, and blemishes.
   d) After 15 minutes, remove the cotton compresses.
   e) The Dr. Jacquet massage movements are given for 5 minutes.

Note: If the client comes to the salon for weekly treatments, squeezing and extracting of blemishes will be done only by the esthetician. If the client cannot come to the salon on a regular basis, because of school, vacation, or work schedules, the client should be taught how to do the following: When pimples are ripe for extracting, they will have a light yellowish head in the center. Wrap thin strips of cotton moistened in astringent around the forefingers. The sides of the blemish can be gently squeezed and lifted until the infectious material is expelled. The pressure must come from the fingertips and not the fingernails. If the blemish is not easily cleansed or drained with gentle squeezing of the surrounding skin, this indicates that the blemish is not ready for extraction and should be left alone. To force squeezing of a blemish will only invite the spread of infection into the surrounding tissues. If the blemish drains, the gentle pressure may be continued until clear fresh blood is seen. The cotton strips on the fingers are changed after the cleansing of each blemish. Following the extraction procedure, the face is cleansed with a clean cotton pad that has been saturated with astringent.

f) A mask for acne-prone skin is applied for the recommended length of time.

g) The mask is removed with cool water and cotton pads.

h) The skin is patted dry with facial tissue.

i) A treatment cream especially formulated for acne skin is applied.

> **Note:** The client should be reminded that a "flare-up" or worsening of the condition may occur before the skin starts to look better. This is because the infection is escaping from below the surface of the skin, now that the follicles are being cleared. The face should not be cleansed more than two to three times a day as this tends to irritate the condition and overstimulate the sebaceous glands. Gradually with salon and consistent home treatments, the skin will be restored to its normal functioning. The client must follow instructions exactly, if results are to be achieved.

Disincrustation

Disincrustation is a process that softens and emulsifies grease deposits and blackheads in the follicles. When machines are used in facial treatments, disincrustation is performed with galvanic current. When machines are not used in the facial treatment, disincrustation is achieved by applying cotton strips or compresses that have been saturated with disincrustation lotion. The compresses are applied to areas that are oily and have enlarged pores, blackheads, and pimples (Figs. 16.8 and 16.9).

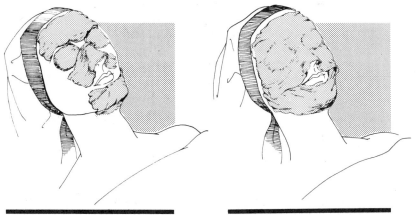

16.8—Cotton strips have been saturated with disincrustation lotion and applied to an oily "T" zone.

16.9—Cotton compresses have been saturated with disincrustation lotion and applied to an entire oily skin surface. Large eyepads are applied to the eye area before the compresses are applied.

The client is placed under an infra-red lamp (when available) for approximately 7 to 10 minutes. If the infra-red lamp is used, it should be placed at a far enough distance to keep the compresses warm without drying them out. It is best to use a commercial disincrustation lotion, which can be purchased from a beauty supplier that carries products for the professional esthetician. When a commercial lotion is not available, a simple substitute disincrustation lotion can be made by mixing 1 level tablespoon of bicarbonate of soda with 1 pint distilled water.

When the compresses are removed, the Dr. Jacquet massage is usually performed as the next step. This is followed by the extraction of blackheads and whiteheads, and the cleansing of pimples.

Facial Treatment for Couperose Skins

Couperose skin is skin that has broken capillaries and, therefore, the following rules must be observed:

1. Do not use an infra-red lamp in the treatment of couperose skin.
2. Ice should not be used on couperose skin.
3. Mild skin lotion, not astringent is used for couperose skin.
4. No strong massage movements are used on coupersose skin.

Masks for Couperose Skin

Commercially prepared masks may be used or a mask may be prepared as follows: One part kaolin powder to one part zinc oxide powder (USP grade only). These ingredients can be found in most drugstores.

Mix the ingredients with a moisturizer, mineral oil, or a protection fluid to form a paste in a consistency that will spread well. This mask will calm and soothe the skin and help diminish redness.

PROCEDURE
1. Prepare the client.
2. Sanitize hands.
3. Cleanse the client's face.
4. Analyze the skin.
5. Apply a cotton compress mask of warm coltsfoot or mint herb tea. Leave the mask on for approximately 10 minutes.

> **Note:** Coltsfoot (also called wild ginger) aids in the constriction of small blood vessels, soothes irritated tissue, and reduces swelling. The tea is prepared by steeping 1 teaspoon of the herb in 1 cup of boiling water for 30 minutes. The tea is then strained. Mint leaves soothe, strengthen, and tone the skin. Mint tea is prepared by steeping 1 teaspoon of the herb in 1 cup of boiling water for 20 minutes and the tea is then strained. Both herbs can be found in a health food store.

6. Apply the massage cream and proceed with Massage #1. Concentrate on gentle piano movements. No strong massage movements are done on a couperose skin.
7. Remove the massage cream.

> **Note:** Treatments will vary depending on the location of the couperose condition so as to prevent further damage to the skin. On an oily skin, disincrustation is done with cotton compresses. Expelling of pimples and blackheads (if done at all) must be done with extreme care on areas where it will cause no further damage to the skin.

8. Massage #2 is given.
9. The special mask is applied.
10. The mask is removed.
11. Mild skin-freshening lotion is applied with a wet cotton pad or a sponge.
12. A protection fluid is applied.
13. The treatment is completed.
14. The cleanup procedure is completed.

> **Note:** The client should be reminded that it is important to protect the skin at all times. Washing the face with hot water then splashing with cold water, rubbing ice cubes on the face, or other extremes of hot and cold should be avoided. If the client lives in a cold climate and enters warm buildings from out-of-doors, it is helpful to place the hands over the face for a few minutes to break the shock of the sudden change in temperature. A makeup foundation will serve as an added protection. The foundation will also help to conceal the couperose condition.

The esthetician should advise the client as follows:

1. Be sure the client knows how to care for couperose skin at home.
2. Remind the client to protect the skin from extreme changes in temperature.
3. Suggest that the client analyze his or her diet to be sure that only healthful foods and beverages are consumed.
4. Give instructions on how the "piano" movements are to be done at home. (See Massage #1 in Chapter 14.)
5. Suggest a foundation and/or protective cream or lotion.
6. Suggest that the client add Vitamin P (also known as bioflavonoids and almost always accompanies natural Vitamin C) to his or her diet.

The Epidermabrasion Treatment

The term *epidermabrasion* should not be confused with *dermabrasion*, which deals with deeper layers of the skin and must be done by a dermatologist.

The epidermabrasion treatment is sometimes called cosmetic peeling or skin thinning. The treatment can be given with or without the use of machines. The treatment cream often contains enzymes that have the ability to dissolve and decompose the dead cells on the surface of the skin. The treatment cream may also contain pumice powder that works as a mild abrasive to remove dead surface cells.

The primary purpose of the peeling treatment is to remove dead surface cells, to uncover follicles (pores) that have been blocked by cellular buildup, and to help prevent the formation of blackheads and other skin blemishes. Skin texture and color are both improved by this treatment. The skin feels smoother, follicles appear smaller, and the number of blackheads are reduced. An additional benefit is that the outer layer of the skin is more easily moisturized after the dry, hard surface cells are removed.

The epidermabrasion treatment is especially popular in winter when the skin becomes dry and flaky. It is an excellent alternate treatment, which benefits most skins. The treatment can be given on skin with minor blemishes but should not be done on acne skin, or on areas heavy with broken capillaries. It is up to the esthetician to use discretion when giving epidermabrasion treatments.

The concept of epidermabrasion (peeling or thinning) of the skin is not new. Pumice, almond meal, and other coarse materials have been used since ancient times to polish and cleanse the skin. The skin must always be thoroughly cleansed before the epidermabrasion treatment. The treatment stimulates the skin to produce new cells more rapidly by increasing the blood supply to the surface of the skin. The theory is that when the surface cells are removed, the skin's metabolism is increased, and since the skin has to replace the dead cells, it will work harder. Normally, skin cells are renewed approximately every 28 days. New cells rise to the surface as old ones are sloughed off. As a person ages, the cells may not be removed evenly. Therefore, epidermabrasion is particularly beneficial to most skins that have begun to show signs of aging.

PROCEDURE FOR THE EPIDERMABRASION TREATMENT

1. The face is cleansed using the normal cleansing procedure.
2. The skin is analyzed.
3. The warm vapor mist or warm wet towels may be applied to the face to soften dead surface cells for easy removal.
4. A thin layer of the epidermabrasion (peeling) cream is applied and left on the face for 10 to 15 minutes or until nearly dry. If the cream is allowed to become completely dry, it will be harder to remove. (See Fig. 16.10.)
5. To remove the epidermabrasion (peeling) cream, a rolling motion is done with one hand over the other, starting at the neck and moving over the chin, cheeks, upper lip, nose, and forehead. A shampoo cape can be placed over the client's chest with the back of the cape tucked under the client's head and over the head rest. The cape will catch the treatment particles as they flake off the face. (See Fig. 16.11.)

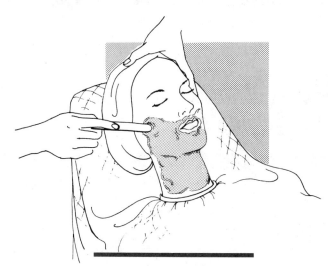

16.10—A thin layer of epidermabrasion cream is applied.

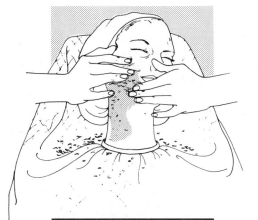

16.11—The epidermabrasion
treatment cream is removed. The
shampoo cape is arranged to catch
the particles.

6. The face is sprayed or wiped with a wet pad or sponges moistened with astringent or skin freshener.
7. Massage #2 is given with a treatment cream formulated especially for the client's skin condition.

> **Note:** Massage #1 is not given in this treatment.

8. A mask is applied and left on the face for approximately 7 to 10 minutes.
9. The mask is removed and the face is sprayed or wiped with a wet cotton pad or sponges that have been sprinkled with astringent or skin freshener. The face is blotted with tissue.
10. The application of protection fluid (moisturizer) is the final step in the epidermabrasion treatment.

QUESTIONS DISCUSSION AND REVIEW

FACIAL TREATMENTS WITHOUT THE AID OF MACHINES

1. Why is it important to know how to perform a facial without the aid of a machine in the salon?
2. List the benefits of steaming the face.
3. Give two alternate treatments for dry and/or dehydrated skin.
4. Can the wax or epidermabrasion treatment be used for oil dry skin as an alternate?
5. When treating combination skin, is all the skin on the face given the same treatment?
6. How often should a client who you are treating for acne come in for treatments?
7. What is disincrustation?
8. What rules must you follow when working on couperose skin?
9. What is another name for cosmetic peeling or skin thinning?
10. When should the epidermabrasion treatment not be given?

Electricity, Machines, and Apparatus for Professional Skin Care

LEARNING OBJECTIVES

After completing this chapter, you should be able to:

❶ Explain and demonstrate how to use the magnifying lamp, the skin scope, and the Wood's lamp.
❷ Explain the facial vaporizer and why it is used.
❸ Demonstrate the brushing machine and explain its importance.
❹ Explain why the galvanic current is used.
❺ Define high-frequency and its benefits.
❻ Demonstrate and explain the vacuum and spray machine.
❼ Explain and demonstrate the electric mask and treatment mitts.
❽ Explain electricity and safety practices.
❾ Explain light therapy.

INTRODUCTION

As men and women have become more concerned with grooming, beauty, health, and the effects of pollution on the skin, their interest in scientific skin care has grown. This increasing interest on the part of the public has led to the increased use of machines in professional skin care treatment.

Although facials can be given without the use of machines, utilizing these specialized pieces of equipment lets the esthetician give better service and present a more professional operation to the public. There are many different types of equipment used for facial treatments. Some are more valuable than others. Not all the types will be used for every facial.

The Magnifying Lamp

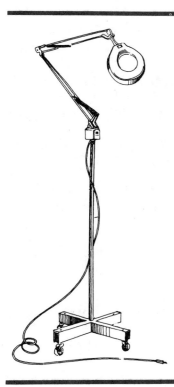

The magnifying lamp is one of the most important tools at the esthetician's command. It provides magnification and glare-free light to aid the esthetician in detecting tiny imperfections when analyzing the skin. The use of the magnifying lamp assures the client that his or her skin is being examined thoroughly and, therefore, will receive the correct treatment for the skin condition. The lamp is especially helpful when extracting blackheads and whiteheads, and cleaning out pimples. The lamp gives a professional look to the salon and also adds professionalism to the treatments.

The magnifying lamp may also be used to provide light when the magnifying lens is not being used. The esthetician will often turn out the overhead light in a facial room once the treatment has started. This adds a more relaxing atmosphere to the facial room.

Magnifying lamps use cool fluorescent lights, usually protected by a translucent plastic shield. When the lamp is placed directly over the client's face for analysis or manual extraction, his or her eyes should be protected with eyepads.

Some models have a clamp that mounts the magnifying lamp to a table. There is also a model that mounts to a wall. The most common lamp in service, however, is the floor standing model (Fig. 17.1).

17.1—Magnifying lamp

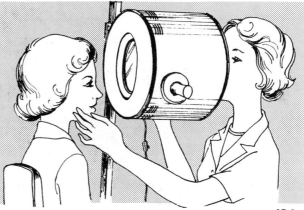

17.2—Skin scope

The Skin Scope

The skin scope is an elaborate magnifying lamp used for analyzing the skin (Fig. 17.2). It has a one-way magnifying mirror allowing the esthetician to scan the client's skin, while at the same time allowing the client to see his or her reflection in the magnifying mirror. A circle of lights set behind frosted glass surrounds the mirror and lights the face very well. Although it is expensive, the skin scope is impressive and adds a professional touch to the consultation. (*See Color Plate 19.*)

The Wood's Lamp

The Wood's lamp was developed by Robert Williams Wood, an American physicist. It has been used in the medical profession to help diagnose such skin conditions as ringworm.

The Wood's lamp is used by the esthetician to help analyze skin conditions (Fig. 17.3). It works on the principle that different skin conditions show different colors when viewed under the deep ultra-violet light of the lamp. The lamp works best when used in a totally dark room. The ultra-violet rays let the esthetician analyze the surface and deeper layers of the skin to determine skin type and proper treatment of the client. Blemishes that are barely visible to the naked eye can be seen readily under the Wood's lamp. Different skin conditions will show up in varied shades; for example, the thicker the skin, the whiter the fluorescence will be. The following are some examples of skin conditions and their appearance under the Wood's lamp.

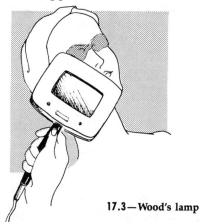

17.3—Wood's lamp

SKIN CONDITION	WOOD'S LAMP INDICATION
Thick corneum layer	White fluorescent
Horny layer of the skin and dead cells	White spots
Normal and healthy skin	Blue-white
Thin skin without enough moisture (dehydrated)	Purple fluorescent
Dehydrated skin	Light violet
Hydrated skin	Bright fluorescent
Oily areas of the face and comedones	Yellow or sometimes pink
Pigmentation and dark spots	Brown

A healthy scalp and hair will show up as a pale grayish violet color. Dandruff will appear as white specks. Nails have a bright white fluorescence.

If there is any doubt that a formula has been changed it will show up on a comparison test under the Wood's lamp, as identical cosmetic formulations have the same fluorescence.

> **Caution:** The Wood's lamp should not be allowed to overheat. Avoid direct contact between the bulb and skin. Neither the client nor the esthetician should look directly into the light source while the lamp is being used.

The Facial Vaporizer

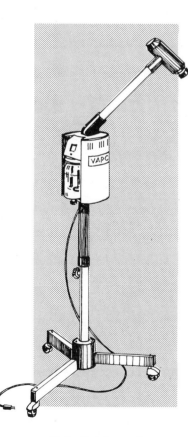

17.4—Facial vaporizer

The facial vaporizer is considered by many estheticians to be the most important electric apparatus used in the field of esthetics (Fig. 17.4). The benefits of the lukewarm vapor mist are many when diffused on the skin's surface. They include the following:

1. The vapor mist softens dead surface cells so they can be sloughed off during Massage #1 and/or during the brushing procedure.
2. The warm, humid mist aids in opening the follicles so that they can be properly cleansed.
3. The vapor penetrates deep into the follicles to soften deposits of grease, blackheads, makeup, and dirt so that this debris can be removed with ease.
4. The vapor mist helps the pores to eliminate toxins.
5. The vapor mist temporarily softens superficial lines.
6. The vapor mist increases blood circulation by causing the blood vessels to expand.
7. The action of the vapor improves cell metabolism.

The vaporizing is done on the skin after it has been cleansed and analyzed. Vaporizing done over massage cream will not penetrate the skin because the cream acts as a barrier to the mist.

The reservoir holding the water that makes the vapor mist is made from glass or metal. The manufacturer's instructions will include the amount of water to be used in the vaporizer.

Distilled or filtered water should be used in the vaporizer to prolong the life of the machine. The use of tap water may eventually cause malfunction of the machine, due to calcium and mineral deposits.

Some models will turn off automatically when the water has reached a low level. If the model has a glass reservoir and no automatic turn off, it is important to check the water level several times during the day. If the water level is allowed to get too low, the glass will burst. Some models have an automatic timer. Most models require approximately 10 minutes for the water to heat and send out a flow of vapor. It is important to turn the machine on at the beginning of each treatment so that the vapor will be ready when it is needed.

When preparing to use the vapor, the head of the apparatus should be turned away from the client's face, until the mist has an even flow. If the machine makes a gurgling sound or starts to spurt water, this may indicate that the machine has been filled with too much water. The machine should be turned off and some of the water drained.

In some models the rubber hose leading from the reservoir to the head of the vaporizer may become twisted or slack and this may also cause the water to spurt.

Once the machine has a steady mist flowing, it may be turned toward the client's face. The vapor should be set approximately 16 inches from the client's face so that as the vapor travels through the air, it cools to the proper lukewarm temperature (Fig. 17.5). The lukewarm water will prevent the skin from perspiring. If the skin is allowed to perspire, water is drawn from the skin and dehydration is increased.

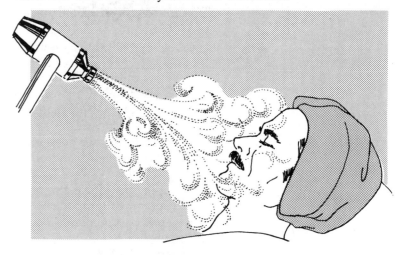

17.5—The vapor should be set approximately 16 inches from the client's face.

For skin with large couperose areas, the vaporizer is moved a few inches farther from the face so that the vapor is cooler. For a thick or oily skin, the machine may be moved closer to the face. The distance between the vaporizer and the client's face can vary a few inches, as some models have a stronger mist. Directions for the use of the vaporizer should be studied carefully and followed. During the vaporizing, the client is told to keep his or her eyes closed. No eye pads are used because the vapor mist is beneficial to the eye area.

> **Note:** Air conditioners, fans, and ventilating systems should be adjusted so as not to interfere with the steady flow of the vapor.

CARE OF THE VAPORIZING MACHINE

The reservoir and heating elements should be cleaned once a week by filling the machine with a solution of distilled water and white vinegar (1 cup white vinegar to 1 quart water), and allowed to stand overnight. The reservoir is emptied and rinsed then stored until ready for use.

> **Note:** In the European method of facial treatments, some models of the vaporizing machine have an ozone generator incorporated in the head of the apparatus. Ozone is a form of oxygen used as a disinfectant. As vapor passes the generator, it is charged with ions of electricity. This imparts each vapor droplet with the same electrical charge. Since like electrical charges repel one another, the droplets are prevented from coming together. This changes the consistency of the vapor into a cloud-like mist that flows over the client's face. This ionized mist is believed by many estheticians to have an antibacterial action that is beneficial to the skin. Check with applicable regulatory agencies such as the Department of Health and the Cosmetology State Board concerning the use of ozone in your area.

The Brushing Machine

The brushing machine is manufactured in several sizes and shapes. Some models are held completely in the hand, while others are floor standing models. Yet another consists of a unit that is part of several units, which are stacked one on top of the other. Some refer to this type as a mobile unit. The brushing machine comes with small brushes that rotate at different speeds. The brushes come in different sizes and vary in texture from soft to coarse. Some are made for use on the body and others for use on the face. (*See Color Plate 21.*)

A coarse brush is sometimes used on thick or oily skin. A soft brush is better for a dry or delicate type of skin, and most estheticians prefer to use a soft brush on all skin types.

The purpose of the brushing is to slough off the dead cells, and to remove any dirt and grime that clings to the surface of the skin. Before any brushing is done, the skin is cleansed with either viscose sponges or cotton pads. The face is vaporized or steamed with warm, moist towels to soften the dead surface cells so that they can be more easily removed. The vaporized face is then given Massage #1.

Massage #1 removes some of the dead surface cells, and the brushing is a continuation of the cleansing process (Figs. 17.6–17.8). Following Massage #1, the skin is cleansed of the massage cream and a lotion cleanser is applied to the skin. The brushing is started on the neck, continued to the jaw, chin, cheeks, upper lip, nose and forehead. Swirling on the skin thousands of times per minute, the brush creates an excellent massage for the skin. It stimulates and cleanses the skin while giving a very light exfoliation. Brushing is beneficial and is used on all types of skin with the exception of acne skins. Brushing could irritate the acne and possibly spread infection.

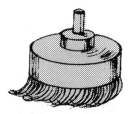

17.6—If too much pressure is applied to the brush, the bristles will bend.

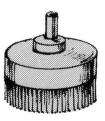

17.7—For the best results in the removal of dead surface cells and other debris, less pressure should be applied so the bristles remain straight.

On skins that have broken capillaries, the brush may be used very lightly over the area. In cases of severely broken capillaries, brushing is avoided.

If no massage is given, brushing follows the application of warm towel compresses or the vaporizer apparatus. The brushing machine assures a more thorough cleansing of the skin since the bristles of the brush can loosen dirt and grime embedded in the skin, where a sponge or cleansing pad cannot reach.

Some machines are designed with more than one speed. When using this type of machine, slow brushing speeds are used on dry and sensitive skins, and faster speeds on skins that are coarse and thick. Following each treatment the brush should be thoroughly cleaned by washing with soap and water. The brush is then placed in a small bowl of alcohol for about 20 minutes to be sure it is sterilized. When not in use, clean brushes are stored in a dry sterilizing cabinet. Before using the brush on the skin, it should always be moistened with water to soften the bristles. A tissue is held over the brush after moistening and the machine is turned on at a slow speed for a few seconds in order to remove excess moisture.

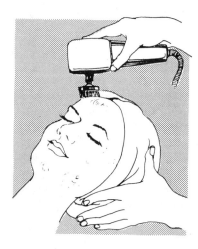

17.8—The brushing machine is used in a facial treatment.

Note: There are brushing machines manufactured for home use. However, these brushes are not the same as those used in salon treatments given by a professional esthetician. When equipment designed for home use is used in the salon, it detracts from the professional image of the salon.

The Galvanic Current Machine

The galvanic current machine has two important functions during a facial treatment. (*See Color Plate 22.*) One is to soften grease and sebum deposits, making them easier to remove. The process is called disincrustation (dis-in-krus-**TAY**-shun). The second function is to introduce water soluble treatment products into the skin. This process is called iontophoresis (eye-on-to-fo-**REE**-sis) (Fig. 17.9).

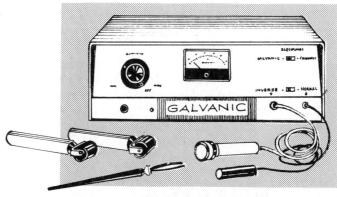

17.9—The galvanic machine

Galvanic current is a low level and direct current (D.C.). Chemical changes are produced when this current is passed through certain solutions containing acids and salts. Chemical effects are also produced when a galvanic current is passed through the tissues and fluids of the body (Fig. 17.10).

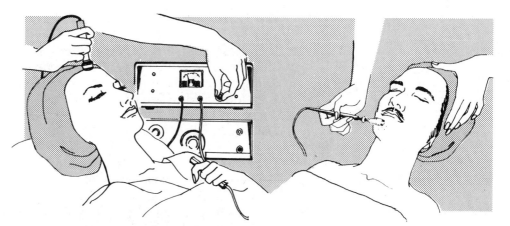

17.10—These illustrations show different attachments for the galvanic machine that are used for disincrustation and ionization.

TEST FOR POLARITY   When using galvanic current, there are two poles or terminals, a negative (−) and a positive (+). Different polarity is used for different functions. Polarity means having the ability to determine the direction of flow of a direct or galvanic current. Before applying the galvanic current, the esthetician should know which is the positive pole and which is the negative pole. Most galvanic current machines have a polarity indicator. If necesary, polarity can be tested as follows:

1. Separate the tips of the two conducting cords and immerse them in a glass of water to which a dash of salt has been added. Turn up the current. As the water is ionized many small bubbles will accumulate at the negative pole and fewer larger bubbles will appear at the positive pole.
2. Place the tips of two conducting cords on moistened litmus paper. The paper under the positive pole will turn red, while the paper under the negative pole will turn green or blue.

The effects of the positive pole on the body are the opposite of those produced by the negative pole.

POSITIVE POLE (ANODE)	NEGATIVE POLE (CATHODE)
Produces acid reaction.	Produces alkaline reaction.
Soothes nerves.	Stimulates nerves.
Decreases blood supply.	Increases blood supply.
Hardens tissues.	Softens tissues.

The positive pole may be used:

1. To close the follicles (pores) after the facial treatment.
2. To decrease redness, as in mild acne.
3. To prevent inflammation after comedone and blemish treatment.
4. To force acid pH solutions, such as astringent, into the skin.

The negative pole may be used:

1. To stimulate the circulation of blood to dry skin.
2. To force disincrustation lotion (alkaline pH solution) into the skin.

▶ **Caution:** Do not use the galvanic current over an area having many broken capillaries.

PHORESIS   Chemical solutions can be forced into unbroken skin by means of a galvanic current. This process is called *phoresis* (fo-**REE**-sis).

CATAPHORESIS   Cataphoresis (kat-uh-fo-**REE**-sis) is the use of the positive pole (anode) to introduce an acid pH product such as an astringent solution into the skin.

ANAPHORESIS   Anaphoresis (an-uh-fo-**REE**-sis) is the use of the negative pole (cathode) to force an alkaline pH product such as disincrustation lotion, into the skin).

Disincrustation

Disincrustation describes a process that softens and liquifies grease deposits, which are accumulations of sebum in the follicles. This sebum is usually filled with dead cells, makeup and grease. In order to do the disincrustation treatment, an alkaline solution is used to penetrate the follicle and dissolve the debris. For example, if you have heavy grease on your hands, you would use a soap, which is alkaline, to dissolve the grease. Disincrustation works in much the same way to dissolve the grease deposits in the pores. The disincrustation solution acts as a liquid type of soap. Disincrustation solutions are carefully formulated and are available from beauty supply manufacturers who carry products for estheticians. If the solution is not available, a simple formula can be prepared by mixing 1 level tablespoon (15 milliliters) sodium bicarbonate (household baking soda) with 1 pint (0.47 liter) distilled water.

HOW THE POSITIVE AND NEGATIVE POLES WORK   During the disincrustation process, the positive pole is held in the client's hand when the machine is turned on. The disincrustation solution is applied to a cotton pad or vicose sponge that is attached towards the negative pole. The negative pole is slowly glided over the client's skin (Fig. 17.11). The alkaline disincrustation solution will be attracted to the positive pole in the client's hand. The current is turned to its lowest point (amperage) before the negative pole is placed on the client's face. The client holds the positive electrode in his or her hand. The negative electrode holding the disincrustation lotion is placed on the chin and the rheostat is gradually turned clockwise to increase the intensity of the current. The client will usually experience a metallic taste in the mouth. The client will also feel a slight prickling sensation, which indicates that the current is strong enough. Do not increase the current once the prickling sensation is felt. These harmless sensations should be explained to the client.

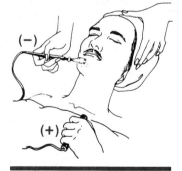

17.11—The negative (active) pole is slowly glided over the client's skin while he or she holds the positive (indifferent) pole in his or her hand during the disincrustation step.

Before moving the electrode from the chin to another area such as the cheek, the milliamperemeter is turned back to zero and the current is increased in the new area of the face, until the client once again feels the prickling sensation. The reading on the milliamperemeter will often vary, as the skin may be more sensitive in some areas than in others.

To further understand what happens inside the pore during disincrustation, try to imagine a bar of butter in its solid state being placed in a frying pan. When the heat is turned on, the butter will dissolve. In this treatment, the galvanic current and disincrustation lotion is the heat that dissolves the grease deposits in the follicles. This is an important step in the treatment of oily acne skin. Since dry or aging skin does not have an abundance of oil, it is usually not necessary to use the disincrustation treatment for those types of skin. For combination skin, disincrustation is used on the oily areas only, such as in the "T" zone. The amount of time spent doing the disincrustation part of a facial treatment will depend on the condition of the skin. If just the forehead, nose, and chin are treated, 5 to 7 minutes will be sufficient. If the skin is oily or acned, 10 minutes may be required. Smaller areas of the face may take as little as 3 to 4 minutes.

It is important to remove all traces of massage cream and cleanser from the skin before starting the disincrustation treatment, because the disincrustation lotion will emulsify the products and may force them deep into the follicles.

Following the disincrustation process, the Dr. Jacquet movements are used. This is followed by suction, and then whitehead and/or blackhead extraction. The suction lifts the debris out of the skin, helps to loosen blackheads and makes it easier for the esthetician to expel them with a minimum of pressure.

Ionization (Iontophoresis)

Ionization (iontophoresis) is the forcing of a solution or cream into the skin. In this procedure, the esthetician holds the positive pole (anode) on the client's face and the client holds the negative pole (cathode) (Fig. 17.12). Just as the positive pole attracts an alkaline solution from the negative pole, the negative pole will attract an acid solution from the positive pole.

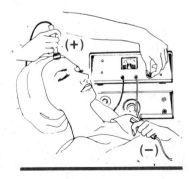

17.12—The esthetician holds the positive pole on the client's face and the client holds the negative pole for the cataphoresis procedure.

A cotton pad or viscose sponge is saturated with a mild sodium chloride solution, commonly known as salt. Just a pinch of salt dissolved in a few ounces of water is sufficient. This step assures that there is an acid pH solution on the positive pole that will come in contact with the client's face, and it will attract the positive current toward the negative pole being held in the client's hand. The ions of electricity from the positive pole will pass through a moisturizing cream or lotion that has been applied to the client's face and assure deep penetration of the product into the skin.

> **Note:** In order for the ionization to work properly, the cream or lotion applied to the face must be water soluble (O/W), such as a moisturizer or vanishing type cream. Heavy creams that do not dissolve in water (W/O), and leave an oily film on the skin, will not penetrate due to the product's large molecular structure.
>
> Manufacturers of products used by estheticians will often indicate on the package whether the negative or the positive pole should be used with that product. This indication is symbolized by a + (positive) or a − (negative) sign on the package.

IONTO ROLLERS   Another method of ionization is to use a set of metal rollers known as *ionto rollers* (Fig. 17.13). These rollers may come with the machine or they may be purchased separately as an accessory. One roller is attached to the negative pole and the other to the positive pole. The client does not hold either pole. After the cream or lotion has been applied to the skin, the esthetician places the rollers on the skin. When a rolling movement is made over the skin, ionization is achieved. The rolling movement should be very slow (Fig. 17.14).

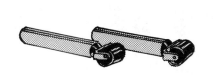

17.13—Ionto rollers

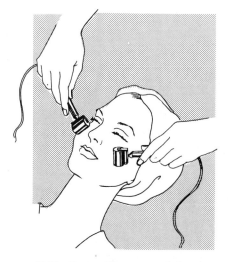

17.14—Ionto rollers are used for ionization on top of skin.

If the cream or lotion on the face has an acid pH, the current flowing through the roller that is attached to the positive pole will cause penetration of ingredients of the product. Should the cream on the face have an alkaline pH, the negative roller will penetrate the product. In either case the face is only receiving penetration on one side. To insure penetration on both sides of the face, the rollers should change hands after 3 to 5 minutes, so that each side of the face receives equal penetration.

In recent years some galvanic machines have been designed so that there is equal penetration from both rollers at the same time. This eliminates the changing of rollers from hand to hand and saves time. Some models of the galvanic machine necessitate the use of a double layer of gauze or cheesecloth that has been saturated with a mild chloride solution (common salt). This is placed over the product to be penetrated. The ionto rollers are then slowly rolled over the fabric (Fig. 17.15). The fabric prevents the metal rollers from coming into contact with the skin and eliminates any chemical irritation to the skin. Many galvanic machines have such low amperage that the ionto rollers are used directly over the product without any irritation to the skin. There are also ionto rollers that have been treated or coated with material. When in doubt, reread the instructions and if necessary, consult the manufacturer or place of purchase.

IONTO MASK An attachment sometimes used with the galvanic machine is an *ionto mask* (Fig. 17.16). The mask is made of spongy material and covers the entire face and chin. It is used for penetration of products and/or disincrustation and must be wet when in use. Instead of having the client hold an active pole, a wet pad is placed under the client's shoulder, and small metal plates are inserted into the mask. (*See Color Plate 23.*)

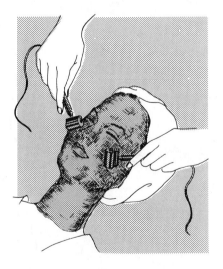

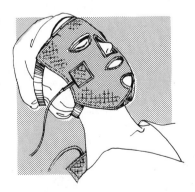

17.15—Ionto rollers are used for ionization on top of gauze or cheesecloth.

17.16—The ionto mask is used for ionization.

BLEACHING PIGMENTATION SPOTS

For clients with pigmentation discoloration of the skin, the following treatment has proved to be quite effective for bleaching out or lightening these spots. After the face has been thoroughly cleansed, blackheads removed, and prior to the application of the treatment cream and the mask, do the following:

Cut a juice orange in half and insert the conducting cord of the positive pole into the orange, piercing the peel. Place the negative pole in the client's hand. Turn the machine on. Begin tapping the skin with the orange as you turn the rheostat to increase the current. When the client begins to feel a tingling sensation, the current is strong enough. Rub the orange over the area of the skin that has the pigmentation blotches for approximately 5 to 7 minutes. The acidity from the juice of the orange, with the help of the galvanic current, will penetrate the skin and in most cases lighten the pigmentation blotches (Fig. 17.17). Wipe the face with a wet cotton pad or sponge. Blot with tissue and continue with the rest of the facial treatment. This treatment is more effective on clients who come to the salon on a regular basis.

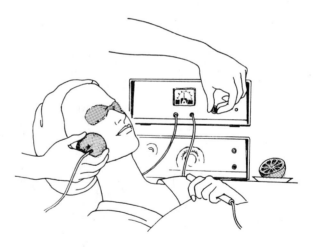

17.17—An orange is used to bleach pigmentation spots with the use of galvanic current.

Note: Do not use lemons for this treatment as the acid is too strong for the skin.

High-Frequency Machine

The high-frequency machine generates a current characterized by a high rate of oscillation (Fig. 17.18). This current is also known as *Tesla Current*. The action of this current is thermal, or heat-producing and germicidal. Because of the rapid oscillation of the current, there are no muscular contractions caused. The physiological effects are stimulating.

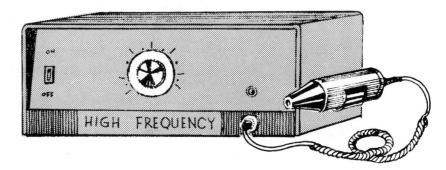

17.18—A high-frequency machine

ELECTRODES

The *electrodes* of the high-frequency machine are generally made of glass. They come in a variety of shapes and sizes. Four types are generally used by estheticians. The most frequently used is the mushroom-shaped electrode.

The *mushroom-shaped electrode* is used in circular motions on the face and neck (Fig. 17.19).

The *horseshoe-shaped electrode* is used in upward strokes on the client's neck (Fig. 17.20).

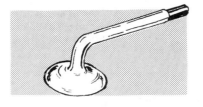

17.19—Mushroom-shaped electrode

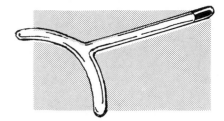

17.20—Horse-shoe shaped electrode

The *roller electrode* is used in a back and forth rolling movement over a cosmetic product that has been applied to the face (Fig. 17.21).

The *indirect electrode* is held in the client's hand (Fig. 17.22).

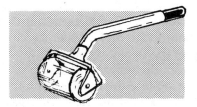

17.21—Roller electrode

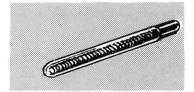

17.22—Indirect electrode

As the current energizes the glass electrode, tiny sparks are emitted. When the high-frequency current energizes the glass electrodes, they glow with a violet light. This is not to be confused with ultra-violet radiation. When the glass electrode contains neon gas, it will light up an orange-red color. Many estheticians believe that the orange-red light from the electrode is infra-red, producing more heat and deeper penetration. Actually the violet and orange-red rays produce approximately the same benefits.

Psychologically, the warmer color may benefit the client.

> **Note:** Quartz electrodes have been used on acne-prone skin. These electrodes contain a small amount of mercury, which increases the germicidal action on the skin. These electrodes have been banned for use in the United States.

BENEFITS OF HIGH-FREQUENCY   High-frequency current offers a number of benefits.

1. It stimulates circulation of the blood.
2. It increases glandular activity.
3. It aids in elimination and absorption.
4. It increases metabolism.
5. Germicidal action occurs during use.
6. It generates heat inside the tissues.
7. It aids in deeper penetration of products into the skin.

USE OF HIGH-FREQUENCY

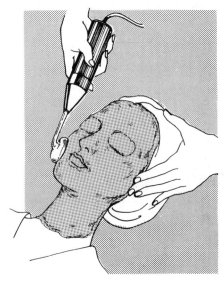

17.23—**For the direct current application, the esthetician holds the electrode and applies it over the client's skin.**

All treatments given with high-frequency should be started with a mild current, and gradually increased to the required strength. The length of the treatment depends upon the condition to be treated. For a general facial treatment, approximately 3 to 5 minutes should be allowed. There are two general methods of using the high-frequency current.

1. *Direct current application*—The esthetician holds the electrode and applies it over the client's skin (Fig. 17.23). In facial treatments, the electrode is applied directly over the treatment cream or mask. Direct application of the high-frequency current will have a sedative effect, because of the heat generated in the facial tissue. Oily and acne skins benefit from the germicidal action of the high-frequency current. It is necessary to place the forefinger on the stem of the electrode each time it is lifted or placed on the client's face or neck to prevent unpleasant sensations.

2. *Indirect application*—The client holds the electrode while the esthetician massages the area being treated. At no time is the electrode touched by the esthetician. To prevent shock, the current is turned up after the client is holding the electrode firmly in his or her hand. The current is turned down before the electrode is removed from the client's hand. Indirect application of the current has both a toning and stimulating effect on the skin.

When using high-frequency, start movements on the neck and work upward to the jaw, cheeks, chin, nose, and forehead. For proper use of the machinery, follow the manufacturer's instructions.

SPARKING

The skin will be stimulated when sprayed with a shower of sparks, which occurs when the electrode is held a fraction of an inch from the skin's surface. (The rheostat should be turned to a low position.) If the client seems apprehensive about the sparks, the treatment may be applied through a small, dry, cotton towel. Nylon or other synthetic fabric should not be used. The sparks will travel through the fabric and the treatment will be less dramatic. Sparking a pimple after the skin has been cleansed and follicles cleansed out, will destroy germs and bacteria and will aid in drying and healing the blemish. To prevent shock, the current is turned on after the electrode is on the client's face; or the esthetician's forefinger can be placed on the stem of the electrode and removed once the electrode is placed on the skin's surface. The finger is again placed on the stem before lifting the electrode from the client's skin.

Note: The client must not come in contact with any metal object. Clients should remove jewelry from hands and arms.

▶ | **Caution:** High-frequency current should not be used when the client is pregnant nor on clients who may have a pacemaker. In using high-frequency with skin lotions, never use a lotion with alcoholic content. If it is desirable to use this type of lotion, the high-frequency is used first, and the lotion applied after the application of the high-frequency has been completed.

The Spray Machine

The *spray machine* is also called an atomizer. The spray has many features when used in a facial treatment. It helps achieve a thorough cleansing of the skin's surface, is cool, soothing and has a pleasant fragrance. The bombardment of spray is used to flush out the pores, especially after suction and squeezing of blackheads and pimples. This is done almost in the same manner as a garden hose is used to flush debris from the cracks and crevices of a sidewalk. The spray rinses the skin and also helps restore the skin's acid mantle. (*See Color Plate 20.*)

 | **Note:** Although the suction and spray may be two separate machines, they are usually combined in one machine with both spray and suction functions.

A plastic spray bottle is filled with two parts distilled water and one part astringent or skin lotion. The container is filled approximately two-thirds of the way to the top. Estheticians often prepare two bottles of the spray liquid, one with astringent for normal or oily skin and one with mild skin lotion for mature, dry and/or sensitive skin.

The spray stimulates nerve endings and activates cell metabolism. It should be used on broken capillaries for a longer period of time. The spray creates an excellent light massage that exercises and strengthens the capillary walls by causing them to expand and contract. If the treatment calls for a lengthy spray, as is necessary for dehydrated or mature skins, the client will feel more comfortable if a towel is placed around the shoulders. Tissue may be used to fill in the area on both sides of the neck. This prevents moisture from dripping down onto the neck. The client should be handed a face cuvette (face bowl) when available to catch the excess spray, or tissue can be placed across the chest to protect the client's body from the spray (Fig. 17.24).

If sponges are used to cleanse the skin at the beginning of the facial treatment, instead of applying the astringent or skin lotion to the sponges, the face is rinsed with the spray. A sponge is held in the free hand to blot

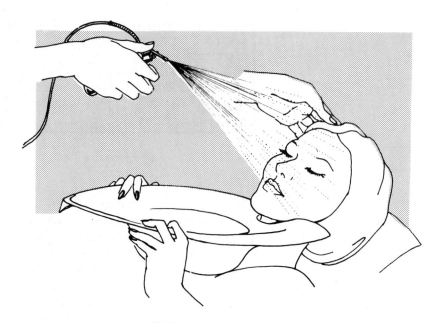

17.24—The client is holding a cuvette (facial bowl) during the facial spray procedure.

any excess spray. Distilled water is recommended for all atomizers and sprays because regular tap water contains minerals that will eventually clog the opening of the spray apparatus and can cause it to malfunction.

The spray is to be used:

1. As the second step to cleansing when sponges are used at the beginning of the treatment.
2. After suction and squeezing of blackheads and pimples.
3. After the mask is removed.

The Suction Machine

The suction machine is helpful in deep-pore cleansing of the skin. It acts much like a miniature vacuum cleaner to suction out deeply embedded dirt, grease and other impurities. The suction machine also gives a deep penetrating massage and draws blood to the surface of the skin. The blood provides nourishment and oxygen to the cells and carries away toxins. Massage is eliminated in a mini or short type treatment when the suction machine is used because the machine provides adequate stimulation of the skin (Fig. 17.25).

The suction machine may be used on all skin types except in areas that are heavily couperosed (broken capillaries). On an oily skin, the suction is always performed after disincrustation and/or the Dr. Jacquet movement.

The main function of the suction machine is to draw impurities and debris from the pores and follicles, but it is not strong enough to dislodge most blackheads. However, following the vacuum step, blackheads and grease deposits will be more easily extracted with manual pressure.

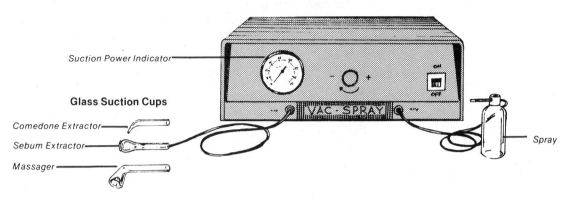

17.25—This model of the vacuum-spray machine has an indicator showing the strength of suction being used and uses glass suction cups.

When treating acne skin, the suction cup does not slide over the skin as it does on unblemished skin. Instead, a spot suction can be applied directly over a blemish. Some machines have a pulsating action that can be turned off and on (Fig. 17.26). The pulsating motion of this model can be used for spot suction. The pulsating action of the suction cup will be beneficial to skin that is lined or wrinkled. It will not cause the lines and wrinkles to disappear but it will activate the circulation of the blood and draw moisture to the surface of the skin.

Suction cups come in different sizes and are made of either glass or metal. Some models have a dial to control and regulate the suction strength. In other models the suction control is in the handle that holds the suction cup. The glass suction cups have a hole that the finger is placed over when the machine is in operation. When the finger is released the suction is broken. A thin film of cleansing lotion is placed on the skin to act as a buffer and to allow the cup to glide over the skin during the treatment. This helps to prevent pulling of the skin.

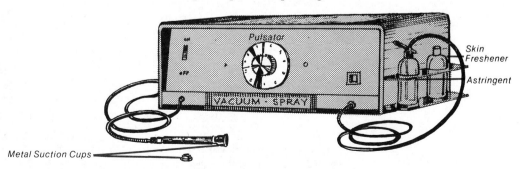

17.26—This model of the vacuum-spray machine uses metal suction cups and has a dial for regulating a pulsating action when desired.

When the skin is thin, dry, or aging, a light suction is used. A stronger suction may be used on an oily skin. The strength of the suction should be adjusted and can be tested on the esthetician's inner arm or hand to be sure the vacuum is right for the type skin that is being treated. The suction treatment is not recommended for skins that are suffering from rosacea, as the suction tends to cause the affected areas to become inflamed. Suction cups come in different sizes for various areas of the face. Two cups are usually sufficient. The larger cup is used to vacuum the neck, jaw, cheeks, and forehead. (See Figs. 17.27–17.30.) The smaller cup is used to vacuum the chin and the area between the nose and lip and the space between the eyes and the sides of the nose. (See Figs. 17.31–17.33.) The smaller cup has less vacuum power while the larger cup can build up to more vacuum power.

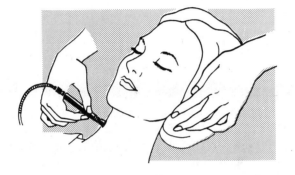

17.27—The suction starts at the center of the neck, moving outward.

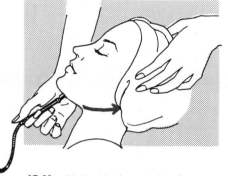

17.28—Suction is done under the chin, starting in the center and moving outward along the jawbone.

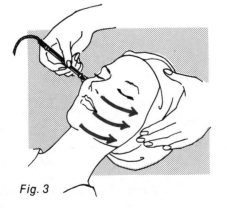

Fig. 3

17.29—Suction is done on the cheeks, starting on the chin and moving outward toward the ear.

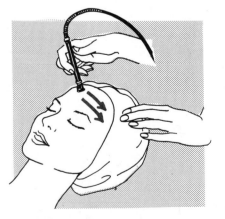

17.30—Suction is done on the forehead. Start in the center, moving outward toward the temple.

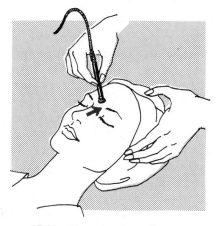

17.31—Change to a smaller suction cup and vacuum between the eyebrows.

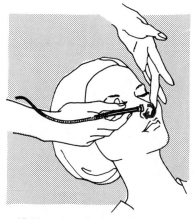

17.32—With the smaller suction cup, vacuum the nose. Support the nose with your free hand to avoid bending the nose.

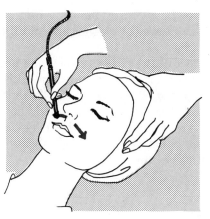

17.33—Continue with the smaller suction cup and vacuum the area between the nose and lips. Starting directly under the nose, work outward to the corner of the mouth.

CARE OF THE SUCTION MACHINE

If too much cleanser is applied to the face, it can be drawn into the machine or compressor and cause a breakdown. When a thin film of lotion cleanser is on the face it will gather around the rim of the cup and the debris that is pulled from the pores will cling to the lotion. After the treatment, the suction cup is removed, washed with soap and water, and placed in a bowl containing alcohol or in a dry sterilizing cabinet until needed. Some glass suction cups have an area where a small piece of cotton can be placed as a filter. To keep any type of material from going up into the suction machine, it should be turned off immediately after use.

Following the suction treatment the face is wiped with a clean cotton pad or sponge that has been sprinkled with a few drops of astringent. You will often see pollution and stale makeup which have been drawn from the pores on the pad. This debris on the pad will show the client the value of the suction treatment.

The Electric Pulverizer

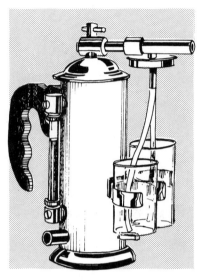

17.34—Electric pulverizer

The *electric pulverizer* is by far the most unique of all atomizers and sprays. It is widely used in Europe by most estheticians. The spray carries plant extracts, herb teas, skin fresheners and astringents to the face in a very fine mist. The mist is excellent for treating dehydrated, mature and couperose skins. The mist can be used warm to increase the blood flow to the skin's surface, and thus nourish the cells, or it can be used cool for couperose skin.

The Electric Pulverizer is filled ¾ full with distilled water. A glass gauge on the side of the pulverizer indicates the water level. Over-filling will cause the boiling water to spurt.

Two removable glass beakers are attached to the side of the pulverizer. The smaller beaker is to catch any drippings that might fall from the mouth of the spray. The larger beaker holds the solution to be pulverized.

A plastic tube dips down into the larger beaker to draw up the solution to be pulverized, where it will mix with the jet of steam coming from the boiler (Fig. 17.34).

Prepare the client by handing him or her a face cuvette or drape the body with a towel or plastic cape. Stuff tissue on each side of the client's neck or place a towel around the neck to catch any dripping solution.

The back of the client's chair may need to be raised a few degrees in order to keep the atomizer upright. This will not be too disturbing to the client as the spray is used near the end of the treatment.

The pulverizer will take approximately 3½ minutes to heat before the spray is ready. When ready, a hissing sound is heard. The distilled water inside the boiler will not spray until the plastic tube is dipped into the solution to be pulverized.

THE ELECTRIC PULVERIZER SPRAY The large beaker is filled with the desired plant extract, herb tea, astringent or skin freshener. When using astringent or skin freshener, mix ⅓ astringent or freshener to ⅔ distilled water. Preparation of the electric pulverizer can be done before the treatment starts or while the mask is on.

The Carbonic Gas Spray

The *carbonic gas spray* is a metal apparatus that producues a high-powered spray used mainly for oily and acne skins. Because of the high power of the spray, it has a deep-pore cleansing action that can increase the acidity deep in the pores and thus help protect the skin against germ penetration. The spray gives a stimulating massage to the surface of the skin, and when used on an acne skin will not spread infection.

The carbonic gas spray is used on the face directly after blackhead extraction and/or the cleansing out of blemishes. If the esthetician is not going to clean out blemishes and extract blackheads, then the carbonic gas spray will be used following the suction machine.

PREPARING THE CARBONIC GAS SPRAY

There are two basic models of carbonic gas spray. The difference in each model is the manner in which the liquid is charged with carbonic gas (CO_2).

The carbonic gas spray is prepared by filling the metal tank with distilled water that has been mixed with ½ ounce astringent. The carbonic gas spray apparatus holds 6 ounces of liquid. It should be filled to three-fourths full, which is 4½ ounces of fluid. The fluid used to fill the carbotom spray can be prepared in a measuring cup: one half ounce of astringent to 4 ounces of distrilled water. The top of the spray is screwed on tightly. The liquid is then charged with carbon dioxide gas (CO_2) (Fig. 17.35).

The Model A sprayer charges the liquid with CO_2 cartridges, which may be purchased at most drug or department stores. These are the same gas cartridges that are used to make carbonated water at home. The cartridge of carbonic gas is inserted into the cartridge holder and screwed to the top part of the carbonic spray. Twist the cartridge holder tightly until a hissing sound is heard. When the hissing sound stops, the container has been charged and is ready for use (Fig. 17.36).

For model B, the carbonic gas spray is prepared in the same manner as model A, with one exception. The liquid is charged with the CO_2 gas in a different manner. This model comes with a metal tank that holds the carbon dioxide gas. This tank is used in place of the CO_2 cartridges used in model A (Fig. 17.37).

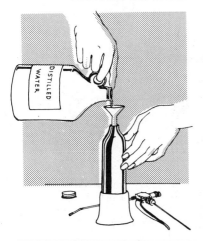

17.35—Preparing the carbonic gas spray

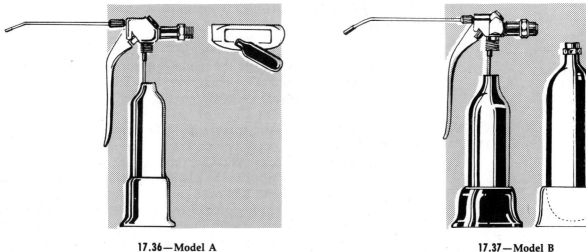

17.36—Model A   **17.37**—Model B

When the tank that comes with the carbonic gas spray runs out of gas, it is recharged with carbon dioxide gas. To recharge the tank, it will be necessary to rent a tank of dry carbon dioxide gas from a private gas company, which can be located by checking the yellow pages of the telephone book (Figs. 17.38 and 17.39).

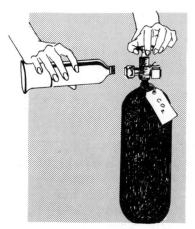

17.38—Recharging the tank

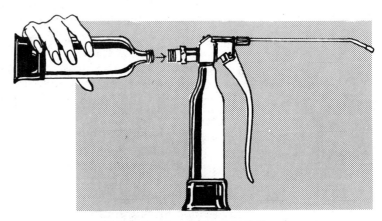

17.39—The newly charged tank is screwed to the carbonic gas spray. The gas from one tank will charge the water in the other tank.

> **Note:** If the carbonic gas spray is manufactured in Europe, a special adapter is usually needed to connect the two tanks. This is due to the difference in the manufacturing of American and European fittings. When the tank is being filled, a hissing sound is heard. When the sound stops, the tank is filled.

Most busy salons prefer to use the model B method of charging the carbonic spray because it is less expensive per use. The rented tank of gas should last the average salon several months.

HOW TO USE THE CARBONIC GAS SPRAY   The benefits of the carbonic spray should be explained to the client. Because of its power the spray will produce a strong tingling sensation on the face. For this reason, eye pads with the center twist should be used to protect the eyes. Never surprise the client with the spray. The first time the spray is used on a client, it should be tested on the client's hand to familiarize him or her with the force of the spray. The client is handed a face cuvette or a shampoo cape may be placed across the client's chest and back of head. A tissue is placed across the chest and on both sides of the client's neck to prevent excess spray from dripping onto the neck.

The spray is held approximately 20 inches from the client's face and three or four circles are made around the client's face with the spray (Fig. 17.40). The face is blotted with tissue and the esthetician may then proceed with the next step of the treatment.

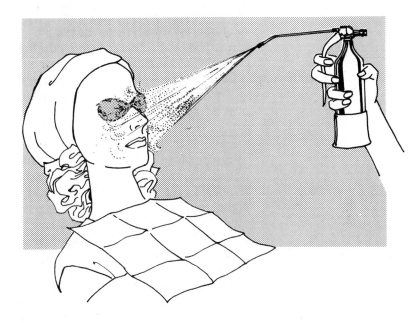

17.40—Carbonic gas spray in use

The Electric Mask

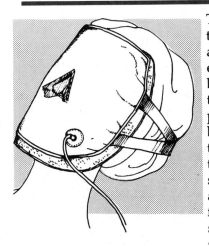

17.41—Electric mask

The *electric mask* is one of several methods used for deep penetration of the skin (Fig. 17.41). The mask produces heat at a comfortable temperature, and is used to help soften the skin for deep-pore penetration. The electric mask can be used on dry or oily skins depending on the products being used with the mask. For dry skin a moisturizer or deep-penetration treatment cream is used. The heat and warmth of the mask will help the product to penetrate deeper into the skin. For oily, acne, or problem blemished skin, the electric mask can be used with disincrustation solution to soften and liquify grease deposits. The mask is not used on a face that has a great percentage of broken capillaries. If the client has a thin, sensitive skin or areas with broken capillaries such as on the cheekbones, a fairly thick piece of moist cotton is placed over that area to protect it from the heating pad. The electric mask is also excellent for a combination skin that has an oily "T" zone and areas that are dry. The disincrustation solution is applied to the oily areas of the skin with a wet cotton compress and the treatment cream for dry skin is applied to the dry areas.

In this way a specialized treatment for each condition is accomplished at the same time. A treatment cream is always applied directly to the skin. After the product has been applied to the face, a tissue (with a hole in the center for the nose) is placed on the face. The nostrils must not be covered. A wet terry cloth (also with a hole cut out for the nose) is placed over the tissue. The precut terry cloth will usually come with the mask or it can be made from inexpensive terry wash cloths. The cloth must always be washed and sterilized after use. The electric mask is applied over the terry cloth. The electric mask should be turned on about 5 minutes before use so that it is warm when placed on the face.

The mask must be secured in place. Some models have a band that ties around the back of the head to hold the mask close to the face, while others have a U-shaped band that is placed over the surface of the mask to hold it in place. After application, the mask is left on the face for approximately 7 minutes. The mask produces warm, moist heat that opens the follicles and allows deep penetration of the products. After removal of the mask, dry skin will appear moist and superficial lines will soften. If the electric mask was used for disincrustation, suction and extraction of blackheads will follow. Some companies make attachments for the electric mask. One is for the neck and fits like a collar. Another attachment fits under the jaw. These attachments are also used to apply moist heat.

Should it be necessary for the esthetician to leave the facial area while the mask is in place, a timer should be set to let the client know that he or she is not being neglected. While the electric mask is on the face, most estheticians will take advantage of these few minutes and fill out the client's cards and records.

▶ **Caution:** To prevent the mask from burning out, it should be turned off immediately after use and disconnected from the wall plug.

Treatment Mitts

Treatment mitts are electrically warmed and heat is controlled by a thermostat. They are used as an added accessory and are optional as part of the salon's list of treatments. The mitts add a touch of luxury and pampering for the client, who may be conscious of the appearance of his or her hands (Fig. 17.42).

While the client is having a facial treatment, the hands are massaged with a small amount of treatment cream or hand lotion and the hands are slipped into a plastic liner and the warm treatment mitts. The warmth helps the beneficial cream to penetrate the skin leaving the hands smoother and softer. The warm hand treatment also soothes and helps to relieve pain in the hands that may be caused by an arthritic condition. The plastic liner must be washed after each treatment.

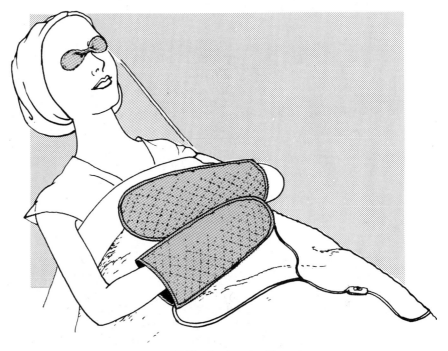

17.42—Treatment mitts

Electricity

Electricity, and its beneficial effects, have long been recognized to be of value, provided it is used intelligently and safely. It can be used to supply light and heat and to operate electrical appliances, all for the advantage of the esthetician and the client.

Although the exact nature of electricity is not yet completely understood, its generating sources and effects are known. It is generally believed that electricity is a form of energy, which when in motion, produces *magnetic*, *chemical*, or *heat* effects.

ELECTRICAL CURRENT A current of electricity is a stream of *electrons* (negatively charged particles) moving along a conductor.

ELECTRIC WIRE An electric wire is composed of twisted fine metal threads (conductor) covered with plastic, rubber, or silk (insulator or nonconductor).

CONDUCTOR A conductor is a substance that readily transmits an electric current. Most metals, carbon, the human body, and watery solutions of acids and salts are good conductors of electricity.

NON-CONDUCTOR A non-conductor or insulator is a substance that resists the passage of an electric current, such as rubber, silk, dry wood, glass, cement, or asbestos.

FORMS OF ELECTRICITY   Two forms of electricity are employed, namely:

1. *Direct current (D.C.)* is a constant and ever-flowing current, traveling in one direction.
2. *Alternating current (A.C.)* is a rapid and interrupted current, flowing first in one direction and then in the opposite direction.

CONVERTER AND RECTIFIER   If necessary, one type of current can be changed into another by means of a converter or rectifier.

The converter is an apparatus used to convert a direct current into an alternating current. A rectifier is used to change an alternating current into a direct current, and is necessary to generate galvanism.

CIRCUIT   The complete circuit of electricity is the entire path traveled by the current from its generating source, through various conductors (wire, electrode, or body), and back to its original source.

FUSE   A fuse is a safety device that prevents the overheating of electric wires. It will blow out because of overloading (too many machines, apparatus, or appliances on one wire), or due to a short circuit. To re-establish the circuit, electrical apparatus should be disconnected before inserting a new fuse.

Precaution—When replacing a blown fuse make sure to:

1. Use new fuse with proper rating.
2. Stand on a dry surface.
3. Keep hands dry.

If an electrical appliance goes out of order while in operation, the plug should be pulled, and if necessary, an electrician called.

Electrical Measurements

Electrical measurements are expressed in terms of the following units:

VOLT   The volt is a unit of electrical *pressure*.

AMPERE   The ampere is a unit of electrical *strength*.

OHM   The ohm is a unit of electrical *resistance*.

An electrical current flows through a conductor when the pressure is sufficiently great to overcome the resistance offered by the wire to the passage of the current. According to *Ohm's law*, the strength of a current (amperage) equals the pressure (voltage) divided by the resistance (ohm).

MILLIAMPERE   Instead of the ampere, which is too strong, the milliampere, 1/1000th part of an ampere, is used for facial treatments. The milliamperemeter is an instrument for measuring the rate of flow of an electric current.

Electrical Devices

JACK   A jack is a fitting device, often found on the end of an electrical cord. It is inserted into a receptacle on the apparatus.

PLUG   The plug is the part of an electrical cord that connects the apparatus by inserting into an electrical outlet or socket.

POLARITY CHANGER   The polarity changer alters the direction of the current.

CONDUCTING CORDS   Conducting cords carry the current to the electrodes.

ELECTRODE   The electrode serves as a conductor and applicator of electricity to certain areas of the body.

RHEOSTAT   The rheostat regulates the strength of the current used.

MILLIAMPEREMETER   The milliamperemeter is an instrument for measuring the rate of flow of an electric current.

Safety Practices in Electricity

Use only one plug to each outlet. Overloading may cause a fuse to blow out (Fig. 17.43).

To disconnect current, remove plug without pulling cord. Never pull on cord as the wires may become loosened, and may cause a short circuit.

Examine cords regularly. Repair or replace worn cords to prevent short circuiting, shock, or fire (Fig. 17.44).

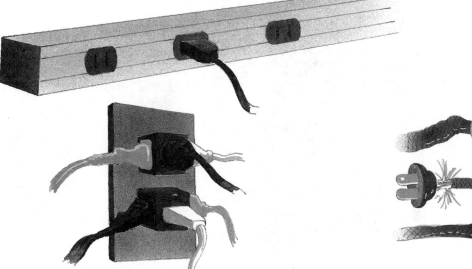

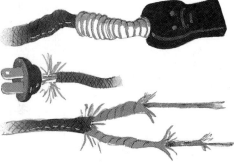

17.43—Use only one plug to each outlet. Overloading, as in bottom illustration, may cause a fuse to blow out.

17.44—Examine cords regularly.

▶ **Caution:** Keep a flashlight at top of steps, so you won't stumble down a dark stairway. Using your flashlight, open the fuse box and examine each fuse to locate the "dead" one. When you replace a burned-out fuse, touch only its rim. Never put a coin in the fuse box instead of a fuse.

Be sure to have some good fuses on hand. To test a fuse, use a flashlight battery and bulb (or the bulb assembly), and a piece of wire. If the fuse is good, the bulb will light.

In an emergency, turn off main switch to shut off electricity for entire salon or building.

When replacing a blown-out fuse (Fig. 17.45), make sure to:

1. Use a new fuse with proper rating.
2. Stand on a dry surface.
3. Keep hands dry.

Circuit breakers are now the most commonly used device for protecting electrical circuits (Fig. 17.46). When there is an overload condition, the switch or breaker simply moves automatically from the "on" to the "off" position. To reset, first switch off or unplug whatever appliances were being used on the circuit. Open the door of the circuit breaker panel to see which of the breakers has moved to the "off" position. Keep in mind that the breaker switch does not always move all the way to the "off" position, but slightly away from the "on." To re-establish power, move the breaker switch all the way to the "off" position then snap it back to the "on" position. Close the circuit breaker door. Resume the use of the appliance. If the circuit breaker again shuts off power, then it is likely that there is a short in the appliance being used, or the circuit is overloaded with too many appliances.

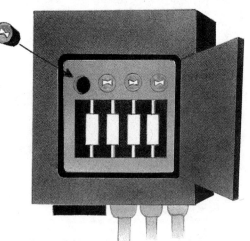

17.45—Carefully replace blown-out fuses.

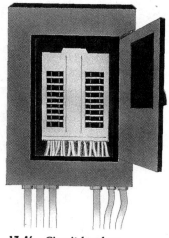

17.46—Circuit breakers automatically disconnect any current to a defective appliance.

Light Therapy

Light therapy (**THERR**-uh-pee) refers to treatment by means of light rays. Light or electrical waves travel at a tremendous speed—186,000 miles per second.

There are many kinds of light rays, but in salon work we are concerned with only three—those producing heat, known as *infra-red rays*; those producing chemical and germicidal reaction, known as *ultra-violet rays*; and visible lights, all of which are contained within the spectrum of the sun.

If a ray of sunshine is passed through a glass prism (**PRIZ**-um), it will appear in seven different colors, known as the *rainbow* or *spectrum*, arrayed in the following manner: red, orange, yellow, green, blue, indigo and violet. These colors, which are visible to the eye, constitute the *visible rays*, comprising about 12 percent of sunshine.

Scientists have discovered that at either end of the visible spectrum are rays of the sun which are *invisible* to us. The rays beyond the violet are the *ultra-violet rays*, also known as *actinic* (ack-**TIN**-ick) *rays*. These rays are the shortest and least penetrating rays of the spectrum, comprising about 8 percent of sunshine. The action of these rays is both chemical and germicidal.

Beyond the red rays of the spectrum are the *infra-red rays*. These are pure heat rays, comprising about 80 percent of sunshine (Fig. 17.47).

Natural sunshine is composed of 8 percent ultra-violet rays, 12 percent visible light rays, 80 percent infra-red rays.

Properties of Infra-Red Rays:	*Properties of Ultra-Violet Rays:*
1. Long wave length	1. Short wave length
2. Low frequency	2. High frequency
3. Deep penetrating power	3. Weak penetrating power

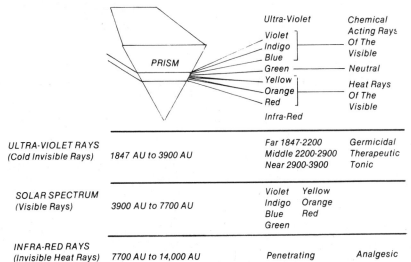

17.47—Dispersion of light rays by a prism

How Light Rays Are Reproduced

A *therapeutic* (**THERR**-uh-pew-tick) *lamp* is an electrical apparatus capable of producing certain light rays. There are separate lamps for infrared and for ultra-violet rays.

There are three general types of *ultra-violet lamps*: The glass bulb, the hot quartz, and the cold quartz.

The *glass bulb lamp* is used mainly for cosmetic or tanning purposes (Fig. 17.48).

The *hot quartz lamp* is a general all-purpose lamp suitable for tanning, health, cosmetic, or germicidal purposes (Fig. 17.49).

The *cold quartz lamp* produces mostly short ultra-violet rays. It is used primarily in hospitals (Fig. 17.50).

Infra-red rays give no light whatsoever, only a rosy glow when active. Special glass bulbs are also used to produce infra-red rays.

The *visible rays*, or *dermal lights*, are reproduced by carbon or tungsten filament in clear glass bulbs. They produce white light, or in colored bulbs, red or blue colors.

The client's eyes should always be protected with wet cotton pads, which may be sprinkled with witch hazel solution, and placed on the eyelids during light-ray treatments. The esthetician and client should always wear safety eye goggles when using ultra-violet rays.

> **Note:** Though rarely used in the facial salon, the use of ultra-violet rays should be understood by the esthetician. Check with your state board of cosmetology regarding the use of ultra-violet rays in your state.

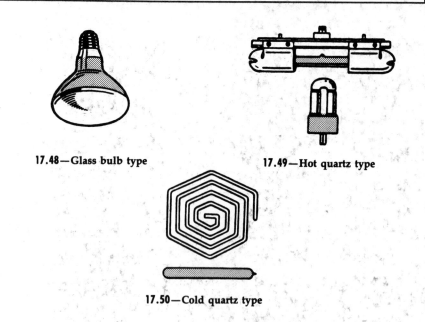

17.48—Glass bulb type

17.49—Hot quartz type

17.50—Cold quartz type

Ultra-Violet Rays

Ultra-violet rays are invisible rays. Their action is both chemical and germicidal. Plant and animal life needs ultra-violet rays for healthy growth. In the human body, these rays produce changes in the chemistry of the blood and also stimulate the activity of body cells.

EFFECTS OF RAYS   Ultra-violet rays increase resistance to disease by increasing the iron and vitamin D content and the number of red and white cells in the blood. They also increase elimination of waste products, restore nutrition where needed, stimulate the circulation, and improve the flow of blood and lymph (limf).

The slightest obstruction of any kind will hinder ultra-violet rays from reaching the skin. Consequently, the skin must be entirely cleansed before being subjected to ultra-violet rays.

HOW TO APPLY RAYS   Ultra-violet rays are the shortest light rays of the spectrum. The farther they are from the visible light region, the shorter they become. The longer ultra-violet rays tend to increase the fixation of calcium in the blood. If the lamp is placed from 30 to 36 inches away, few of the shorter rays will reach the skin, so that the action is then limited to the effect of the longer rays.

The shorter rays are obtained when the lamp is within 12 inches from the skin. These rays are not only destructive to bacteria, but to tissue as well, if allowed to remain exposed for too long a period of time.

Average exposure may produce redness of the skin, and overdoses may cause blistering. It is well to start with a short exposure of 2 or 3 minutes, and gradually increase the time to 7 or 8 minutes.

Caution: The esthetician and client must wear eye goggles to protect their eyes.

Skin tanning is the result of exposure to ultra-violet rays, which stimulate the production of pigment, or coloring matter, in the skin.

Sunburn may be produced by ultra-violet rays in various degrees; however, for cosmetic purposes, only a first degree sunburn is given. This is manifested by a slight reddening, appearing several hours after application, showing no signs of itching, burning, or peeling. Overexposure produces more severe burns, which are destructive to the tissues.

Infra-Red Rays

Generally speaking, *infra-red rays* produce a soothing and beneficial type of heat, which penetrates for some distance into the tissues of the body.

Use and effect of infra-red rays on exposed area:

1. Heats and relaxes the skin without increasing temperature of the body as a whole.
2. Dilates blood vessels in the skin, thereby increasing blood flow.
3. Increases metabolism and chemical changes within skin tissues.
4. Increases the production of perspiration and oil on the skin.
5. Relieves pain.
6. Aids in deeper penetration of products into the skin.

HOW TO APPLY INFRA-RED RAYS   The lamp is operated at an average distance of 30 inches, depending on the wattage of the bulb (Fig. 17.51). When the lamp is used for the purpose of keeping the product on the face from turning cold, it may be set at a further distance. Wet cotton pads, which may be sprinkled with witch hazel solution, are placed over the client's eyelids.

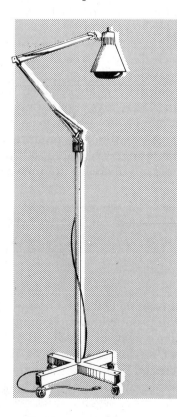

17.51—Infra-red lamp

Use of Visible Light

The psychological value of color has long been used in creating moods or atmosphere. Rooms decorated in warm colors, such as red, deep pink, brown, orange, or yellow, tend to stimulate or create a feeling of warmth and coziness. Rooms decorated in cool colors, such as green, blue, white, and pastels, tend to create a feeling of coolness and relaxation. We have been conditioned since birth to associate certain colors with different actions. Colored lights, such as red and blue, are used in facial salons during some stages of facial treatments for their psychological effect on the client. Blue light suggests coolness, sterile conditions, and is conducive to relaxation. During certain stages of a treatment, such as when the mask is left on the face for several minutes, the esthetician may set the mood by turning off all lights, except for the colored light fixture.

Other Apparatus Used in Facial Treatments

In addition to the electrical machinery discussed in this chapter, estheticians may find certain nonelectrical equipment useful. These include:

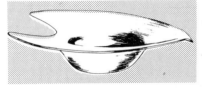

17.52—Face cuvette

- Face cuvettes to protect the client from spray during the treatments (Fig. 17.52)
- An adjustable facial chair for the client and a utility table with a swing-out tray for keeping supplies and treatment products close at hand (Fig. 17.53)
- A stool for the esthetician to use during the facial treatment (Fig. 17.54)

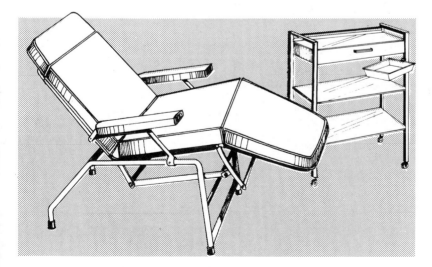

17.53—Facial chair and utility table

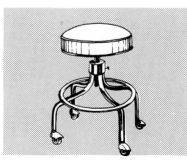

17.54—Esthetician's stool

Machines for Skin Care not a New Concept

An ad appeared in "American Hairdresser" magazine in 1937 (Fig. 17.55). The ad showed a practitioner vacuuming the pores during a facial treatment with a suction machine that was the forerunner of today's modern suction machine. The wall plate produced different currents used for face treatments including galvanic current used for disincrustation and ionization and high-frequency current used for stimulation and deep penetration. The machines shown in this ad were manufactured in the United States of America.

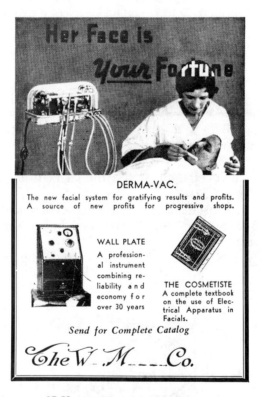

17.55—Machines are not a new concept in skin care but their use is currently being revived. Some have been improved in design and function.

QUESTIONS DISCUSSION AND REVIEW

ELECTRICITY, MACHINES, AND APPARATUS FOR PROFESSIONAL SKIN CARE

1. Why do estheticians use magnifying lamps?
2. Who developed the Wood's lamp?
3. What color will thin dehydrated skin appear as under the Wood's lamp?
4. List the benefits of the vaporizer.
5. How far away should the vapor nozzle be set from the client's face?
6. What is the mixture that is used to clean the reservoir and heating elements of the vaporizing machine?
7. What is the purpose of the brushing machine?
8. How should you cleanse the brushes of the brushing machine after each use?
9. What are the two functions of the galvanic current during a facial treatment?
10. When does a galvanic current have a chemical effect?
11. Give another name for the negative pole and positive pole.
12. What is the primary action of the high-frequency current?
13. List the different types of electrodes of high-frequency machines and where they can be used.
14. List the benefits of high-frequency.
15. In a general facial treatment, how long should high-frequency be applied?
16. What are the three methods of using the high-frequency current?
17. What is the purpose of the vacuum-spray machine?
18. What is another name for the spray machine?
19. List some benefits of the spray.
20. What skin type will the electric pulverizer benefit most?
21. What type of skin is the carbonic gas spray mainly used on?
22. What cautions should be taken when using the carbonic gas spray?
23. When would you not use the electric mask?
24. What is an electrical current?
25. What is a conductor?
26. What are two safety devices that prevent the overheating of electric wires?
27. How is the current measured in most facial treatment machines?
28. What is a polarity changer?
29. What does a rheostat do?
30. Why should you examine cords regularly?
31. What is light therapy?
32. What are the three forms of light rays used in salons?
33. Natural sunlight is composed of what percentage of ultra-violet, visible, and infra-red rays?

CHAPTER 18

Facial Treatments with the Aid of Machines

LEARNING OBJECTIVES

After completing this chapter, you should be able to:

❶ Demonstrate different facial procedures with the aid of machines.
❷ Explain which skin type each facial is for and their benefits.
❸ Discuss how to advise your clients on a home care regimen.

INTRODUCTION

The facial treatments in this chapter are accomplished with the aid of various modern machines. Machines help the esthetician to give treatments that are, in some cases, more thorough than can be achieved using only the hands. For example: Galvanic current will aid in dissolving grease deposits in the follicles so they may be removed easily. Machines have various functions that aid in giving treatments for different skin conditions. Machines alone will not assure the success of facial treatments, but in the hands of a professional esthetician, machines can be valuable aids in keeping the skin healthy and attractive.

Machine Facials for Normal Skin

In Chapter 11 it is explained how a normal skin will benefit from maintenance treatments that help to keep it healthy and attractive. Regular care will assure that normal skin will continue to function in a normal way.

PROCEDURE

1. Prepare the client.
2. Sanitize your hands.
3. Cleanse the client's face.
4. Analyze the face. (Use eyepads and the magnifying lamp.)
5. Vaporize the skin for approximately 10 minutes to open pores for deep cleansing and to soften dead cells for easy removal.
6. Proceed with Massage #1.
7. The massage cream is blotted off with a tissue. This is followed by cleansing the face with a wet cotton pad or sponges that have been sprinkled with 10 to 15 drops of skin-freshening lotion.
8. A thin layer of cleanser is applied to the face, avoiding the eye area. The brushing machine (with a soft brush) is used for approximately 2 minutes.

Note: The cleanser is left on the face for the next step (suction).

9. Suction is done over the face and neck.
10. The skin is cleansed with a cotton pad or sponges that have been moistened with skin-freshening lotion.
11. The face is sprayed well and blotted with tissue.
12. The treatment cream or lotion is applied. Deep penetration is done by one of the following methods:
    a. Galvanic ionization
    b. Application of the electric mask
    c. High-frequency current procedure
    d. Massage #2
13. Following the deep penetration step, the mask for normal skin is applied. The mask is left on for approximately 10 minutes.
14. The mask is removed with wet sponges or the cotton compress mask.
15. The face is sprayed.
16. The face is blotted with a tissue to remove excess spray.
17. Protective fluid is applied.
18. The treatment is completed.

ALTERNATE TREATMENT PROCEDURE

A good alternative for the client with a normal skin would be the epidermabrasion treatment.

Facial Treatment for Dry Skin with the Aid of Machines

There are three classifications of dry skin and the treatments for all three are basically the same. The difference in treatments will be in the products used. Dry skin is classified as one or all of the following:

1. Oil-dry—lacking sebum
2. Dehydrated—lacking moisture
3. Mature dry—aging

Most manufacturers produce special treatment creams or lotions for oil-dry and dehydrated skin. When the skin is oil-dry, the main objective is to stimulate the sebaceous glands to produce the natural sebum the skin needs. For a dehydrated skin the stimulation may not be as necessary, but it will be necessary to use products that help the skin to retain the moisture it needs. A dry skin is often thin and delicate. Therefore, all massage movements, as well as suction or brushing, must be done gently.

> **Note:** A client with dry skin may be using a cream for dry skin with no apparent improvement in the condition of the skin. The esthetician can explain that the dry surface of the skin is due to a barrier of dead cells, makeup, or dirt and other debris that keeps the skin from being lubricated properly. To lubricate the skin and relieve dryness, it is necessary to remove this layer of debris and moisten the inner layers of the skin so that the products can work effectively.

PROCEDURE
1. Check to be sure the vaporizer is ready for use.
2. Prepare the client.
3. Sanitize hands.
4. Cleanse the client's skin with a lotion cleanser formulated for dry skin.
5. Analyze the skin. (Use eyepads and the magnifying lamp.)
6. Vaporize the skin for approximately 10 minutes.
7. Do Massage #1.

> **Note:** The vaporizer may be left on during all or part of Massage #1. It is important when treating a thin skin, that the massage cream is soft enough to spread easily over the face. The cream allows the hands to glide over the surface of the skin without pulling.

8. The massage cream is blotted off with a tissue. This step is followed by cleansing the face with a wet cotton pad or sponges that have been sprinkled with 10 to 15 drops of skin-freshening lotion.

9. A thin layer of cleanser is applied to the face. Avoid the eye area. The brushing machine (with a soft brush) is used for approximately 2 minutes.

 Note: The cleanser is left on the face for the next step (suction). Disincrustation is not done on dry skin.

10. The suction is done gently and is always lighter on a dry or delicate skin than on an oily or thick skin.
11. The skin is cleansed with a cotton pad or sponges that have been moistened with skin-freshening lotion.
12. The face is sprayed thoroughly and blotted with tissue.
13. The treatment cream or lotion is applied. Deep penetration is done by one of the following ways:
    a. Galvanic ionization
    b. Application of the electric mask
    c. High-frequency current procedure
    d. Massage #2
    e. Warm wax mask
14. Following the deep penetration step, the mask formulated for dry skin is applied. The mask is left on for approximately 10 minutes.
15. The mask is removed with wet sponges or the cotton compress mask.
16. The face is sprayed. The warm, electric pulverizer spray is excellent for dehydrated skin and should be used when it is available.
17. The face is blotted with a tissue to remove excess spray.
18. Protective fluid is applied.
19. The treatment is completed.

 Note: The client should be advised to drink plenty of water and other healthful liquids to provide moisture for the skin from within.

ALTERNATE TREATMENT PROCEDURE

1. Following the application of the treatment cream, the warm wax mask may be applied. The warm wax mask is used for deep penetration.
2. After the wax mask is removed, the face is sprayed thoroughly. The warm electric pulverizer spray may be used, especially if the skin is dehydrated and dry.
3. Following the spray, the skin is blotted with tissue.
4. Protection lotion is applied.
5. The treatment is completed.
6. The cleanup procedure is completed.

Facial Treatment for Mature (Aging) Skin with the Aid of Machines

Aging is a natural process and the esthetician is limited in overcoming the effects of aging on the skin. However, proper treatment at home, and in the salon, using specially formulated products can bring about significant improvement in a short time. In many cases, the aging process can be slowed down, superficial lines diminished, and the skin given a more healthy, youthful appearance.

PROCEDURE

1. Check the vaporizer to be sure it is ready for use when needed.
2. Sanitize hands.
3. Cleanse the client's face.
4. Analyze the client's skin. Use eyepads and the magnifying lamp.
5. Vaporize the skin for approximately 10 minutes.
6. Proceed with Massage #1.

> **Note:** It is important that all massage movements on a mature skin be gentle, so as not to stretch the skin.

7. Remove the massage cream with tissue, followed by cleansing with a wet cotton pad or sponges that have been sprinkled with skin-freshening lotion.
8. Do a light suction over a thin film of cleansing lotion that has been applied to the entire face and neck.
9. Cleanse the face with a wet cotton pad or sponges that have been moistened with skin freshener.
10. Spray the face thoroughly and blot with tissue.
11. Apply a special treatment cream and proceed with Massage #2. One of the following deep-penetration procedures may be used after Massage #2:
    a. High-frequency current
    b. Galvanic ionization
    c. Electric mask
    d. Warm wax mask
12. Following the deep-penetration step, the mask formulated for dry and/or mature skin is applied. The mask is left on for approximately 10 minutes.
13. The mask is removed with wet sponges or the cotton compress mask.
14. The facial spray is used. The warm, electric pulverizer spray (if available) is excellent for a mature skin.
15. The face is blotted with tissue to remove excess spray.
16. Protective fluid is applied.
17. The treatment is completed.

> **Note:** The client should be advised to drink plenty of water and other healthful fluids to provide moisture for the skin from within.

ALTERNATE TREATMENT
1. Following the application of the treatment cream (Step 11), the warm mask is used for deep penetration.
2. After the wax mask is removed, the face is sprayed thoroughly. Otherwise, the electric pulverizer spray may be used, as this is excellent for mature, dry skin.
3. Following the spray, the skin is blotted with tissue.
4. Protection lotion is applied.
5. The treatment is completed.
6. The cleanup procedure is completed.

Note: If time permits, giving Massage #2 and applying the warm wax mask is permissible. However, it is unwise for the client to become accustomed to an extended treatment. It is best to adhere to a schedule and do what can be done within the time allotted for the treatment.

Facial Treatment for Oily Skin with the Aid of Machines

The major problem with an oily skin is that it contains oil and grease, which attract dirt. The dirt becomes trapped beneath the surface of the skin where it can cause infection. This debris is the start of pimples and acne. During the treatment for oily skin, the accumulation of dead cells, dirt, and other debris must be softened, the follicles opened, and the excess oil and dirt removed. Deep-cleansing treatments help to normalize the production of sebum by the sebaceous glands and remove the debris that so often causes infection. Once the follicles are cleansed and unplugged (as in the extraction of blackheads), the sebum can flow more easily to the surface of the skin where it can be cleansed away.

Note: When the skin is extremely oily, as is often the case of a young adult, Massage #1 may be eliminated and the extra time used for a thorough disincrustation and extraction of blackheads and whiteheads. In this type of treatment, the Dr. Jacquet movements are done over the oily areas of the skin.

PROCEDURE FOR OILY SKIN TREATMENT
1. Check the vaporizer to be sure it is ready when needed.
2. Sanitize hands.
3. Cleanse the skin with lotion cleanser followed by astringent.
4. Analyze the skin. Use eyepads when the client is under the magnifying lamp.
5. Vaporize the skin for 10 minutes.
6. Proceed with Massage #1.
7. Remove the massage cream.
8. Apply a thin film of cleansing lotion and proceed with the brushing procedure on the neck and face.

9. Remove all traces of massage cream and cleansing lotion. Use a wet cotton pad or sponges that have been sprinkled with astringent.
10. Proceed with disincrustation on all areas that are oily and have open follicles, blackheads, and whiteheads. Disincrustation can be done with galvanic current or the electric heating mask.

> **Note:** The vaporizer may be left on the face and neck during all or part of Massage #1, the electric brushing, or the disincrustation. This is done at the discretion of the esthetician.

11. The Dr. Jacquet movements are performed following disincrustation in the oily areas, and where there are open follicles and blackheads.
12. A thin layer of cleansing lotion is applied and the suction procedure is done over the face and neck.

> **Note:** At this point in the treatment, the skin has been softened, the follicles opened with a vaporizer or warm, moist towels, and the dead cells have been removed from the surface of the skin with the brushing apparatus. Blackheads and grease deposits have been softened and melted by disincrustation and the suction has loosened the debris in the follicles. Now the blackheads and debris in the follicles can be expelled with a minimum amount of pressure.

13. Complete the extraction of blackheads, whiteheads, and other debris.
14. Cleanse the face with a wet cotton pad or sponge that has been sprinkled with astringent.
15. Spray the face with one part astringent to two parts of distilled water. (The carbonic gas spray may be used if available.)
16. Apply a treatment cream, preferably one that is water-soluble and formulated for oily skin.
17. The deep penetration may be done by using any one of the following:
    a. High-frequency current
    b. Galvanic ionization
    c. Electric mask
    (Steps 16 and 17 are optional.)
18. Apply the specially formulated mask. If the treatment cream that is being used is water-soluble, the mask formulated for oily skin may be applied directly over the treatment cream.
19. The mask is removed with sponges or the cotton compress mask.

> **Note:** When the skin is very oily and if the weather is warm, the protection fluid may be omitted if the client prefers.

20. The face is sprayed with a mixture of two-thirds water to one-third astringent.
21. Protection lotion is applied to the face and neck.
22. Complete the treatment.
23. Complete the cleanup procedure.

> **Note:** The client will usually realize that the esthetician can remove a great deal of the debris from the skin during the first treatment. Improvement should be seen following the first treatment and the client will be eager to see further improvement. The client should be reminded that there are too many follicles on the face to thoroughly cleanse them all during one treatment. The skin does not become blemished overnight, and it will take time and patience to rid the skin of blackheads and the accumulation of debris. The client should be advised of correct home care for his or her skin, in order to gain the greatest benefit from the salon treatments.

Facial Treatment for a Combination Skin with the Aid of Machines

When treating a combination skin, each area of the face and neck are treated for the problem in that particular area. For example, if your client has an oily "T" zone (forehead, nose, and chin) and the rest of the face and neck are dry or normal, you would apply a mask for oily skin on the oily "T" zone and a mask for dry or normal skin in the areas that are dry or normal.

PROCEDURE

1. Check the vaporizer to be sure it is ready when needed.
2. Sanitize hands.
3. Cleanse the skin and follow with a mild astringent.
4. Analyze the skin, using eyepads on the eyes while the client is under the magnifying lamp.
5. Vaporize the skin.
6. Proceed with Massage #1.
7. Remove the massage cream with tissue, followed by a cleansing with a wet cotton pad or sponges that have been sprinkled with skin freshener.
8. Do the brushing procedure.
9. Do the disincrustation procedure on the oily areas only.
10. Proceed with the Dr. Jacquet massage in the areas that are oily with open pores and blackheads.
11. Apply a thin film of cleansing lotion over the face and neck and proceed with the suction procedure.
12. Remove blackheads with light pressure.
13. Spray the face with one part astringent to two parts distilled water.
14. Blot the face with tissue.

15. Apply a light-textured treatment cream or fluid. Deep penetration is done by using any one of the following:
    a. Electric mask
    b. Galvanic ionization
    c. High-frequency current
    d. Massage #2
16. Following the deep-penetration procedure, a mask for dry and normal areas is applied. A mask formulated for oily skin is applied to oily areas of the face.
17. Remove the mask.
18. Spray the face thoroughly and blot.
19. Apply protection fluid or lotion.
20. Complete the treatment.

Facial Treatment for Acne (Problem-Blemished) Skin with the Aid of Machines

The client with an acne skin condition will need to be educated on how to care for his or her skin with home treatments, as well as receiving specialized treatments in the salon. Proper cleansing of the skin is of vital importance. The client should be told not to cleanse the skin too often, because excessive cleansing tends to irritate an acne skin and overdries the surface. Theoretically, overcleansing the skin stimulates the sebaceous glands to work harder to replace the oil that has been removed. Washing the skin with too much soap and water not only dries the surface but destroys the skin's acid mantle, which fights germ penetration. It may take 20 minutes or more for some skin to replace the acid mantle. During this time the skin is left unprotected and vulnerable to germ penetration.

COUNSELING THE CLIENT   The client will usually have questions about the severity of an acne condition. He or she may ask how many treatments will be required to achieve results, and how much a series of treatments will cost. If the acne condition has persisted for months or even years, it will be more difficult to clear. Acne requires more frequent treatments than other skin conditions. It is desirable to have the client come to the salon for treatments once or twice a week if at all possible.

It is estimated that if an acne condition has persisted for less than a year, it will usually take three months of treatments, providing the client comes to the salon at least once a week. Twice weekly would be better. If the client has had the acne condition for one or more years, it will take longer to clear. Estimate this way: Three is added to the number of years the client has had the acne condition; this equals the approximate number of months the condition will take to clear with treatment. If the client has had acne for 2 years, it is estimated that it will take 5 months of treatments to clear the condition. If the client has had acne for 7 years, three is added to seven, indicating that it will take approximately 10 months of treatments to clear the condition satisfactorily.

PROCEDURE FOR GIVING THE ACNE TREATMENT

For sanitary reasons, only cotton pads are used throughout the treatment for acne skin. The cotton compress mask is used to remove the treatment mask. Massage #1 and Massage #2 are eliminated in the treatment for acne skin. On a skin with only a few minor blemishes, Massage #1 may be given, working around the blemished areas.

1. Check the vaporizer to be sure it is ready when needed.
2. Prepare the client.
3. Sanitize hands.
4. Cleanse the client's skin with lotion cleanser followed by astringent.
5. Analyze the skin.
6. Vaporize the skin.
7. Proceed with disincrustation on all areas of the skin that have open follicles, blackheads, and pimples. This procedure will take approximately 7 to 10 minutes.
8. Proceed with the Dr. Jacquet massage.
9. Proceed with spot suction.
10. Extract blackheads and clean out pimples.
11. Cleanse the face with wet cotton pads that have been sprinkled with astringent.
12. Spray the face with one part astringent and two parts distilled water.

> **Note:** The carbonic gas spray is used (if available) to flush out the follicles and stimulate tissues. The spray helps the solution of distilled water to penetrate for deep acidity and to protect against germ penetration.

13. Blot the face with tissue if necessary.
14. Apply treatment cream for acne skin. The deep penetration of the product is done by one of the following methods:
    a. High-frequency current (preferred for its germicidal action)
    b. Galvanic ionization
    c. Electric heating mask
15. Apply mask for acne skin. If the treatment cream is water soluble, the mask may be applied directly over the treatment cream.
16. Remove the mask with the cotton compress mask.
17. Do a final spraying of the face.
18. Apply acne protection lotion.
19. Complete the treatment.
20. Complete the cleanup procedure.

> **Note:** When acne begins to appear, the skin naturally fights harder to clear the condition, but after acne has persisted for several years, the skin seems to adapt to acne as a normal function. For this reason, it takes longer for the skin to function again in a healthy manner. It is important to inform the client that in the beginning treatments, the skin may have a "flare-up" and appear to worsen. This is no cause for alarm as it is a sign that the infection is working its way to the surface of the skin.

Special Acne Facial Treatment with the Aid of Machines

When the client has a severe acne condition, it is important to start a series of treatments that will not cause undue irritation, but will be soothing to the skin. The client should be advised that it will take a number of treatments before the clogged pores (follicles) and blemishes can be cleansed and healed. Results will require the client's cooperation, using at-home and salon treatments in order to soften the surface of the skin so that the infection, which is being held down in the skin, can escape to the surface and be removed.

The esthetician's main objective is to soften the surface of the skin and clean out large, infectious pimples that have yellowish caps, which are ready to be extracted. When it is necessary to open a blemish, a sterilized needle, or blood lancet is used to prick the blemish. No facial massage or brushing is done when giving the special acne treatment.

PROCEDURE FOR THE SPECIAL ACNE TREATMENT

1. Everything that is to be used during the special acne treatment must be ready before the treatment begins. The vapor machine is turned on to be sure it is ready when needed.
2. Prepare the client for treatment.
3. Sanitize hands.
4. Cleanse the skin with cleansing lotion followed by astringent. Use cotton pads only.
5. The skin is analyzed carefully.
6. Vapor is used on the face for 10 minutes.
7. The disincrustation procedure is started. If vaporizer is used, it may be left on during the disincrustation procedure. Galvanic current, in this treatment, is kept low, as the skin is sensitive. Disincrustation should take approximately 7 to 10 minutes. The Dr. Jacquet movements are not done during the first few treatments on strong acne skin, as the skin may be too sensitive.
8. Spot suction may be done over the blemished and clogged areas.
9. Blackheads are extracted and pimples are cleansed.
10. The skin is sprayed with a solution of one part astringent to two parts distilled water or the carbonic gas spray may be used.

11. The treatment cream is applied. Eyepads are placed over the client's eyes and a high-frequency or an infra-red lamp is used to aid deep penetration of the cream into the skin.
12. The acne treatment mask is applied. If the treatment cream is water-soluble, the mask is applied directly over the treatment cream.
13. The mask is removed with a wet cotton compress mask.
14. The face is sprayed with the astringent and water solution.
15. The acne protective lotion is applied to the face.
16. The treatment is completed.
17. The cleanup procedure is completed.

Home Facial Care for Acne Skin

Acne is not considered a disease but is a manifestation of changes that take place in the body, especially during adolescence. Proper care of the skin and good health habits will do much to prevent the onset of acne, but once acne gets a start, it must be kept under control to keep the condition from worsening. With today's knowledge of the skin and its functions, acne can be controlled and in most cases, cleared, providing proper treatment is received. The client should be told that it takes time, patience and cooperation to achieve results. It is important that the client maintain a strict home care regimen in addition to salon treatments. The client must avoid picking and squeezing blemishes if the spread of infection is to be controlled.

The following guide for home treatment of the skin will help the client to control acne as well as help the esthetician to clear the condition sooner.

PROCEDURE FOR HOME FACIAL TREATMENT

1. Every morning and evening, the face should be cleansed with moist cotton pads; first with cleansing lotion, then with astringent. After the morning cleansing, a protective lotion for acne is applied. In the evening after cleansing, a night treatment cream or fluid formulated for acne skin should be applied.
2. At least twice a week the following home facial is given.
   a. Prepare the disincrustation lotion by mixing 1 tablespoon of baking soda (bicarbonate of soda) in 1 pint of distilled warm water. Commercial disincrustation lotion should be purchased from the salon if available.
   b. Cleanse the face with cleansing lotion followed by astringent.
   c. Place cotton compresses that have been saturated in the disincrustation solution over the areas of the face that have enlarged follicles, blackheads, and blemishes.
   d. After 15 minutes, remove the cotton compresses.
   e. The Dr. Jacquet massage movements are given for 5 minutes.

Note: If the client comes to the salon for regular weekly treatments, squeezing and extracting of blemishes will be done only by the esthetician. If the client cannot come to the salon on a regular basis, because of school, vacation or work schedules, the client should be taught how to do the following: When pimples are ready for extracting, they will have a light yellowish head in the center. Wrap thin strips of cotton moistened in astringent around the forefingers. The sides of the blemish can be gently squeezed and lifted until the infectious material is expelled. The pressure must come from the fingertips and not the fingernails. If the blemish is not easily cleansed or drained with gentle squeezing of the surrounding skin, this indicates that the blemish is not ready for extraction and should be left alone. To force squeezing of a blemish will only invite the spread of infection into the surrounding tissues. If the blemish drains, the gentle pressure may be continued until clear fresh blood is seen. The cotton strips on the fingers are changed after the cleansing of each blemish. Following the extraction procedure, the face is cleansed with a clean cotton pad that has been saturated with astringent.

 f. A mask for acne-prone skin is applied for the recommended length of time.
 g. The mask is removed with cool water and cotton pads.
 h. The skin is patted dry with facial tissue.
 i. A treatment cream especially formulated for acne skin is applied.

Note: The face should not be cleansed more than two to three times a day as this tends to irritate the condition and overstimulates the sebaceous glands. Gradually, with consistent salon and home treatments, the skin will be restored to its normal functioning. The client must follow instructions exactly if results are to be achieved.

Facial Treatment for Couperose Skin with the Aid of Machines

The client may not know the meaning of "couperose" skin or its causes. It may be helpful to explain that a couperose skin condition is usually found in thin, dry, delicate, and mature skins. The condition is commonly known as broken capillaries. The condition is characterized by a weakening of the capillary walls. Delicate skin can be affected by harsh weather—extremes of sun, wind, heat, or cold. Highly spiced foods and alcoholic beverages may also contribute to a couperose condition. Adding foods rich in vitamin P to the diet (found in the rind and white pulp of citrus fruits) is helpful in strengthening the capillary walls. In some cases medical attention is needed before facial treatments can be given. When giving a treatment for couperose skin, the esthetician must remember to exercise extreme care and to work with a light touch when proceeding with the various steps of the treatment. Treatment will vary depending upon the location and intensity of the couperose condition. The presence of a couperose condition will alter treatment routines to prevent further damage to the skin.

PROCEDURE

1. Prepare the client for the treatment.
2. Sanitize hands.
3. Cleanse the client's skin.
4. Analyze the skin.
5. Vaporize the skin.

> **Note:** The vaporizer must be kept at a further distance from couperose skin so that the vapor will not be too warm. Fast changes from cold to warm or hot temperatures are not recommended for couperose skins.

6. Do Massage #1, avoiding strong movements. Gentle "piano" movements are recommended (Steps 5 and 8 of Massage #1). End the massage by stroking downward on the jugular vein (Step 13 of Massage #1). Tapping movements are avoided on couperose areas.
7. Remove the massage cream.
8. Do a light brushing over the face avoiding the heavily couperose areas. No suction is done on couperose areas and any squeezing or expelling of debris from the skin must be done with extreme care.
9. Massage #2 or mild high frequency may be used. Avoid couperose areas.

> **Note:** Wax or electric masks are not used in this treatment.

10. Apply the special treatment mask. (See pages 256–257.)
11. Remove the mask with sponges or the cotton compress mask.
12. Spray the face. Use the electric pulverizer spray if available.
13. Complete the treatment.
14. Complete the cleanup procedure.

> **Note:** The client should be reminded that it is important to protect the skin at all times. Washing the face with hot water then splashing with cold water, rubbing ice cubes on the face, or other extremes of hot and cold should be avoided. If the client lives in a cold climate and enters warm buildings from out-of-doors, it is helpful to place the hands over the face for a few minutes to break the shock of the sudden change in temperature. A makeup foundation will serve as an added protection. The foundation will also help to conceal the couperose condition.

HOME CARE REGIMEN   The esthetician should advise the client as follows:

1. Be sure the client knows how to care for couperose skin at home.
2. Remind the client to protect the skin from extreme changes in temperature.
3. Suggest that the client analyze his or her diet to be sure that only healthful foods and beverages are consumed.
4. Give instructions on how the "piano" movements are to be done at home. (See Massage #1, Chapter 14.)
5. Suggest a foundation and/or protective cream or lotion.
6. Suggest that the client add vitamin P (also known as bioflavonoids and almost always accompanies natural vitamin C) to his or her diet.

QUESTIONS   DISCUSSION AND REVIEW

FACIAL TREATMENT WITH THE
AID OF MACHINES

1. Discuss the machines that are generally used when giving a facial treatment for combination skin.
2. Discuss how machines are helpful when giving a facial treatment for oily skin.
3. When giving a facial treatment for oily skin, when is the Dr. Jacquet method used?
4. Discuss the length of time it may take to clear (common, not acute) acne skin.
5. What is happening to the skin when there is a "flare-up" following a facial treatment for acne skin?
6. Why is it important to insist that the client follow a specific home care regimen?
7. What type of implement is used to open a blemish when it is ready to be extracted?
8. Name the three classifications of dry skin.
9. Why is a warm wax mask beneficial to dry skin?
10. When giving a treatment for oily skin, why does the esthetician sometimes eliminate Massage #1 and Massage #2?

CHAPTER 19

Removing Unwanted Hair

LEARNING OBJECTIVES   *After completing this chapter, you should be able to:*

❶ Explain the history of electrolysis and why training is so important.
❷ Discuss the shortwave method and the preparation of the client and the machine for this method.
❸ Explain the different methods of temporary hair removal, including tweezing, chemical depilatories, soft and hard wax.

INTRODUCTION

Unwanted hair on the body is often a problem for both men and women. As an esthetician, you will be able to offer a valuable service by advising your clients of the most appropriate method to either conceal or remove unwanted hair effectively. All methods will be discussed in this chapter.

Electrolysis, the only permanent method of hair removal, requires additional special training to become proficient in this service. This method destroys the hair papilla and prevents regrowth. There are temporary methods such as shaving, tweezing, and the use of depilatories. These methods must be repeated at regular intervals as new hair grows out.

Electrolysis

Unwanted hair could not be removed permanently until 1875, when Dr. Charles E. Michel, an ophthalmologist, used an electric current directed through a thin wire to remove ingrowing eyelashes. When he found that the lashes did not grow back, he suggested that this method could be valuable in removing unwanted hair from the face.

A few dermatologists tried Dr. Michel's method, but the process was so slow and tedious that it could not be used to any great extent.

In 1916, the multiple needle machine was developed, and electrolysis became a practical aid to beauty. The demand for treatments grew—slowly at first, and then more rapidly when the shortwave method was introduced. This newer method was much faster, requiring less time to clear hair from an area. Thus, permanent removal of heavy growths on large areas, such as arms and legs, became practical.

General Information

The electrologist deals with the skin, and an inefficient or unskilled operator could cause irreparable damage. Therefore, every electrologist must be thoroughly trained, both in the theory and in the practice of electrolysis. This means that he or she must use live models to practice on, under the supervision of an instructor, until proper skills, certification (if required), and confidence are achieved.

Machines—Many shortwave machines have safety factors. They are automatically timed and FCC (Federal Communications Commission) approved. Pain is reduced to a minimum by rapid shut-off current.

Areas that may be treated—The lips, cheeks, chin, eyebrows, hairlines, underarms, and the body

Areas that may not be treated—The eyelids, inside of the ears, nostrils or moles. Do not treat clients who have conditions such as diabetes, those who have pacemakers, those taking hormones, or clients who are pregnant. The only exception is when a physician authorizes treatment.

Causes of unwanted hair—The growth of excessive hair is due to hormonal imbalance in the body. No one knows the exact cause, although some authorities agree that heredity often determines those persons inclined toward excessive hair growth. Certain drugs, pregnancy, and weight problems are known to influence hair growth.

Definitions

Electrolysis is the process of removing hair permanently by means of electricity. The term "electrolysis" has become synonymous with both the multiple-needle galvanic method and the more modern single-needle shortwave method.

An *electrologist* is a person trained and licensed to give electrolysis treatments for permanent hair removal.

Epilation (ep-i-**LAY**-shun) is the removal of hair by the roots. This is done by waxing, tweezing, and electrolysis.

Hypertrichosis (high-pur-tri-**KO**-sis) is a growth of hair in excess of the normal. It is a Greek word, combining *hyper* (meaning "over") and *tricho* (meaning "hair").

Hirsuties (hur-**SUE**-shee-eez) is excessive hairiness.

Hirsutism (**HUR**-sewt-izm) is the presence of excess hair on areas where it is not normally expected.

The following terms are synonymous with shortwave electrolysis:

Thermolysis (thur-**MOL**-i-sis)   Alternating current

Diathermy (**DYE**-uh-thur-mee)   Radio frequency

High-frequency

Permanent Methods of Hair Removal

Methods of permanent hair removal are the galvanic, single or multiple needle method, the blend method, and the more modern shortwave method.

1. The galvanic method destroys the hair by decomposing the papilla (the source of nourishment for the hair) through the use of direct current.
2. The blend method decomposes the papilla with the simultaneous use of galvanic current and low-intensity high-frequency current.
3. The shortwave method destroys the hair by coagulating the papilla through the use of heat.

SHORTWAVE METHOD   The shortwave method is faster than other hair removal methods and is most commonly used. The majority of all permanent hair removal treatments today are performed by the shortwave method.

Equipment and Supplies   Everything needed for a treatment should be ready and at hand. Here is a checklist of essential equipment and supplies:

Shortwave machine	*Antiseptic lotion and powder*
Magnifying light	*Sunglasses or eyepads to protect the client's eyes*
Treatment chair for client	*After-treatment lotion*
Chair for electrologist	*Tweezers or forceps*
Sterile cotton	*Tissues*

Preparation of the Client   Seat the client comfortably in a reclining position. Place a clean towel or tissue under the head and have another tissue handy for disposal of hairs as you remove them. Sanitize the area of the body or face to be treated, using a cotton pad that has been saturated with an antiseptic. Use only sanitized tweezers and needles.

Preparation of the Machine   Turn the machine to "on." Adjust machine according to the manufacturer's instructions and analysis of area to be treated. Turn timer control to "automatic." Refer to chart provided with the machine.

Plug in the foot pedal and place it in a comfortable position. Adjust the electrologist's chair or stool to the desired height.

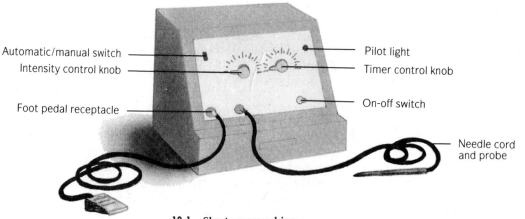

Automatic/manual switch
Intensity control knob
Foot pedal receptacle

Pilot light
Timer control knob
On-off switch
Needle cord and probe

19.1—Shortwave machine

The quicker the current is shut off the less sensation the client will feel, therefore, the timer should be set at the shortest time interval. When the need arises to use more current, increase the intensity slightly until the hair is easily removed, using as little time as possible. This is known as the *flash method*. All good shortwave machines are FCC (Federal Communications Commission) approved.

The machine is automatically timed, thus eliminating human failure, or the necessity for the electrologist to keep watch on the time.

The depth of insertion of the needle will vary with the coarseness of the hair and the area of the body being treated.

Hair grows at different angles on various parts of the face and body. Figures 19.2–19.4 show the usual angle of hair growth on the neck and throat, the chin, the side of the face, and the body.

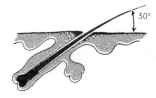

19.2—Hair growing at a 30° angle on the neck.

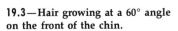

19.3—Hair growing at a 60° angle on the front of the chin.

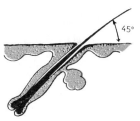

19.4—Hair growing at a 45° angle on the face.

Analysis Before beginning the treatment, the electrologist should carefully analyze the area to be treated. The following factors should be noted:

1. *Oil and moisture level*—Skin having a healthy level of moisture and natural oil will be easier to treat.
2. *Abrasion or irritations*—The area to be treated should be free of any condition that could cause infection or slow healing after treatment.
3. *Diameter of hair to be removed*—Many electrologists suggest tweezing two to three samples in the area to be treated. Grasp the hair at the skin level with the tweezers and firmly remove in the direction of the hair growth. Examine the hair, noting the diameter of the tweezed hair and the depth of the root.

The needle used should equal the diameter of the tweezed hair, and be as long as the hair from the skin level to the bottom of the root. If the needle selected is too large, it will not penetrate to the follicle for permanent hair removal. If the needle is too small, the treatment will be painful and less effective.

Inserting Needle into Follicle
Hair grows at an angle to the surface of the skin. Insert the needle alongside the hair and slide it into the follicle alongside the hair root (Fig. 19.5). In making insertions, it is important to carefully observe the angle or slant of the hair follicle before inserting the needle.

The slant of follicles varies from 15 to 90 degrees (.26–1.6 rad). Some follicles are curved and can present difficulty during treatment (Fig. 19.6). Force should not be used because the side wall of the follicle might be pierced and the current may not reach the papilla.

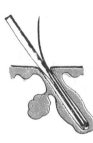

19.5—Needle inserted correctly.

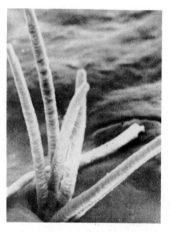

19.6—Follicle with multiple hairs

After you have inserted the needle, depress the foot pedal. The current goes on and shuts off automatically. Never depress the foot pedal while you are inserting the needle. Remove the needle and slide the hair out gently with tweezers. If it does not glide out easily, reinsert the needle a second time and use the flash method previously outlined. If the hair still does not glide out easily, remove it forcibly with tweezers and treat again during subsequent treatments.

After-Treatment Procedure
After the treatment, turn the machine off. Saturate sterile cotton pad with a special after-treatment lotion and press it gently on the area that has been treated. This cools and soothes the skin and closes the pores from which the hair has been removed.

When the lotion has dried, gently press on an antiseptic powder using sterile cotton. Antibiotic cream is often used to prevent infection.

Regrowth
It takes 8 to 13 weeks for the hair to grow from the papilla to the surface of the skin. When the client has been tweezing regularly, the hair tweezed one week is not the hair tweezed the preceding week, but hair that was tweezed many weeks before. Due to distorted follicles, sometimes caused by tweezing, waxing, or natural causes, it is not always possible to destroy the papilla with the first treatment, and the hair will grow again. The regrowth will vary. Usually not more than 10 percent of the hairs that are

in the anagen (growing) phase will grow back. A slightly higher percent of the hairs in the catagen (resting) phase will grow back. Regrowth may be as high as 20 to 25 percent in cases of distorted or multiple follicles. Additional treatment will be required for permanent removal.

Important Reminders

1. Clients should be told that sometimes, after a treatment on legs or arms, tiny scabs may appear. These soon drop off leaving the skin normal and healthy. Application of a special after-treatment lotion will hasten the healing process.
2. Hands, implements, and the area to be treated must be carefully sanitized.
3. Never remove hairs from an area where the skin shows signs of eruption, abrasion, or inflammation.
4. Do not remove hair from warts or moles.
5. Never use force when inserting a needle.
6. Do not treat hairs that are too close together.
7. Do not treat children without parental and medical permission.
8. Instruct the client on how to care for the skin after treatment. Advise the client not to pick or tamper with the skin.
9. Cosmetics should not be applied to the treated area for at least 24 hours.
10. Remind the client to stay out of the sun for a few days to avoid irritation.

Another Method of Hair Removal

Another method for the removal of unwanted hair that is being used in salons, employs the use of electrically charged tweezers (Fig. 19.7). This technique, considered to be painless to the client, is known by various commercial names depending on the manufacturer of the machine.

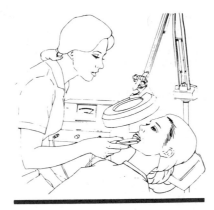

19.7—Removing hair with the electrically charged tweezer.

The electrically charged tweezers are used to grasp a single strand of hair. Hair is not a good conductor of electricity. The hair is used as a dielectric material to transfer thermal radio frequency energy to the germinal matrix of the hair root for at least 30 seconds. It is claimed that the germinal matrix is caused to detach from the papilla allowing the hair to slide out painlessly.

The process of clearing any area of hair is slow, as no more than 2 hairs can be removed per minute.

The FDA (Federal Food and Drug Administration) has determined that electronic tweezers cannot be advertised as a method of permanent hair removal.

> **Note:** Dielectric is a term applied to a nonconducting material that transmits electricity by induction, not by conduction.

Temporary Methods of Hair Removal

Shaving may be preferred when the annoying hairs cover a large area, such as in the armpits and on the arms and legs. A shaving cream is applied before shaving off the hair.

An electric razor may also be used. The application of a preshaving lotion will help to reduce any irritation.

Tweezing is commonly used for shaping the eyebrows and for removing undesirable hairs around the mouth and chin. (For the complete eyebrow tweezing procedure, see Chapter 25.)

HAIR LIGHTENING   To lessen the visibility of unwanted hair, you can lighten it by applying an oil bleach mixed with two parts of peroxide.

Procedure   Apply mixture thoroughly to the hair with a tint brush or swab. Repeat application to keep the lightener wet until the hair has lightened to desired shade.

Lightening time varies from 15 to 50 minutes, depending on the color and texture of the hair. Dark, coarse hair takes more time than fine, lanugo (lah-**NOO**-goh) hair, which is softer and lighter.

Remove lightener; then apply an emollient cream.

DEPILATORIES   Depilatories belong to the group of temporary methods for the removal of unwanted hair. There are physical (wax) and chemical types of depilatories.

CHEMICAL DEPILATORIES The *chemical depilatories*, available as a cream, paste, or powder (mixed with water into a paste), are generally used to remove hair from legs.

A skin test is advisable to determine whether the individual is sensitive to the action of this type of depilatory.

To give such a test, select a hairless part of the arm, apply a portion of the depilatory according to manufacturer's directions, and leave it on the skin from 7 to 10 minutes. If, at the end of this time, there are no signs of redness or swelling, the depilatory can be used safely over a large area of the skin.

Procedure The cream or powder depilatory may be used as follows:

1. The cream type is applied as it comes from the container, while the powder type is mixed, according to the directions of the manufacturer, to form a smooth paste.
2. After the skin has been cleansed and dried, a thick layer of the depilatory is applied over the area where the hair is to be removed.
3. Surrounding skin may be protected with vaseline.
4. Depending on the thickness of the hair, the depilatory is retained from 5 to 10 minutes or according to manufacturer's instructions.
5. Then, the depilatory and hair are washed off with warm water.
6. Finally, the skin is patted dry and a soothing cream or lotion is applied.

SOFT WAX HAIR-REMOVAL TREATMENT Wax hair-removal treatments have become more popular as a salon service in recent years, due to the introduction of soft liquid wax, which is easier and quicker to use and makes hair removal in large areas of the body more efficient. There is little discomfort to the client as there is only a momentary smarting on the surface of the skin when the wax is pulled off. Hair growth is often stopped after several epilation treatments. Since hair does not grow at the same speed, some hair reaches the surface of the skin faster than others. This method makes the area appear more sparse and is an advantage over shaving or the use of depilatory creams. For example, when hair is shaved or removed by a depilatory, it is removed at the skin line or surface, and within a few days of hair growth, all the hair can be seen at the surface of the skin and the stubble can be felt. When hair is removed by epilation, it grows back without a stubble.

The product used for hair removal is referred to by some manufacturers as "soft depilatory wax," or "liquid hair remover." Regardless of what the product is called, it achieves the same results. Follow manufacturer's instructions for the use of the product.

How to Prepare the Skin for the Wax Treatment Cleanse skin of all oil and makeup, using cotton pads that have been saturated with astringent or witch hazel. Some manufacturers recommend dusting the area to be waxed with talcum powder. The talcum powder absorbs any moisture or oil residue, helping the hair to adhere to the wax.

Materials Needed for the Wax Treatment

In addition to the cleansing pads and astringents for cleansing the skin, a few other basic items will be needed.

1. A heating unit for heating the wax—Several models are thermostatically controlled. Electric waxing pots keep the wax at the proper temperature during the treatment. The wax can also be heated in a double boiler (a pan set over a pan of boiling water).
2. Wood spatulas for applying the wax to the skin
3. Orangewood sticks—These are excellent for applying wax to the area around the eyebrows where hair removal is desired.
4. Muslin fabric or other specially manufactured fiber strips—These materials are usually available from the beauty supply house where you purchase the wax. The strips are precut. However, if the material is unavailable, unbleached muslin can be purchased from a fabric store. Cut muslin into strips approximately 3 inches wide by 6 inches long (7.62 centimeters by 15.24 centimeters).
5. A medicated, soothing lotion will be needed to apply to the skin following the wax treatment.

> **Note:** Begin heating the treatment wax before the client enters the treatment area so that it is ready when needed. The client should change into a salon gown because the wax is extremely difficult to remove if it gets on clothing.

Safety Precautions

To prevent burning the skin, test the temperature of the wax before applying it to the client's skin. Take a small amount of the wax onto a spatula and test it against the back of your hand.

Be sure the wax does not come in contact with the client's eyes or any area where it is not supposed to be used.

Do not use a wax depilatory over warts, on moles, on abrasions, or on irritated or inflamed skin.

For clients who cannot tolerate heated wax, a *cold wax method* of hair removal is also available. This technique has all the advantages of hot wax and comes in ready-to-use form. Cold wax is applied at room temperature. Use a spatula to spread the wax evenly on in the direction of the hair growth. Press a thin strip of cellophane or cotton cloth to press the wax down so that it adheres correctly. Hold the skin taut with one hand while taking hold of the strip with the other hand. With one fast movement, pull the strip against the hair growth to remove the wax with the hair adhering to it.

Procedure for the Wax Hair-Removal Treatment

When removing hair from any part of the body, such as the face, arms, legs, back, and abdomen, always apply the wax in the direction of the hair growth. On some areas of the body hair will grow in different directions. For example, the hair on the upper lip grows in one direction on one side of the lip and another direction on the other side. In this case, each side of the upper lip is waxed separately, and the wax is removed in the opposite direction of the hair growth.

When you are ready to apply the wax, dip the spatula into the liquid wax and scrape one side of the spatula against the side of the melting pot, or on a scraping bar that comes with some of the melting pots. This leaves the liquid wax on one side of the spatula. Quickly place the spatula on the skin at a 45 degree angle (never flat on the skin). Then draw the spatula over the area of the skin to be treated in the direction of the hair growth, allowing the liquid wax to flow smoothly.

Don't apply the wax over a larger area than can be covered by the muslin or fiber strips. Once the wax is applied to the skin, the muslin strip is placed directly over the wax and smoothed with the hand in the direction of the hair growth. This allows the hair that is bonded to the wax to adhere to the fabric strip. Leave enough free edge on the strip (approximately 1 inch or 2.5 centimeters) so that you can grasp it with your fingers. Place your hand on the skin to hold it firmly. When working on large areas, such as the arms and legs, slap the area several times lightly with the hand that was holding the skin taut immediately after pulling the strip from the skin.

Light slapping will help relieve any momentary smarting of the skin. Never slap the face. After the first treatment, the area where hair has been removed will become less sensitive.

It is important, when pulling the strip back (in the opposite direction of the hair growth), that the hand remain as close to the skin as possible. This forces the follicle to open and allows the hair bulb or root to be removed more easily.

The strip that is used to remove hair can be used two or more times before it needs to be replaced by a fresh strip. After the hair has been removed, if any trace of wax remains on the skin, it can be removed easily by taking a used strip of fabric and pressing the wax side over the wax that is on the skin. When the strip is pulled away, the wax will be lifted from the skin.

When the desired area has been cleansed of unwanted hair, apply a soothing antiseptic lotion to the area.

Note: If the client has been shaving an area or using a chemical depilatory, ask the client to discontinue the practice at least 2 to 3 weeks prior to the wax treatment. This will allow the hair to grow long enough to become bonded with the wax during the treatment. In some instances, when the hair is extremely short, the liquid wax may be applied against the direction of the hair growth. The smoothing of the fabric over the area is also done against the direction of the hair growth. This enables the short hair to stand up so that it is easier for the wax to bond to the hair. If, after waxing an area, a few stray hairs still remain, remove the strays with a tweezer, instead of rewaxing the area.

Procedure for Removing Unwanted Hair from the Legs with Soft Wax

1. While holding the spatula at a 45 degree angle, apply a thin film of wax to the area being treated. Draw the spatula in the direction of the hair growth. (See Fig. 19.8.)
2. Stretch the muslin strip directly over the wax application. Allow enough free edge of the fabric for the hand to grasp for removal. (See Fig. 19.9.)

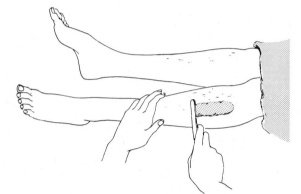

19.8—Apply wax.

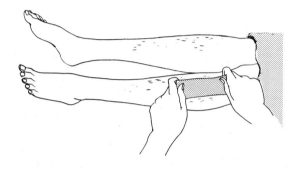

19.9—Place muslin strip over wax.

3. Smooth the fabric strip in the same direction as you applied the wax to assure bonding of the hair and wax to the strip. (See Fig. 19.10.)
4. Grasp the free edge of the strip tightly with one hand while holding the other hand against the skin to hold the skin taut. Quickly pull the strip in the opposite direction of the hair growth. Be sure that the hand pulling the strip remains close to the skin. The area covered by the strip should be clean and free of hair. (See Fig. 19.11.)

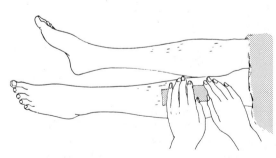

19.10—Smooth the strip over the wax.

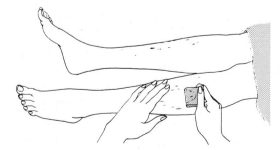

19.11—Remove the strip.

5. Continue the procedure until the entire area is free of unwanted hair. (See Fig. 19.12.)

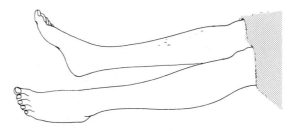

19.12—The result will be an area free of unwanted hair.

Procedure for Removing Underarm Hair with Soft Wax

When the underarm has not been shaved for sometime, it will be necessary to clip the hair leaving the hair long enough to bond to the wax.

1. Because the underarm is sensitive, remove the hair in three or more small areas. Apply the wax in each area in the direction of the hair growth. (See Fig. 19.13.)
2. Apply wax to a small area of the underarm. (See Fig. 19.14.)
3. Press the strip to the wax and quickly remove it by pulling in the opposite direction to the hair growth. (See Fig. 19.15.)
4. The underarm is left smooth and clean. (See Fig. 19.16.)

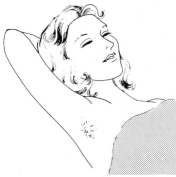

19.13—Remove the hair from the underarm in three or more small areas at a time.

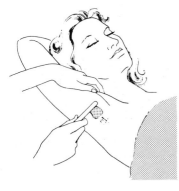

19.14—Apply wax to a small area in the direction of the hair growth.

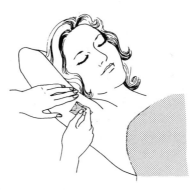

19.15—Press strip to the wax and remove in the opposite direction to the hair growth.

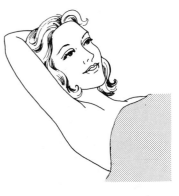

19.16—Result

Procedure for Removing Hair from Upper Lip with Soft Wax

1. The most common area for hair removal in the salon is the upper lip. The hair on the upper lip usually grows in two (or more) directions. (See Fig. 19.17.)
2. Apply the wax with a spatula to one small section of the lip at a time, in the direction of the hair growth. (See Fig. 19.18.)
3. Press the muslin or fiber strip to the wax and smooth in the same direction the wax was applied. (See Fig. 19.19.)
4. Grasp the free edge of the strip tightly with one hand while holding the other hand against the skin to keep it taut. Pull the strip quickly in the opposite direction of the hair growth. Be sure the hand pulling the strip remains close to the skin. (See Fig. 19.20.)
5. The area treated should be clean and free of unwanted hair. (See Fig. 19.21.)
6. Continue the wax treatment procedure until the entire area is free of unwanted hair. (See Fig. 19.22.)

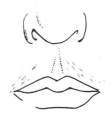

19.17—The hair on the upper lip grows in two or more directions.

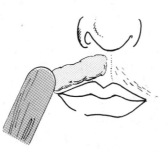

19.18—Apply wax with spatula to a small area in the direction of hair growth.

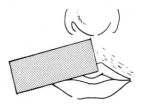

19.19—Press strip to the wax.

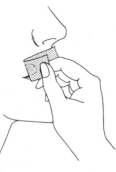

19.20—Remove in the opposite direction to the hair growth.

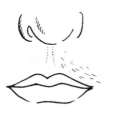

19.21—The treated area will be free of unwanted hair.

19.22—Result

HARD WAX DEPILATORY The hard wax may be applied over such parts of the body as the cheeks, chin, upper lip, nape area, arms, and legs. For many years, hard wax was prepared by mixing rosin and beeswax to the desired consistency. Mineral oil and paraffin wax were sometimes added. Hard wax now comes in flat, rectangular bars that vary in size and weight. The wax is brittle and can be broken off in the amount needed for individual treatments, then melted either in a thermostatically controlled wax-melting pot or in a double-boiler pot on a heating plate.

Procedure for Wax Application
1. Remove clothing from area to be treated. Have the client sit in a comfortable position.
2. Clean the area to be waxed with a cotton pad saturated with astringent.
3. Lightly talcum the surface of the skin.
4. Melt the wax in a thermostatically controlled electric wax pot or in a small pot over a heating plate. The pot should be removed from the heating plate when the cake of wax is about two thirds melted. Stir the wax until the consistency is thick but flows from the spatula.
5. Test the temperature and consistency of the heated wax by applying a small amount on the inside of your wrist. The wax should not be so hot as to be uncomfortable.
6. Spread the warm wax evenly over the skin surface with a spatula, following the same direction as the hair growth.
7. Allow the wax to cool until semihard.
8. Quickly pull off the adhering wax against the direction of the hair growth.
9. Gently massage the treated area.
10. Apply an emollient cream or antiseptic lotion to the treated area.

▶ | **Caution:** Always test the wax for temperature before applying it to the client's skin. Never allow wax to run into eyes or onto areas where the treatment is not being given. Never use a wax depilatory on warts, moles, abrasions, or on irritated or inflamed areas of the skin.

THE USE OF HARD WAX FOR EYEBROW REMOVAL When only a few stray hairs are to be removed from the eyebrows, it is best to use tweezers. When a client has thick, unruly brows, with excess hair growing outside the normal browline, the shaping of the eyebrow can be done faster by first waxing the excess hair surrounding the brow, then using tweezers to finish the shaping of the eyebrow. This method of hair removal can be accomplished with either hard or soft liquid wax. The following procedure for hair removal is done with hard wax.

Procedure for Removal of Brow Hair

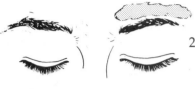

19.23—Apply wax to a small area in the direction of hair growth.

1. Apply the wax to a small area surrounding the brow in the direction of the hair growth. Be sure the wax is applied thicker at the edge that will be grasped between the thumb and forefinger for removal. The wax is applied to the area directly above the eyebrow. The wax is ready for removal when you can leave a fingerprint in the wax without having it stick to the finger. (See Fig. 19.23.)

2. Grasp the thicker edge of the wax with one hand while holding the other hand against the skin to keep it taut. Pull the wax strip quickly in the opposite direction of the hair growth. Keep the hand that pulls the wax strip close to the skin. (See Fig. 19.24.)

3. Repeat the same procedure for cleaning the area between the brows. (See Fig. 19.25.)

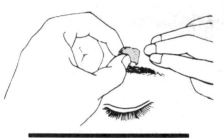

19.24—Pull the wax strip quickly in the opposite direction of hair growth.

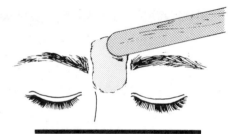

19.25—Clean the area between the brows.

4. Use the tweezers to finish the shaping of the eyebrows. (See Fig. 19.26.)

5. The brow area is cleaned of excess hair, making the brows a more attractive frame for the eyes. (See Fig. 19.27.)

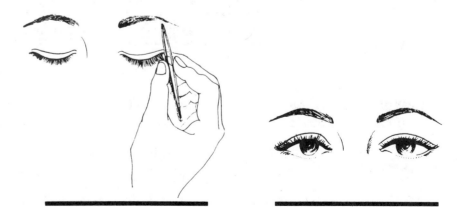

19.26—Shape the eyebrows with a tweezer.

19.27—Result

QUESTIONS DISCUSSION AND REVIEW

REMOVING UNWANTED HAIR

1. Define electrolysis.
2. Define epilation.
3. What is a depilatory?
4. Which type of hair removal results in hair growing back with a blunt stubble?
5. Which type of temporary hair removal treatment is commonly used to remove hair from large areas such as the arms and legs?
6. What are the advantages of using the wax method to remove thick, unruly eyebrows?
7. When removing unwanted hair by the use of a wax treatment, is the wax applied and removed against or in the direction of the hair growth?
8. After hair removal, how much time does it usually take for the hair to grow from the papilla to the surface of the skin?

Enemies of the Skin, Aging Factors, and Cosmetic Surgery

CHAPTER 20

LEARNING OBJECTIVES

After completing this chapter, you should be able to:

❶ Discuss the effects of the environment on the skin.

❷ Explain what clients can do to help protect their skin.

❸ Discuss the enemies of the skin, explaining how they can damage the client's skin.

❹ Describe what plastic surgery is and how it can help some of our clients.

❺ Discuss how to handle the needs of clients who have already undergone cosmetic surgery.

INTRODUCTION

Taking care of the skin should start at an early age, because once the skin has been neglected, it is more difficult to improve its appearance or to undo damage that has been done by neglect. Facial treatments and proper makeup techniques can help maintain the health and attractiveness of the skin for a lifetime.

Loss of the skin's elasticity, and the body's biological changes in midlife may cause the fine lines and wrinkles on the face and neck to become more prominent. Persons with light, thin, and dry skin tend to develop lines and wrinkles at an earlier age than do persons whose skins are oily, thick, and dark.

The skin shows signs of age faster than any other organ of the body. As the body's protective covering, the skin is vulnerable to attack and is subject to daily wear and tear. This is why the skin requires regular and daily care throughout its lifetime, if it is to remain healthy and retain its youthful appearance.

Effects of Too Much Sunlight on the Skin

Overexposure to the sun is harmful to the skin. The ultra-violet rays of the sun not only penetrate the epidermis of the skin, but also the dermis, where it affects living cells. One of the skin's main defenses against too much sun is its ability to tan. Suntan is a shield set up by the skin to help prevent the sun's rays from causing damage to underlying tissues. It is important when suntanning to do so gradually, in order for the skin to set up its protective mechanism.

People whose skins have been overexposed to sunlight during their younger years generally start to show signs of age between the ages of 38 and 45. This is partially due to structural damage that affects the skin's elasticity. People who have not overexposed their skin and were cautious when suntanning, will generally have younger looking skin. Once the skin has lost its elasticity, it cannot be restored. You might compare the skin's loss of elasticity to loss of elasticity in a garment. For example, if you purchase identical elasticized garments and wash one in hot water 50 times and the other in cold water 50 times, the garment washed in cold water will hold its shape far better than the one washed in hot water. The heat deteriorates the elastic and there is no way it can be restored to its original firmness. The excessive heat of the sun acts on the elasticity of the skin in the same way that hot water acts on an elasticized garment.

Many people feel that a deep tan is a mark of good health but over-exposure can be harmful and sometimes fatal. The ultra-violet rays of the sun are strongest at midday. Therefore, it is better to limit tanning sessions to mornings and midafternoons when the sun is not so strong. It is better to take the sun for short periods to start, then increase the time each day until the desired tan is acquired. The skin should be protected by a good sunscreen oil or lotion. Always read instructions included with suntanning products. The directions often suggest a test patch before the product is used all over the body. A test patch is usually done on a small area of skin on the wrist. If there is any reaction such as redness, itching, or a tingling sensation, the product should be washed off the wrist and not used. Artificial suntanning products must also be used with caution.

SUNBURNS CAN BE DANGEROUS Most sunburns involve the superficial layers of the skin and may be uncomfortable for a few days while they are healing. For this degree of sunburn, a soothing lotion may be all that is needed. Deeper degrees of burns, if not properly treated, can lead to more serious complications. A physician should treat a severe sunburn without delay.

FRECKLES Freckles are caused by an excess of pigmentation in the skin that becomes darker after overexposure to the sun. To keep freckles from becoming more intense, a good sunscreen lotion should be applied to exposed areas of the skin before going into strong sunlight.

Air Pollution

The air pollution that affects the skin has been brought about by automobile exhaust, smoke, and other impurities being put into the air. The chemical reaction of pollutants can be devastating to the health and appearance of the skin. Sulfur-containing compounds are among the most common pollutants in the air. When the polluted air comes in contact with the skin, it is partially converted to sulfuric acid, which is dehydrating and harmful to the skin. Areas of the body that are protected by clothing remain younger looking longer, whereas, the face and hands, which are constantly exposed to the outside environment, age the fastest (Fig. 20.1). For example, if you were unable to see a person's face and hands and you were to examine the skin on an unexposed area, such as the arm, you would not be able to tell if the skin was that of an 18 year old or a 48 year old person.

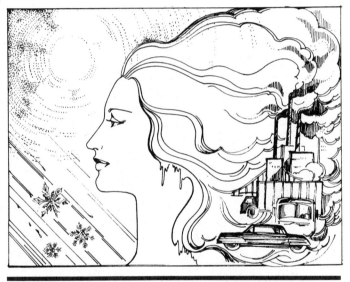

20.1—The face is in direct contact with environmental enemies of the skin. These enemies include overexposure to the sun, harsh weather conditions, and pollution in the air. Protective lotions and cleansing facial treatments can help to protect the skin from these environmental enemies.

In many of the major cities of the world, such as Athens, Greece, treasured outdoor objects that have remained intact for over 2,000 years are now deteriorating due to pollutants in the air. Two of the best ways to combat this environmental enemy of the skin is to keep the skin thoroughly and properly cleansed to remove pollutants, and to physically protect the skin by the application of protective lotions. Makeup foundation also helps protect the skin.

The photographs in Figure 20.2 dramatically show how skin that is protected from environmental enemies, such as pollution and overexposure to the sun, will remain young looking years longer.

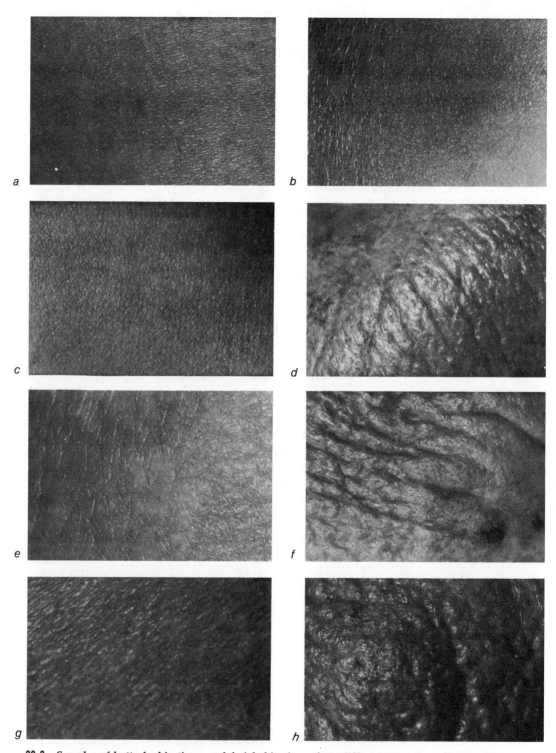

20.2—Samples of buttock skin tissue and facial skin tissue from different age groups: Photographs on the left are of buttocks; on the right, of faces *a* and *b*: 2-year-old girl; *c* and *d*: 49-year-old woman; *e* and *f*: 77-year-old woman; *g* and *h*: 80-year-old woman. (*Photographs reprinted courtesy of J. Bedford Shelmire, Jr., M.D., Author of* The Art of Looking Younger, *St. Martin's Press, New York.*)

Other Enemies of the Skin

The skin can be affected by excessive use of drugs, alcohol, and tobacco smoking. It can also be affected by too frequent a gain and loss of weight, by excessive massage, and by the unwise use of gadgets and products. If the client confides that he or she is overindulging in alcoholic beverages, taking drugs, smoking excessively, or doing anything that may damage the skin, the esthetician can discourage the client by pointing out, tactfully, the harmful effects of these habits on the skin.

ALCOHOL
Heavy intake of alcohol overdilates the blood vessels. If continued over a long period of time this can weaken capillary walls. When the blood expands, the weakened capillary walls can burst, causing unsightly splotches in the sclera (white) of the eye or underneath the skin. Alcohol also draws water out of the tissues and leaves the skin dull and dehydrated.

DRUGS
Drugs of various kinds may have an adverse effect on the skin and should be taken only as prescribed by a physician. Studies of the effects of drugs on the skin show that some drugs interfere with the intake of oxygen, which the body needs for healthy cell growth. Tranquilizers, amphetamines, barbiturates, heroin, marijuana and similar drugs can cause dryness and allergic reactions, and often aggravate existing problems, such as acne.

TOBACCO
In addition to warnings about diseases, such as cancer and heart disease, which are caused or aggravated by excessive smoking, it is also reported that smoking contributes to premature aging and wrinkling of the skin. Nicotine causes small blood vessels and capillaries to contract, which decreases the blood circulation to the skin and deprives it of essential nutrients and oxygen. In some cases, excessive nicotine in the system can cause a yellow cast to the skin.

FREQUENT WEIGHT GAIN AND LOSS
To keep the body healthy, an individual should maintain his or her normal weight. As excess weight is gained, the skin stretches to accommodate the extra pounds. When weight is lost too rapidly, as in the case of crash diets, the skin does not have time to adjust to the changes in the underlying facial muscles. This causes premature wrinkling and sagging of the skin. Overweight clients should be advised to lose weight gradually under the supervision of a physician.

EXCESSIVE MASSAGE
Massage is good for the skin if done properly by a trained esthetician. However, constant rubbing and pulling, or wrong massage movements can weaken the collagen fibers, resulting in wrinkling of the skin. The client should be advised to always use gentle upward movements when cleansing the skin. Mannerisms such as tugging, pulling, or pushing the facial muscles should also be avoided. Facial exercises that include exaggerated facial expressions may contribute to premature wrinkling and lining of the skin. Biting the inside of the cheeks and pursing or biting the lips should also be avoided.

Gadgets and Overrated Products

In recent years, there has been an increase in high-priced gadgets and overrated cosmetics that some manufacturers and distributors claim will prevent or erase lines and wrinkles on the face and neck. Such advertisements can be misleading. The Federal Food and Drug Administration endeavors to control the production of gadgets and products that have no valid use, that may be potentially harmful, or that are backed by false and misleading claims. Although the manufacturers and/or the distributors offer a money-back guarantee with the purchase of a gadget or product, the client should be cautious. Science has not yet found miraculous shortcuts to skin health and beauty (by way of gadgets or unproven products) that will erase lines and wrinkles once they have formed. Proper diet, rest, and good health habits, along with everyday care of the skin, are still the best preventative measures against wrinkles and other signs of aging.

The Theory of Physiognomy

The first associations between appearance and character and personality were made by people many centuries ago. The ancient Greeks devised a canon (an established rule or judgment) as a means of determining ideal proportions of the human face and body. *Physiognomy* (fiz-ee-**OG**-nuh-mee) is the study of the face and features as related to the character or disposition of an individual. The ancient Greeks used it as a guide for artists in creating harmonious proportions and to serve as a basis for comparison (Fig. 20.3). Painting, drawings, sculpture, and in more recent times, photography help us to study concepts of attractiveness or unattractiveness throughout the ages.

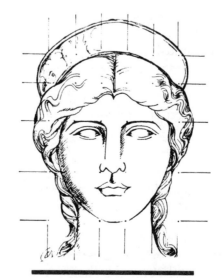

20.3—Ancient Greek sculptures and artists established a "canon" or rule of judgment as a means of determining facial proportions.

It is important to realize that what may appear to be beautiful to people in one part of the world may appear to be the opposite to people somewhere else. Customs play a big part in how people perceive themselves and others. For example, scarring, tatooing, and forms of mutilation of the face and body are considered to be marks of beauty in some parts of the world. However, the desire for good health is universal.

FACIAL PROPORTIONS

A working knowledge of the dimensional relationship between one facial feature and another helps us appreciate the differences in individual faces. Few people have perfect facial proportions, and without the imperfections that give distinction to the face, everyone might look alike. Makeup and hairstyle help women to compensate for small imperfections while men use hairstyles, beards, and mustaches to improve their appearance. Attractiveness is not dependent upon perfect facial features. However, some people do have plastic surgery to improve the proportion of some feature(s) of their face.

The horizontal diameter of the face is divided into three equal sections. The first section starts at the forehead and extends to a line that is even with the top of the eyebrows. When the hairline is very high, the hair can be arranged to achieve pleasing proportions. When the hairline is low, the hair can be styled to conceal the hairline, or styled to make the forehead appear higher. The second section extends from the eyebrows to the tip of the nose. The third section is from the tip of the nose to the tip of the chin.

The vertical diameter of the face is divided into five equal sections. Each section is about the width of one eye, with space approximately the width of one eye between the eyes. Lips and eyebrows measure slightly more than the width of one of the sections (Fig. 20.4).

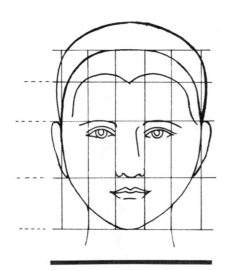

20.4—The horizontal and vertical diameter of the face divided into equal sections.

In profile, the face is divided into equal sections. The lines at the top of the eyebrows and the base of the nose are on line with the top and lobe of the ear (Fig. 20.5).

Figures 20.4 and 20.5 show how larger or smaller eyes, noses, lips, and heavier or thinner brows add distinctive character to the face.

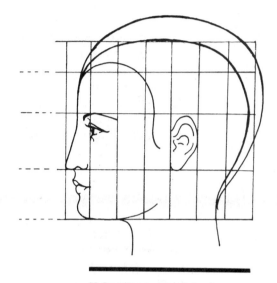

20.5—The profile of the face divided into equal sections.

APPEARANCE AND SELF-ESTEEM

It is not unusual for a person to become dissatisfied with his or her appearance for no particular reason. How one feels about one's physical appearance has a lot to do with self-image and self-acceptance. For example, a person with a poor self-image may feel that an unusual feature detracts from his or her appearance, while, on the other hand, a person with a good self-image will consider the unusual feature a part of his or her individuality. There are cases where the changing of a facial feature (by cosmetic surgery) will improve the appearance of the person and increase his or her self-esteem. Congenital problems, such as a harelip (a fissure of the upper lip), can be corrected by surgery.

People who have been injured or disfigured in accidents, in fires, or by disease may be left scarred or deformed. They not only suffer extreme physical pain but psychological pain as well. Intensive studies have shown that self-image and self-confidence are restored when a person's appearance is restored to normal.

It was during World War I (1914–1918) that reconstructive surgery became recognized as part of the rehabilitation of the wounded. Since that time, outstanding progress has been made in the techniques of plastic (also called reconstructive or cosmetic) surgery. Plastic surgery today is a special area of medical science that benefits people both physically and psychologically.

APPEARANCE AND PERSONAL TRAITS
Television and movies use popular concepts of beauty and ugliness in the portrayal of different characters. Quite often you will see the villian made up to look abnormal in some way. Whereas, the heroine or hero is a more attractive character. For example, we may see a witch with a crooked nose and a chin covered with warts. Her hair is stringy and her hands are knotty with long clawlike nails. This combines the concept of ugly and bad. In contrast, another character (the princess) is shown to be well-groomed, with perfectly proportioned features and endowed with good traits. From such portrayals it is easy to see how some people (especially children) can become conditioned to relating physical characteristics with personality traits. In recent years, this type of portrayal, especially in children's literature, has been discouraged. Most people are aware that perfect or imperfect features are not the only criteria by which we judge the character or beauty of an individual.

The Characteristics of Age as Seen in the Face

All living things go through the process of aging from birth to death. Aging cannot be prevented, but the signs of aging can be controlled to a certain degree. The signs of aging differ from person to person and some people retain a youthful appearance longer than others. This is mostly due to heredity, to the individual's state of health, and to skin care. Men and women undergo similar aging processes.

The skin ages due to the deterioration of the elastic tissue. In most cases, the skin becomes dry (dehydrated), and liver spots (small brown spots) and small broken capillaries appear. A dermatologist should be consulted when removal of spots or broken capillaries is desired. Any lesion or abnormal condition of the skin should be given immediate medical attention.

Most people accept aging with grace and dignity. However, they want to retain their youthful appearance as long as possible and welcome the esthetician's suggestions for keeping the skin healthy and attractive. Premature aging can be prevented to some degree by daily skin care, a well-balanced diet, and other good health habits.

People who guard their health and give the skin daily care will retain a youthful appearance longer. It is usually around the age of 35 that fine expression lines begin to appear around the eyes, the mouth, and on the forehead. Women can use subtle makeup to conceal the signs of aging, but too much makeup will only call attention to lines in the face (Fig. 20.6).

By 45 years of age, the expression patterns on most faces begin to deepen around the mouth, the eyes, and on the forehead. The skin shows loss of elasticity, especially around the eyes. A double chin may start to show and the neck may begin to appear crepy in texture (Fig. 20.7).

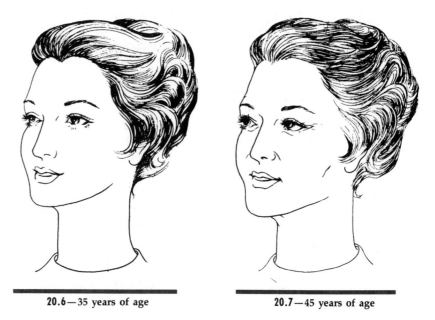

20.6—35 years of age   **20.7**—45 years of age

By the age of 55, the skin becomes looser and the folds and sagging tissue around the eyes more pronounced. The cheekbones appear to be more prominent and the naso-labial (nose to mouth) folds will be more distinct. An overweight person will likely notice the formation of a double chin (Fig. 20.8).

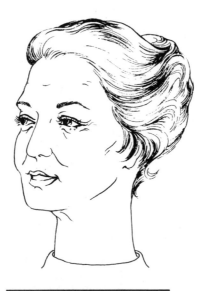

20.8—55 years of age

As we age, the skull may remain the same or start to shrink while the skin continues to grow. This causes the skin to sag. By age 65 to 70, the contours of the face change and there are deeper folds and lines due to loss of muscle tone. The skin of the cheeks and jaw becomes flabby and the nose and chin usually appear to be more prominent. Drooping tissue around the eyes causes them to appear smaller. Lines on the neck deepen and skin becomes loose and crepy (Fig. 20.9).

By age 75 and into advanced age, all expression lines and folds in the face deepen. The head shrinks, causing increased sagging of skin and underlying muscles. The small lines that have been forming on the face become more prominent. During advanced age, the aging process continues so that each year the face gradually becomes older looking. Some people become more attractive as they mature, as the signs of aging add character and expression to the face (Fig. 20.10).

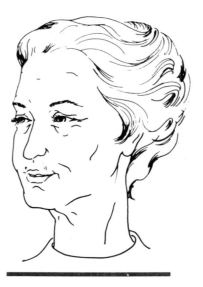

20.9—70 years of age

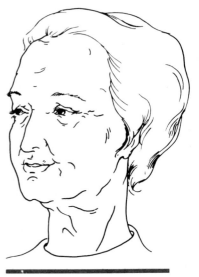

20.10—75 years of age

Plastic (Cosmetic) Surgery

Plastic (cosmetic) surgery involves complex medical procedures, which in no way involve the esthetician. However, some knowledge of the subject will help the esthetician to recognize the problems he or she can handle and those which a medical doctor must treat. The client may come to the salon for treatment of such problems as pouches under the eyes, drooping or puffy eyelids, sagging skin due to loss of elasticity, double chins, lines and furrows in the skin, and other signs of aging. It is better to tell the client honestly what can and cannot be accomplished by facial treatments. The esthetician should not mislead the client into believing that these conditions can be eliminated by facial treatments. The client may ask advice about plastic surgery to improve the condition. The esthetician should encourage the client to consult with his or her personal physician, who will be in a position to recommend a qualified surgeon.

The client may request facial treatments following plastic surgery. The skin can be kept healthy and attractive with proper treatments. For example, if the client's skin is oily and has blackheads before surgery, it will still be oily and prone to blackheads following surgery. Surgery removes the excess skin but does not change the condition of the skin. When the client has undergone surgery, the esthetician must be certain that healing is complete before treatments are given. When there is any doubt about the client's readiness for facial treatments, the client's physician should be consulted.

The following information about plastic (cosmetic) surgery has been included in this chapter to acquaint you with the medical terms for various procedures. Although you will not be involved directly with any type of surgery, plastic surgeons and dermatologists often employ estheticians or have occasion to recommend them so it will be to your advantage to understand the surgeon's work.

RHYTIDECTOMY   Unlike most of the other plastic surgery procedures, which were developed at one time or another in Europe, *rhytidectomy* (rit-i-**DECK**-tuh-mee), the face-lift, was developed in the early 1900's reputedly by Dr. Charles Conrad Miller of Chicago. He was considered a quack and a genius, an embarrassment to the American medical profession of his time, yet a man who today is considered one of the fathers of modern cosmetic surgery. Dr. Miller performed not only face-lifts but also such unheard-of surgical procedures as reducing large mouths, narrowing wide nostrils, and creating dimples, whose location on the face he selected "after having the patient smile."

In 1912, Madame le Docteur Suzanne Noel, a Parisian physician with an interest in dermatology, read in the newspapers that an aging French actress had just returned from a tour in the United States, where she had undergone an extraordinary operation on the scalp that had restored her youth. The news, as Madame Noel wrote late in a book about esthetic surgery, excited her so much that she begged the actress to allow her to examine the scars. It turned out that the actress had undergone something similar to today's mini-lift. Madame Noel immediately put aside dermatology and dedicated herself completely to surgery—the face-lift had thus crossed the Atlantic.

Since Madame Noel's day, though surgery has become bolder and the results more striking, not much has been added to the technique of face-lift. To reassure her patients of their progress, she even thought of preoperative and postoperative photographs, a practice all modern plastic surgeons follow. It is an unwritten law that photographs should always be taken: They are the surgeon's—or the patient's—best evidence, in case of a malpractice suit, of what the operation was all about. In general, however, the surgeon needs preoperative photographs to discuss the possible improvements with the patient, and later takes them to the operating room as a guideline during surgery.

Ear surgery, nose surgery, and oral surgery are far more intricate matters than a face-lift, involving as they do, alterations to the very framework of the face. The face-lift's purpose is just the opposite: to "tidy up" the face without altering its configuration, and in this lies the challenge.

In the face-lift, the surgeon is concerned primarily with the skin; the nose, the chin, the ears, the jaws and the scalp are landmarks around which he works, using them as points of reference and as anchorage for the sutures. The first thing the surgeon must decide when planning an operation for an aging face is whether to perform a rhytidectomy (standard face-lift), a *blepharoplasty* (**BLEF**-uh-ro-plas-tee) (correction of wrinkles around the eyes), or both. In the latter case, he further has to decide whether to perform them in a single session and which to do first. Also to be taken into consideration is whether the excess skin in the lower lid is indeed a defect of the lid and not part of the sagging of the cheek; in which case the face-lift alone might take care of it. Finally, in the case of a pronounced double chin or extremely loose skin on the neck, a standard face-lift may not be enough, and a *submandibular lipectomy* (sub-man-**DIB**-yoo-lur li-**PECK**-tuh-mee) (correction of the chin) might be required in addition to or instead of the face-lift.

The choice of whether to perform the operations in one session depends, in part, on the endurance of both the patient and the surgeon. Also, the temporary swelling caused by an eyelid correction could mislead the surgeon about the actual condition of the rest of the face.

A standard face-lift starts with an incision in the hair-bearing scalp, about 3 centimeters above the "widow's peak" along a small strip of scalp. The incision proceeds downward in front of the ear, parallel to a little crease, which is usually present, and curves around the earlobe. It continues upward and then sharply back, reaching into the neck hairline, along a second strip of scalp.

The second step is to separate the skin from the superficial subcutaneous tissue, starting from the back of the ear and proceeding toward the jaws, taking care not to injure the facial nerves, the muscles, or the blood vessels. On the temples the surgeon must undermine a little deeper in order not to damage the hair follicles.

Often the surgeon gathers the subcutaneous tissue upward and backward toward the ear, and sutures it firmly to the fascia (the tissue protecting the facial muscles), which has become as inelastic as the aging skin. Over this smoother ground, the surgeon gently rotates and redrapes the skin. Two key sutures are placed near the ear, one slightly above it, the other behind it, and the excess skin is cut off. The incision in front of the ear is the last one to be closed. The surgeon rotates the skin upward without pulling it, cuts off the excess skin and sutures it delicately in place. The same is done on the other side of the face, once the surgeon has assured himself or herself of the symmetry.

Some surgeons favor general *anaesthesia* (an-es-**THEEZH**-uh), but many prefer a local anaesthetic combined with an intravenous *analgesic* (an-al-**JEE**-zick). For one thing, the general anaesthesia tube might conceal a portion of the face and mislead the surgeon in his judgment of the face's overall condition.

A firm dressing that exerts a slight pressure is placed over the face, with cotton pads around the ears; these are removed after 48 hours. The sutures in front of the ears are usually removed after 3 to 5 days; those behind the ears are not touched for at least 10 to 12 days (Figs. 20.11–20.13).

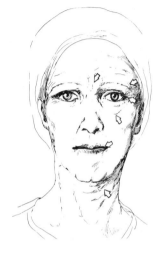

20.11—A woman approximately 60 years old about to undergo the following cosmetic surgery and adjunct procedures: rhytidectomy (face-lift); blepharoplasty (eyelid correction); submandibular lipectomy (chin correction); dermabrasion or chemical peel of the upper lip; injections of liquid silicone in the frown lines and other expression lines, such as those above the eyebrows and those encompassing the mouth (see page 352 for explanation of silicone injections); insertion of a solid silicone implant into the chin.

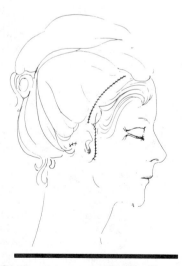

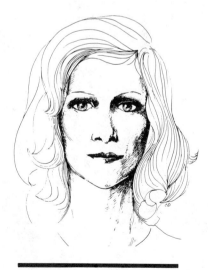

20.12—The same woman shortly after surgery. In practice of course, each procedure—except for rhytidectomy and blepharoplasty, which are sometimes performed in one session—takes place at a different time.

20.13—The same woman after recovery, which is completed approximately 6 weeks after surgery, but can vary considerably, depending on the individual.

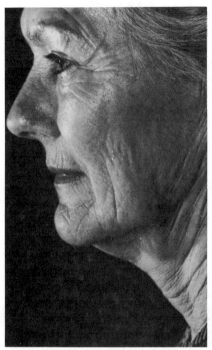

Figures 20.14–20.17 are dramatic before and after photographs, all of the same woman, which illustrate the results that can be achieved by cosmetic surgery. Notice in the before photographs the crepiness of the skin and the loss of elasticity around the mouth, jawline, and especially on the neck. Excess skin and fat deposits have formed pouches under the eyes. A heavy naso-labial crease extends from the flare of the nostrils down to the outside corner of the mouth.

The after photographs have been taken one year following the cosmetic face-lift. Notice the dramatic results, especially on the jawline and neck. The line extending from the flare of the nostrils to the area completely surrounding the mouth is firmer and softer. Droopiness on the upper eyelids has been improved and fatty deposits and loose skin underneath the eyes, which formed the pouches, have been eliminated. The overall effect of the surgery has left the skin tighter and firmer and the client looks years younger.

(Photos courtesy of Sherrell J. Aston, M.D., F.A.C.S., New York, NY)

20.14—Before—side view

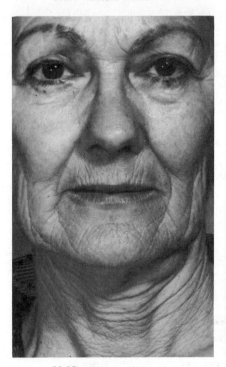

20.15—Before—front view

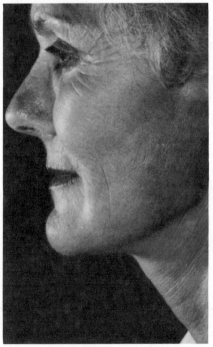

20.16—After—side view

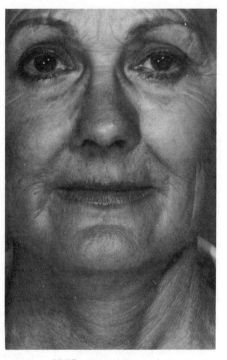

20.17—After—front view

BLEPHAROPLASTY   The technique of this plastic surgery procedure, which is often performed in conjunction with a face-lift, is quite simple: It consists of removing an ellipse of skin from the upper eyelid and then a small strip of skin from the lower, with an incision on the outer side coinciding with one of the "crow's feet." Finally, once the surgeon has made sure that the corrections on the lids of one eye match those on the other, he or she sutures the incisions with silk and nylon threads.

What is not simple, though, is deciding on the length of the incisions, drawing a steady curve, and measuring the exact amount of skin to be removed. Too little would not correct the defect; a few millimeters too much and the eye might look distorted or, worse, not be able to close properly. Also, inside both the upper and the lower lid are three pockets of fatty tissue lying next to one another; any combination of these little lumps can protrude as the result of a weakening of the membrane that contains them, giving the eye a tired, old look, even in young people. In correcting the eyelids, therefore, some of this protruding fat must also be trimmed. And again, removing the exact amount is of enormous importance, especially from the lateral pocket in the lower lid. An overcorrection would create an unattractive depression (Figs. 20.18 and 20.19).

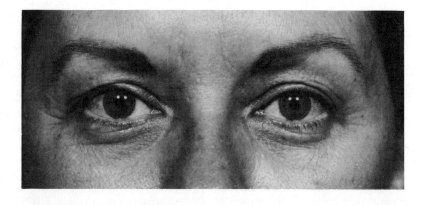

20.18—Before—Note how the upper lids of this 50-year-old woman are drooping with the right lid resting on the eyelashes. She has pouches and puffiness underneath the eyes. *(Photo courtesy of Sherrell J. Aston, M.D., F.A.C.S., New York, NY)*

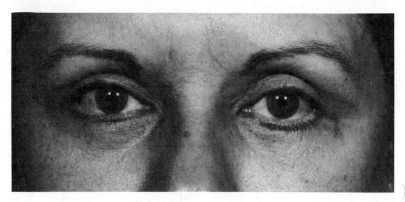

20.19—After—You can see how corrective surgery has eliminated the excess skin overhanging the eyelids. Squint lines at the outer corners of the eyes have been softened and the fatty deposits (puffiness) underneath the eyes have been eliminated. *(Photo courtesy of Sherrell J. Aston, M.D., F.A.C.S., New York, NY)*

Sometimes cutting excess skin from the upper eyelids is not enough; even before planning a blepharoplasty, a surgeon must decide whether the defect is indeed in the upper lid or rather in a drooping eyebrow. The latter can be elevated by excising a modified ellipse (wider toward the temple) directly above the brow, with the final suture line lying within the brow's upper line. But for eyelids suffering from chronic *edema* (retention of liquid) there is very little that can be done at all: The puffiness will reappear shortly after the operation.

For these operations, most surgeons prefer local anaesthesia combined with preoperative sedatives. The operation lasts about 1½ hours, and the sutures are usually removed after 4 or 5 days; however, if the scars are not completely healed, a special adhesive tape is applied across them for a few additional days.

Procedure

1. Pockets of fat are present underneath the skin in the upper and lower lids. Any combination of these little lumps can protrude as the result of a weakening of a membrane that contains them. An ellipse of skin to be removed in order to elevate a drooping eyebrow is marked in surgical ink. (See Fig. 20.20.)
2. The ellipse of skin is excised, and the wound is sutured along the eyebrow. The excess skin of the upper eyelid is marked with surgical ink. (See Fig. 20.21.)
3. The excess skin and fat in the upper eyelid are removed, and the wound is sutured. (See Fig. 20.22.)
4. The excess skin of the lower lid is cut below the lash line and undermined. The protruding fat is delicately trimmed, and after painstaking measurements, the excess skin is excised. (See Fig. 20.23.)
5. The final stage of the operation: The suture line in the upper eyelid coincides with the lid's natural fold and with one of the natural creases about the eyes. The one in the lower lid is partially disguised by the lashes and, again, by a natural crease. (See Fig. 20.24.)

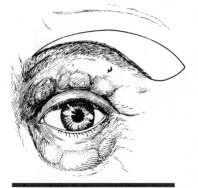

20.20—The skin to be removed is marked.

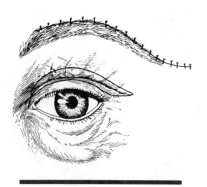

20.21—The skin is excised.

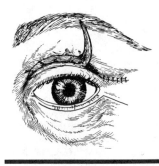

20.22—The skin is removed.

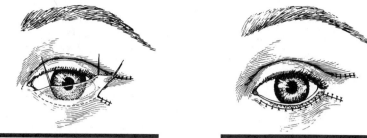

20.23—The skin is cut.   **20.24**—The final stage

> **Note:** All drawings and information about rhytidectomy, blepharoplasty, rhinoplasty, dermabrasion, and chemical peel are reprinted from *The Encyclopedia of Health and Beauty*, by Simona Morini, Copyright © 1975. Reprinted by permission of the publisher, The Bobbs-Merrill Company, Inc., New York, NY.

RHINOPLASTY

Rhinoplasty (**RYE**-no-plas-tee)—plastic surgery of the nose—can reduce the size of, straighten, build up, lengthen, shorten, scoop out, tilt up, or tilt down a "wrong" nose. It can do everything from reconstructing tissue and bone to correcting the slightest malfunction in breathing, smelling, or uttering a vocal sound.

The most popular operation, so common that many people immediately associate it with fleshy-nosed teenagers, is *reduction* rhinoplasty. The actual steps of this operation are relatively easy for an expert plastic surgeon. The difficulty lies in deciding just how much to remove and how much to retain. It is this decision, measured within sixteenths of an inch, that makes rhinoplasty one of the most delicate and, at times, unpredictable operations ever undertaken (Figs. 20.25–20.27).

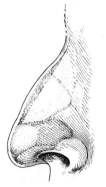

20.25—A long and hooked nose, with slightly too fleshy nostrils and a large tip. Visible is the bone segment of the nose bridge and the upper and lateral cartilages. Indicated is the amount of cartilage to be shaved off in order to correct the profile. The dotted line near the nose tips indicates where the cartilage is cut in order to slim the tip.

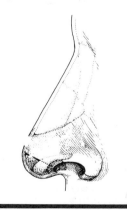

20.26—The dotted lines indicate, respectively, where the cartilage is cut in order to shorten the nose and where the nostrils are narrowed.

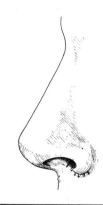

20.27—The operation is completed. With the exception of the nostrils, surgery is performed from inside the nose.

Surgery is performed from inside the nose and under a local anaesthetic painlessly administered after the injection of a *barbiturate* whose effects last only a short while. This prevents the patient from bleeding as much as he or she would under general anaesthesia, and keeps the face looking natural during the operation, thus providing a guide for the surgeon, who constantly has to consider the future relationship of the nose to the face.

Usually, the nose tip is reshaped first. Second, the hump of the bridge is removed. And third, the septum (the sheet of cartilage dividing the nose lengthwise) is cut shorter or straightened and, particularly in thick-skinned, hooked noses, also scooped out to compensate for the inevitable telescoping of the skin over a suddenly shortened framework.

Excision of a triangle from the septum tilts the nose; excision of a rectangle shortens it; excision of a trapezoid shortens and tilts it; excision of an ellipse repairs a hanging columella (the midline tissue between the tip and the floor of the nose) (Fig. 20.28).

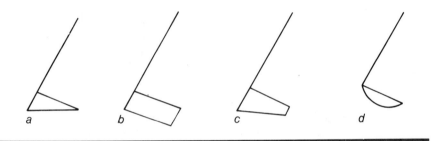

20.28—Excision of a triangle (a) from the septum tilts a nose; excision of a rectangle (b) shortens it; of a trapezoid (c) shortens and tilts it; of an ellipse (d) repairs a hanging columella—the tissue between the tips and the floor of the nose.

To narrow the nose, the surgeon performs a carefully designed fracture of the bone plates and presses them, often with his thumbs, into a new, slender position. Usually, the last step is the suturing of the mucosa (the nose lining), which requires extremely light stitches. However, sometimes the very last step, necessary only in case the lowering of the bridge has made the nose wings collapse, requires a triangular or diamond-shaped excision at the base of each nostril that will draw the wings together, leaving only two barely visible scars.

Reduction rhinoplasty is a 45-minute operation followed by 1 week of bandages. The dreaded black-and-white aftereffect and the swelling vary greatly according to the patient's skin and healing capacity. It varies also with the skill of the surgeon; particularly if he or she narrows the nose. A knowledgeable handling of the bones is important to avoid bruises and to prevent the bones from resuming their previous position.

Augmentation rhinoplasty, a less common but more dramatic procedure, is required for a nose twisted or flattened by an accident, for an abbreviated nose with an exaggerated upward-tilted tip and large soft-edged nostrils, or for a nose overly trimmed by previous surgery.

Through an incision within one of the nasal passages, the surgeon dissects a pocket straight along the depressed bridge in which he or she later inserts an implant to build up the bridge. A sliver from the patient's hipbone or rib cartilage, or else a piece of *silicone* rubber provides the implant. The implant is carved with great precision so as to fit exactly where the nose is depressed, thereby avoiding later shifting. On the upper surface, which will become the new contour of the nose, it is adjusted to fit the patient's face. If the tip also needs support, the implant is L-shaped and is inserted through an incision in the columella or the lower part of the septum.

The operation is followed by a few days of *antibiotic* therapy, 5 days in the hospital, and biweekly checking of the bandages until the incision has healed—3 or 4 weeks in all.

> **Note:** The esthetician should be able to discuss plastic surgery intelligently with a client; however, no advice should be given. Only a qualified surgeon can determine the needs of the individual who seeks plastic (cosmetic) surgery.

Dermabrasion

Dermabrasion (dur-muh-**BRAY**-zhun) is a cosmetic surgery technique that consists of sanding the skin—usually of the face—with a rotating wire or steel brush. Dermabrasion is used to smooth scars, to reduce surface irregularities, and to even out ridges and other aftereffects of acne or chickenpox. It is also helpful in removing so-called *traumatic* tattoos— foreign material that is sometimes driven into the skin during an accident. (Esthetic tattoos are more difficult to eradicate with this technique, because the pigment is located much deeper within the skin.)

Irregular scars can often be improved by dermabrasion, which equalizes the margins and eliminates elevations. Fine wrinkles, such as the "pruning" that appears around the mouth with aging, can also be improved, even if only temporarily.

Dermabrasion is carried out with a motor-driven instrument, the dermabrader, which revolves at a high speed and is controlled by varying the pressure on a foot pedal. Attached to the dermabrader is a tiny cylinder of sandpaper or wire brush. The cylinders of sandpaper are available in several sizes: The larger ones are used for sanding broad flat surfaces, while the smaller ones help in planing narrower surfaces, such as around the nose. The wire brush is needed for *deep* planing; for more *superficial* sanding, a smooth cylinder, called diamond fraise, is used.

Local anaesthesia is achieved by freezing the skin with ethyl chloride. This method temporarily hardens the skin and yet preserves its usual surface contour. The effect of ethyl chloride, however, is so short that abrasion can be performed only a few square centimeters at the time. Other local anaesthetics have the disadvantage of altering the skin configuration, and when used, the doctor marks the ridges and depressions with surgical ink so that they can be identified.

Bandages are applied and the patient can go home, if not out in the world, per doctor's orders. After a few days, a crusty surface develops, which is then smeared with some mineral oil or cold cream to help remove the crust and lubricate the surface beneath, which tends to be dry. The crust will shed in about 1 week, leaving a pink surface—the new layer of epidermis that has formed over the raw dermal surface—which soon fades, depending on the patient's type of skin. Powder and makeup can be applied after the abraded surface has healed, but it is important to wash the area well each day and to lubricate it. Direct or indirect sunlight should be avoided for several months after abrasion because it may produce discolorations and dark, uneven spots.

The face and scalp respond better to dermabrasion than any other area of the body. The back of the hands do moderately well, while the chest and upper and lower arms do poorly, as do legs and feet. People with dark skin do not profit much from dermabrasion, as the treated areas often become darker than the normal adjacent skin.

Still, dermabrasion is a sound and often extremely successful procedure. Improvement is achieved because once the dermis—the inner layer of the skin—has been thinned by this technique, it never regains its original thickness. And the new layer of epidermis that grows over it is considerably smoother and more even-colored than the old one (Figs. 20.29 and 20.30).

Chemical Skin Refining

The chemical peel is a procedure (often used as an alternative to dermabrasion) in which a caustic substance is applied to the face in order to burn the skin's outer layer (the epidermis), and part of the adjoining inner layer (the dermis). The purpose is to eliminate a rough, sun-damaged, large-pored, freckled, or blemished skin and restore to it a healthier, younger texture. The removal of a portion of the dermis stimulates the growth of new tissue and helps promote a partial rebuilding of the skin. When it heals, the dermis is slightly thicker, firmer, and more resilient, thus plumping up the skin and eradicating fine wrinkles. When the epidermis regrows, it becomes completely and extraordinarily smooth and small-pored.

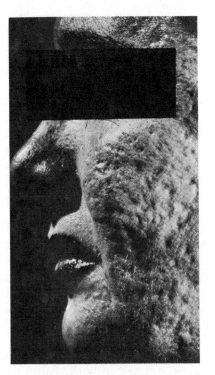 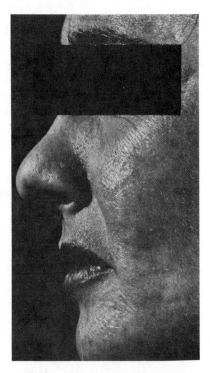

20.29—This woman's face has been left with severe acne scars and pits.

20.30—After dermabrasion treatments, the scars and pits have been almost eliminated. *(Photos courtesy of Norman Orentreich, M.D., New York, NY)*

The chemical peel has only a limited usefulness in treating the problems of aging tissue, because it tightens loose skin only slightly. But after a face-lift, which improves the general contour of the face, a chemical peel is ideal to smooth out the fine wrinkles on the upper lip, the forehead, and the eyelids, which are generally unaffected by a face-lift.

As a rule, women with fair skin, fine creases, and only slightly sagging skin are ideal candidates for a chemical peel. Those with a more olive complexion may be less satisfied, because the treated areas of the skin could turn a lighter or darker shade than the surrounding skin.

The caustic substance used for a chemical peel is a solution of phenol (or chloracetic acid), distilled water, a few drops of croton oil, and liquid soap. The solution is administered with ordinary cotton applicators, with care taken to apply it only to the areas where it is needed. Special care is to be taken around the eyes to prevent it from splashing on the conjunctiva, the delicate membrane that lines the eyelids and covers the eyeball.

Before the treatment, the patient is given a mild sedative to ease or relieve the solution's burning sensation; this burning rapidly subsides, however, because of the local anaesthetic property of phenol. For several minutes the skin appears white, as if frosted, then turns dark red. Waterproof adhesive tape is applied over the treated area and left in place for approximately 48 hours (the longer it remains, the deeper the penetration of of the peeler), then carefully removed. An antiseptic powder is dusted on and reapplied several times during the following 24 hours, while a thick crust forms. About 1 week later, the crusts will lift, leaving a pink-colored skin that pales down in about 6 to 12 weeks. But the maximum benefit of a chemical peel is fully realized only after 4 to 5 months, during which time a person should not expose the skin to either direct or indirect sunlight.

The entire face must be treated initially, to avoid contrasting areas, but local touch-ups may be needed later. If unskillfully performed, a chemical peel could cause toxic reactions, scars, blotchy discolorations of the skin, or an unattractive ruddiness due to an abnormal enlargement of small blood vessels. But even when the peel is entirely successful, "the skin never looks entirely normal again," as Dr. Bedford Shelmire, Jr., writes in *The Art of Looking Younger*:

> The new skin often has a slightly artificial look about it, as though it might be of some synthetic material. This is due to the fact that the regenerated portion of the inner layer consists entirely of scar tissue and therefore lacks the tone and pliability of the original article. It is also much less durable than normal tissue.

However, the overall improvement of the skin after a professionally performed chemical peel is often so astonishing that scores of women (and men) gladly exchange a leathery, splotchy, wrinkled face for one that is ever so slightly artificial looking.

Injections to Smooth Lines and Eliminate Wrinkles

Scientists are constantly searching for ways to maintain the health and attractiveness of the skin, as well as to repair skins that have been damaged by disease or accidents. Silicone injections to plump up the skin and to fill in crevices have been given by some specialists. The injection of any serum into lines and wrinkles causes a reaction that produces a swelling (edema) of the area. This puffing or swelling of the skin fills out the lines and wrinkles, but as soon as the swelling goes down, the lines and wrinkles usually reappear. Silicone injections have not been approved by the FDA, and their legality remains in question.

Collagen Injections

The flexibility of the skin is due to a microscopic network of fibers (collagen) made up of proteins and elastin. These fibers are woven together like threads in fabric and act as a framework into which cells and blood vessels can grow. In young looking facial skin, the collagen network is intact, so the skin is smooth and soft. Over time, this network can weaken, and as it does, so does its support of the skin. As a result, the skin begins to lose its shape and resiliency.

TREATMENT FREQUENCY

Skin also begins to look older (usually around 45 to 50 years of age) because the sebaceous glands and sweat glands begin to decrease their activity. The result is drying of the skin from lack of moisture and lubrication (Fig. 20.31).

Collagen, a natural animal protein is used in a process called replacement therapy and must be done by a physician. The collagen is injected into the tissue where it plumps up or "fills" the underlying skin layer and gives a smoother appearance.

The physician gives a skin test to determine if the patient is sensitive to the collagen and advises the patient regarding the potential benefits or possible treatment reactions.

Collagen is incorporated into some skin care products, especially in moisturizing creams. Collagen is "hydrophilic," that is, it is a good binder of water, therefore, it helps to reduce the amount of moisture lost by the skin.

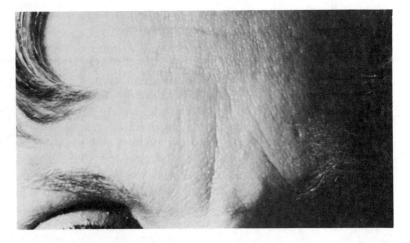

20.31—Frown lines and small lines on the forehead are noticeable before treatment with collagen. *(Photo courtesy of the Collagen Corporation (Zyderm Collagen), Palo Alto, CA)*

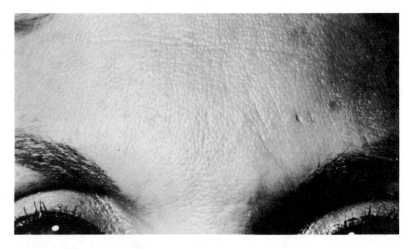

20.32—Following the collagen treatment, the forehead appears smoother and the face more youthful. *(Photo courtesy of the Collagen Corporation (Zyderm Collagen), Palo Alto, CA)*

Generally, patients receive a series of injections (at least 2 weeks apart) into the uppermost layers of the skin. Improvement is seen in two to four sessions depending on the problem area to be treated. Clinical evidence suggests that patients choose to receive a touch-up treatment within 6 to 24 months of their original treatment series (Fig. 20.32).

Collagen used to soften age-related lines is similar to the collagen in your own skin. It can be incorporated into the tissue so that it cannot be distinguished from the surrounding skin.

Retin-A

Retin-A, the trade name for the drug *tretinoin* (tre-**TIN**-o-in), or *retinoic* (ret-i-**NO**-ick) *acid*, is a derivative of vitamin A. It was developed as a topical ointment to be used as an acne treatment, and has been very effective for this purpose.

It was noted that patients using the drug also benefited in other ways. Their skin became smoother, more flexible, and thicker. This led to some dermatologists prescribing it as an anti-aging agent that would also remove wrinkles and fine lines from the skin. There is considerable evidence that Retin-A does work effectively, especially on fair-skinned people who have sun-damaged skin.

There are some concerns about the safety and effectiveness of Retin-A. As a topical cream, the product does cause some side effects, including irritation, dryness, and peeling. A sister drug, iso-tretinoin, marketed under the trade name, Accutane, was developed as an orally ingested medicine to cure severe cystic acne. Accutane, however, is known to cause birth defects. While Retin-A is not chemically identical to Accutane, the FDA urges caution in its use until more data is available. In fact, some believe that if Retin-A is used chronically, it could potentially increase the chance of skin cancer.

Retin-A is available only through a doctor's prescription. Because of the potential side effects, it should be used with a suitable moisturizer and should be used only under a doctor's supervision. As a drug, it may not be used by estheticians on their clients. Estheticians may, however, discuss the pros and cons of the product with clients and suggest that they discuss the subject with their physicians.

QUESTIONS   DISCUSSION AND REVIEW

ENEMIES OF THE SKIN, AGING FACTORS, AND COSMETIC SURGERY

1. Why does the skin usually start to age faster when approaching or during the midyears of life?
2. Why is too much sun harmful to most skins?
3. How does air pollution harm the skin?
4. Explain how the excessive intake of alcohol can be harmful to the appearance of the skin.
5. How does the rapid loss of weight affect the skin?
6. Explain why taking too many drugs can be harmful to the skin.
7. Discuss chemical face peeling.
8. What is dermabrasion?
9. Discuss the canon of beauty and why it was devised by the Greeks.
10. Discuss how plastic (reconstructive, cosmetic) surgery can benefit the individual.
11. What is the medical name for a face-lift?
12. What is the medical name for plastic surgery on the nose?

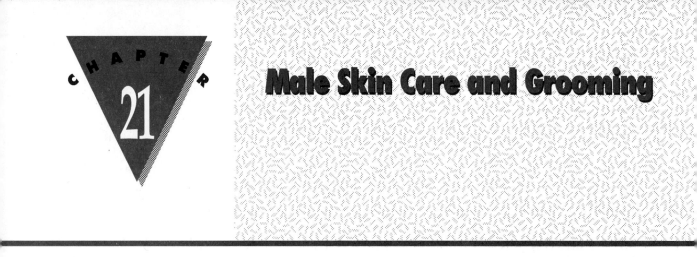

CHAPTER 21

Male Skin Care and Grooming

LEARNING OBJECTIVES

After completing this chapter, you should be able to:

❶ Discuss how men differ from women in their facial needs.
❷ Explain the different services you can offer to your male clients.
❸ Discuss and demonstrate the skin care procedures used on male clients.
❹ Describe skin care products designed for men and skin care regimen for men.

INTRODUCTION

For the most part, the science of esthetics has focused on servicing the needs of women. Women have long been the primary users of skin care services and products. The field has, historically, been dominated by females, both as practitioners and as clients. This has been true partly because of an emphasis on skin care as a beauty aid as well as a health aid, and partly because women have been more concerned with their looks than have men. Also, men have considered skin care as a feminine pursuit.

This attitude is changing, however. More and more, men are becoming concerned with good grooming and becoming aware of the health aspects of making sure their skin is cared for properly. This is an important consideration for the professional esthetician. Simply put, servicing the skin care needs of the male population means significantly more opportunity for business for those estheticians who can take care of the needs of this segment of their clientele.

The skin care needs of men do differ from those of women to some extent, but these differences are not so great that the moderately well-equipped and staffed salon will be unable to adapt to them.

Gender Differences in Skin

There are significant physical differences between males and females that extend beyond the obvious differences in the sex and reproductive organs. Because of their physiology, men tend to grow larger and are stronger and faster.

Men have a larger, more dense bone structure and have as much as 20 percent more muscle mass. Women, however, have more fatty tissue than men and the distribution of fat cells throughout the body is different. In men, fat tends to be evenly distributed, while in women, it tends to be concentrated around the breasts, hips, and buttocks. It is because of these differences in muscle and fat that women tend to be more susceptible to cold than men.

Some of these differences in muscle-mass structure and fat distribution are caused by hormonal differences, specifically in testosterone levels in men, which cause increased muscle mass and widen the shoulders, and in estrogen levels in women, which widen the hips and increase fatty tissues.

When it comes to skin, however, there are few differences. The basic skin structure is the same for both men and women. The differences that do exist are more in the line of tendencies rather than structural differences. A man's skin is made up of the same five layers of epidermal tissue and the same two layers of dermal tissue as that of a woman's skin. The skin of both sexes contains the same vast number of cells and sensory receptors for heat, cold, pain, and touch.

A man's skin, however, tends to have larger sebaceous glands and, thus, produces more sebum than a woman's skin; men's glands also produce it longer in life. The female hormone, estrogen, influences sebum production. After menopause, women's sebum production slows considerably. There is no corresponding reduction of sebum production in men. Therefore, older men will tend to have oilier skin than older women. In general, men will tend to be more prone to acne skin conditions than women because of a greater production of sebum.

Men perspire because of the effects of heat more than women do. A man's skin also tends to be more acidic than a woman's skin, and tends to be coarser and thicker, as well. The most evident difference, however, in so far as the esthetician will be concerned, is in the matter of facial and body hair.

Although men and women have the same number of hair follicles, men grow thicker, coarser hair on their faces and bodies, because of their higher testosterone levels. Beard hair is extremely abrasive and tough, and grows at a rate of more than 5 inches per year.

Men's Skin Care Needs

Men need to care for their skin no less than women do. In particular, men need facial treatments because they tend to work under harsher conditions. That is, they tend to get dirtier than women because of exposure to grease and oil in the workplace and greater exposure to pollution because they don't have the barrier effect of makeup that women have.

Because they produce more sebum, men also tend to have a more acne-prone skin than women do; this condition also requires care. The scraping action of daily shaving automatically exfoliates their faces, so there is less need to remove dead skin cells during a facial treatment. However, the same scraping action causes irritation, which can be a major problem in men's skin care. Where an acne skin condition is present, shaving can also cause inflammation and abrasions, as well.

Men have not been conditioned to care for their skin. The typical regimen for a man is to wash his face with a harsh bar soap, lather it with a shaving cream, shave, quickly rinse off the cream, then splash on an alcohol-based shaving lotion. Clearly, this does not represent an ideal situation for healthy skin.

Teaching the values of skin care is probably the esthetician's first priority when working with male clientele. It is important to show men that proper skin care is effective and a valuable aid to health and good grooming.

Services for the Male Client

The esthetician can offer male clients virtually the same full range of services offered for women. These include cleansing the skin, treating some skin conditions (such as acne), moisturizing and normalizing the skin, selling skin care products and instructing men on skin care regimens for home use.

Hair removal services, either by hot waxing or by electrolysis, are also valid services for men. The salon can offer a wide range of these services for men, including eyebrow shaping and trimming, and removal of excess body hair.

The same machinery and equipment can be used effectively for men, although more careful choices of products may be necessary and the salon atmosphere will have to be considered.

Many men are ill at ease in an environment that they perceive to be "for women only," such as a salon. The atmosphere in the salon should be more unisex in nature to prevent intimidating male clients.

In addition to making the salon environment more comfortable for everyone, it should also offer a degree of privacy. This means treatment rooms and changing facilities should be private.

The salon atmosphere should always be cordial and professional. The salon should be clean, warm, well-lit and well-equipped. The staff should be friendly and competent. Remember, performance is generally more important to men than is appearance.

Skin Care Products for Men

By and large, the same products can be used for male clients as are used for female clients. High-quality cleansers, toners, astringents, moisturizers, masks, and other treatment products work just as effectively on male skin as on female skin. In addition to these types of products, the esthetician may also want to stock shaving creams, after-shave lotions, and colognes.

A number of companies manufacture skin care products formulated for men. These tend to be lighter, and less complicated chemically, and are designed to promote maximum soothing and healing of freshly shaved skin. These products usually do not contain perfumes or fragrances. Except for these ingredients, they are, in fact, not that much different from the products developed for women. It is not necessary to keep separate stocks of products for use in the salon during facial treatments, but it may be profitable to stock men's skin care products for retail sales.

Before choosing products for use or resale, check with the manufacturers and wholesalers of the products and learn as much as possible about the ingredients, what they do, and how well the products measure up to the makers' claims.

Skin Care Procedures for Men

With few exceptions, the same procedures and techniques are used in giving facial treatments to men as are used for women. Consultation and analysis, cleansing, vaporizing, disincrustation, suction, manual extraction, massage, mask application, and moisturizing and normalizing the skin are all important steps.

If possible, have the client shave before coming in for the facial treatment. This will minimize problems with beard stubble. If the client has a beard, treatment will be limited to hairless areas, such as the forehead, nose, and possibly the cheeks.

CONSULTATION AND ANALYSIS   Education starts here. This is where you begin teaching the male client about the value of facial treatments. Conduct the consultation in as private an environment as possible. Discuss fully all of the treatment steps that will be given.

For analysis and treatment, the client should remove his shirt and undershirt and put on a salon gown. The gown, however, should not be frilly and feminine, but should be more like a kimono-type salon robe. (See Fig. 12.2, in Chapter 12.) His hair should be covered.

Carry out the analysis as with female clients. Inspect the skin under a magnifying lamp and use the Wood's lamp (if available). Determine the client's skin type, and develop a treatment regimen accordingly. If the client has shaved before coming in, analysis and treatment can begin. Unlike analysis on female clients, it will not be necessary to precleanse the skin to remove makeup.

All of the steps involved in deep-pore cleansing of the skin, massage, mask application and moisturizing and normalizing the skin will be virtually the same for men as for women. See the chapters covering these topics for full procedural steps.

SHAVING   Quite often a man will come to the salon because his face is irritated, chapped, chafed, or raw in some areas. These conditions are usually brought about by shaving too closely and by using irritating, alkaline shaving products, such as foam from an aerosol can. These conditions can usually be corrected in approximately 3 to 4 days.

To prevent irritation, the client should be advised to use the following procedure when shaving:

1. Use an adjustable razor that has been adjusted to low. This low setting will prevent the blade from scraping the skin. The adjustment setting may be changed during the shave to a higher degree for certain areas but should remain on low for irritated and sensitive areas, such as the neck and chin.
2. Recommend that the client purchase brushless shaving cream. The product comes in jars or tubes, and the client may prefer to try small sizes first, as there are several brands on the market. He may find one more satisfactory than another. Brushless shaving cream is nonirritating, softens the beard, soothes and lubricates the skin, and some brands are mildly antiseptic. In addition to instructing the male client about proper shaving practices, facial treatments should be given to cleanse follicles and clear blemishes. The face should be clean-shaven before the facial treatment, unless the male client has a stylized beard or mustache.
3. After-shave lotions act in the same way as an astringent or skin-freshening lotion. Men may select a mild after-shave lotion or use witch hazel. A highly fragranced lotion may be irritating to some skins. When the skin is dry and sensitive after shaving, a moisturizing lotion may be applied. Some men enjoy an after-shave talcum powder, which also soothes the skin and tones down excessive shine. For the man who feels he needs added color, there are bronzing gels and sticks that can be applied to even complexion color and give a healthy glow or sun-bronzed effect to the skin.

During the consultation the esthetician can demonstrate and/or show products that will be beneficial to the client's skin. Many companies specialize in toiletries for men. Emollient, hydrating, and moisturizing lotions are just as important for the care of a man's skin as for a woman's.

POST TREATMENT CONSULTATION   Take the opportunity to ask the male client for his reactions to the treatment, especially if it is his first, and point out the results of the treatment he has just finished. Discuss how he can care for his skin at home. Point out the problems with "skin care as usual" and show him why he should not use a harsh bar soap on his face. Explain the advantages he will gain by using skin care products especially formulated for his skin type.

Male clients, if treated properly with regard to their particular needs, can be a valuable source of income for the esthetician.

QUESTIONS DISCUSSION AND REVIEW

MALE SKIN CARE AND GROOMING

1. What attitudes toward skin care are men developing?
2. How does muscle structure differ between men and women?
3. How does the distribution of fat differ between men and women?
4. What differences are there between male skin and female skin?
5. What is the typical way men care for their skin and why is it a problem?
6. What services can the salon offer to male clients?
7. How should the salon environment be to appeal to male clients?
8. How do skin care products for men differ from those for women?
9. What is the single most important aspect with respect to male skin?
10. What differences in treatment techniques are used for male clients?

Esthetics and Aromatherapy

LEARNING OBJECTIVES

After completing this chapter, you should be able to:

❶ Discuss the history, manufacture, and use of fragrances from ancient times to the present.

❷ Describe the characteristics of various fragrances and how essences are obtained from natural and synthetic sources.

❸ Discuss the therapeutic value gained from the extracts of herbs, plants, teas, flowers, and fruits.

INTRODUCTION

Aromatherapy is a type of beauty care in which aromatic essential oils from herbs, flowers, fruit, and plants of all kinds are used as active, functional ingredients in various beauty preparations and treatment procedures. These essential oils are basic ingredients in fine perfumes and cosmetic fragrances. However, in aromatherapy, their aromatic qualities are incidental; it is their functional effect as moisturizers, emollients, cleansers, stimulants, relaxers, soothers, softeners, and nourishers that is valued.

Aromatherapists use essential oils in two ways: either as ingredients in creams, lotions, sprays, massage and bath oils, or as vapors. When vaporized, they reach the skin directly in a very diffusive form.

Aromatherapy is also concerned with psychological effects and the altering of emotional states. Relaxation and tranquility are the emotional states that are considered necessary to attain and maintain health and youthfulness.

Aromatherapy dates back to ancient times and is a therapeutic technique using natural aromatic substances in treatments. The ancients used aromatherapy in their medical and personal grooming practices. They considered oils especially valuable and used them in embalming, for medicinal purposes, to fumigate homes, and as part of their toilet preparations. They knew how to use plant extracts as anesthetics as well as for other medicinal purposes.

A Brief History of the Use of Fragrances

In ancient times, pleasant-smelling incense, herbs, and fragrances in the form of oils, colognes, toilet water, and perfume were widely used. Many passages in the Bible and other ancient writings refer to incense and the influence of fragrances. The Egyptians used fragrances lavishly, both in their ceremonies and for curing diseases. They also scented their skins by rubbing aromatic essences and oils into their skin. When the tomb of Tutankhamun was opened in 1922 after more than 3,000 years, receptacles for fragrances were found among the treasures. The Hebrews also mastered the art of perfumery, and ancient Greeks introduced the art of manufacturing fragrances to the Romans. Fragrances were associated with their gods and goddesses and fresh flowers and essences were used extravagantly.

India abounds with a variety of flowers and fruits and the people of India created aromatic resins and other forms of fragrances.

Fragrances in China date back to the earliest written records. The Chinese are credited with discovering the use of musk, which they believed to have healing powers. Flower arranging is considered an intricate art in Japan. The Japanese people love fragrances and are known to use them lavishly.

Germany, France, England, Spain, Italy, and other countries all have fascinating histories regarding the various fragrances they discovered and/or manufactured. All of these countries encouraged the art of perfumery. Kings, queens, and other royal persons used fragrances in the form of sachet, oils, colognes, perfumes, scented water, pastes, powders, and pomades. These fragrances were used to scent bodies, clothing, jewelry, furs, gloves, and the interiors of homes and castles.

Modern day aromatherapy can have positive psychological benefits. It is mainly used in the salon to induce relaxation. Herbal masks and aromatic essences facilitate cellular nutrition and reproduction of cells. The power of essences in healing has been recognized in the treatment of insect bites. Clove, thyme, sandlewood, and lavender are a few of the essences that have antiseptic actions.

Modern department stores, pharmacies, boutiques, and salons offer a wide variety of fragrances for both men and women. Fragrances are described according to a particular characteristic. The following are some basic terms that help us to identify different categories of fragrances.

FLORAL   This term applies to one flower such as a rose, lilac, lily-of-the-valley, jasmine, or magnolia.

FLORAL BOUQUET   This fragrance may be light or heavy and is a combination of fragrances so that no one flower stands out.

ORIENTAL   These fragrances are often blends of spices and give an impression of incense. This does not mean that oriental fragrances are overpowering; they should be tried on in order to get the full benefit of their unique blends.

MODERN BLENDS   These fragrances combine substances that enhance one another so that the fragrance may not be identified as any one substance.

SPICY BLENDS   Cinnamon, clove, vanilla, ginger, and other spices are used to create a spicy bouquet of fragrance.

FOREST OR WOODSY BLENDS   Sandlewood, rosewood, and cedar are some herbs and plants that are used to create distinctive fragrances. Like all other fragrances, they must be tried on to be fully appreciated.

FRUITY BLENDS   These fragrances are based on the fresh smell of fruit such as peaches, limes, and lemons. Some of the popular fragrances for men combine the scent of herbs, spices, and citrus.

Both men and women have different emotional responses to fragrances and it is helpful to try on a fragrance before purchasing it. Perfume departments encourage sampling of fragrances and salespersons are usually trained to help the customer select a fragrance that will be pleasing. Fragrance should be tried on the skin and the alcohol allowed to evaporate before you determine the appeal of the fragrance.

Fragrance and the Psyche

Fragrance was used by many ancient civilizations to influence the mind. They found that fragrances used on the body or inhaled, produced a profound effect on thoughts and emotions. Modern science has investigated the sense of smell and there are a number of theories about how and to what degree we can detect pleasant and unpleasant odors. It is clear that we have an immediate response to odorous substances. Repulsive odors can make us physically ill while pleasant odors can raise our spirits and eliminate feelings of depression and lethargy.

Fragrances, pleasant and unpleasant, are a part of our everyday experiences. Fragrances can change moods, remind us of past experiences, and enliven our environment in numerous ways. Studies have been done on the effects of specific odors on the mind and the body. In some people, the powers of perception become more acute when they smell pleasant odors, and they are better able to deal with emotional problems. Basil, peppermint, jasmine, and citrus oils are thought to relieve depression. Some fragrances seem to have an effect on the nervous system, but how different fragrances work on different emotions is not completely understood. The use of carefully chosen essences can put a person into a harmonious state of mind.

Our minds are influenced and often controlled by our five senses: sight, touch, hearing, taste, and smell. Of these five senses, the sense of smell is thought by some to be the most powerful. Surveys have revealed that people want pleasant fragrances in cosmetics, toilet products (such as soap), laundry products, room sprays, and mouthwashes. Manufacturers are aware of the impact that a fragrance can have on the sale of products: If a product doesn't smell good it will not sell as well. Colors, seasons, scenes, and even places, have been translated or interpreted into fragrances. For example, a room deodorizer may bring visions of fresh pine trees, an orange grove, or a garden of lilacs. We may take a trip in our minds by way of fragrance to almost any place. In recent years, we have seen the growth of scratch and smell advertising. A colored photograph of a beautiful rose can be scratched and behold—it smells like a fresh rose. There is no doubt that fragrance will continue to influence our moods, our attitudes, and our personalities. We should try to be aware of the many ways in which fragrances influence our thoughts and feelings and how we react to different fragrances.

How Aromatic Essences Are Obtained

Oils and essences used in fragrances that come from all over the world, are obtained by distillation of the root, bark, stem, seed root, or flower of a plant or tree, depending on where the fragrant part is located.

The fragrant oils and/or essences may be extracted by five methods.

1. Distillation
2. Extraction by solvent
3. Expression
4. Enfleurage (en-floo-**RAHZH**)
5. Maceration (mas-ur-**AY**-shun)

Distillation uses steam or boiling water to separate the water and fragrant oils.

Extraction by solvent is achieved by placing the plant material in a container with the solvent (ether or petroleum). The solvent penetrates the plant material and when it leaves the material, fragrant oil is retained.

Expression: This is a method where the essential oils are pressed out of the substances. For example, the oils are pressed from the skin of fruits in this way.

Enfleurage: This is a method where fat is used to absorb essential oils from the natural substances. This is done by placing layers of flower petals or other substances on frames that have been spread with fat.

Maceration: This is a process using hot fat. The flower petals or other substances are plunged into hot fat, which absorbs the essential oils.

Aromatic essences are of different colors, feel slightly oily, are insoluble in water, and are soluble in alcohol. Gums, resins, and animal secretions are also used in the art of perfumery.

Substances Used in the Manufacture of Fragrances

Animal Products—Certain oils from animals are used as fixatives in the manufacture of fragrances. Some animals are hunted in their native habitat, while others are raised domestically. Some animals are in danger of becoming extinct. One of these is the civet cat, which is found in Africa. This animal secretes a specific type of oil that has a strong odor that acts as a protection for the animal in the same manner that the skunk repels other animals. Civet cat oil is valued as a fixative in some expensive fragrances. Musk oil is also widely used in perfumery and comes from the gland of the male musk deer. This animal is a native of Tibet and China. Domestic musk oil is obtained from the beaver and muskrat. Ambergris is used as a fixative in fragrances and comes from the sperm whale.

This is a list of some natural products used in fragrances:

Flowers—Rose, lilac, jasmine, magnolia, orange blossoms

Seeds—Caraway, almond

Bark—Cinnamon, cascarilla

Leaves—Bay, thyme

Woods—Sandlewood, rosewood, cedar

Fruits—Lemons, peaches, strawberries

Spices—Nutmeg, clove

Salicylic (sal-i-**SIL**-ick) *acid* is found in the leaves of wintergreen, the flowers and leaves of yarrow, and the bark of sweet birch. Frequently used in acne treatment products, salicylic acid is antiseptic and dissolves the dead cells on the surface of the skin.

Chlorophyll (**KLOR**-uh-fil) is the green coloring matter that is responsible for *photosynthesis* (fo-to-**SIN**-thi-sis) in plants. It is used in the treatment of various lesions and tissue damage to reduce swelling and pus formation. It is also used in deodorants.

Any essence or oil mixed with liquids should be used with caution because it is not uncommon for some people to be allergic to these substances.

In recent years, chemists have been able to identify various odors and produce them synthetically in the laboratory.

Fragrances can be synthetic, but when fragrances are used in cosmetic products, natural plant oils are preferred, since they are more beneficial when applied to the skin. For example, the fragrance of spices may be duplicated, but the spices in their natural form will be mildly antiseptic when used on the skin.

Herbs and Other Substances

The following is a list of some of the many herbs, plants, teas, flowers, and fruits whose extracts, when applied to the skin in a compress, spray, or mask, have therapeutic value.

AROMATIC Substances having an agreeable odor and stimulating qualities:

Nutmeg	Golden rod
Fennel	Lavender
Mint	Majoram
Ginger	Rosemary
Sassafras bark	Sage

ANTISEPTIC Agents used for destroying or inhibiting bacteria (putrefactive or pathogenic):

Clove	Eucalyptus
Heather	Lavender
Olive leaves	Sandlewood
Sassafras bark	Thyme
Peppermint	

ASTRINGENT Agents that contract organic tissue and reduce discharges or secretions:

Comfrey root	Elm leaves
Horse chestnut	Lemon
Lettuce	Magnolia bark
Nettle	Oak bark
Wild plum	Radish
Rhubarb	Sage
Sandlewood	Shepherd's purse
Sumac	Witch hazel
Strawberry leaves	Alum root (extremely astringent)

STIMULATING Substances that have stimulating qualities:

Eucalyptus	Fennel
Rosemary	Thyme
Magnolia bark	Lavender
Mistletoe	Spearmint
Wintergreen	Sandlewood

CALMING AND SOOTHING The following are substances that have a calming and soothing effect on the skin:

Almond	Comfrey root
Hollyhock	Camomile flowers
Balm	Pansy plant
Lettuce	Jasmine
Whitepond lily root	Majoram
Wild daisy	Ginseng

> **Note:** See Chapter 13 for instructions for applying cotton compress masks. See Chapter 15 for formula for herbal jelly masks.

CLEANSING Substances known to have exceptional cleansing action:

Lovage root	Milfoil
Lemongrass	Witch Hazel
Geranium leaves	

EMOLLIENT Agents used externally to soothe and soften the skin:

Almond	Aloe
Comfrey root	Hollyhock
Figs	Olive leaves

HEALING   Agents used for their healing qualities:

Peppermint	Milfoil
Camomile flowers	Elder flowers
Rosemary	Lovage root
Comfrey root	Aloe
Pansy plant	Wild daisy

MOISTURIZING   Substances used for their moisturizing qualities:

Orange blossoms	Camomile flowers
Rose leaves	Rose petals
Rose hips	White willow bark

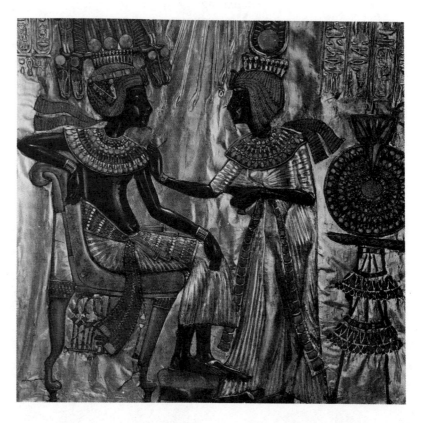

22.1—This panel is from the gold throne of the Egyptian King Tutankhamun. Discovered in 1922, the artifacts found in the King's tomb date back to the 14th century B.C. This scene shows the Queen anointing the King with aromatic oils on what is believed to be his coronation.

QUESTIONS   DISCUSSION AND REVIEW

ESTHETICS AND   1. Define aromatherapy.
AROMATHERAPY   2. Discuss the history of aromatherapy and the use of fragrances.
3. Name the seven basic categories of fragrances.
4. Discuss how fragrances are thought to affect the human psyche and evoke emotional responses.
5. Discuss the five ways aromatic essences are obtained.
6. Name three herbs that are said to have exceptional antiseptic action.
7. Name two of the most widely used natural animal fixatives used in the manufacture of fragrances.
8. Discuss the various substances such as herbs, spices, plants, teas, flowers, and fruits that are said to have specific qualities and therapeutic values. For example: Some aromatic substances having an agreeable odor are nutmeg, rosemary, and sage. Which substances have the following qualities?

Antiseptic
Astringent
Stimulating
Calming and soothing
Emollient
Healing
Moisturizing

Advanced Topics in Esthetics

CHAPTER 23

LEARNING OBJECTIVES

After completing this chapter, you should be able to:

❶ Discuss phytotherapy, its use, and the precautions in using it.
❷ Explain advanced massage techniques, such as reflexology and lymphatic drainage.
❸ Describe the different water therapies that can be used in a specialized salon.
❹ Discuss algae treatments and body wraps and how they are used in the salon.
❺ Describe the procedure for a chemical peeling.

INTRODUCTION

Over the course of his or her career, the esthetician will encounter techniques and technologies that will allow for significant career expansion, as well as new business opportunities for the salon. To take advantage of these developments, it will be necessary for the esthetician to further his or her education.

New products and advanced techniques are being introduced constantly. Some of these, such as advanced massage techniques and the use of herbs, will be directly applicable to the esthetician's practice. The esthetician should be conversant with a variety of advanced topics and techniques and be able to discuss them with clients.

There is a fine line between salon care and medical applications. Although the esthetician is a licensed professional in the beauty and health care industry, he or she is not a medical doctor and must be careful not to cross the line. There are limits to the services that can be offered in the salon. Generally, any product used may be administered *only* externally, with the exception of serving herb teas *for refreshment only*, without discussing their health benefits.

This chapter serves as an introduction to some of these new technologies. Each of these subjects is *complex* and *requires considerable study and practice* beyond the discussions here.

Also, even though each topic is discussed separately here, it is necessary to keep in mind that, in many cases, the treatments are used in conjunction with each other. So, for example, a treatment in a hydrotherapy tub may combine aromatherapy or phytotherapy with lymphatic drainage massage.

Phytotherapy

Phytotherapy (figh-to-**THERR**-uh-pee), or the use of herbs to treat various disorders, is one of the oldest arts and sciences known to humanity. They have been used, in one form or another, without interruption from ancient times to the present day, where they still play an important role in everyday life, whether used as spices, as ingredients in cosmetics, or as medicines.

Herbal therapy is related to aromatherapy, in that both use the same base ingredients. Aromatherapy, however, utilizes just the essential oils from the plants. Herbal therapy uses either the flowers, leaves, or roots of the plants.

Hundreds of different herbs are used. Together, they offer many benefits and have many useful properties. They also have valuable antiseptic and disinfectant properties. Generally, herbs have three functions when used medicinally. They detoxify, or cleanse the body; they normalize, or correct imbalances in bodily functions; and they build, or strengthen organs of the body.

Virtually all types of skin care products will contain some herbal ingredients. Aloe vera, for example, is used in body lotions and beauty creams. Arnica is used in massage and slimming creams. Burdock is used in night creams, while marigold is used in day creams. Cornflower and elder are used in eye creams. Yarrow and wild pansy are used in skin cleansers. The list is almost endless.

Herbs work because they contain active ingredients—chemicals that give them these properties. Like any chemical product, they should be used with caution and used in moderation. The amounts used in commercial preparations will be safe, as long as the manufacturer's instructions are followed. When using any product, the esthetician should become thoroughly familiar with all of the ingredients used in the preparation, especially the active ingredients, such as herbs. There are many good books on herbal remedies available. The esthetician should read some of them and have them available for reference.

Although the esthetician can make his or her own herbal preparations and use them as herbal treatments with clients, it is better from the standpoint of liability and effectiveness that he or she stick with commercial preparations. If the esthetician chooses to make his or her own herbal preparations, they must be limited to external use and must be used with caution.

There are a number of ways to prepare herbs. *Infusions* (in-**FEW**-zhunz) and *decoctions* (de-**COCK**-shunz) are made by steeping the herb in boiling water (in the case of an infusion) or by boiling the herb in water (in the case of a decoction). Herb teas are infusions. The resulting liquid may be applied to the skin with cotton pads or cotton compress masks, or as a *fomentation* (fo-mem-**TAY**-shun), made by soaking a towel in the liquid and wrapping it around the part of the body to be treated.

Tinctures are made by soaking the herb in alcohol, which extracts the active ingredient from the plant. A tincture is applied to the skin in the same manner in which infusions or decoctions are.

To make a *poultice*, crush the herb and mix it with a hot liquid or other substance to make a paste. The poultice can be applied to the skin directly or put into a hot, moist towel and wrapped around the part to be treated. *Ointments* are made by mixing the herb with petroleum jelly to make a thick cream or salve, which is spread on the area to be treated. Poultices and ointments are more effective than fomentations because they use more of the active ingredient contained in the herb.

Advanced Massage Techniques

The benefits of massage may be extended far beyond those discussed in the chapter on massage in this book, through the use of advanced massage techniques that stimulate and detoxify major organs and nerve centers in the body. Two of these techniques are reflexology and lymphatic drainage massage. Although each requires advanced training and study, both types of massage are practical for application in the salon. Reflexology, especially, may be offered as an additional service during a facial treatment, while the client has on a mask or is steaming.

REFLEXOLOGY *Reflexology* (**REE**-flecks-ol-uh-jee) is a system of massage that balances the inner organs of the body. Manipulations are primarily of the feet, although hands may also be massaged. The theory of reflexology holds that reflex points in the extremities correspond to various organs and parts of the body. Massage pressure at the reflex point energizes the organ or body part, detoxifying it and bringing it into balance, thereby improving its function. So, for example, the tips of the toes energize the sinuses. The heels energize the sciatic nerve. (See Fig. 23.1.)

Reflexology is an energy-based form of massage. Nerve impulses are a form of electrical energy, which flow within the body in specific patterns and constitutes the body's vital life force. The body is a polar organism; that is, the energy flow has both a positive side and a negative side, and completes a circuit. There are 10 meridians (lines or energy pathways) of energy in the body, five on each side. The extremities, the five toes and the five fingers on each side of the body, are the end points of these meridians.

Disorders within the body block the flow of energy and cause an imbalance. Pressure on the end point of the meridian, in either the foot or the hand, corrects the blockages and rebalances the system. Pressure at the end of any meridian affects all of the organs and muscles that lie along that meridian.

At the same time, internal disorders cause the toxins to crystalize and form deposits at the extremities. The pressure of a reflexology massage

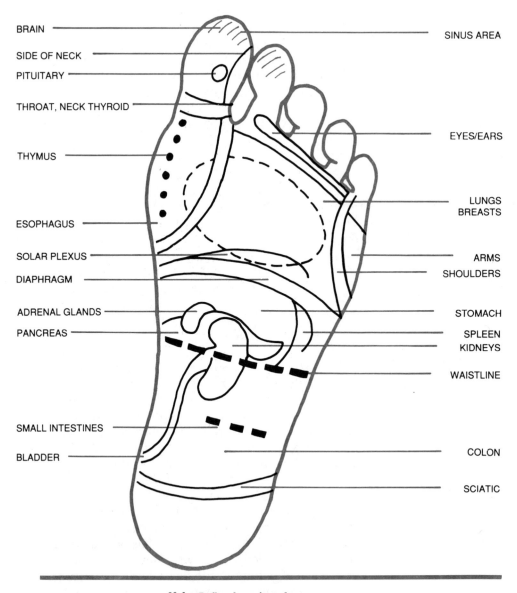

23.1—Reflexology foot chart.

crushes these deposits and puts them back into the circulatory and excretory systems to be flushed out of the body.

Thus, reflexology accomplishes a number of objectives: It balances the energy flow of the body, eliminates blockages, and it detoxifies the body, by removing waste products and toxins. In addition, reflexology massage improves circulation and relaxes the body.

Although requiring special training and practice, reflexology services can be offered in the salon. They require no specialized equipment. Since the massage is usually conducted on the client's feet, it can be given while he or she is relaxing under the mask or during steaming, without disturbing the facial service.

As with any massage treatment, communication is vital. It is important that the client knows what the treatment will entail and what will happen. However, there should be no talking during the massage.

The client should be lying on the facial chair with his or her spine as straight as possible to keep the meridians straight. He or she should be relaxed. Both the client and the esthetician should be comfortable during the massage. The client's hands should be apart, to prevent a "short circuit" in the energy flow.

The reflexology massage always starts on the left foot, which is the negative pole, and ends on the right foot, which is the positive pole. No massage cream or lotions should be used. The foot should be dry. Creams and lotions may cause the esthetician's hands to slip and misapply pressure. They also interfere with the "feel" of the pressure. "Feel" is a very important consideration.

The technique for a reflexology massage is important. The pressure points are relatively small and precisely located. The energy points must be stimulated properly and all vital spots must be touched.

Before starting, relax the client's left foot by grasping it in both hands and gently rotating it and bending it back and forth. Using the tips of the thumbs and fingers, apply constant pressure to each pressure point, beginning at the toes and working back to the heel. Keep the pressure on any point brief. Do not glide the fingers over the skin. Apply pressure cautiously to avoid hurting the client. The pressure will, however, be somewhat stronger than with a facial massage. If the client feels pain or anxiety, stop the treatment. After finishing the left foot, repeat the process on the right foot.

As with any massage procedure that detoxifies, the client may feel ill as the toxins work their way out of the body. Therefore, don't overdo any single treatment. It is far better to conduct a series of shorter massage sessions than to try to completely clean out the body with one long session.

▶ **Caution:** Do not conduct reflexology massage on diabetics or on people with heart or circulatory problems. Do not massage pregnant women without written consent from their physicians.

LYMPHATIC DRAINAGE MASSAGE

Lymphatic drainage massage is a system of massage that helps move waste matter through the body through the lymphatic system, thus detoxifying the body. It is a full-body massage technique that is structure-based, rather than energy-based, like reflexology. The system works with gentle pressure and stroking along the main circulation channels of the lymphatic system.

As discussed in Chapter 5, the lymphatic system is the waste disposal and drainage system for the body tissues. It is a separate circulatory system that consists of lacteals, lymphatic capillaries (which join larger lymphatic vessels and serve as drains), and lymph glands, or nodes (which act as filters and produce lymph). The lymph, which is derived from blood plasma, circulates through the system, carrying nutrients from the blood to the cells and carrying off waste products from the cells. The lymphatic system may be considered as a bridge between the digestive tract and the blood vessels.

The lymphatic system roughly parallels the blood capillary and venous-system channels. Most of the lymph, from the lower extremities, the pelvis, the stomach, and the left side of the body, funnels back into the bloodstream through the thoracic duct. Lymph from the upper part of the right side of the body funnels through the right lymph duct into the veins at the base of the neck. There are a large number of one-way valves in the lymph vessels to keep the lymph flowing in only one direction.

The human body contains large numbers of lymph nodes. Although they are spread throughout the body, there are large concentrations of the nodes behind the knees, in the armpits, and in the groin area.

Unlike blood, which is pumped through the body by the heart, the lymphatic system has no mechanism to pump lymph through the body. Some lymph flow occurs because of contractions in the vessels, but most flow comes from the pumping action caused by muscular contractions. Consequently, lymph flow is not as rapid as blood flow.

Lymphatic drainage massage increases the lymph flow and speeds up the natural detoxification process of the system. It stimulates the system and rejuvenates cellular function, which, in turn, affects the health of the skin. Like any treatment that detoxifies, it must be done carefully and in moderation. The client may feel nauseous or may undergo increased urine flow on initial treatment because of the toxins being driven out of the body.

This type of massage, while suitable for inclusion in the list of services offered by a full-service salon, does require specific training. It offers many benefits in skin care, and is useful in treating acne and similar skin disorders. Unlike reflexology, which may be offered as an additional service during a facial treatment, lymphatic drainage massage is a separate service. It requires no special equipment, other than a sturdy massage table and suitable draping cloths.

The client will be resting on the massage table. He or she will be undressed, but should be appropriately draped. Apply pressure and stroke gently in the direction of lymph flow; that is, from the extremities inward, toward the major ducts. Keep pressure light to avoid damaging the lymph channels. Use a massage cream to reduce friction and allow the hands to move smoothly. In many cases, essential oils may be used.

> **Caution:** Do not use lymphatic drainage massage on pregnant women, diabetics, or persons with heart or circulatory system conditions.

Water Therapies

There are a number of water-based treatments that are beneficial in skin care and may be offered as special services by the skin care salon. Most of these are spa treatments and require highly specialized and expensive equipment and extensive training.

The therapies may be grouped into *thalassotherapy* (tha-lass-o-**THERR**-uh-pee) treatments and *balneotherapy* (bal-nee-o-**THERR**-uh-pee) treatments. Both are similar. Thalassotherapy, however, utilizes sea water and products from the sea. Balneotherapy, on the other hand, utilizes fresh water. Treatments in either case include hydrotherapy tub treatments, Scotch hose treatments, saunas, and steam baths.

In *hydrotherapy* (high-dro-**THERR**-uh-pee) *tub treatments*, the client relaxes in a tub of hot water, sea water in the case of thalassotherapy or fresh water in the case of balneotherapy, while jets of water and air bubbles provide a gentle massage action. The air bubbles stimulate the lymphatic system. The water jets stimulate the deeper tissues.

In the *Scotch hose treatment*, the client stands at the end of a long, narrow shower stall while the therapist sprays jets of hot water, either sea water or fresh water, up and down the spine and the main lymphatic channels.

Saunas and *steam baths* promote perspiration and increase the elimination of toxins from the body.

All of these treatments detoxify and relax the body. They all can provide beneficial treatments for skin care. Since they utilize heat or hot water, however, they should be used with care.

> **Caution:** Do not use on pregnant women or on people with high blood pressure or heart or circulatory disorders.

Algae Treatments

Although the various water therapies may be beyond the scope of most salons, the esthetician may still use some of the techniques of thalassotherapy, by utilizing various *algae treatments*. Algaes, products from the sea, are effective cleansers and revitalizers of skin. These products contain all the minerals in sea water, but in a much more concentrated form. They remineralize and rehydrate the skin and contain phytohormones, which work the same way as essential oils and herbs. They also help detoxify the body.

In algae pack treatments, the algae is mixed with water to form a paste. The client lies face down on the treatment table and the paste is applied along the spine and covered. Heat lamps keep the paste warm. The algae paste is normally left in place for 30 to 45 minutes, then rinsed off. The algae wrap may be used on other parts of the body, as well; as a facial mask or in leg wraps, for example.

Algae products are available from a number of manufacturers in various forms, including powders, liquids, and gels. They are high in vitamins and minerals, and thus provide good nutrition for the skin. However, they are also rich in iodine, and should not be used on clients who are allergic to shellfish.

Body Wraps

Body wraps are another service that can be performed by the esthetician. Like algae packs, they require some specialized training, but a minimum of specialized equipment, and will be administered as a separate service. They may be used in conjunction with other services, such as thalassotherapy, lymphatic drainage massage, or steam or sauna treatments.

There are a number of benefits to body wraps. They help to improve circulation and elimination, to detoxify, or to temporarily recontour the body; and they help to reduce fat deposits. Almost any part of the body can be wrapped. The most common treatment is leg wrapping, for removal of localized fatty deposits and body recontouring; however, the arms, breasts, abdomen, hips, and buttocks may also be wrapped.

In general, all body wrap treatments follow much the same procedure. The client lies down on the treatment table and the esthetician applies the treatment product to the part to be wrapped. Then, the esthetician covers the body part and treatment product with either a plastic sheet wrapping material, such as plastic wrap, or with contour tapes (wide cloth tapes similar to elastic bandages). Moist or dry heat may then be used to keep the wrap warm. The client rests for a period of time, up to 1 hour. Then the part is unwrapped and the treatment product is removed.

The treatment product may be an algae or herbal preparation, a slimming or moisturizing cream, or another product, depending on the result desired.

The plastic sheet material is wrapped snugly, but not tightly, around the body part. It holds in heat and moisture and helps the treatment product work. The plastic is used when the esthetician wants to detoxify, increase elimination, or increase circulation.

Contour tapes must be wrapped more tightly than the plastic wrap, but not tight enough to cut off circulation or to make the client uncomfortable. These tapes are used when the esthetician wants to recontour the body.

The client should be kept warm and relaxed throughout the treatment.

▶ | **Caution:** Do not use body wraps on pregnant women or on clients with high blood pressure, heart or circulatory disorders. As with algae packs, make sure the client is not allergic to shellfish before using algae, or other products from the sea, as a treatment product. If there is doubt about a product's safety, conduct a patch test on the client's skin.

Cellulite

Cellulite (**SEL**-yu-ite) is the name given to those localized deposits of fat, water, and waste materials, which seem to collect around the hips, thighs, and buttocks. This type of fat, according to experts in the beauty-care industry, is a highly specialized form of fat that resists elimination by diet and exercise. It is a different kind of fat, one that is caused by imbalances in the system, which cause the fat cells to combine with water and toxic waste materials, forming semihard, gel-like masses, which accumulate under the skin. The result: the bulgy, rough, orange-peel appearance of the skin in the affected areas.

Cellulite is typically a women's problem. Men do not have cellulite-like deposits, mostly because their hormonal balance is different and their fat distribution is different.

Cellulite is a controversial topic. Although widely accepted as a concept by the beauty industry, its existence is not accepted by the medical community. Many doctors doubt that there is any such substance known as cellulite. They have found no scientific evidence that identifies a separate type of fat, bound up with waste materials. The physical laws that govern the science of physiology, they believe, do not allow such a substance to be possible. They believe that cellulite is a fat deposit, just like any kind of fat deposit, and can be removed only by diet and exercise programs that reduce fat levels throughout the body. They doubt the ability of any products, body wraps, or other treatment procedures to remove these localized deposits.

In view of the controversy, the esthetician should be very careful not to make claims that treatments will substantially recontour or reshape the body and eliminate cellulite. At best, he or she can only suggest that the client will see temporary changes resulting from a body wrap. Body wraps, however, are valuable as a method of detoxification and increasing circulation and elimination, especially when used in conjunction with lymphatic drainage massage, herbal therapy, or aromatherapy.

Salon Chemical Peeling

The *salon chemical peeling* is a procedure in which a formula is applied to the skin that causes the epidermis to peel in the same way a deeply sun-burned skin would peel. This is considered an advanced treatment and should only be done by a skilled and experienced esthetician who has made a special study of the process.

The chemical peel is not a new treatment. In an article in *Beauty Culture Magazine*, written by J. Howard Crum, M.D. in the early 1930's, it was explained that skin peeling was not a recent development as many had thought, nor was it magic. Skin peeling is simply the application of a certain formula with the expectation of certain results just as you might apply certain lotions and expect certain benefits.

The salon chemical peeling is not to be confused with the "epidermabrasion" treatment described in Chapter 16, which often contains enzymes that have the ability to dissolve and decompose the dead cells on the surface of the skin or the medical peeling described in Chapter 20, which is known as chemosurgery and removes the entire epidermis and the upper layers of the dermis.

One of the major benefits of the salon chemical peeling is that it makes the skin produce *biostimulins*, a substance that helps the cells survive. In the 1930's, Vladimir Filatov, a member of the Academy of Medicine in the USSR and Director of the Institute of Ophthalmology in the Ukraine, discovered that living cells, when subjected to great stress, will struggle for life by producing biostimulins. The shock and trauma caused to the skin by the salon chemical peeling induce the skin to fight back by producing these biostimulins. Think of biostimulins as the healthiest cells your body can produce. Now think of these cells moving forward from deep in the skin toward the surface. As the cells move forward, collagen fibers are strengthened, excessive oiliness is normalized, follicles that have been blocked by cellular buildup are uncovered, rough textured skin will look smoother and shallow lines are softened. The skin will feel tight and acne infection deep in the skin will race forward to the surface because it cannot live in an area that has been flooded with biostimulins.

The following is a good example of how biostimulins work. When a person has an operation such as the removal of the appendix, the stitches are usually removed within 2 to 4 days, the incision already beginning to heal. However, a scab on the knee will take 3 to 4 weeks to heal. Why? The operation is a shock to the body, whereas the scab on the knee is not. Biostimulins are manufactured in the area of the trauma, which speeds healing. The scab on the knee is not a trauma or emergency to the body so no biostimulins are manufactured and the healing process is slow.

The formula for the salon chemical peeling comes in both a cream or liquid form. The formula contains a combination of chemical ingredients such as resorcinol, sulfur, phenol and salicylic acid. The liquid formula is applied with a cotton swab while the cream formula is applied with a wooden or plastic spatula. As many as 10 applications of the liquid are applied during a single visit to the salon. The cream formula requires 1 to 4 applications applied on consecutive days. Each application is left on the skin for 90 minutes. The number of applications will depend on several things such as whether or not the skin has acne, the thickness and texture of the skin, and the experience and discretion of the esthetician.

The salon will generally charge more for the cream formula because of the time spent with the client. It is not unusual for the salon to charge $500 or more for the salon chemical peeling when the cream formula is used.

After the peeling formula is applied, the client will feel a burning sensation for approximately 5 to 10 minutes. This can be relieved by fanning the skin. On the first day the skin will look like it has a sun burn. On the second day the skin will look like it has a sun tan and it will feel tight. On the third day the skin will have a deep sun tan look, the surface will be very taut and the skin will feel like parchment paper. It will be difficult to move the face or open the mouth wide. By the end of the third day or on the fourth day the skin will start to peel around the mouth. The skin will continue to peel for days five, six and sometimes day seven. When the peeling is completed the skin will have a younger more radiant look.

The client must be advised to avoid direct sun light for the first month following the peeling and to use a sun screen with an SPF of at least 15 when going outside. (*See Color Plates 24–29.*)

▶ | **Caution:** Because salon chemical peeling is a controversial treatment it should only be done by an esthetician with training in its procedure.

QUESTIONS DISCUSSION AND REVIEW

ADVANCED TOPICS IN ESTHETICS

1. Why should the esthetician be aware of advanced techniques?
2. What must the esthetician keep in mind with some of the advanced techniques?
3. What is phytotherapy?
4. How is phytotherapy different from aromatherapy?
5. What three functions do herbs have?
6. Why should the esthetician use commercial herb preparations?
7. What is reflexology?
8. How does reflexology work?
9. What sets reflexology apart from the other techniques discussed in this chapter?
10. What is lymphatic drainage massage?
11. How does lymphatic drainage massage work?
12. What is the difference between thalassotherapy and balneotherapy?
13. Name two water therapy techniques.
14. Why are algae products useful?
15. What do body wraps do?
16. What are two materials used in body wraps and why are they used?
17. What is cellulite?
18. Why is cellulite controversial?
19. What is chemical peeling?
20. What is one of the major benefits of chemical peeling?

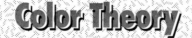

Color Theory

LEARNING OBJECTIVES

After completing this chapter, you should be able to:

❶ Discuss color psychology and how colors can affect emotions.
❷ Explain how skin gets its color and define the different skin colors.
❸ Explain color harmony and how combining colors can help with choosing clothing and cosmetic colors.

INTRODUCTION

Knowing how to make the most of color can be a tremendous confidence booster. When clothing designers start working on creative ideas for a specific fashion season, they consider line, design, and balance, all of which are important factors when creating attractive fashions. The weight and texture of the fabrics used must be carefully selected so the design of the garment can be a success. Possibly the most important of all decisions is the choice of color or color combinations for the finished garment. Faulty lines can be overlooked by the buyer but if the color isn't attractive there isn't much chance that the sale will be made.

The client who comes to the salon is not always aware of the importance of color selection in makeup. She may be wearing the wrong foundation, eye makeup, cheek- and lipcolors. Skin color is classified as light, pale, medium, deep, or dark and any of these skin colors will have undertones of color. In order to select the individual's most becoming foundation colors, skin tones should be studied carefully. All other makeup used on the client's face should be in harmony with the color of the eyes and hair. In addition, the client may want to wear lipcolor and nail polish that matches, coordinates, or picks up a color in the wardrobe.

Color Psychology

It is interesting to study how color was discovered and used since our primitive beginnings. For example, red was associated with life-giving blood and fire. You can imagine why early people associated black with the darkness of night and yellow with the brightness of day. White is a symbol of purity, while purple is the color worn by persons of royal status. Different societies came to attach different significance to colors. It is difficult to name any color that cannot be associated with something that we have experienced as either pleasant or unpleasant. We seem to instinctively like or dislike certain colors, but the color specialists say we tend to dislike a color because of some unpleasant incident we may have forgotten. We do know that people feel happier when surrounded by certain colors. Some color experts say that the colors we use in our homes are definite indications of personality traits. For example, people who surround themselves with cool colors such as green and blue may be expressing their desire for peace and tranquility. People who use an abundance of bright colors such as red, orange, and yellow are usually people who love gaiety and who are outgoing. Can you think of ways in which you use color to express yourself? We often hear people describe a mood in color terms. Someone may feel "blue" or "green with envy." A coward may be described as "yellow" and a bank account may be in the "red."

COLOR AND EMOTION It is interesting to note how frequently poets refer to color to express emotions. They particularly relate color and emotion with the changes of the seasons. Imagine the first blossoms of spring bursting forth in a rainbow of color to delight the eye and lift the spirits. Imagine the lush, rich colors of fruits and vegetables ripening in the summer sun. As summer turns to autumn, imagine the trees and the landscape turning into a symphony of warm red, yellow, brown, green, and gold. A winter scene treats our eyes to a sparkling contrast as the earth rests under a blanket of freshly fallen snow.

You may not realize to what extent we are affected by color, but when you awaken on a dull, gloomy morning, you probably will reach for something bright and cheerful to wear. You have probably noticed also, that even though you know food is fresh, well-prepared, and delicious, unless the color is what you expect it to be, you will likely pass it by. We have become so accustomed to foods being of a certain color, that food processors often add color just to please the eye. It is interesting to note how often we can find labels stating that artificial color has been added to food.

How Skin Gets Its Color

Human skin contains four types of pigment: melanin, hemoglobin (oxygenated and reduced), and carotenes. Melanin is the dark brown or black pigment that is responsible for hair, skin, and eye coloring. It is the most potent pigment and is what causes the skin to become darker as it tans. The cells that produce melanin are called melanocytes and are considered to be identical in all races. A square inch of skin on an adult contains approximately 60,000 melanocytes. It is known that the depth of melanin in the skin can affect the color of the skin, but scientists are still studying melanin and its structure.

Hemoglobin is the pigment that gives red blood cells their color. When hemoglobin is oxygenated (combined with oxygen) it produces a healthy color to the skin. When the hemoglobin is lacking oxygen, or is oxygen-reduced, the skin takes on a pale or bluish color. Some diseases, exposure to chemicals, drugs, intense cold, and other factors can cause the skin to change color. For example, anything that produces dilation of the blood vessels will cause the skin to appear redder.

Carotenes are pigments that give a yellow tone to the skin. A yellow cast can be caused by eating too many foods that are yellow or orange (oranges, carrots, etc.). This condition is known as carotenoderma. Jaundice is a condition that causes discoloration of tissues and body excretions resulting from bile pigments in the blood. The whites of the eyes, as well as the skin, take on a yellow cast.

When the pigments of the skin are unevenly distributed, the skin will have lighter and darker areas, such as freckles. Darker skin contains more melanin granuals and will tan more quickly than light skin. Certain diseases interfere with the production of melanin and can cause the skin to become blotchy. Any change in the normal color of the skin should be brought to the attention of a dermatologist. There are no known permanent ways to change the basic color of the skin. Tanning or the use of cosmetics are temporary, but can be useful in balancing uneven color.

ALBINISM   An albino is a person who has melanocyte cells that do not produce melanin. Therefore, there is a lack of color in the person's skin, hair, and eyes. The hemoglobin shows as pink in the eyes and some other parts of the body. *Albinism* is rare and is not restricted to any one race.

Skin Colors Defined

1. *White skin*—The lightest human skin is without color pigmentation. A person or other living creature without color pigmentation is called an albino. Generally a person who is an albino will have a milky,

translucent skin, white or colorless hair, and eyes with a pink or blue iris and deep red pupils. This is a rare condition.

2. *Light creamy skin*—This is a fair skin which may have light creamy or slightly pink undertones. Persons with this skin type are sometimes referred to as "Nordic." This term pertains to the tall, blond-haired subdivision of the Caucasian ethnic stock. These people came mainly from North Western Europe. However, a person may have a light skin and dark hair or light hair. When selecting clothing colors we generally select them to complement the skin first, then the hair and eye colors.

3. *Golden skin*—This skin has a definite yellow cast if light, and if tan, it has a golden tone. Generally, we think of people with yellow or golden skin as being of the yellow race (Mongoloid) but this is not always true. Many people have a yellow or golden skin tone.

4. *Pink skin*—A pink skin can be faintly pink, light, or florid. A florid skin has a ruddy color (flushed with redness). People from different ethnic groups may have red undertones in their skin. North American Indians generally have red undertones in brown or tanned skin.

5. *Tan skin*—You have noticed that some people have what can be described as tan skin. However, tan skin can range from light to dark brown. The undertones of tan skin can be predominantly red or yellow, or the skin can be more clearly brown.

6. *Olive skin*—This skin color is said to resemble the color of an olive. It is described as having a dull, yellowish green color or a somewhat brown complexion tinged with yellow green. Sometimes this greenish undertone is difficult to detect. Generally the person with olive skin will also have dark hair.

7. *Brown skin*—Brown skin may range from light to dark and it may be classified as clear brown, light, medium, or dark, or with red or yellow undertones. A fair-skinned person may get a tan and he or she should select clothing colors to be compatible with the undertones of the tan.

8. *Ebony*—Ebony is the name of a wood that is almost black but not jet black. A dark skin may range from dark olive, dark brown, deep yellowish-brown and deep reddish-brown. When selecting colors for dark-skinned people, it is important to study the undertones of the skin. Colors should bring out the richness of the complexion tones. Intense red and yellow can be cooled by wearing cool colors that reflect into the face.

The Basics of Color Harmony

Colors can be combined in many ways. (*See Color Plate 31.*) If you understand these basic principles, it will be easier to select colors that enhance personal coloring. The color wheel is used to explain the following principles of color harmony (Fig. 24.1).

The primary colors are red, yellow, and blue. From these three basic colors, all other colors are created.

The secondary colors are created by mixing equal amounts of two of the primary colors.

Example: Yellow + blue = green
Red + yellow = orange
Blue + red = violet

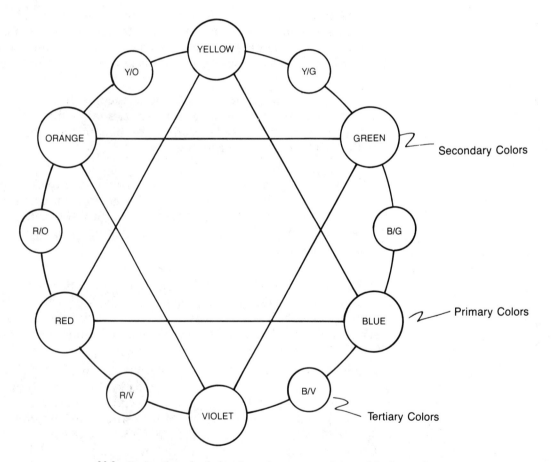

24.1—Basic color wheel showing primary, secondary and tertiary colors.

Tertiary colors are achieved by mixing a secondary color and a primary color in equal amounts. (An intermediate color is thus achieved.)

Example: Yellow + green = Yellow/green or chartreuse
Green + blue = Blue/green or turquoise
Violet + red = Red/violet or plum

By further mixing various amounts of color with black or white, numerous fashion colors are created. These are quite often named after the seasons of the year, fruits, vegetables, flowers, inanimate objects, and living things.

Some examples are:

Forest green	Metallic gold	Chinese red
Earth brown	Autumn gold	Cloud gray
Rose red	Lemon yellow	Steel gray
Peacock blue	Emerald green	Midnight blue

COMBINING COLORS   Learning to combine colors successfully is an asset when choosing clothing and cosmetic colors. The following is a review of color terms.

Hue — A color as the eye perceives it. We have learned to identify colors by name as we see that color. Red is seen as red.

Value — The lightness or darkness of a color. Light red, medium red, dark red, etc.

Intensity — The brightness or dullness of a color. A bright red would seem more intense in shiny satin than in dull wool.

Shade — Having a low color value, or the darkness of a color. A shade of red is darker than a tint.

Tint — Having high color value, or the lightness of the color. Light pink is red to which a greater percentage of white has been added.

Here are some terms used by artists, decorators, and designers to describe color harmonies.

Monochromatic color scheme — *Mono* means "one," *chroma* means "color;" thus monochromatic means one color, or a monotone. This is a single color with variations of lightness and darkness. The use of one color (hue) in a costume, with different values and intensities is called a monochromatic color scheme; for example, a brown and beige costume.

Analogous color scheme—This is achieved by use of three colors that lie adjacent to each other on the color wheel. These are neighboring colors, each containing some of the primary color. Costume example: A blue suit (primary color), a green print blouse containing turquoise and turquoise jewelry. For best results the colors should vary in intensity.

Triadic color scheme—This is a combination achieved by using three colors that are equal distances apart on the color wheel. Costume example: A print, plaid, or pattern containing various shades and tints of blue, red, and yellow. You often see these colors combined on a neutral background.

Complementary color scheme—This is achieved by combining two hues that are directly opposite on the color wheel. Red and green are complementary colors that intensify one another. Example: Bright red hair is enhanced by a green costume and green eye makeup.

WHAT COLORS DO   *Colors advance or recede*—Bright colors advance and make the covered area appear larger. Dull and dark colors recede and make the covered area appear smaller. This color rule can be applied to conceal, or to create an illusion. If a person's figure is large, dark and dull colors will make the figure appear smaller. If a figure is small, a bright or light color will make the figure appear larger. Light emphasizes, dark minimizes.

Colors reflect other colors—Some colors tend to reflect back more color than they take away. For example, a red scarf near a ruddy complexion will make the face appear redder. A bright yellow would tend to emphasize the yellow in a skin with predominantly yellow tones.

Color will steal color—Bright blue placed beside light or pale blue will make the pale color appear less colorful. Thus, the darker and brighter color will steal color from a lighter color. A person with blue eyes can intensify the eye color by wearing a lighter blue than the blue eye color. A darker blue worn near the face would make the eye color appear lighter in contrast.

COLOR HAS TEMPERATURE   Colors are classified as warm or cool. Some colors can be both warm or cool depending on the shade, tint, lightness, or darkness of the color. Some colors combine better with others. The following basic guide by no means limits color combination possibilities. Sometimes unlikely color combinations can be striking.

Pink—We think of pink as being a warm, rosy color, but a pastel (tint) is cool looking. When more red is added to white, the pink becomes warmer. Pink is flattering to most skin tones unless the skin is ruddy and the pink unusually bright. Pink combines well with other shades and tints of pink, blue, black, green, yellow, gray, orange, purple, brown, beige, and white.

Blue—Blue is a cool color and is complementary to most skin tones. Lighter blues enhance darker skins while darker blue brings out color in a lighter skin. Blue combines well with almost all other colors. Examples are: pink, green, soft yellow, light blue, deep purple, red, gold, white, black, beige, and brown.

Purple—Pale tints of orchid and lavender are cool looking. Darker shades with red (plum) undertones are warmer and more dramatic colors. Purple is not kind to blemished or reddish skin tones, and should be studied carefully against the skin. Purple combines well with pink, white, gray, soft blue, beige, black, and pale yellow.

Green—Almost all greens are members of the cool family. An exception is bright yellow-green. The greater the percentage of yellow added to the green, the warmer the color. Green is easy on the eyes and flattering to most skin tones. Bright green can intensify red in the skin but blue greens are cooling and generally attractive colors for light- or dark-skinned people. Green combines well with other greens, blue, yellow, orange, beige, brown, white, and black.

Brown—A member of the warm family, brown is kind to almost all complexion tones. Other reflecting or accent colors can be worn near the face if the skin is dark brown. Brown combines well with green, beige, blue, pink, yellow, orange, gold, white, and black. Beige is usually thought of as cool especially if it is clear (bone) beige. Some beige will have a yellow undertone. Tan containing quite a lot of brown is considered warm. Beige and tan combine well with yellow, orange, gold, green, navy blue, pink, black, white, and red.

Red—Red is a warm, exciting color, easy for most people to wear. Be cautious of the undertones of a specific tint or shade, as they may not be kind to a ruddy complexion. Freckles will look darker when red is reflected into the face. Red combines well with many other colors. Among them are black, white, beige, gray, pink, blue, navy, green, and yellow.

Black—Black is considered a neutral color and combines well with all other colors. A black costume can create a startling contrast for light skin and light or dark hair. When the skin and hair are dark, a color contrast near the face acts as a frame or highlight for the face.

White—White is considered a neutral color. White is easy to wear but be cautious of the undertones of white. Some materials reflect a beige or yellow undertone while other materials will appear to be slightly blue or pure white. White combines well with all other colors.

Gray—Gray is a cool neutral color that combines well with many other colors. Gray combines well with warm colors such as yellow, red, orange, and gold.

To select colors for clients that will harmonize and not clash, it is important to take hair color, lipcolor, and skin tone into consideration. The Color Key Chart (*Color Plate 30*) has grouped colors according to warm and cool shades to help you.

Selecting Cosmetic Colors

FOUNDATION AND POWDER During the cleansing of the skin and the skin-type analysis, you can study the undertones of the client's skin. When selecting a foundation, you may need to try several shades before finding one that blends well with the natural skin tones of the client's face and neck. Foundation should be selected to enhance the client's natural coloring, but foundation may match the skin or a color can be selected to tone down excessive ruddiness or pink in the skin. Test the foundation color by applying a few dots to the client's jawline. Blend the foundation upward on the jaw and down onto the neck. The makeup should blend with the natural skin tones and leave no line of demarcation. Once the correct color has been determined, blend the makeup over the entire face. Skin tones often change in the seasons and the client may need to change foundation color if she or he has acquired a tan, or if a tan is fading.

When used, face powder may be translucent (colorless) or matched to the color of the foundation. Some makeup artists use powder that is the same color as the foundation or they select a powder that is slightly lighter or slightly darker to achieve a particular effect. However, translucent powder remains the favorite because it does not change color on the skin.

EYEBROW PENCIL AND BRUSH-ON COLOR An eyebrow pencil with a fine lead will enable you to improve natural brows by using the pencil to make them appear fuller or to give them a more defined arch and a more attractive color. The pencil can be used to cover small scars and other imperfections in the eyebrow. If you are a beginning makeup artist, you will find it helpful to practice sketching eyebrows on your own hand. Practice until you can sketch realistic-looking brows. Try combining powder and pencil in light and dark shades. The pencil colors are generally light, medium, and dark brown, charcoal and black, titian (red-brown), and gray. These colors coordinate with natural hair colors. Dark brown and charcoal coordinate well with dark brown and black hair. Gray is used with "salt and pepper" (gray and black) hair. Titian (red-brown) or light brown will look best with red hair. Eyebrow color that is too dark appears harsh on light-skinned clients. Dark-skinned clients with black hair may prefer a soft charcoal pencil but black may be used. Pencil color should not be applied so heavily that it looks like a crayon has been rubbed over the brows. Powdered eyebrow color is brushed on for a natural look and is more suitable for brows that require no corrective work.

EYELINE COLORS   A thin line of color drawn above the upper lashes or drawn into the upper and lower lashes is used to accent the eyes. When the use of eyeliner is in fashion, the most popular colors (brown, black, charcoal) are those that match the natural lash colors or the mascara color. White, navy, purple, blue, green, gold, and silver are high-fashion colors that are also used as eyeliner colors.

EYESHADOW AND EYECOLOR   The purpose of eye makeup is to enhance the beauty of the eyes and to conceal imperfections. For example, the bone above the eye may protrude so that it makes the eye appear sunken. This space can be minimized by using brown shadow (the natural pigment color of the skin). When the space between the eye and the brow is too small or narrow, a highlight (skin tone or white) will make the space appear larger and will emphasize the eye. In recent years a wide range of colors have been added to the basic brown, blue, and green eye shadow shades. It is very fashionable to use a combination of several colors to accentuate natural eyecolor. Eye-makeup colors may match or contrast with the color of the iris of the eye or the clothing color. Most manufacturers of eye makeup provide color charts that show various color combinations.

LIPCOLOR (LIPSTICK)   A lip-lining pencil or a brush is used to outline the lips. Lipcolor is then brushed within the outline. The pencil or brush can be used to correct or change the natural outline of the lips, but should not be exaggerated. Light-skinned clients usually find dark lipcolors too harsh. Dark-skinned clients are able to wear deeper and more vivid colors. Very pale lipcolors create a chalky look on dark skin. Fashion often dictates a lighter or darker lipcolor depending on seasonal clothing colors and styles. Sometimes two or more lipcolors are used to create a special effect. The modern makeup artist will have to be abreast of fashion changes and should also develop a keen eye for color in order to determine the most appropriate and fashionable makeup colors for the client. Cosmetic manufacturers usually provide charts that show the current fashion names as applied to new makeup items. Fashion magazines are also a good source for seasonal makeup innovations. Once you have learned to apply an attractive makeup to any type of face, it will be easy to use your imagination and creativity in applying different makeup color combinations.

Guide to Selecting Makeup Colors

SKIN TONE	FOUNDATION
Cameo (white)	Light beige or peach to add a touch of color
Ivory (pink or beige)	Natural beige or a rosy beige
Golden (light to medium)	Beige or matching
Peach (creamy tone)	Peach or beige undertone
Pink (florid)	Soft beige to tone down too much red in the skin
Tan (ruddy or reddish-brown)	Natural or beige to tone down too much red
Tan (clear brown, light to dark)	Match or coordinate with natural skin tones
Olive (brown with greenish undertones)	Beige to even color
Copper (tan with golden red undertones)	Medium to dark beige to tone down too much red
Brown (light, medium, and dark brown)	Match or coordinate with natural skin tones
Ebony (darkest brown to black)	Match or coordinate with natural skin tones

POWDER

Powder should be translucent, color coordinated, or it may match the foundation.

> **Note:** Cheekcolors and lipcolors need not match but they should coordinate to blend well with the foundation colors. Contouring shades are light to dark brown and are selected to coordinate with the natural pigment colors of the skin. For example, contouring powder in a shade or two darker than the color of the skin will blend well with most foundations.

Guide to Selecting Eye Makeup Colors

EYECOLOR	EYESHADOW	SHADING	HIGHLIGHTS	LINER AND MASCARA
Light, medium, deep blue, or violet	Brown Blue Violet Mauve	Brown Navy Green Charcoal	Ivory White Pale yellow Pale pink	Black Charcoal Brown Navy
Blue green	Grey Navy	Charcoal Black	Beige	Dark green Bright blue
Blue grey	Silver Gold			Silver Gold
Green	Turquoise	Brown	Ivory	Black or charcoal
Hazel	Green	Charcoal	Pale pink	Dark brown
Brown	Brown	Green	Peach Light pink	Dark blue or navy
Dark brown	Mauve	Navy	Light yellow	Dark green
Black	Taupe Gold	Charcoal	Beige Silver	Silver Gold

> **Note:** The makeup artist will experiment with color combinations to achieve the desired results. Generally, colors of the same color family are used for a more natural look. For example, brown eyeshadow, shaded with a deeper brown, highlighted with beige will create a pleasant contrast. Dark brown liner and mascara will further enhance this combination of basic colors. Startling color contrasts are usually preferred for evening.

Cheekcolors (Rouge or Blushers)

Colors used on cheeks need not match lipcolors or nail polish; however, they should be coordinated. Garish color contrasts should be avoided. For example, if the cheekcolor has an orange undertone, then the lipcolor should also have a hint of orange rather than a plum or blue red, which would not harmonize.

Guide to Lipcolors Coordinated with Hair Color

HAIR COLOR	LIPCOLORS
Blonde, white, silver, and grey	Soft pink, lilac, pale orange, soft wine-red, clear red, soft earthtones
Light auburn and golden red	Apricot, soft orange, soft rust, golden peach, soft pink, coral, clear red
Dark auburn or copper	All the above colors; may be slightly deeper than for lighter hair
Light to dark brown	Beige tones, clear red, coral, true pink, rose-red, wine-red, plum, soft orange, strawberry-red
Dark brown to black	All of the above colors; may be slightly deeper than for lighter hair

Note: When selecting lipcolors, the color of the skin must be considered first. The deeper or brighter the lipcolor the more emphasis will be placed on the mouth. The lighter the skin and hair, the brighter the lipcolor and cheekcolor will appear on the skin.

QUESTIONS DISCUSSION AND REVIEW

COLOR THEORY
1. What is meant by color psychology?
2. What are the three types of pigment in our skin?
3. What is albinism?
4. Name the eight basic categories of skin colors from lightest to darkest.
5. Name the three primary colors and how they are mixed to form secondary colors.
6. How are intermediate or tertiary colors formed?
7. What is hue?
8. What is value?
9. How do colors advance or recede?
10. How are colors classified?
11. What must you consider when selecting a foundation for your client?
12. Where would you test foundation to determine if the color is right for your client?
13. What can be used to cover small scars and other imperfections in the eyebrows?
14. What are the most popular colors of eyeliners?
15. What is the purpose of eyecolor?
16. What can be used to correct a lipline?

CHAPTER

25

Professional Makeup Techniques

LEARNING OBJECTIVES *After completing this chapter, you should be able to:*

❶ Discuss how to be a successful makeup artist.
❷ Explain how to set up a makeup area in the salon.
❸ Demonstrate how to analyze a client's facial shape and features before the application of makeup.
❹ Demonstrate how to properly shape and tweeze brows.
❺ Explain and demonstrate the different cosmetics used when applying makeup and the purpose of each.
❻ Explain and demonstrate the different types of artificial lashes and the procedure for each.

INTRODUCTION

By way of paintings, sculpture, photographs, and many excellent books, we can journey back into history to study the fascinating makeup practices from past to present day. We find evidence that almost all cultures, since early times, have used some form of face and body adornment. The modern day makeup artist provides a valuable service to clients who want to learn to apply makeup artistically. Makeup should always be applied with an eye for enhancing the client's good features while diminishing unflattering ones.

The Professional Makeup Artist

The makeup artist's first concern is with making any woman look her best for daytime or evening, and to be able to recommend the right products for the woman's individual skin type and coloring. Some men may request some types of makeup for television appearances, for photographs, or other occasions.

Some of the most talented people are not always born with a natural artistic talent; like anything else, the art of makeup application requires patience and practice. To be successful as a makeup artist, it is not only important to be able to apply makeup artistically, but to be able to interest the client in purchasing cosmetics.

Sales Ability

The salon or department store will usually pay an artist a salary with a commission on sales. If one artist does an average makeup but has a large volume of sales, he or she will be more valuable to the salon than someone who can do a better than average makeup but is weak in selling.

The makeup artist who does demonstrations in a department store will, in most cases, give complimentary makeup applications. This is done to attract attention to the cosmetics department and to increase the sale of products. It is important for the artist to know how to apply makeup skillfully, to stimulate the customer's desire to purchase products for home use. The salon artist must be aware of new trends and be able to apply the latest makeup styles when it is requested by the client. The main objective when applying makeup is to help the client whether naturally attractive or not, to improve her appearance.

SUCCESS RULES OF MAKEUP ARTISTS To be successful as a makeup artist, it is important to observe the following rules:

1. Be honest with the client and tactful when discussing skin care and makeup problems.
2. Demonstrate what various products can do for the client without false flattery and exaggerated promises.
3. Never pressure the client or make her feel uncomfortable. This is a sure way to lose her confidence.
4. Suggest that she return to your salon when she needs to replenish her cosmetics. If she likes the makeup, she will become a regular customer.
5. Don't lead the client to believe that makeup will make her resemble a famous model or star, but do compliment her on her own individual good features, while minimizing any unattractive features she may have.

6. Always be sure that your own appearance, manner, and speech reflect the profession that you are representing.
7. Never make derogatory remarks about competitors or their products. Build the client's interest and confidence in you by giving excellent service and selling good products.
8. Be sure that every service is given in the most sanitary and professional way.
9. Remember that the client is interested in her own improvement. Educate your client on her skin type, color enhancements, and how to work with her natural assets.
10. Don't brag, but don't be timid about your accomplishments. If you are recognized for your accomplishments, word will soon get around. If you have certificates and other items of recognition, such as trophies, by all means display them. Just as most doctors display certificates for patients to see, clients are also interested in your credentials and your accomplishments.

Furnishings for the Makeup Area

The atmosphere in the salon and in the makeup area should be pleasant. Most salons will have an attractive display case in the reception area so that it can be seen by clients as they come and go for the various services. Displays stimulate interest and can lead to increased sales (Fig. 25.1). The

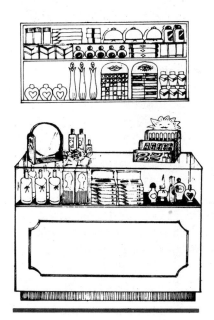

25.1—A combination cosmetic cabinet: The top part of the cabinet is used to display cosmetics and the lower part for storage of the more frequently used items.

makeup area and all materials used to apply makeup should be well-organized and spotlessly clean. The client will not be impressed by dusty display cases and used items strewn on the makeup counter. When the client wishes to sample cosmetic items, such as lip and cheek colors, she must be provided with clean, sanitary brushes or applicators, and tissues to remove the cosmetics if desired (Fig. 25.2).

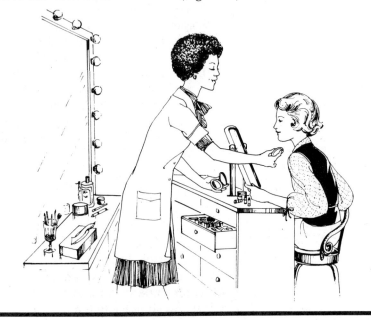

25.2—A makeup station or counter used for professional makeup should have drawers for additional storage of items frequently used or sold. The top of the station should be easy to clean after each makeup.

SEATING THE CLIENT IN THE MAKEUP CHAIR

A makeup chair that has a headrest is most comfortable for the client and makes it easier to hold the head steady during the makeup application. It is especially important that the head is held steady during the application of the lip and eye makeup. The makeup should not be done while the client is lying down, as direct overhead light will often flush out shadows that otherwise would be corrected by the makeup artist. The face (especially the full face) tends to flatten when the client is in a reclined position. This makes it difficult to do corrective makeup on some areas of the face. If the back of the chair is adjustable, it may be tilted back, but at no more than a 45 degree angle. The height of the chair should be comfortable for the client as well as for the makeup artist. Professional chairs have a footrest, but if the chair has no place to rest the feet, a foot stool should be provided. The makeup artist should learn to work from one side of the client only. It is considered unprofessional to move from one side of the chair to the other when applying makeup. Whether the chair is adjustable or not, it should be at a height at which the makeup artist can apply the makeup without uncomfortable stooping or bending.

STORAGE OF COSMETICS AND SUPPLIES

Most salons have a dispensary and additional storage space for supplies. All materials used for makeup should be kept separate and well-organized. The makeup area from which the makeup artist works should be clean and neat. Items that are reusable must be sterilized and placed in a clean container until ready for use.

LIGHTING THE MAKEUP AREA

The makeup area in a salon need not be elaborate, but it should be attractively appointed and set up for maximum efficiency. A well-lighted makeup mirror is one of the most important items, because without adequate lighting, the artist will be working under a tremendous handicap. Incandescent light bulbs produce red and yellow light rays and, when used alone, give a warmer and more flattering color. Fluorescent bulbs produce green and blue rays which tend to be cool and harsh. In some salons, a combination of incandescent and fluorescent bulbs are used to balance the light.

THE MAKEUP MIRROR

Some makeup mirrors are designed so that the finished makeup can be viewed under incandescent light and again under only fluorescent light, which is the type of lighting used in most places of business. It is helpful to explain to the client that some makeup colors change drastically under certain lighting conditions. The client may not realize that the makeup she wears for one occasion may not be suitable for another.

The ideal makeup mirror is one that resembles a theatrical makeup mirror: Bulbs surround the mirror on three sides only. Lighting on the underside of the mirror causes unnatural light on the face and generates too much heat on cosmetics that are placed near them. Use nothing stronger than 40 watt bulbs. The heat of higher watt bulbs will be too intense. Fifteen 40 watt bulbs would equal 600 watts, which is sufficient light. It is ideal to have a rheostat (dimmer) to be able to simulate different lighting conditions. When the mirror is surrounded by incandescent bulbs, the light is softer and more flattering. Thus, the makeup artist's job becomes easier. Most professional makeup is done for a client's indoor activities and, therefore, should not be done in natural daylight (Fig. 25.3).

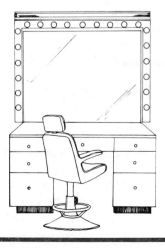

25.3—The makeup mirror

SUPPLIES FOR PROFESSIONAL MAKEUP

Check List:

Eyebrow tweezers

Sponge-tipped applicators

Cotton-tipped applicators

Facial tissue

Silk cosmetic sponges

Cotton

Headbands and clips for moving hair off the face

Manicure scissors for trimming eyelashes

Spatulas

Small cups or glasses for blending makeup

Cleansers

Astringent and skin-freshening lotion

Assortment of foundations in colors for various skin tones

Moisturizer and/or protective lotion

Assortment of cheekcolors (blushers)

Assortment of lipcolors (lipsticks)

Assortment of eyebrow pencils in various colors

Eyeshadows (color) in various colors and textures

Mascara in basic colors (black, brown, navy blue)

Eyelash curler

Assortment of artificial eyelashes and lash adhesive

Cover cream or stick for corrective makeup, concealing blemishes, lines, and dark circles under the eyes.

Shading powders and/or creams for highlighting and shading of facial contours

A makeup cape, if one is needed, and tissue to place next to the client's skin under the neck of the cape

An assortment of brushes (Fig. 25.4)

A makeup kit (Fig. 25.5)

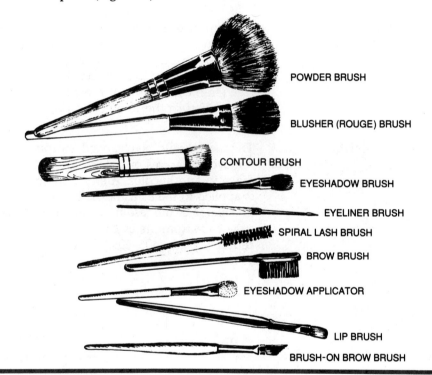

POWDER BRUSH

BLUSHER (ROUGE) BRUSH

CONTOUR BRUSH

EYESHADOW BRUSH

EYELINER BRUSH

SPIRAL LASH BRUSH

BROW BRUSH

EYESHADOW APPLICATOR

LIP BRUSH

BRUSH-ON BROW BRUSH

25.4—Makeup brushes

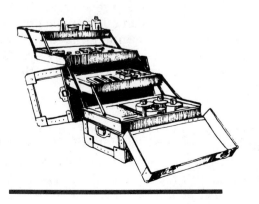

25.5—A well-stocked makeup artist's kit is used for makeup that is done outside the salon. Some clients may have the makeup artist do makeup for weddings, fashion shows, club demonstrations, and for special occasions.

Preparing the Client for the Makeup

When the client is having a makeup only, it is not necessary to have her change into a salon gown, unless she wishes to do so. Since headbands around the head tend to flatten the hair, the hair may be pinned back with hair clips. Some makeup artists like to use a small makeup cape; others prefer tucking tissue around the neckline of the client's clothing. The client may be wearing expensive clothing and it is courteous to ask if she would prefer changing into a salon gown.

If the client is having her hair done on the same day she is having the makeup application, then the makeup is done after the hair has been dried and before final curling or styling. If makeup is applied before the shampoo or before the client goes under the dryer, the makeup will be disturbed. When the hair has been set so that some of the hair is on the face (side curls, bangs), the hair should be pinned back carefully so as not to disturb the line of the original style.

PREPARING THE SKIN FOR MAKEUP   The face should be cleansed thoroughly with cleanser and astringent to remove any traces of stale makeup. Care must be taken to remove all eye makeup and lipcolor. A small amount of moisturizer or protective lotion is applied to the face and neck. Excess moisturizer is blotted with a tissue. The shape of the face may now be determined. Now is the time to tweeze stray hairs from the eyebrows and shape them. (See eyebrow shaping procedures, pages 406–409.)

Analyzing the Client's Facial Features and Shape of Face

When applying makeup, it is important to try to make the most of the client's attractive features while minimizing features that are out of proportion or unattractive in relation to the rest of the face. Learning to see the face and features and determining the best makeup for the individual takes practice. The beginning artist will often have an unsteady hand when applying makeup, especially eye colors and lipcolors. However, diligent practice and experience are the best ways to master makeup application.

THE OVAL-SHAPED FACE   The oval-shaped face with well-proportioned features has long been considered to be ideal, but all face shapes are attractive when makeup is applied properly. What counts most is that the client's individuality is enhanced. For the beginning makeup artist, it is helpful to study the basic face shapes and, after some experience, it becomes easier to look at a face and know almost instinctively what to do.

The artistically ideal proportions and features of the oval-shaped face are used to form the basis for corrective makeup application. It is divided into equal thirds lengthwise. The first third is measured from the hairline to the point between the eyebrows where they begin. The second third is measured from the eyebrows to the end of the nose. The last third is measured from the end of the nose to the bottom of the chin.

The ideal oval-shaped face is approximately three-fourths as wide as it is long. The distance between the eyes is the width of one eye.

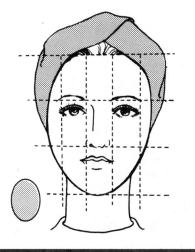

25.6—The oval-shaped face

THE ROUND-SHAPED FACE   The round-shaped face is usually broader in proportion to its length than is the oval-shaped face. It has a rounding chin and hairline.

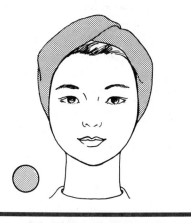

25.7—The round-shaped face

THE SQUARE-SHAPED FACE   The square-shaped face is composed of comparatively straight lines with a wide forehead and square jawline.

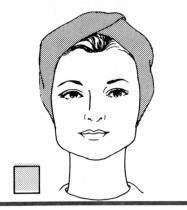

25.8—The Square-shaped face

THE PEAR-SHAPED FACE   This face is characterized by a jaw that is wider than the forehead.

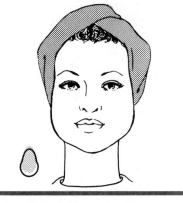

25.9—The pear-shaped face

THE HEART-SHAPED FACE   The heart-shaped face has a wide forehead and a narrow, pointed chin.

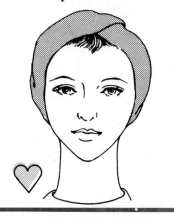

25.10—The heart-shaped face

THE DIAMOND-SHAPED FACE   This face has a narrow forehead. The greatest width is across the cheek bones.

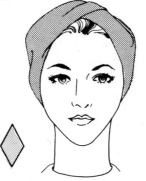

25.11—The diamond-shaped face

THE OBLONG-SHAPED FACE   This face has greater length in proportion to its width than does the square- or round-shaped face. It is long and narrow.

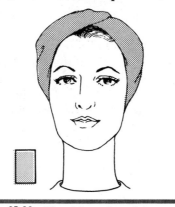

25.12—The oblong-shaped face

COMBINATION FACE SHAPES   It is not uncommon to look at a face and be unable to determine the exact shape. The features within the shape of the face make a difference. The eyes may be close set, the nose short and wide, and the lips thin or thick; or the features may be the opposite. Once you know how to use corrective makeup to enhance the various features, each part of the face can be given the attention it needs.

UNEVEN FEATURES   Few people have perfect faces but all faces are interesting. It is not uncommon for one eye to be larger than the other, and it is rare to find eyebrows exactly alike. When looking into a person's face, we are usually unaware of these small differences, because we see the entire face as a whole and not one feature. However, some people feel self-conscious about uneven features and appreciate knowing how to use makeup to equalize proportions of the face. When the features are crooked or out of balance, then makeup can be used to balance the features.

Grooming the Eyebrows

A picture or painting takes on a more interesting look when it is well-framed. The same is true of the eyebrows, as they act as a frame for the eyes. Eyebrows help to set the expression of the face, and well-formed brows add balance to the face while accenting the eyes.

When shaping the eyebrows, it is best to keep them as natural as possible. Some brows only require the removal of a few stray hairs. There are times when brows are improved by reshaping. Extremely heavy brows can be waxed to remove excess hair and then shaped by tweezing. Brows should be tweezed out one hair at a time in the direction that the hair grows. In most cases, the client's brow should be shaped so that it starts over the inside corner of the eye. A pencil may be used to determine the exact point to start the tweezing.

TWEEZING THE BROWS To determine where tweezing should begin, align a pencil from the inner corner of the eye to the side of the nose. Hair growing between the eyebrows from this point should be tweezed out.

The pencil is placed vertically so that it passes across the outer edge of the iris of the eye. Where the pencil crosses the brow should be the highest point (apex) of the brow.

The pencil is held from the corner of the nose on a line that passes the outer corner of the eye. This will determine the minimum length of the outward taper of the brow. (See Fig. 25.13.)

Tweeze out brow hairs in the direction in which they grow. (See Fig. 25.14.)

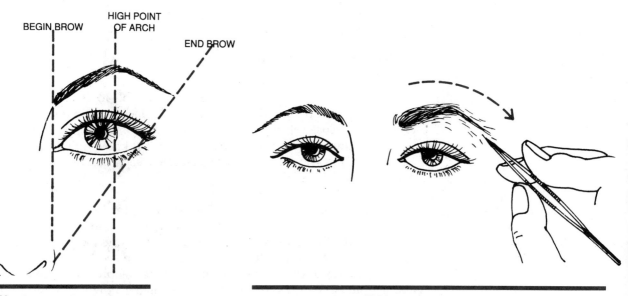

BEGIN BROW HIGH POINT OF ARCH END BROW

25.13—Correct points for tweezing the brows

25.14—Remove hair in this direction.

EYEBROWS CAN CHANGE FACIAL EXPRESSIONS

Well-shaped eyebrows add character to the face. It is interesting to see how actors, for example, use their eyes and brows to portray emotion.

When the eyebrows are too thin and highly arched, they give the face a surprised look that draws attention to the brows rather than to the entire face (Fig. 25.15). When brows are too widely spaced and slanted downward at the outer ends, they give the eyes a vacuous stare (Fig. 25.16). When brows are too heavy and too close together, they give the impression of frowning or that the person is displeased (Fig. 25.17).

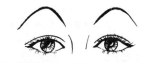

25.15—Thin and highly arched eyebrows

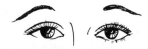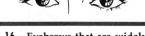

25.16—Eyebrows that are widely spaced and slanted downward

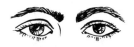

25.17—Eyebrows that are heavy and close together

The distance between normally set eyes is the width of one eye (Fig. 25.18). For close-set eyes, tweeze the eyebrows so that the distance between them equals the width of one eye. Start tweezing over the tear duct rather than over the corner of the eyes (Fig. 25.19). Wide-set eyes will seem closer together if the eyebrows are tweezed to the distance of one eye-span from the other (Fig. 25.20).

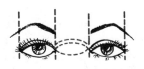

25.18—Normally set eyes

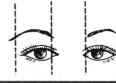

25.19—Close-set eyes

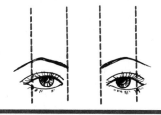

25.20—Wide-set eyes

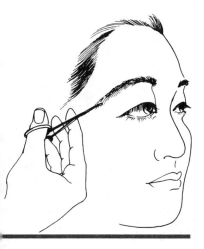

25.21—Shaping brows that grow in a downward direction with cuticle scissors

Some people have brows that grow in a downward direction. This is especially common with Asian people. When shaping brows of this type, a small cuticle scissor is used to clip the hair underneath the brow. It is interesting to note that when brow hair grows in a downward direction, eyelashes will usually tend to grow downward, too. Straight lashes can be curled with an eyelash curler before mascara is applied (Fig. 25.21).

PROCEDURE FOR TWEEZING THE BROWS   The brows are tweezed only enough to create a flattering frame for the eyes. To cause as little discomfort to the client as possible during tweezing, do the following:

1. Soften the brows by applying a small amount of oil or cleansing cream.
2. Hold the skin taut where the brow is to be tweezed.
3. Pull the hairs out in the direction in which they grow.
4. After tweezing, apply a cold, wet cotton compress that has been sprinkled with a few drops of witch hazel or astringent.

EYEBROW COLOR   There are two basic products used for making up the brows. These are pencils and pressed powder, which is applied with a brush. The pencil may be a mechanical type with refillable leads (thin or regular) or a wood type brow pencil. When color is applied to the brows with a pencil, the pencil should have a fine point. It will be necessary to keep a pencil sharpener at the makeup station. The makeup artist may use either a pencil, the dry brush-on color, or both. Pencil and brush-on colors come in a variety of shades, such as light, medium, and dark brown auburn, charcoal, and black. To prevent the brow color from becoming overpowering or harsh, the color selected is usually a shade lighter than the natural color of the brows. If the brows are extremely light (blonde) a deeper shade of color may be applied.

Procedure   1. Before the application of eyebrow color, an eyebrow brush is used to brush away any makeup on the brows. The brows may be brushed upward and then across in the direction of the hair growth. (See Fig. 25.22.)
2. Brow color should be applied with light hair-like strokes. When brows are sparse, a finely pointed pencil is used to sketch in fine, hair-like strokes to resemble real brow hair. At first this takes practice in order to create the illusion of real brow hair. (See Fig. 25.23.)

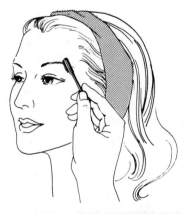

25.22—Start by brushing makeup on the brows.

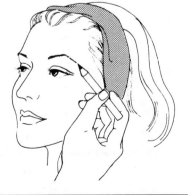

25.23—Apply hair-like strokes with a pencil.

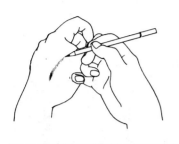

25.24—Practice sketching eyebrows.

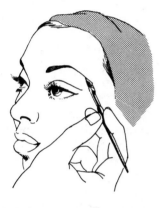

25.25—Brush on brow color.

3. The beginning makeup artist may wish to practice sketching eyebrows on the back of his or her hand until it becomes easy to sketch natural-looking brows. (See Fig. 25.24.)

4. Brush-on brow color is easy to apply and works well when little corrective work needs to be done on the brows. (See Fig. 25.25.)

5. Once you have determined where the high point, or apex, of the brow should be, it is easy to reach this point by starting the brow-color application on the underside of the brow. Stroke the color in a straight line directly up to the high point of the brow, then sweep the color outward toward the temple. Once the high point has been achieved, fill in the rest of the brow. (See Fig. 25.26.)

6. Keep in mind that for most clients, the brow will start directly above the inside corner of the eye and extend no farther outward than an imaginary line from the nostril past the outer corner of the eye. For a more dramatic or evening effect in eye makeup, the brow is sometimes extended outward. This is especially true when the eyeshadow or color has also been extended outward for a more dramatic effect. (See Fig. 25.27.)

7. Once the brow color has been applied, the brows are brushed lightly with a clean brow brush to remove excess color and give a soft, natural look to the brow. (See Fig. 25.28.)

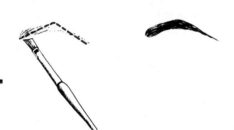

25.26—Stroke the color up to the high point of the brow and outward.

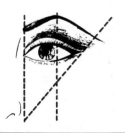

25.27—The brow will start at the inside corner of the eye and extend outward. The length will be determined by the effect the client wishes.

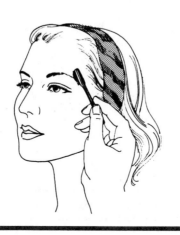

25.28—Brush excess color from the brow.

Foundation

When applying foundation to the face, think of an artist preparing a canvas. The entire surface should be made to look flawless before other colors are applied. To achieve this flawless look, the makeup artist uses foundation. In areas that need coverage (corrective makeup) such as circles under the eyes or blemishes, corrective creams or cover sticks are used.

The color and type of foundation that is appropriate for the client's skin is selected. The purpose of the foundation is to make the skin appear flawless and even in color. An easy way to select foundation color is to hold a few shades (in their containers) near the skin and select the one that is closest in color to the client's skin (Fig. 25.29). Apply a small amount of foundation on the jawline to make sure it is a harmonious color and will blend with the natural tones of the face and neck. No lines of demarcation should be seen. It is sometimes necessary to blend two foundations to get the desired shade. For example, if one shade is too light and another too dark, the two shades together can be blended to achieve the proper tone. Blend foundation in a small container with a cotton-tipped swab. This container of custom-blended foundation should be kept until the makeup is completed, in case additional foundation or corrective coloring is needed during the makeup.

The cotton-tipped swab is used to test a dot of the makeup on the jawline while blending, until the desired shade is achieved. It is not uncommon for the client to purchase the two foundations so that she can custom blend them at home (Fig. 25.30).

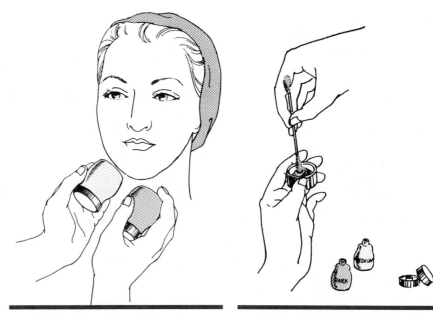

25.29—Select a foundation color that is closest in color to the client's skin.

25.30—Two foundations are sometimes blended to achieve the desired shade.

> **Note:** Don't try to change the natural color of a client's skin with foundation. The purpose of the foundation is to even the skin coloring and to give a more flawless look. There are exceptions, such as when a client's skin is too florid (red) and a beige foundation color will tone down the red. Generally, makeup is not applied on the neck because it will soil the collar or neckline of the client's clothing.

Foundations come in different textures, such as liquid, cream, stick, and cake form. The most popular makeup foundation is the liquid type. It gives good coverage, is easy to apply, and gives a healthy, natural look to the skin. Liquid foundation can be used successfully on almost all types of skin, because the base of the liquid foundation is usually an emulsion of water and oil that spreads easily. It is sometimes referred to as a water-base foundation. Souffle (lightly whipped) makeup is light in texture and comes in jars or aerosol cans. Like the liquid foundation, it can be used on all types of skins. It is sometimes formulated to give extra coverage without feeling heavy on the face. This is due to the airy, whipped texture.

An oil-based foundation is heavier in texture than water bases or souffle foundations. It feels oily to the touch and only a small amount is needed to give good coverage to the entire face. The container should be shaken before use, as the oil separates from the pigment. Cream and stick foundations are heavy in texture with an oily feeling. They give excellent coverage. Cream and stick foundations are often used for theatrical makeup. A more natural, light-textured look can be achieved if the makeup is applied with a damp sponge. Cream foundation is usually too heavy for oily skin. Cake foundation is a dry makeup that must be applied with a damp sponge. It gives good coverage and is also often used as theatrical makeup by models and television actors (male and female) who must work under hot lights.

APPLYING THE FOUNDATION

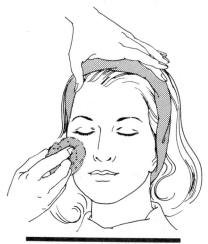

25.31—A sponge is used to apply makeup foundation.

The foundation may be applied with the fingers or a makeup sponge (Fig. 25.31). The sponge helps to give the makeup a sheer natural look, and the makeup can be blended around the hairline easily. It is important that the sponge be neither too wet nor too dry, or the makeup will streak. The sponge is moistened in water and the excess water is then squeezed out.

The sponge is then placed in a tissue and squeezed again so that it contains just the right amount of moisture. The foundation is applied to the face (forehead, nose, cheeks, and chin) with the sponge and blended until it is smooth and even in color. After the makeup has been applied, more coverage may be needed in some areas of the face, such as around the nose. In this case, a small amount of the foundation can be applied with the fingers. The extra coverage will blend in with the thin, sheer film of foundation already on the face. Foundation should be applied to the eyelids and to the lips when corrective work is needed.

Basic Corrective Makeup

After the foundation is applied, it is important to step back to view the client's face to decide if corrective work will be needed. A cover-up or corrective cosmetic (lighter in shade than the foundation) is applied to soften deep creases running along the sides of the nose down to the corners of the mouth, and to diminish dark areas; and the darker shades are used to minimize puffy or light areas. Cover sticks come in light, medium, and dark shades (Figs. 25.32 and 25.33).

For coverage of blemishes or other discolorations, the cover-up cosmetic should match the foundation as closely as possible. The corrective makeup can be applied with the fingers, but a brush does a better and more professional job. The edges of the coverage cosmetic should be blended into the foundation so there is no contrast in color (Figs. 25.34 and 25.35). (For more extensive corrective makeup see pages 426–431.)

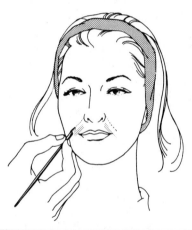

25.32—A pointed brush is used to apply the cover-up cosmetic to naso-labial folds (smile lines).

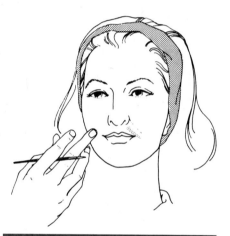

25.33—The coverage is patted with the fingers to blend it with the foundation.

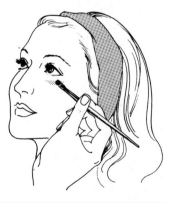

25.34—A brush is used to apply corrective, cover-up cosmetics underneath the eyes.

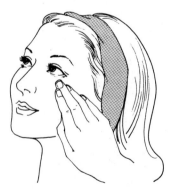

25.35—The coverage is then patted with the fingers until it is blended with the foundation.

Face Powder

The main purpose of powder is to set the foundation and give the face a velvety, soft matte finish. Facial flaws are less prominent and makeup will last longer when powder is applied over the foundation. Translucent powder is the most versatile and is most frequently used by makeup artists. Some powders come in colors such as rose, tan, rachel, beige, etc.; but colored powder often tends to give the face an unnatural or "made-up" look. The disadvantage of colored powder is that it can turn "orangy" when it absorbs the oils from the foundation or the skin. These problems are avoided when colorless (translucent) powder is used.

APPLYING FACE POWDER

1. Powder may be applied to the face with a soft powder brush. However, it is important to use a clean brush for each client. Many professional makeup artists use clean cotton puffs for powder application. (See Fig. 25.36.)
2. To apply powder, press a clean cotton puff into loose translucent powder. Excess powder on the cotton is placed on the palm of the hand. (See Fig. 25.37.)
3. To apply powder to the face, press the cotton puff against the face. Don't use wiping motions, as this will disturb and partially remove the foundation and corrective makeup. Too much powder around the eye area may accent superficial lines. Very little or no powder is needed in this area. When powder is applied around the eyes, it must be pressed on gently to set the makeup and to avoid accenting fine lines. After the loose powder has been applied (pressed) over the entire face, the excess is brushed away with the cotton puff or powder brush. (See Fig. 25.38.)
4. Another method of setting makeup around the eyes is to press a tissue gently to the area. The tissue will absorb excess oil. (See Fig. 25.39.)

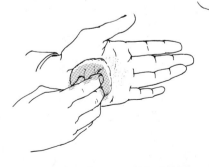

25.36—Applying powder with a soft brush

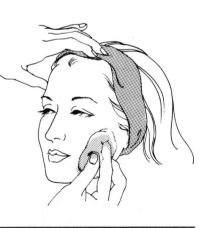

25.37—Removing excess powder from cotton puff

25.38—Applying powder with a cotton puff

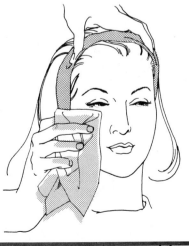

25.39—Setting makeup around the eye with a tissue

SETTING THE MAKEUP   A clean cotton pad may be dipped in cold water and the excess water squeezed from the pad. The pad is then pressed gently over the face to remove a "powdered look" and to set the makeup. Loose powder would be used for the initial makeup but the client may use pressed (compact) powder for touching up the makeup.

Cheekcolor

Some people call it rouge or cheekcolor, others call it blush-on; some use cream, others use powder. No matter which one you use or what name you give it, cheekcolor adds the look of health.

Apply color to the cheeks, never going below the nose. Sweep the color up and out into the hairline below the temples. Blend it so there is a healthy blush to the cheeks.

The first cheekcoloring material widely used was called "rouge" and came in a limited choice of colors. Modern cheekcoloring cosmetics come in a wide range of colors in gels, creams, sticks, powders, and liquids. The most popular form is the dry, brush-on type. This type of cheekcolor is called a "blusher." Cheekcolor applied on the cheekbone will give the face a lift. Cheekcolor that falls below the tip of the nose will drag the face down. In most cases, the cheekcolor is applied no closer to the nose than the center of the eye. The exception would be when the face is very full or wide. The cheekcolor is then brought closer to the nose to create the illusion of thinness. Keep the color away from the hairline. On a thin, long face the cheekcolor is applied on the outer part of the face to give the illusion of width. Blend the color into the hairline. The color is brushed upward and outward toward the temples to the hairline. The color should be so well-blended that it appears to be the woman's own natural coloring.

APPLICATION OF CREAM BLUSH   Cream cheekcolor is applied with the fingertips in several quick pressing and patting motions in the area where color is desired. The edges are then carefully blended with the fingertips.

A softer and more natural effect is achieved when the cream blush is applied directly over the foundation, and then set with translucent powder. To prevent the cheekcolor from fading, a dry blusher is applied over the cream blush after the translucent powder has been applied. This application of color on color will hold for many hours without fading.

CHEEKCOLOR AND FACE SHAPES   1. For the round-, full- or square-shaped face, the cheekcolor is brought closer to the sides of the nose but no lower than the tip of the nose. The color is brushed upward but not into the hairline. The aim is to create the illusion of slenderness. (See Fig. 25.40.)

2. A good basic rule is to apply the color no closer to the nose than the center of the eye, and no lower than the tip of the nose. The color is swept upward toward the temples. This will work well on almost everyone. (See Fig. 25.41.)
3. For the long thin face, color applied toward the outer sides of the cheeks will create the illusion of greater width. The color is blended no lower than the tip of the nose. (See Fig. 25.42.)

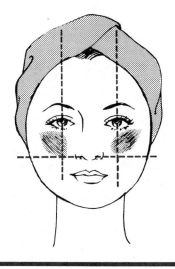

25.40—Cheekcolor application for the round/full/square-shaped face

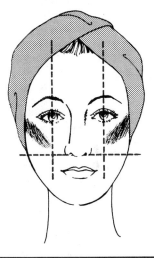

25.41—Cheekcolor application for the oval-shaped face

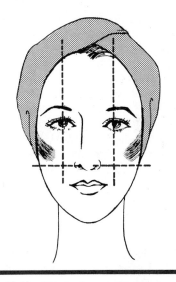

25.42—Cheekcolor application for the long/thin face

Eye Makeup

EYESHADOW   It is helpful to find out what the client prefers in eye makeup colors. The choice of color should be based on what makes the client attractive, rather than current fashion fads. However, the client will not want to wear any eye makeup that makes her appear outdated.

Eyeshadow comes in a variety of colors and textures, such as powders, pencils, creams, and liquids. The most popular eyeshadow is the pressed powder type. The color is often chosen to accentuate the client's eyecolor or to coordinate or match with her clothing color. Turquoise will often be flattering to the mature woman with white or silver hair, while women with red or deep auburn hair will usually prefer green, navy blue, or brown.

Procedure for Applying Eye Shadow

1. With a brush or sponge-tipped applicator, apply the color at the base of the lashes up to the crease line of the eyelid. Sometimes a deeper eyeshadow pencil color is desired in place of the eyeliner; this color can be smudged near the base of the upper and lower lashes to create a softer look. (See Fig. 25.43.)
2. In the crease of the lid, apply a darker contouring color, such as navy blue, dark green, brown, or charcoal. Brown is the most frequently used contouring color, as it adds depth and is flattering to most skin tones. The contouring color should become lighter as it is blended closer to the eyebrows. (See Fig. 25.44.)
3. Directly under the brow, apply a highlighting color such as ivory, pink, white, light beige, or soft yellow. The lighter color is blended into the contouring color leaving no line of demarcation. The colors should

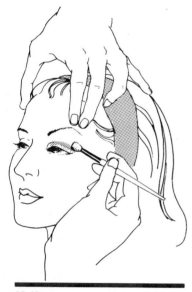

25.43—Apply the color at the base of the lashes up to the crease line of the eyelid.

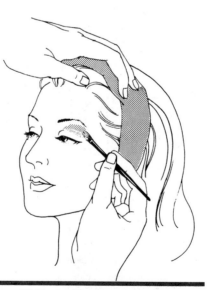

25.44—In the crease of the lid, apply a darker contouring color.

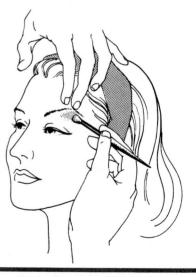

25.45—Directly under the brow, apply a highlighting color.

seem to flow one into the other in a soft rainbow effect. As fashion colors change, the makeup artist should experiment with new styles in makeup and new color combinations. The best place to find new fashion trends in makeup is to observe models in fashion magazines. It takes imagination, a light hand, an eye for color and style, and lots of practice to do beautiful eye makeup well. (See Fig. 25.45.)

4. After eyeshadow (color) has been applied to the eyelid, have the client look directly ahead. If the color has disappeared under a fold of skin, the shadow will have to be applied higher up on the lid. (See Figs. 25.46–25.49.)

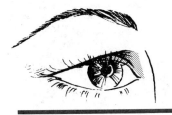
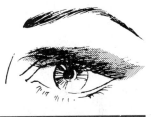

25.46—The eye with the shadow applied just on the lid

25.47—The eye with the shadow applied slightly higher on the lid

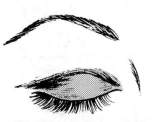
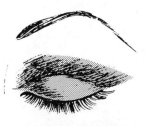

25.48—The fold of the eyelid with no color showing

25.49—The eye after color has been brushed higher on the lid

5. The basic rules to remember when applying eyeshadow are (Fig. 25.50):
   a. The main fashion color (blue, green, plum) is applied on the eyelid.
   b. The shading color (brown, charcoal, navy) is applied in the crease of the eyelid.
   c. Highlighting is done underneath the brow.

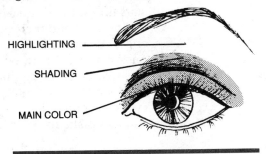

HIGHLIGHTING

SHADING

MAIN COLOR

25.50—Eyeshadow application

LINING THE EYE   Although some women prefer a touch of eyeshadow and mascara as their only eye makeup, many women feel that eye makeup is incomplete without eyeliner. Eyeliner does make a difference when it is applied properly. Liner accentuates the eye, changes its shape, and makes the eyelashes appear thicker. Liner comes in a variety of colors, but the most popular and most natural liners are dark brown and soft black. Liners are available in dry cake (that must be moistened before use), soft pencil, and liquid form. The cake liner is preferred by most makeup artists (Figs. 25.51 and 25.52).

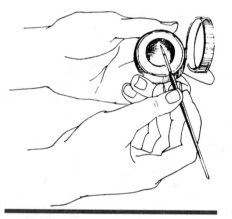

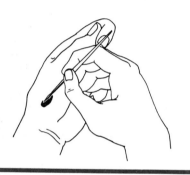

25.51—Liquid and cake liner are applied with an eyeliner brush. It is easier to achieve a finer line when a finely pointed eyeliner brush is used. Water is mixed with dry cake liner.

25.52—The right consistency is achieved by blending the eyeliner on the ball of the thumb.

Basic Eyeliner Application   The eyelids should be dry and free of oil before the liner is applied.

1. With the client looking downward, place one or two fingers on the eyelid to help hold the eye steady in case the client blinks.
2. Draw a fine line as close to the base of the lashes as possible. (See Fig. 25.53.) When the line is about two-thirds across the width of the eye, start lifting the line slightly. (See Fig. 25.54.)
3. To line the bottom lid, keep the liner only on the outer half of the lid and close to the lash growth. Cotton-tipped swabs are used to correct mistakes or to clean off excess liner.
4. The two ends of the liner should not be brought together. The small open space at the outer end of the eye makes it look larger. When the eye is surrounded entirely by a rim of liner, the eye will appear smaller and the makeup will look too harsh and theatrical. (See Fig. 25.55.)

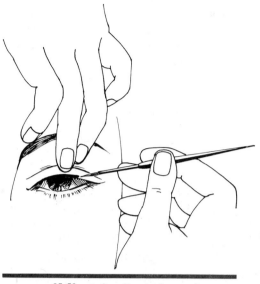

25.53—A fine line is drawn close to the base of the lashes.

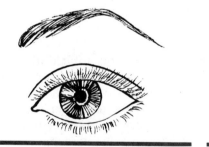

25.54—The correct application of eyeliner with the end slightly extended

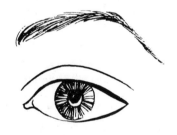

25.55—The eye completely rimmed with liner causes the eye to appear smaller and the makeup too obvious.

EYELINER STYLES

The purpose of eyeliner is to accent the eyes in much the same way that a frame is used to accent a beautiful painting or photograph. Fashions in eye makeup may change from season to season, but fashion can be enjoyed without following fads, which are not attractive on all women. The majority of women prefer a conservative eye makeup for daytime wear and a more glamorous look for evening or special occasions. The beginning makeup artist will learn by experimenting with different styles in makeup and determining what is most appropriate and becoming for each client.

The Natural Look

When the client wants just a touch of eye makeup, a very fine line may be drawn into the base of the upper lashes. The line is not extended beyond the corner of the eye and no line is drawn on the lower lid (Fig. 25.56).

25.56—The natural look

The Daytime Well-Groomed Look

For the woman who wants a little more eye makeup for daytime wear, a line may be drawn from the inner corner of the eye and extended slightly beyond the outer corner of the eye. The line is lifted at the outer corner to give the eyes a more open look and to make the eyelashes appear thicker (Fig. 25.57).

25.57—The daytime, well-groomed look

Evening and Special Occasion Makeup

Eyeliner for evening is applied to make the eyes appear more glamorous. A line is drawn from the inner corner of the eye and is made wider over the pupil of the eye, when looking straight ahead. The line is tapered very thinly as it reaches the outer corner of the eye. A small space is seen between the upper and lower lines. This makes the eyes appear larger and brighter. For evening, some women like a colored liner such as dark green or navy (Fig. 25.58).

25.58—Evening and special occasion makeup

The Exotic Eye

The exotic eye is usually almond or oblique in shape. To enhance almond eyes or to make round eyes appear to be almond shaped, a line is drawn from the inner corner of the eye and becomes wider from the center of the lid to the outer corner of the eye. The upper and lower lines may be extended upward and the space filled in. To achieve a less obvious effect, eyeshadow may be used to give a lift to the outer corner of the eyes (Fig. 25.59).

25.59—The exotic eye

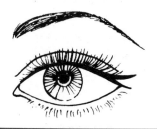

THE USE OF MASCARA A great many women prefer using only a touch of mascara for day makeup, while others will use liner, shadow, and mascara for day and evening wear. The purpose of mascara is to make the lashes look thicker, longer, and darker. The lashes create a luxurious frame for the eyes, making them appear larger and brighter. Mascara comes in cake, cream, and liquid form. The wand-type mascara that is brushed on, is the most popular type. Mascara colors are usually dark brown and soft black, but other colors, such as navy blue and green, are available.

▶ **Caution:** To keep the eyes free of debris and bacteria, replace a container of mascara every six months.

Mascara Application
1. When applying mascara to the upper lashes, the client is asked to look down. The lid is lifted with the fingers for easier application. A thin coat of mascara is applied to the top and then to the underside of the lashes. It is better to build the thickness of the mascara with several light applications, rather than to apply a heavy coat with one application. A clean brush is used to remove excess mascara. (See Fig. 25.60.)
2. To apply mascara to the bottom lashes, the client is asked to look up. The bottom lashes are shorter, so it will be easier to apply the mascara with just the tip of the brush. Move the brush back and forth across the lashes, then straighten them with the tip of brush. (See Fig. 25.61.)

▶ **Caution:** For sanitary reasons, use disposable wands when applying mascara to clients.

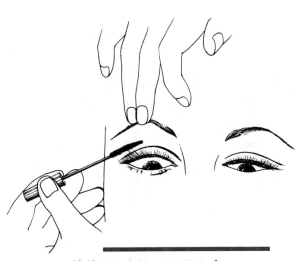

25.60—Applying mascara to the upper lashes

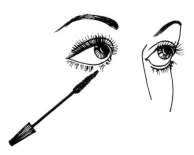

25.61—Applying mascara to the bottom lashes

Curling Eyelashes   When eyelashes have no sweep or curl, they can be curled with an eyelash curler. Position the eyelash curler on the top lashes and gently press and release the curler several times. Straight lashes are curled before the application of mascara. (See Fig. 25.62.)

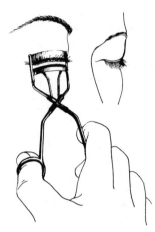

25.62—Curling eyelashes

Makeup for the Lips

The expression of the mouth and the lips lend character to the face. Lip makeup can add or detract from the beauty of the face. It is better to wear no lip makeup at all than to wear the wrong color or lip makeup that is poorly applied. Lipcolor (lipstick) should add a look of softness to the mouth. Lipcolor can be used to conceal defects and to shape the lips so they are harmoniously proportioned with the other features of the face.

The lips should be clean and dry before starting the lipcolor application. If corrective work is to be done, foundation and powder are usually applied to the lips before the application of the lipcolor to help conceal the outline of the lips. For sanitary reasons the same lipstick should not be used from one client's mouth to another.

It is more professional (and a sanitary precaution) to take scrapings of the lipcolor on a small metal spatula, which serves as a palette. (See Fig. 25.63.) The makeup artist picks up the lipcolor on the lip brush just as an artist picks up paint on a brush. (See Fig. 25.64.)

The spatula is also used to blend two shades of lipcolor together to achieve desired effects.

It is helpful when selecting lipcolors to hold different shades of lipstick near the client's mouth to help you determine which shade of lipcolor will harmonize best with the over-all look of the makeup. (See Fig. 25.65.)

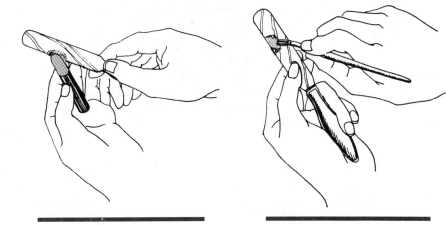

25.63—Place a scraping of lipcolor on a metal spatula.

25.64—Pick up the lipcolor with a lip brush.

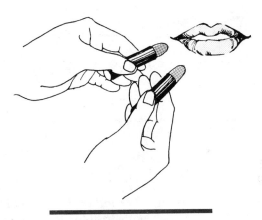

25.65—Hold different shades of lipcolor near the client's mouth to determine the best shade.

PROCEDURE FOR APPLYING LIPCOLOR

The client should be asked to relax, stretch, and part her lips into a slight smile. Some makeup artists find it helpful to use the little finger on the chin to steady the hand while applying the lip line and brushing on color. Apply lipcolor to the upper lip first. Start the line at the corner of the mouth away from you. Draw the line toward the center of the lip. Draw the line from the corner near you to the center of the lip to meet the other line. Be sure the upper curves of the lips are even. Follow the same application procedure for the lower lip. Lips may be outlined with either a lip pencil or brush. The color of the lip-pencil lead should match or coordinate with the lipstick that is to be applied. Usually the lead will be deeper in color. The makeup artist will often use a brown shade for more dramatic effects.

When the lip brush is used to outline the lips, the bristles are flattened so that only the edge of the bristles and the tip of the brush are used to line the lips. The flat side of the brush would make the line too thick. (See Fig. 25.66.)

After the lips have been outlined in the desired shape, the lipcolor is filled in. The lips may be blotted if desired, and a gloss applied to give a moist look to the lips. (See Fig. 25.67.)

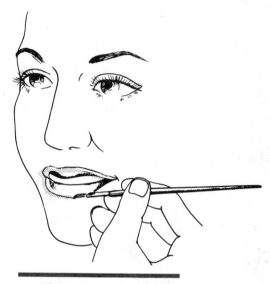

25.66—Outlining the lips

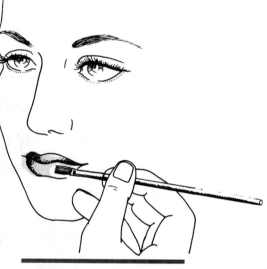

25.67—Filling in the lips with lipcolor

CORRECTIVE TECHNIQUES FOR THE LIPS

1. *Thin lower lip*—The curve of the lower lip can be lined and filled in with lipcolor to balance with the upper lip (Fig. 25.68).

25.68—Thin lower lip

2. *Thin upper lip*—Use lipcolor to build the curve of the upper lip to balance with the lower lip (Fig. 25.69).

25.69—Thin upper lip

3. *Thin lips*—Increase the size of both upper and lower lips by outlining and filling in color to make the lips appear fuller. Be cautious when the lips have definite natural lines. To go over natural ridges of the lips will tend to look too contrived (Fig. 25.70).

25.70—Thin lips

4. *Cupid bow lips*—The Cupid bow means that the upper lips are quite pointed. The points can be filled in with lipcolor by widening the sides of the lips (Fig. 25.71).

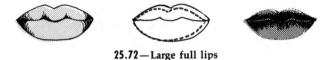

25.71—Cupid bow lips

5. *Large, full lips*—Line lips by staying within the natural lip line. Use lipcolors that are not too bright or that do not attract attention. Also do not use a glossy lipstick, but rather, use a matte finish (Fig. 25.72).

25.72—Large full lips

6. *Small mouth and lips*—A small mouth can be made to look larger and lips fuller by outlining and building out the sides of both the upper and lower lips with color (Fig. 25.73).

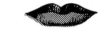

25.73—Small mouth and lips

7. *Drooping corners*—Lipcolor and liner can be used to build up the corners of the mouth and minimize the drooping corners (Fig. 25.74).

25.74—Drooping corners

8. *Uneven lips*—Outline the lips so that both upper and lower lips are even and attractively shaped. Fill in color (Fig. 25.75).

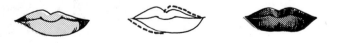

25.75—Uneven lips

> **Note:** Keep in mind that lips and mouths lend character to the entire face. Study the contours of the individual lips and apply lipcolor to enhance rather than to change.

Contouring and Corrective Makeup

There is no mystery to facial contouring when you remember that the application of a lighter cosmetic emphasizes and a darker cosmetic will minimize a facial feature. Unless corrective makeup is done carefully, the shadowing will appear as dirty spots on the face. Shading powder is usually easier to use than liquid or cream cosmetics, as it can be dusted lightly over foundation and powder without smearing or spotting. Professional models use shading powder almost exclusively. However, the choice is up to the makeup artist.

Some makeup artists like to do the corrective or contouring part of the makeup by using a lighter and darker foundation, others use a tawny or brown blush shading powder with a brush. The beginning makeup artist should experiment with various types of cosmetics until he or she feels confident in doing corrective makeup. When foundation is used for highlighting and shadowing an area of the face, it is applied before the powder application. When a contouring powder makeup is used, it is applied after the translucent powder. A face may need no corrective makeup, but some features are enhanced by subtle contouring (Figs. 25.76–25.78).

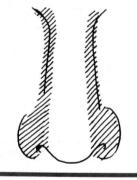

25.76—When the nose is too wide, the sides may be shaded and the bridge lightened.

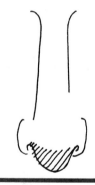

25.77—When the nose is too long, the underside is shaded.

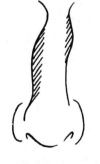

25.78—When the nose is crooked, straight lines of shading can be applied to the sides and a straight line of highlighting to the center of the nose. This creates the illusion of a straight nose.

CORRECTIVE MAKEUP   The correction of flaws and blemishes on the skin, such as dark circles under the eyes and deep expression lines that extend from the flare of the nose to the corner of the mouth, are corrected after the foundation has been applied. Most makeup artists will do the corrective work first and apply the foundation later. However, this tends to disturb the corrective makeup underneath as foundation cannot be applied over a corrective cream without moving the cream. Better coverage is achieved by applying cover-up stick or cream over the foundation. Corrective cover sticks come in different shades, usually light, medium, and dark.

CORRECTIVE MAKEUP FOR THE EYES

Dark Circles   Circles or dark shadows under and around the eyes can be minimized by the application of a cover-up makeup. There are a number of factors that may be responsible for dark circles and puffiness around the eyes. Sometimes the condition may be an inherited trait. The condition can be aggravated by too much or not enough rest, eating certain foods, or drinking some types of beverages. The client can be advised to evaluate his or her dietary and other health habits to try to determine what may be contributing to the condition.

Puffy Areas   A puffy area underneath the eyes will appear lighter than the surrounding skin. The lighter cover-up cosmetic can be applied to the darker areas under or around the puffed area. A darker cover-up cosmetic applied over the puffed area will minimize the condition. The two shades of cover-up cosmetic should be blended carefully.

> **Note:** Corrective makeup of this type can be especially beneficial to men and women whose work keeps them in the public eye. Good corrective makeup will help the person to look better in photographs, on the television screen, and when speaking in public.

Use dark foundation or shading powder to minimize the following:

Large or crooked nose	Double chin
Prominent jaw	Protruding forehead
Heavy-lidded eyes	Prominent chin

Use light foundation or highlighting powder to emphasize the following:

Short nose	Small or deep set eyes
Dark circles around the eyes	Long thin neck
Receding chin	Long thin face

HIGH CHEEKBONE LOOK

To make the cheekbones appear more prominent, draw an imaginary line from the corner of the mouth to the middle of the ear.

Shading is applied along this line and no closer to the nose than the outer corner of the eye. (See Fig. 25.79.)

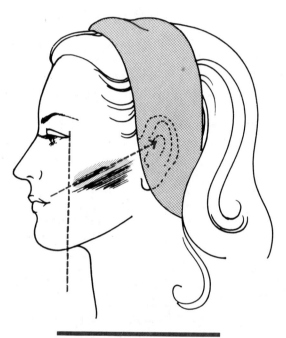

25.79—Makeup application for a high cheekbone look

BIRTHMARKS AND BLEMISHES

A small blemish, such as a mole or a dark-pigmented spot, can be concealed by applying the cover-up cosmetic with a brush. The fingers may be used to tap lightly over the area to blend the cosmetic with the foundation. A large portwine (dark red-wine color) birthmark, scars, and blemishes will require more time and patience to cover adequately. After the foundation is applied, the cover-up cosmetic should be brushed and patted carefully over the area to be concealed. A thin film of foundation may be blended over the concealing makeup, and the entire face powdered lightly. It is important to avoid using so much makeup that it accentuates rather than conceals the problem. The cover stick that is closest in color to the foundation is best for covering blemishes (Figs. 25.80 and 25.81).

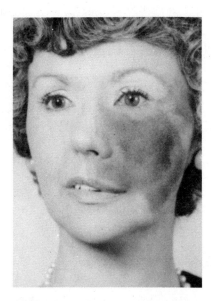

25.80—Before: In this photograph we see a woman with a portwine (deep red) birthmark. She is wearing no makeup. (*Photograph permission of Lydia O'Leary, Inc., New York, NY.*)

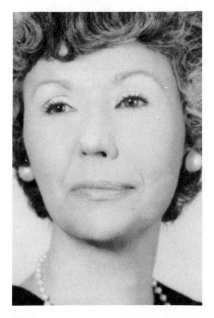

25.81—After: In this photograph we see the same woman after a special makeup foundation has been applied. The makeup was matched to her natural skin tones and skillfully blended to conceal the birthmark. (*Photograph permission of Lydia O'Leary, Inc., New York, NY.*)

THE USE OF HIGHLIGHTING COSMETICS

1. A highlight or lighter foundation applied down the center of the nose will make the nose appear longer and thinner. (See Fig. 25.82.)
2. Dark circles under the eyes can be minimized by the application of a lighter foundation to the dark area. (See Fig. 25.83.)
3. A receding chin will appear to be larger and less receding when a lighter foundation is applied to the area. (See Fig. 25.84.)
4. Deep set and small eyes will appear larger when a lighter foundation is applied between the eye and the eyebrow, and around the eyes. (See Fig. 25.85.)
5. Lighter foundation applied to the sides of a thin neck will make it appear fuller. (See Fig. 25.86.)
6. A long thin face will appear wider and fuller when light foundation is applied to the sides of the face. (See Fig. 25.87.)

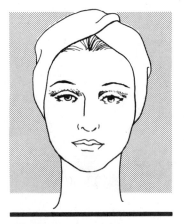

25.82—Highlighting for a wide nose

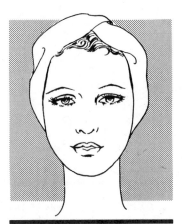

25.83—Highlighting for dark circles under the eyes

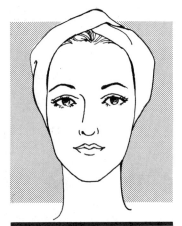

25.84—Highlighting for a receding chin

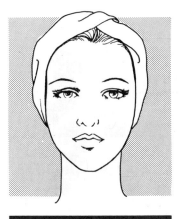

25.85—Highlighting for deep-set and small eyes

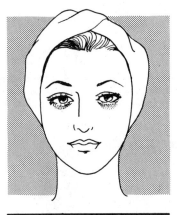

25.86—Highlighting for a thin neck

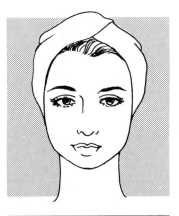

25.87—Highlighting for a long face

THE USE OF SHADING COSMETICS

1. Dark foundation applied to the sides of a wide nose will make it look narrower. (See Fig. 25.88.)
2. A darker foundation applied to the sides of the face or on the jawline will slenderize the face. (See Fig. 25.89.)
3. Apply a darker foundation or shadow to heavy lids or on a prominent area between the brows and eyelids to diminish the area. (See Fig. 25.90.)
4. A double chin will appear to be less prominent when darker foundation is applied to the area. (See Fig. 25.91.)
5. When the chin or face is long, the chin can be made to appear less prominent by the application of a darker foundation. (See Fig. 25.92.)
6. A protruding forehead will appear less prominent when darker foundation is applied to the area. (See Fig. 25.93.)

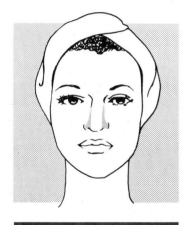

25.88—Shading for a wide nose

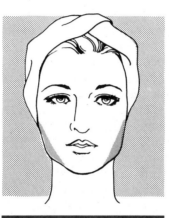

25.89—Shading for a wide jawline or face

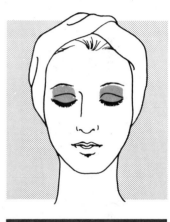

25.90—Shading for heavy eyelids

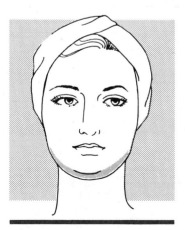

25.91—Shading for a double chin

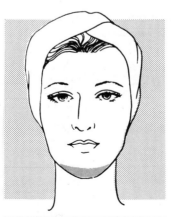

25.92—Shading for a long chin or face

25.93—Shading for a protruding forehead

Special Makeup Techniques for the Black Client

In previous chapters, the care of the skin and selection of cosmetic colors for dark-skinned clients have been discussed. The esthetician should remember that when applying makeup to any face, many of the same techniques apply. The skin is analyzed and given treatments for its specific condition and makeup is selected to enhance the individual's personal coloring of skin, eyes, and hair. Each face is individual and unique, therefore makeup must be personalized for each client. What may look beautiful on one face may be a disaster on another. Many makeup artists mix their own colors from two or more standard makeup colors to achieve the desirable shades. However, most cosmetic manufacturers offer a full range of makeup colors and some manufacturers specialize in makeup for black skin.

Before the makeup application, thoroughly cleanse the face, use an appropriate astringent, and a moisturizer, if needed.

FOUNDATION

When selecting a foundation for black skin, color is important. Foundations formulated for black skin have less coverage than foundations formulated for very light skin. This is due to the foundation containing little or no titanium dioxide, a chemical compound used in makeup to give good coverage. When makeup containing titanium dioxide is used on dark skin, it tends to give an "ashy" appearance to the skin. Black skin generally requires less foundation coverage because the same imperfections that are quite visible on a light skin are harder to see on a dark skin. When selecting a foundation, the color should be tried on the jawline and blended to be sure it is compatible with the individual's personal coloring.

POWDER

Translucent powder is preferred, but a tinted powder may be used if it does not change color when applied over the foundation.

CONTOUR SHADING AND HIGHLIGHTING

Shading and highlighting of the facial features with corrective or enhancement makeup techniques may be done as effectively on dark skins as on light. However, shading will not be as prominent on deep, dark skins, but highlighting will create interesting planes on the face. (See Fig. 25.94.)

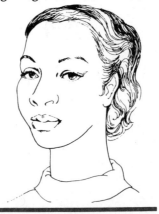

25.94—The purpose of makeup is to enhance the individual beauty of the client. A personalized makeup will add to her sense of confidence in selecting and applying makeup.

PROCEDURE FOR MAKEUP APPLICATION

1. It is important to select a makeup base or foundation that gives radiance to the natural skin tone and covers small imperfections. Translucent powder may be used to tone down too much sheen. (See Fig. 25.95.)

2. Cheekcolor should be applied high on the cheekbones. Deeper colors are usually the most flattering. Be especially cautious of cheekcolors that are light pink or orange. (See Fig. 25.96.)

3. Pastel colors in eye makeup that look right on a light skin will often be too pale and washed out for a dark skin. Eyeshadow should be deeper and brighter in color. For example, a light blue eyeshadow will be best for light skin while a medium bright to navy blue will enhance dark skin and dark eyes. (See Fig. 25.97.)

4. Eyebrows that are already dark should not be darkened with harsh, black pencil. A dark brown or brown-black pencil or brush-on color will be softer and more natural looking. (See Fig. 25.98.)

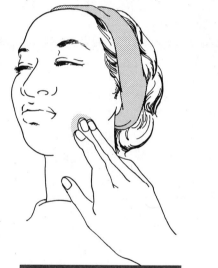

25.95—Select foundation.

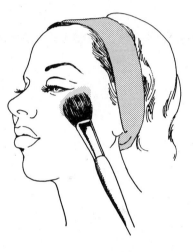

25.96—Apply cheekcolor.

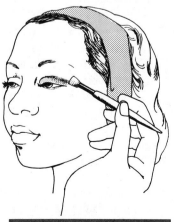

25.97—Apply eye makeup.

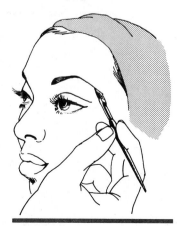

25.98—Fill in eyebrows.

5. Full lips are made more beautiful with the application of the right lip-color. Foundation can be applied over the lips and then a lip line drawn slightly inside the natural ridge of the lips and color filled in. However, any attempt to make a full mouth appear smaller may look too contrived and should be avoided. Pastel pink or orange lipcolors are not as attractive as deeper colors, such as red-brown and burgandy. Lip moisturizers help to keep lips smooth and moist. (See Fig. 25.99.)

6. Many exciting color combinations in makeup are available for black women. Artistic makeup can enhance every woman's beauty and increase her sense of poise. (See Fig. 25.100.)

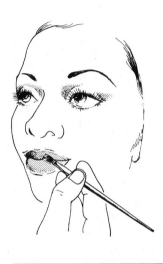

25.99—Apply lipcolor.

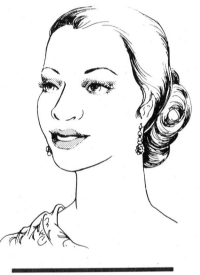

25.100—Finished look

Artificial Eyelashes

In the past, artificial eyelashes were used primarily for theatrical purposes. The average woman did not wear artificial lashes because they were unnatural looking and unacceptable as part of everyday makeup. In the mid 1960's, artificial eyelashes became the new fashion rage. Women were discovering that artificial lashes, when applied correctly, made the eyes look larger and more glamorous. Lashes became available in styles from long and heavy, to light and natural looking. Artificial lashes were made of real or synthetic hair. Today lashes come in a variety of styles (light brown to black) that need little if any trimming. Sometimes it is necessary to snip a few lashes from the outer ends of the lashes so they will fit the contour of the eyelid. Artificial eyelashes make the eyes look larger and more expressive, but they will appear harsh and theatrical unless applied skillfully.

MASCARA Mascara should not be applied to the natural eyelashes before the application of the artificial lashes. The mascara will prevent the client's natural lashes from blending together with the artificial lashes. When mascara is desired, it should be applied after the application of the artificial lashes.

FITTING THE LASHES When the new lashes are removed from the box, there is usually enough adhesive on the base of the lash to allow the lash to cling to the skin long enough to be checked for the correct length from corner to corner. If the lash does not hold on the lid, a small amount of adhesive may be applied to the base of the lash. The lash should not be applied from one corner of the eye to the other, but should start about ¼ inch or less from the inner corner of the eye and end about ¼ inch from the outer corner of the eye.

When the new lash is longer than desired, snip a piece off the outside edge of each lash. (See Fig. 25.101.)

Lashes should be feathered (clipped unevenly) when purchased. However, it may be necessary for the makeup artist to do additional feathering to shorten the lashes. Feathering is done with a pair of straight manicure scissors by cutting into the lash, never straight across them. (See Fig. 25.102.)

To give the eyes a more flattering look, lashes should be feathered so that the longer lash hairs are on the eyelid above the outside of the eye. (See Figs. 25.103 and 25.104.)

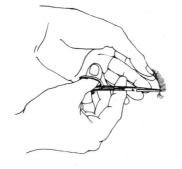

25.101—Trimming the lashes

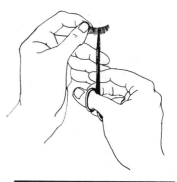

25.102—Feathering the lashes

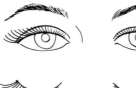

25.103—Lashes feathered incorrectly

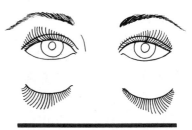

25.104—Lashes feathered correctly

Artificial eyelashes are harder to detect when eyeliner is applied before the application of the artificial eyelashes. Lashes will not adhere well to a penciled liner. The liner may be touched up again after the lashes are applied. (See Figs. 25.105 and 25.106.)

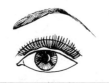

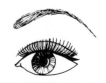

25.105—Right—Eyeliner applied before artificial eyelashes.

25.106—Wrong—Eyeliner applied after artificial eyelashes.

When the client has straight lashes that grow downward, they should be curled with an eyelash curler before the artificial eyelashes are applied. When the natural lashes are not curled to fit the artificial lashes, a separation will be seen between the real lashes and the artificial lashes. (See Fig. 25.107.)

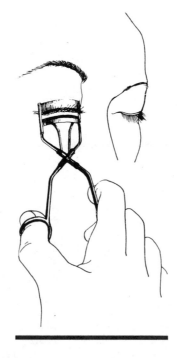

25.107—Curling the client's lashes before the application of artificial eyelashes

LASH ADHESIVE   The best type of adhesive for lashes is surgical adhesive, which may be purchased at most drugstores. The adhesive is applied to the base of the lash with the round end of an eyeliner brush or a toothpick. (See Fig. 25.108.) Adhesive is not applied to the lash directly from the tube, because too much adhesive may spurt onto the lashes. In recent years, manufacturers have produced adhesive in black, but it has proven less practical than the white adhesive. The black is messy to work with and does not adhere as well. The white adhesive can be seen when applied to the base of the lashes, then becomes invisible or transparent as it dries.

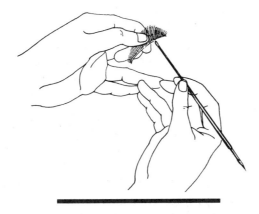

25.108—Applying adhesive to the base of the lash

APPLYING THE LASH   When ready to apply the artificial lashes, ask the client to look down. Hold the artificial lash at one end with the tweezers and the other end with the thumb and forefinger. Center the lash so that it is about ¼ inch in from the inner eye and the outer corners of the eye. Set the lash so that the base is as close to the natural lash as possible. Press the lash down into the client's natural lashes with the tweezers. Be extremely cautious when using the tweezers near the eye. Beginning artists may need to practice a great deal before attempting to apply lashes with tweezers. (See Fig. 25.109.)

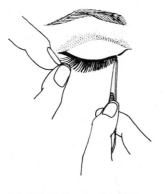

25.109—Applying the lash

APPLYING LOWER LASHES Artificial lower lashes are rarely used; however, a client may request them. Lower lashes should be fine and on an extremely thin base. The lower lashes are trimmed to the desired size and applied as close to the natural lashes as possible. The lashes will usually look best when applied to the outer corner of the lid. (See Fig. 25.110.)

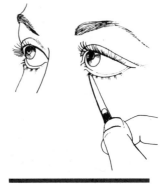

25.110—Apply lower lashes.

CURLING THE FALSE LASH Most lashes have a permanent curl, but if curl needs to be restored, a piece of wrapping tissue may be rolled around a pencil and the lash placed on the tissue with tweezers. (See Fig. 25.111.)

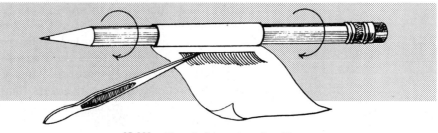

25.111—Place lash on wrapping tissue.

The lash is then rolled onto the pencil. It is important to keep the base of the lash straight so that all the lashes curl around the pencil. Leave lashes rolled around pencil for at least one half hour. (See Fig. 25.112.)

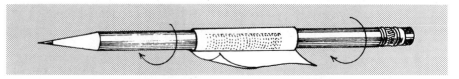

25.112—Roll the lash onto a pencil.

Individual Eyelash Application

Individual eyelash application is the technique of attaching (invisibly) almost weightless, individual eyelashes to the client's own eyelashes.

The artificial lashes are attached to the client's natural eyelashes and become a part of those lashes. They last from several days to several weeks. Due to natural lashes falling out regularly (a few each week), taking the artificial lashes with them, the artificial lashes should be filled in by periodic visits to the salon.

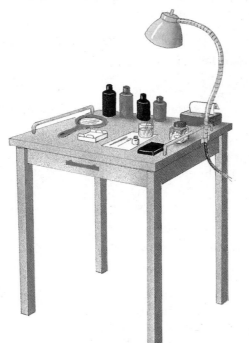

25.113—False eyelash set-up

SUPPLIES REQUIRED FOR ARTIFICIAL EYELASH APPLICATION

1. Alcohol to sanitize metal implements
2. Tweezers
3. Eyelash brush
4. Hand mirror
5. Manicure scissors
6. Tissues
7. Trays of individual eyelashes
8. Eyelash adhesive
9. Adhesive container
10. Eyelid and eyelash cleanser
11. Eyelash remover
12. Manicure or makeup table
13. Adjustable light (gooseneck lamp or magnifying lamp)
14. Makeup or facial chair
15. Headband and makeup cape, if needed.

ALLERGY TEST

Since some people may be allergic to adhesive, it is advisable to give the client an allergy test before applying the lashes. Put a small drop of adhesive behind the client's ear. If there is no reaction after 24 hours, it is safe to proceed with the eyelash application.

LENGTHS OF ARTIFICIAL LASHES

Individual lashes usually come in three lengths: short, medium, and long. Some manufacturers have developed extra-long lashes and extra-short lashes. These different lengths are used by themselves or in combinations in order to achieve certain effects.

1. A natural effect is created when short lashes are mingled with medium-length lashes.
2. A more luxurious effect is created by using a mixture of short- and medium-length lashes with a few long ones added for glamor.
3. A very glamorous effect is achieved by using only long lashes, but it is rare that a client will request this style.
4. The extra-short lashes are used on lower lashes or in combination with others to achieve special effects.
5. Many different effects can be created by various combinations of different-length lashes.

PROCEDURE FOR UPPER LASHES (TOP)

1. Wash and sanitize your hands.
2. Check to see that all required supplies and sanitized implements are on hand.
3. Place the client in the makeup chair with her head at a comfortable working height.
4. Make sure that the client's face is well-lighted. However, for the client's comfort, make sure that the light does not shine directly into her eyes.
5. If the client has not already done so, remove all eye makeup. If the eyelashes are not entirely clean, the adhesive will not adhere properly.
6. Brush the client's lashes to make sure that they are clean and free from foreign matter. Brushing also separates lashes.
7. Discuss with the client the length of eyelashes desired and the effect she hopes to create. Try to create an effect that makes the eyelashes fuller and more attractive, yet not unnatural looking.
8. The esthetician works from behind or slightly to the side of the client, except when applying the bottom lashes.
9. Place a small amount of adhesive in the adhesive container. The adhesive dries very quickly; therefore, only a small quantity should be used at one time.
10. Using the tweezers, remove an eyelash from the tray. Hold the lash as close to the butt (bulb) end as possible. (See Fig. 25.114.)

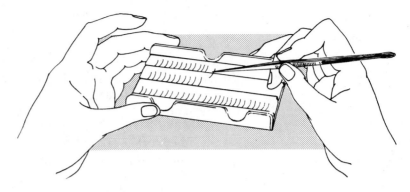

25.114—Remove eyelash from tray.

11. When the lash is free from the tray, move the tweezers past the center of the lash.
12. Brush the under side of the individual lash over the adhesive. (See Fig. 25.115.)

Note: To form an adhesive container, place a small piece of aluminum foil over the open end of a bottle cap.

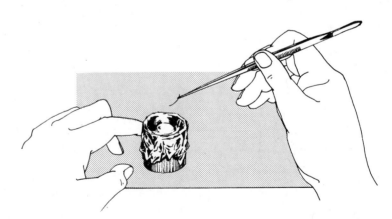

25.115—Apply adhesive.

13. Only a very small amount of adhesive is needed. If too much adhesive is picked up, brush off the excess with your fingertip.

14. If the client wears glasses, place the first lash in the center of the lid. Have the client put her glasses on. If the lash touches the glass, it is too long and a shorter length must be selected. If the lash does not touch, it may be used. (See Fig. 25.116.)

15. It is important to remember that the lash is held in the tweezers at exactly the same angle that it will be placed on the natural lash.

16. If you are right-handed, you will start applying lashes at the outer corner of the left eye, applying the lashes side by side until you reach the inner corner of the left eye. This method will prove to be the most efficient and time saving. The first two or three lashes applied to the outer corner and the last two or three lashes applied to the inner corner of the eye should be short, to give a gradual, more natural build up to the lashes.

17. Start the application procedure by brushing the adhesive from the underside of the individual lash onto the topside of the client's natural lash. Transfer the adhesive to the entire length of the natural lash, starting at the base (the part closest to the lid) and brushing out to the tip.

18. The individual lash is placed on top of the natural lash, as close to the eyelid as possible without actually touching the lid. (See Fig. 25.117.) For efficient performance, the tweezers must be kept free of adhesive.

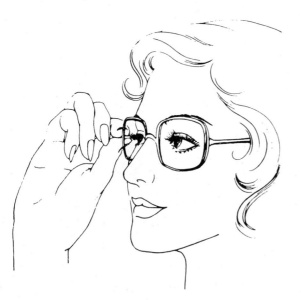

25.116—Be sure eyelashes do not touch glasses.

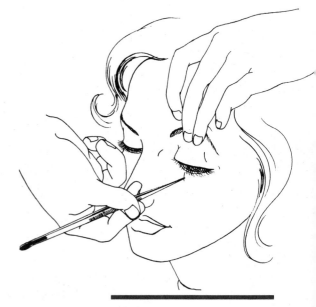

25.117—Place lash on top of natural lash.

19. Start the application of lashes to the other eye by applying the individual lashes to the inside corner of the eye, and continue placing the lashes side by side until reaching the outer corner of the eye.
20. For the inside corners of the eye, it may be necessary to use the thumb of the free hand to gently extend the eyelid and hold it taut. This exposes the natural inside corner of the eye and permits the placing of the artificial eyelash properly. (See Fig. 25.118.)
21. When necessary, the same technique is applied when attaching the outside corner lashes. (See Fig. 25.119.)
22. When attaching lashes in the corners of the eyes, the upper and lower lashes must be kept separated for several seconds to permit the adhesive to dry and prevent the eyelids from sticking together.

Note: If you are left-handed, follow the above procedure, but start at the outer corner of the right eye and work toward the left.

Clients who prefer individual eyelash application often have their lashes cared for by regular visits to the salon. The client should be instructed in how to care for the lashes at home in order to prevent loss of her own natural lashes and to avoid irritation to the eyes.

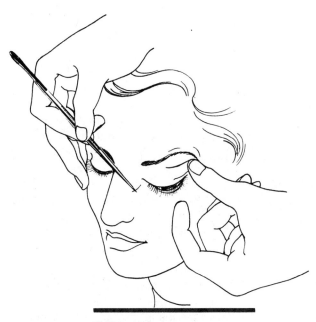

25.118—Pull eyelid taut to apply.

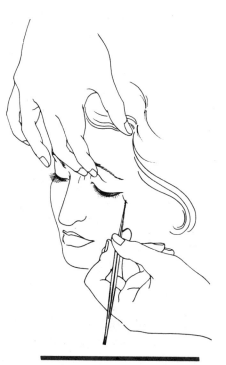

25.119—Attach at outside corner.

PROCEDURE FOR BOTTOM (LOWER) LASHES

The application of bottom (lower) lashes requires a different technique. The procedure is as follows:

1. The client is required to be in a sitting-up position facing you.
2. The client looks upward keeping the eyes open. (See Fig. 25.120.)
3. Only short lashes are used on the lower lids.
4. The procedure for picking up adhesive and applying bottom lashes is the same as for the upper lashes. The lash will curve downward.
5. Have the client hold her eyes open for a few extra seconds to allow the adhesive to dry.
6. More adhesive is used in the application of the lower lashes in order to assure a lasting application.

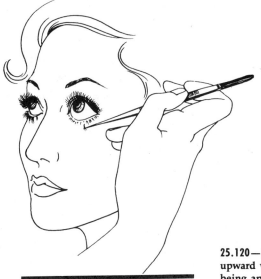

25.120—Have the client look upward while the lower lashes are being applied.

Caution: Clients should be advised that the natural oils from the eyelids tend to dissolve the adhesive. As a result, the lower artificial lashes will not stay on as long as the upper lashes. Lower lashes will begin to fall off about 1 week after application. Many clients will only need to have sparse eyelashes filled in so that they will appear thicker. The client should be advised that oil dissolves adhesive so extra care must be taken when cleansing with cleansing lotions and creams.

PROCEDURE FOR FILLING IN SPARSE LASHES

The individual lashes are angled slightly inward. This technique fills in all the gaps. Then a second set of eyelashes are cemented on top of the first set of lashes. The second set of lashes is also angled inwardly, effectively closing any gaps that may exist. In this way, clients with very sparse eyelashes can enjoy full, luxurious eyelashes.

REMOVING INDIVIDUAL LASHES

If it should become necessary to remove artificial eyelashes, do not, under any circumstances, attempt to pull them off. Pulling off the artificial eyelashes will also pull out the natural eyelashes.

Have the client sit directly in front of you. In order to protect her eyes, place an eye pad, shield, or tissue under her eyelid, with the eyes closed. Saturate a small, soft brush or cotton swab with eyelash remover. Gently brush or swab the eyelash until the adhesive dissolves and the lash can be removed. Or, the client may coat her lashes with baby oil before retiring. The oil will usually dissolve the adhesive overnight.

CARE OF LASHES

There are several disadvantages to the use of individual lashes. The client should be made aware of these disadvantages in advance. After application, the client must take every precaution to see that the lashes are not disturbed. She should not put her face under a shower or submerge her head under water when swimming. She must cleanse around the lashes with cotton swabs making sure not to touch the individual lashes with cleanser. Any light oil or cream, such as in moisturizers, night creams, and cleansers, that comes in contact with the lashes, will cause them to begin to peel off. It is not uncommon for a client who wears individual lashes to loose her own natural lashes when the artificial lashes come off. Very often lashes are lost in clumps. Many estheticians and cosmetologists feel the individual lashes are unsanitary. However, there are clients who wear the individual lashes and have no difficulty at all and will request individual eyelash application.

TEMPORARY APPLICATION AND FLARE-TYPE LASHES

Makeup artists often apply individual lashes with surgical adhesive at the end of a makeup to add fullness and glamor to the client's own lashes (especially for special occasions). The lashes are removed and discarded when the makeup is removed, or they may be left on for an extra day or two if extreme care is taken. In recent years, a new type of individual lash has been introduced on the market, which really is not an individual lash at all, but rather a few lashes arranged in a flare or fan shape. These are excellent to use after the makeup is applied. The lashes are attached with surgical adhesive. Five to seven flare lashes will fill in the client's natural lashes and it can be done quickly with good results (Fig. 25.121).

When a makeup artist applies individual lashes as part of a makeup, he or she should charge more for the makeup.

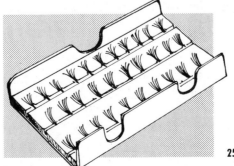

25.121—Flare type lashes

Eyelash and Eyebrow Tinting

An aniline (**AN**-i-leen) derivative should *never* be used for coloring eyebrows or eyelashes; to do so may cause *blindness*. Instead, a harmless coloring agent should be used.

The choice of color is limited to either brown or black. While black is favored in most cases, brown is recommended for very light blonde complexions. Follow the specific directions of the manufacturer when applying the coloring agent.

IMPLEMENTS AND SUPPLIES

Petroleum jelly (Vaseline™)	Bowl of clear water
Lash and brow tinting solutions (Solutions No. 1 and No. 2)	Towels
Stain remover	Cotton and toothpicks (to make applicator swabs)
Bowl of soapy water	Paper eye shields (Fig. 25.122)

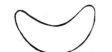

25.122—Paper eye shield

PREPARATION

1. Follow sanitary measures.
2. Place the client in a partially reclining position in the facial chair at approximately a 45 degree angle. *Do not* permit her to lie in a straight position. Such a position would permit the tinting solution to enter the eyes more easily.
3. Place a clean towel across the client's chest.

PROCEDURE

1. Wash lashes and brows with warm, soapy water, using a cotton pledget (a compress or small, flat mass of absorbent cotton). Remove all traces of cosmetic makeup from lashes and brows. (See Fig. 25.123.)
2. Apply petroleum jelly around eyes and on paper eye shields.
3. Adjust eyeshields. Ask patron to look up, adjust shield and close eye gently. Do the same with the other eye.
4. Apply No. 1 solution. Moisten cotton-tipped applicator with solution. Touch tip to towel to remove excess solution. Apply over and under lashes close to skin. Reapply several times. *Break the applicator stick, and discard. Use a fresh applicator stick each time solution is required.* (See Fig. 25.124.)

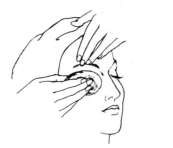

25.123—Wash lashes and brows with cool water.

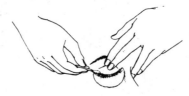

25.124—Apply solution to lashes.

5. Apply No. 1 solution to brows, following natural brow line. Reapply against natural growth, working solution in thoroughly. (See Fig. 25.125.) *Replace cap on No. 1 solution bottle.* (If bottle caps are interchanged, oxidation starts and the liquids lose their value.)

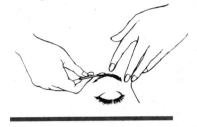

25.125—Apply solution to brows.

> **Note:** Moisten fresh applicator with stain remover and place on edge of towel for future use. Replace cap on stain remover bottle.

6. Apply No. 2 solution to lashes and brows in the same manner as No. 1 solution. If stain gets on skin, use stain remover immediately. *Replace cap on No. 2 bottle.*
7. Remove eyeshields and wash lashes and brows with soapy water, using cotton pledgets.
8. Rinse lashes and brows with clear water and cotton pledgets.

> **Note:** Soapy water for washing lashes and brows is made by adding baby shampoo to a bowl of water.

9. Remove stains with stain remover. Replace bottle cap.
10. Soothe skin with lotion or cream.
11. Clean up in the usual manner.

Help Your Clients to Discover Their Own Unique and Individual Look

THE NATURAL LOOK When doing makeup, a client will often ask for a natural-looking makeup. She means that she wants makeup that cannot be detected, or that it will appear to be her own natural beauty rather than an imposed one. When we speak of something as being "natural," we mean that it is existing in or produced by nature and has not been changed by artificial means. There are women, especially young women, who look their best with little or no makeup. Their main concern is with proper skin care and a well-groomed look. However, what we often take to be natural beauty is often an illusion created by the artistic use of cosmetics. During the consultation, you can determine how the client feels about makeup and how she wants to look. It is better if the client will allow you to use your own ideas in creating her personalized makeup. The more sophisticated client will usually welcome an opportunity to learn some new makeup techniques and try them all before deciding on the look she prefers. If a client expresses objections to certain makeup that you suggest, then it is best to go along with her wishes.

THE PROFESSIONAL WOMAN Millions of women are involved in careers of all types and their makeup and wardrobe needs differ. The woman working in some areas of the fashion industry, the entertainment field, or the beauty business, may want to wear the latest in clothing styles, makeup, and hairstyles. This is the woman who will test your fashion and artistic "know-how." Women in service professions will want to look their best, but will need a practical routine. For example, nurses, doctors, lawyers, policewomen, airline attendants, and pilots, (as well as women in other professions too numerous to mention here) are the women who will want to look fashionable but must be practical. Above all, today's busy women are concerned with having a healthy well-coordinated look from head to foot. A bit more makeup may be needed for some women to achieve their best look for business and social occasions. As an esthetician and/or makeup artist, you must remember that a great many women combine careers with home-making, and women who do not work outside the home are more often than not as beauty-conscious as women with full-time careers. The interest in makeup and other facets of beauty continues to grow, because modern day men and women are concerned with maintaining their good health and appearance. Your job is to satisfy the client's needs so that he or she will keep returning to the salon for products and services. In addition, you will have the satisfaction of knowing that you are providing a valuable service.

A Touch of Glamor

Your first consideration when doing makeup is that it must be suitable for the client's age, her personal coloring (eyes, skin, and hair), the time of day, and the nature of the occasion. Properly applied, glamor makeup enhances and beautifies. You have no doubt seen dozens of "before" and "after" make-overs in magazines and in the salon. These make-overs show that makeup can work magic, especially when glamor touches, such as contouring and artificial eyelashes, are included. A good makeup artist will realize that current glamor makeup trends may be perfect on a model with a flawless complexion and beautiful facial features, but that this same makeup may be grotesque on a not-so-perfect face. Perfection in makeup application comes when you discover how to give your client the feeling that she is radiantly beautiful in her own unique and individual way.

Quick Step-By-Step Makeup Application Practice Routine

The following step-by-step practice routine is designed to help you learn to gain speed and skill as you apply makeup. This routine gives you a quick reference of all you have learned about makeup so far. The beginning artist will find it helpful to keep the step-by-step routine handy while proceeding with a makeup on a classmate. You may wish to time yourself until you are able to give a complete makeup in 30 to 45 minutes.

PREPARATION Be sure to have everything you need for the makeup ready before you start.

1. *Prepare client*—Position the client in the makeup chair and do the necessary preparations, such as pinning back the hair and putting on a makeup cape or tucking tissue into the neckline of her dress.
2. *Sanitize hands*—Sanitize your hands with astringent or alcohol and dry them with a fresh towel or tissue.
3. *Apply cleanser*—Apply the appropriate cleanser to a wet cotton pad (or the fingers, if cotton pads are not available), and cleanse the face. Don't forget to use upward and outward movements. Use a second pad and more cleanser if necessary.
4. *Apply freshener*—Apply skin freshener or astringent with cotton pads.
5. *Apply moisturizer*—Apply protective lotion or moisturizer.
6. *Shape brows*—Shape the eyebrows if necessary.
7. *Apply foundation*—Test for correct foundation color on the jawline and select and apply the appropriate foundation.
8. *Apply corrective*—Apply corrective makeup as needed.
9. *Do contouring*—Do shading and highlighting of features as needed.
10. *Apply cheekcolor*—Cream blush is applied before face powder. Brush-on (dry) cheekcolor is applied after powder.
11. *Apply powder*—If you are using powder-type shading and highlighting cosmetics for corrective work and contouring, they may be applied after the powder. The cover-up may be used over the eyelids to block any discoloration and to form a base for eyeshadow. The shadow will cling to the cover-up cosmetic and make it last longer. If foundation gathers in the small creases under or around the eyes or in lines on the face, a small brush may be used to smooth out the foundation.
12. *Brush brows*—Brush the brows to remove excess powder.
13. *Apply eyeshadow*—Select and apply eyeshadow. Check with the client to see if she has a color preference or discuss your choice of color with her. She may welcome a change.
14. *Finish eyeshadow*—Clean off any excess shadow with a cotton-tipped swab. The client looks down when you apply shadow to the upper lid and she looks up when you apply it to the lower lid. Remember the ABCs of eyeshadow application. The main color goes on the lid, the darker color is applied into the crease, and the highlighting color is applied directly under the brow. Refer to color chart for flattering combinations on page 393 of Chapter 24.

15. *Apply eyeliner*—After the eyeshadow colors are applied, the eyeliner is applied. Most artists will use the cake eyeliner and mix it to the desired consistency. Remember that if you place your forefinger in the center of the eyelid, it will prevent blinking and smearing the liner during application. When the liner is applied about three-fourths across the eye, lift the brush and draw a line inward from the corner of the eye. Make the line slightly higher than the natural corner of the eye. Use cotton-tipped swabs when it is necessary to make corrections.

16. *Makeup eyebrows*—Make short strokes from the inner corner of the brow to the apex, then draw fine strokes downward to where you want the brow to end. Fill in as necessary. When the brows need no penciling, a touch of color can be added with a brush and dry brush-on type color. Eyebrows should be made up to look soft and natural. Harsh, dark, messy brows detract from the beauty of the face. Best colors are light, medium, and dark brown; titian for women with very red or auburn hair and black-brown for women with very dark hair. Sometimes two colors blended together will give the desired effect.

17. *Apply mascara*—Mascara is now applied to give the lashes a more luxurious look. Apply the mascara on the top side, then underneath the lashes. (The eyelid can be held firmly with your forefinger to keep the client from blinking.) Apply mascara to the underside of the upper lashes. Use a clean mascara brush to remove excess mascara and to separate the lashes. Apply a small amount of mascara to lower lashes. To keep mascara from smearing on the lower lid during the application, a cotton-tipped swab may be held beneath the lashes while the mascara is being applied.

> **Note:** Most stores that sell electric razors will stock accessory brushes that are used to clean razors. The small, round, spiral-tip brushes are perfect for cleaning excess mascara from lashes.

18. *Apply lipcolor*—Use the brush or a pencil to outline the lips in their most attractive shape. Brush on the lipcolor and blot the lips if necessary. The client is asked to part the lips and smile slightly during the lipcolor application. Lipstick application should be discussed with the client as you show her some new shades that may be attractive for her. Use a spatula to scrape the lipstick from the tube and then take the lipcolor onto the brush from the spatula. Remember, the client is aware of sanitary practices and no item must ever be used on more than one client unless it has been sterilized. Lip gloss can be mixed on the spatula with the lipcolor so that it will spread more easily and leave a soft moist glow to the lips.

19. *Inspect makeup*—The finished makeup should be inspected and touched up if necessary.
20. *Remove headband*—Remove the headband from the client's hair as well as the cape or tissue.
21. *Allow client to inspect makeup*—Give the client a hand mirror so that she can inspect the finished makeup.

Special Accents for Evening

After you have completed the client's makeup, she may want to know how to intensify or accent her makeup for evening wear. Add a deeper shadow in the crease of the eye, then add a frosted or silvered highlight beneath the eyebrow. A stronger or deeper cheekcolor may be applied and contouring makeup emphasized. A light film of frosted powder may be dusted over the entire face. A deeper lipcolor with added gleam may be applied. Some women like to add silver or gold to the eyelids for evening. Unusual makeup such as painting butterflies around the eyes is called "fantasy" makeup. Though you may not have an opportunity to apply fantasy makeup on a client in the salon, it is good practice in the classroom. It allows you to expand your imagination as you work with colors and shapes.

You the Professional Makeup Artist

Keep in mind as you progress as a makeup artist, that all artists do not follow the same routine for applying makeup, nor do they use the same products. Artists use their creative imagination with each client. The quick step-by-step practice routine presented here may be changed in sequence. If you prefer applying one part of the makeup before or after another, then by all means do so. However, you should remember that your main goal is to apply makeup efficiently and expertly, and to achieve the most beautiful makeup possible for your client. The more you do makeup applications, the more you will discover your own little "tricks" and techniques. You will find that most makeup artists follow the step-by-step routine or a similar routine for practical purposes. For example, it is easy to see why lipcolor is applied after the rest of the makeup. While applying eye makeup, the artist's hand could brush against the lips. It is helpful to learn a definite routine for makeup application first, then experiment until you know exactly what you will do with each face and why you are doing it that way. Never be so sure of yourself that you fail to listen to suggestions offered by other people. You can always learn from them. On the other hand, don't be afraid to develop your own creative imagination.

QUESTIONS DISCUSSION AND REVIEW

PROFESSIONAL MAKEUP TECHNIQUES

1. What are two things that are important to being a successful makeup artist?
2. What is more important to the salon, sales ability or artistic talent?
3. What is the main objective when applying makeup?
4. Why shouldn't you apply makeup to a client who is in a reclining position?
5. Describe the ideal makeup mirror.
6. Briefly explain how to prepare the client's skin for a makeup application.
7. Which facial shape is considered to be ideal?
8. Can makeup be used to help correct uneven features?
9. How would you remove extremely heavy eyebrows?
10. In what direction do you tweeze brows?
11. Why is liquid foundation the most popular?
12. What makeup foundation is often used for theatrical makeup?
13. How would you cover blemishes?
14. What is the most popular form of blush?
15. How should blush color be applied?
16. What effect will cream blush give your client?
17. How is eyeshadow chosen?
18. What does liner do for the eye?
19. What is the purpose of mascara?
20. What chemical compound used in makeup can give an "ashy" appearance to dark skin?
21. Name two basic types of artificial eyelashes.
22. What is the best type of adhesive for eyelashes?
23. Can some women be allergic to adhesive eyelashes?

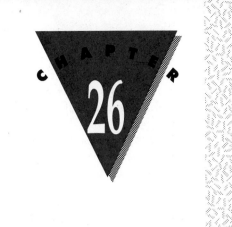

The Salon Business

LEARNING OBJECTIVES

After completing this chapter, you should be able to:

❶ Explain the basic business building blocks and how they relate to successful salon management.

❷ Discuss how to develop a business.

❸ Discuss how to keep employees and public relations.

❹ Explain planning—the physical layout of a salon.

❺ Discuss the average expenses for a salon.

❻ Explain bookings for a salon and record keeping.

❼ Discuss the different types of business ownership.

❽ Discuss the different telephone techniques needed in the salon.

❾ Explain the importance of first aid in the salon.

INTRODUCTION

Personal well-being has never been higher on America's priority list than it is right now in the 1990's. This trend hasn't happened overnight nor will it likely fade away in the foreseeable future. Actually, it's a safe bet to assume that attention to oneself is here to stay.

The significance of this is that many new and lucrative opportunities exist for those in the personal care business, including cosmetology and esthetics. Managing and/or owning a salon is a viable career option for you.

This chapter is devoted to the business principles and marketing techniques that can make the option of owning or managing a personally and financially rewarding experience.

The Challenge

With the potential rewards that come with ownership, come additional responsibility and the need for new skills development. As a salon owner, are you an esthetician first or a businessperson first? Successful operation requires that you be both at the same time.

In essence, you will be learning how to be a businessperson and be teaching associates how to be top professional estheticians; all while building clientele, paying bills, and feeling your way along during the start-up period.

The owner or manager of a full-service or special-service salon must have the proper qualifications. In addition to formal training, working in different types of salons and dealing with a variety of clients, helps build valuable background and experience.

Going into your own business is a big responsibility and not a step to be taken without serious planning. A knowledge of business principles, bookkeeping, business law, insurance, salesmanship and psychology is crucial to the esthetician who aspires to be an owner and/or manager of a salon.

The first-time entrepreneur might consider opening a skin care/makeup department in an already established full-service salon. The benefits include a well-established location with an existing clientele to draw from. Many of the other concerns will be the same as starting a special-service salon from the bottom up. You will need an experienced, well-trained staff, all the necessary equipment (for example, chairs, beds, tables, facial machines, mirrors, tweezers, brushes, cosmetics, etc.), insurance, a business plan, and an innovative advertising campaign.

Basic Business Building Blocks

Three major building blocks constitute the success of a business: costs, revenues (sales), and profit.

Simply stated, your profit is what you make after everyone's been paid. While that may seem to be the most elementary of issues in understanding how to run a business, it is the one issue that causes most business failures.

GETTING STARTED The very first order of business for your operation is to select an accountant. The person must be one that is strictly a "busness" accountant and someone you can communicate easily with on financial matters.

The right accountant for you will take the headaches and heartaches out of practically every financial decision you have to make by merely presenting the "pros" and "cons" in understandable terms. If you choose, your accountant will recommend alternate methods to consider and give recommendations based on your business's status.

You should also select a lawyer to counsel you on business matters including leases, contracts, and local ordinances.

These advisors are well aware of the stress involved in starting a business and will generally negotiate fees to fit your situation. The time and money saved over the life of a business using these services more than compensates for the expense.

COSTS

As part of your business operation, you must always know where your money is being spent. It is always a good idea to apportion your money so that maximum benefit is derived from it.

Costs to operate your own salon break into *fixed* and *variable*. Fixed being costs that are constant for at least a 1 year period (rent, mortgage); variable meaning costs that fluctuate on a monthly basis.

Examples of each might include:

Fixed Costs	*Variable Costs*
• Rent/Mortgages	• Utilities
• Salaries	• Supplies
• Insurance	• Promotion
• Equipment leases	• Postage
	• Taxes

Getting a handle on costs will give you an important insight on how to start and develop the business. You will also know the amount of revenue (sales) you will need to break even or make a profit.

Note: This is one of the areas in which an accountant is an invaluable asset.

REVENUES/PROFITS

Revenues are amassed by selling services and products to customers at *competitive* and *profitable* prices. When you determine specific services and products you can offer, and at what price, you can figure the average weekly and monthly numbers necessary to meet costs and make a profit. This is referred to as business forecasting or projections.

Analyzing your actual business versus your forecast enables you to make good business decisions. For example, adjusting variable costs to capitalize on growth (add personnel, increase supplies, etc.); adjusting variables to neutralize down periods (cut supplies by *x* percent; and rearrange employee schedules, etc.).

Forecast Chart (Expand depth to include most common services)

SERVICES/PRODUCTS	PRICE	NO. PER MONTH	$ TOTAL REVENUE PER MONTH	PER YEAR
One-hour facial treatment	$00	*xx*	$00	$00
Etc.				
Etc.				
Etc.				
Etc.				
Total	(NA)			

Profit Calculator

Total $ Revenue _____ *minus* Total $ Cost _____ *Equals* Total Profit _____

Creating "Your" Salon

After becoming comfortable with the basics of business, the next step is "creating" your salon. This part of developing a business is the most enjoyable, because at this stage, it can be anything you want it to be. There are a few "givens," such as good location and ample parking, which will be discussed in this section in more detail. However, it is here where your creativity takes over and injects the personality and flair that will differentiate your salon from others. You must create the reasons why a customer chooses your salon when all other things apparently are equal, such as price, location, and hours.

LOCATION   A good location will have a population large enough to support the salon. When possible, the salon should be located near other active business places that attract potential clients, such as restaurants, department stores, or supermarkets. Unless you can afford to do a great deal of advertising, it is difficult to operate a successful salon in a low-traffic area. Also, people are drawn to shopping areas where they can make one stop and serve several purposes.

The salon should be clearly visible and "eye catching" in order to attract the attention of people walking or driving by. Avoid too much competition in the immediate area. It is better to locate where no other salon exists.

Study the trading area for potential clients. Find out about the size, income, and buying habits of the area's population. Talk to other business owners to see how they feel a salon would be accepted in the area.

PARKING FACILITIES When selecting a site for a new business or planning to take over an established business, you must consider parking facilities. People hesitate to patronize a business that is inconvenient to reach during bad weather. If possible, locate the salon near public transportation. This will attract clients who do not drive. If your salon is open for evening service, the area should be well-lighted.

PROPERTY LEASES You live with the problems or amenities written into your lease; so it's to your advantage to negotiate everything that is important to you. Short-term (1 year) leases are best, with options to extend. Things to be negotiated include:

- Modification of existing space
- Floor coverings
- Added outlets
- Clean up, maintenance (in salon, policing grounds)
- Water capacity
- Utility costs
- Storage
- Weekend, evening hours

Before signing a lease, review it with your attorney and accountant for advice.

EQUIPMENT LEASES Practically anything you will need can be leased (phones, computers, machines, etc.). More and more, small businesses are becoming "leasers" instead of owners. If you wish to lease equipment, study the terms carefully. Make sure they are in line with your cost projections. Review them with your attorney and accountant.

INSURANCES Various insurances are a must when owning a business. They include fire, liability, employee, theft, occupancy, and equipment extended warranties. Again, your accountant will be of great service in determining the necessities in terms of "required-by-law" and directory coverages.

Your salon's employees will make or break your business (Fig. 26.1). It's imperative that you select them on a basis of several criteria:

- General skill level for the job
- Overall attitude and personality to fit your image
- Doers
- Pleasant to be around (for owner and customers)

Skills can be developed through training. Personality and attitude are traits that rarely change.

Each employee should have formal, initial training as well as an ongoing training regimen.

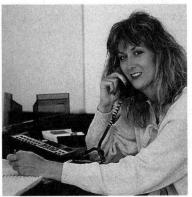

26.1—Salon receptionist

Basic
- Overall goals and mission of the business
- Customer, vendor, visitor interface
- Telephone skills
- Medical—burns, bruises, illness detection; at least one person should be qualified in CPR administration.

Sales
- Every employee is a salesperson. They should suggest add-on services and pre-appointments, however, they should not be overpowering or forceful.

Receptionist
- Secretarial skills, bookkeeping, basic computer skills, bookings, basic financial knowledge

TIPS ON HIRING AND KEEPING TOP PEOPLE

Take the time to write a brief job description for each employee, so they have parameters by which to judge their performance and you have a way to evaluate them for reward or criticism of the efforts they put forth.

Always treat employees with complete dignity doing what you can to help in any job-related issue. Reward for exemplary effort, discuss and guide for efforts not to the standard you both have set by virtue of the job description. Consistency is a must and a responsibility of the owner.

PUBLIC RELATIONS

No matter how small your business, its potential for positive public and community relations is boundless. Make sure you notify local newspapers of your opening, new employees, new services, expansions, and whatever else might be interesting to your customer base.

Join local business associations with the intent to be an active contributor in time and ideas. As your community goes, your business goes.

MERCHANDISING

Merchandising is often a forgotten marketing gem. Generally, an activity or program is planned in conjunction with a vendor or specialist.

Ask your vendors about "free" samples of their product for you to test and, when appropriate, hand them out to customers. Use literature or promotional materials provided by them to explain products and services to your customers.

CUSTOMER SERVICE

Far above any other asset that your business has, is its customers. For any number of reasons, a customer chooses you to perform a service. From the instant the customer enters your salon, impressions and perceptions are formed, creating a positive or negative reaction by the potential client. Your best approach is to always have a positive attitude.

In most business environments, getting first-time customers is fairly easy to do. Keeping them is what will make your business succeed.

Planning the Physical Layout

The layout of a salon takes a considerable amount of planning in order to achieve efficiency and economy (Figs. 26.2 and 26.3).

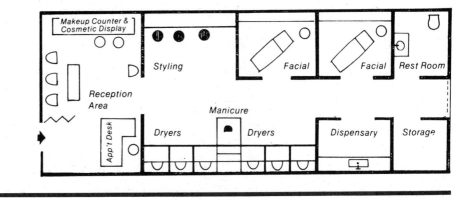

26.2—Full-service salon

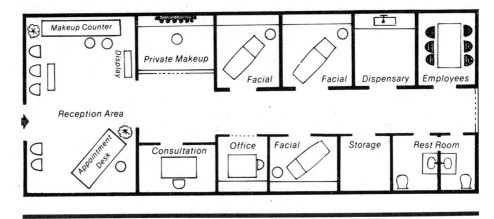

26.3—Facial and makeup salon

The salon should have:

1. Maximum efficiency of operation
2. Adequate aisle space
3. The flow of operational services toward the reception room with amenities such as phone, coffee, magazines, and pleasant music
4. Enough space for each piece of equipment
5. Furniture, fixtures, and equipment chosen on the basis of cost, durability, utility, and appearance. The purchase of standard and guaranteed equipment is a worthwhile investment.

6. A color scheme that is restful and flattering to both males and females (young adult to senior groups)
7. A dispensary and plenty of storage space
8. A clean restroom containing toilet and basin
9. Good plumbing and sufficient lighting for satisfactory services
10. Air conditioning and heating

The reception area should not be overlooked when you plan the layout of your salon. This is the first contact a client has with your establishment, and it sets the tone for the rest of their experience at your salon. An attractively decorated reception area can be one of your best promotional tools, as it immediately makes a client comfortable, and gives the impression that this is a salon that cares about the comfort of its clients. It can also be an eyecatcher for people who pass by and may become prospects for your services.

While proper image is essential to the business, sales efforts and tools must be considered in all planning. Repeat, referral, and add-on sales make the enterprise continue to grow.

Business Operation and Personnel Management

Business problems are numerous, especially when you start a new salon. Contributing causes to salon failures are:

1. Inexperience in dealing with the public and with employees
2. Not enough capital to carry the business through until established
3. Poor location
4. Too high overhead expenses
5. Lack of proper basic training
6. Business neglect and careless bookkeeping methods

The owner or manager must have a business sense, knowledge, ability, good judgment, and diplomacy.

Smooth salon management depends on:

1. Sufficient investment capital
2. Efficiency of management
3. Cooperation between management and employees
4. Good business procedures
5. Trained and experienced personnel in the salon

BE A LEADER OF BEAUTY FASHION

There is no surer way of introducing your services than by using them yourself.

You can be your own best advertisement of the services you perform. In addition, by looking good yourself, you can motivate your clients to do the same.

ALLOCATION OF MONEY Budgeting is essential to good business practices in that it tells you where you are financially, where you are deficient, and where you are on target with the overall plan.

The following figures may be subject to variation in different localities. In large towns and cities items such as rent may run higher, while in small towns rent may be lower and utilities and telephone, higher. *The figures are suggested merely as a general guide.*

Theoretical Expenses for Salons in the United States (Based on total gross income)

	THEORETICAL PERCENT	YOUR EXPENSES PERCENT
Salaries and commissions (including payroll taxes)	53.5	_____
Rent	13	_____
Supplies	5	_____
Advertising	3	_____
Depreciation	3	_____
Laundry	1	_____
Cleaning	1	_____
Light and power	1	_____
Repairs	1.5	_____
Insurance	.75	_____
Telephone	.75	_____
Miscellaneous expenses	1.5	_____
Total expense	85	_____
Net profit	15	_____

You will note that the largest items of expense are salaries, rent, supplies, and advertising. The first three merit your closest attention. The advertising item can be adjusted at your discretion.

When opening a salon it is important to have enough working capital. It often takes time for a new business to build a clientele, so money must be available to take care of necessary expenses. As overhead is met and profits become greater, the budget may be increased to cover more advertising and to expand in other areas.

BOOKING APPOINTMENTS *Booking appointments* must be done with care, for booking can make the difference between success and failure. Services are sold in terms of time on the appointment page. Time, depending on how it is used, may spell either a gain or a loss.

Business Administration

Good business administration demands the keeping of a simple and efficient record system. Records are of value only if they are correct, concise, and complete. Bookkeeping means keeping an accurate record of all income and expenses. Income is usually classified as income from services and income from retail sales. Expenses include rent, utilities, insurance, salaries, advertising, equipment, repairs, etc. The assistance of an accountant will prove valuable. For tax purposes it is imperative to retain check stubs, cancelled checks, receipts, and invoices.

Proper business records are necessary to meet the requirements of local, state, and federal laws regarding taxes and employees.

All business transactions must be recorded in order to maintain proper records. These are required by the owner, or manager, for the following reasons:

1. For efficient operation of the salon
2. For determining income, expenses, profit, and loss
3. For proving the value of the salon to prospective buyers
4. For arranging a bank loan
5. For such reports as income tax, social security, unemployment and disability insurance, wage and hour law, accident compensation, and labor tax

DAILY RECORDS ARE IMPORTANT

Keeping daily records enables the owner, or manager, to know just how the business is progressing. A weekly or monthly summary helps to:

1. Make comparisons with other years
2. Detect any changes in demands for different services
3. Order necessary supplies
4. Check on the use of materials according to the type of service rendered
5. Control expenses and waste

Each expense items bears on the total gross income. Accurate records show the cost of operation in relation to income.

Keep daily sales slips, appointment book, and a petty cash book for at least 6 months. Payroll book, cancelled checks, and monthly and yearly records are usually held for at least 7 years. *Service* and *inventory* records are also important to keep. Sales records help to maintain a perpetual inventory. An organized inventory system can be used to:

1. Prevent overstocking
2. Prevent running short of supplies needed for services
3. Help in establishing the net worth at the end of the year

KEEP CUSTOMER SERVICE RECORDS

A *customer service and care record* should be kept of treatments given and merchandise sold to each client. Such information is the basis for timely suggestions and uniform services, which result in increased sales. For this purpose, use a card file system or memorandum book.

All service records should contain the name and address of the client, date, amount charged, product used, and results obtained. Also, note the client's preference and taste.

Keep a running inventory of all supplies. Classify them as to their use and retail value. Those to be used in the business are *consumption* supplies. Those to be sold are *retail* supplies. Consulting the inventory records indicates which merchandise is most popular, and prevents the running short of any item. In reordering, buy sufficient merchandise that can be used or sold quickly within a reasonable period of time. It is a better policy to have a slight excess rather than a deficiency of supplies.

APPOINTMENT RECORD

The use of a private **appointment record** helps the esthetician to arrange working time to suit the client's convenience. The appointment book accurately reflects what is taking place in the salon at a given time. The esthetician who makes advance preparation can render prompt and efficient service when the client arrives. Besides, waste in time and money is prevented.

Ownership Options and Regulations

A salon may be owned and operated by an *individual*, a *partnership*, or a *corporation*. Before deciding which type of ownership is most desirable, you should be acquainted with the relative merits of each.

INDIVIDUAL OWNERSHIP

1. The proprietor is boss and manager.
2. The proprietor can determine policies and make decisions.
3. The proprietor receives all profits and bears all losses.

PARTNERSHIP

1. More capital is available for investment.
2. The combined ability and experience of each partner make it easier to share work and responsibilities, and to make decisions.
3. Profits are equally shared.
4. Each partner assumes each other's unlimited liability for debts.

CORPORATION

1. A charter has to be obtained from the state.
2. A corporation is subject to taxation and regulation by the state.
3. The management is in the hands of a board of directors who determine policies and make decisions in accordance with the constitution of the charter.
4. The dividing of profits is proportionate to the number of shares possessed by each stockholder.
5. The stockholder is not legally responsible for losses.

BEFORE BUYING OR SELLING AN ESTABLISHED SALON

1. A written purchase and sale agreement should be formulated in order to avoid any misunderstandings between the contracting parties. (Consult your attorney and accountant.)
2. For safekeeping and enforcement, the written agreement should be placed in the hands of an impartial third person, who is to deliver the agreement to the grantee (one to whom the property is transferred upon the fulfillment of the specified contract).
3. The buyer or seller should take and sign a complete statement of inventory (goods, fixtures, etc.) and the value of each article.
4. If there is a transfer of mortgage, notes, lease, and bill of sale, an investigation should be made to determine any default in the payment of debts.
5. Consult your lawyer for additional guidance.

AGREEMENT TO BUY A SALON

An agreement to buy an established salon should include the following:

1. Correct identity of owner
2. True representations concerning the value and inducements offered to buy the salon
3. Use of salon's name and reputation for a definite period of time
4. An understanding that the seller will not compete with the prospective owner within a reasonable distance from present location

PROTECTION IN MAKING A LEASE

1. Secure exemption of fixtures or appliances, which may be attached to the store or loft, so that they can be removed without violating the lease.
2. Insert into the lease an agreement relative to necessary renovations and repairs, such as painting, plumbing, fixtures, and electrical installation.
3. Secure an option from the landlord to assign the lease to another person; in this way, the obligations for the payment of rental are kept separate from the responsibilities of operating the business.

PROTECTION AGAINST FIRE, THEFT, AND LAWSUITS

1. Employ honest and able employees, and keep premises securely locked.
2. Follow safety precautions to prevent fire, injury, and lawsuits. Liability, fire, malpractice, and burglary insurance should be obtained.
3. Do not violate the medical practice law of your state by attempting to diagnose, treat, or cure a disease.
4. Become thoroughly familiar with all laws governing cosmetology and your special field, and the sanitary code of your city and state.
5. Keep accurate records of the number of workers, salaries, length of employment, and social security numbers, for various state and federal laws that affect the social welfare of employees.

 Note: Ignorance of the law is no excuse for its violation.

Summary

Important things to consider when going into business:

CAPITAL
Amount available
Amount required

ORGANIZATION
Individual, Partnership, Corporation

BANKING
Opening a bank account
Deposits, drawing checks
Monthly statements
Notes and drafts

SELECTING LOCATION
Population
Transportation facilities
Transients
Trade possibilities
Space required
Zoning ordinances
Parking

DECORATING AND FLOOR PLAN
Selection of furniture
Floor covering
Installing telephone
Interior decorating
Exterior decorating
Window displays
Electric signs

EQUIPMENT AND SUPPLIES
Selecting equipment
Comparative values
Installation
Labor-saving steps

ADVERTISING
Planning
Direct mail
Local organizations
Newspaper
Radio
Television

LEGAL
Lease, Contracts
Claims and lawsuits

BOOKKEEPING SYSTEM
Installation
Record of appointments
Receipts and disbursements
Petty cash
Profit and loss
Inventory

COST OF OPERATION
Supplies, Depreciation, Rent, Light
Salaries, Telephone, Linen service,
Taxes, Sundries

MANAGEMENT
Methods of building goodwill
Analysis of materials and labor in
    relation to service charges
Greeting patrons
Adjusting complaints
Handling employees
Selling merchandise
Telephone techniques

OFFICE ADMINISTRATION
Stationery and office supplies
Inventory

INSURANCE
Public liability and malpractice
Compensation, Unemployment
Social Security
Fire, Theft, Burglary

METHODS OF PAYMENT
In advance
C.O.D.
Open account
Time payments

**COMPLIANCE WITH
LABOR LAWS**
Minimum wage law
Hours of employment
Minors

ETHICS
Courtesy
Observation of professional trade
    practices

COMPLIANCE WITH STATE COSMETOLOGY LAW governing physical layout of
salon and equipment

LICENSING of salons, salon managers, cosmetologists, and estheticians

Telephone Techniques for the Salon

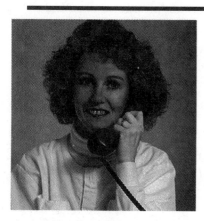

26.4—The telephone is an important part of the salon business.

An important part of the salon business is handled over the telephone. *Good telephone habits* and *techniques* make it possible for the salon owner and esthetician to increase business and win friends. With each call, you have a chance to build up the salon's reputation by rendering service of high calibre (Fig. 26.4).

The telephone serves many useful purposes in the salon, such as:

1. To make or change appointments
2. To go after new business, or strayed or infrequent clients
3. To remind clients of needed services
4. To answer questions and render friendly service
5. To adjust complaints and satisfy clients
6. To receive messages
7. To order equipment and supplies

Your success in using the phone depends to a large extent on the thoughtful effort exerted in observing certain fundamental principles. To the extent that these requirements are fulfilled, the telephone can be a very helpful aid to the success of the salon.

Business in the salon can be effectively promoted over the phone, provided there is:

1. Good planning
2. Good telephone usage

GOOD PLANNING   *Good planning* consists mainly of assigning the *right person* and giving him or her the necessary information with which to do a good telephone job.

An understanding and capable person should be put in charge of telephone calls. He or she should be thoroughly familiar with the prices charged for the various beauty services, and be able to recommend appropriate services to fit the needs of the client. A reliable substitute should be trained to handle the salon's calls when it is necessary for the regular person to be absent.

Next in importance is to have the phone located in a convenient and quiet place. A comfortable seat should be provided. Near the phone, there should be an appointment book readily accessible, client's record cards, a pencil or ball point pen, and a pad of paper. To save time, have available an up-to-date list of telephone numbers commonly used, and a recent telephone directory.

Good business practice requires that the salon's telephone number be freely and prominently displayed on stationery, advertising circulars, newspaper ads, and appointment cards. Business cards should be readily available on the receptionist's desk, and in the reception area. They save clients the trouble of having to look up the salon's phone number, making it easier for them to call your salon.

GOOD USAGE   *Good telephone usage* can best be described as the golden rule of dealing with others as you would have them deal with you. The motto should be *"Phone as you would like to be phoned to."* When put into daily practice, it really means saying or doing the right thing at the right time, and in the right manner.

Good telephone usage requires the application of a few basic principles that add up to *"common sense and common courtesy."*

YOUR GREETINGS   The first thing the caller wants to know is the name of the speaker and the salon he or she represents. The proper way to answer the telephone is to say, "Good morning (afternoon or evening), (your name) speaking. This is (name of your salon)." Following this brief introduction, you may say, "May I help you?"

The first few words you say over the phone immediately register your personality and can lead prestige to the salon. That is why it is so important to greet every caller with a cordial welcome. It shows that you are pleased to receive the call and want to be of service.

BASIC RULES   You, or any person answering the salon telephone, should follow these four basic rules for good telephone usage:

1. Display an interested, helpful attitude, as revealed by the tone of your voice and what you have to say.
2. Be prompt. Answer all calls as quickly as possible. Nothing irritates the caller more than waiting for you to answer.
3. Practice giving all necessary information to the caller. This means identifying yourself and your salon when making or receiving a call. If the requested information is not readily available, be courteous enough to say, "Will you please hold the line while I get the information for you?" Then put the caller on "hold."
4. Be tactful. Avoid saying or doing anything that may offend or irritate the caller. The tactful telephone user is careful:
   a. To inquire as to who is calling by saying, "May I tell Mr. Smith who is calling, please?" or "May I have your name, please?" Refrain from using such blunt questions as "Who's calling?"
   b. To address people by their last names. Make use of such expressions as "Thank you," and "I'm sorry" or "Excuse me."
   c. To avoid making side remarks during a call.
   d. To let the caller end the conversation. Do not bang down the receiver at the end of a call.

YOUR VOICE AND SPEECH

Everytime you telephone someone, you make a definite impression—good, bad, or indifferent. Your voice, what you say, and how you say it are what reveal you to others.

If you want a good telephone personality, then be sure to acquire the habit of:

1. Clear speech
2. Correct speech
3. Pleasing tone of voice

In this way, the other person hearing your voice will readily understand what you are saying.

As a general rule, the most effective speech is that which is correct, and at the same time, natural. A cheerful, alert, and enthusiastic voice most often comes from a person who has these desirable qualities as part of his or her personality.

To make a good impression over the phone, assume good posture; relax and draw a deep breath before answering the phone. Open the mouth, pronounce the words distinctly, use a low-pitched natural voice, and speak at a moderate pace. Clear voices carry better than loud voices over the phone.

If your listeners sometimes break in with such remarks as "What was that?" or "I'm sorry, I didn't get that," it usually means that your voice is not doing its job well. In that event, you should try to find out what is wrong and have it corrected. The more common causes of this condition may be:

1. You are speaking too loudly or too softly.
2. Your lips are too close or too far away from the mouthpiece. They should be about the width of two fingers from the mouthpiece.
3. The pitch of your voice is too low or too high.
4. Your pronunciation is not precise.

PLANNING YOUR TELEPHONE CONVERSATION

Whether it be a friendly chat or a business conversation, list the main points on your pad so you will know what to say. In this way, you will project an image of someone who knows how to handle all types of situations in an efficient manner. The salon will benefit from this image, as clients will obtain a favorable impression of the people who are employed there.

If a client is talking to you in a lengthy conversation, take notes of the main points of the conversation. When you answer, you will be able to address yourself to the points in which the client expressed interest.

EFFECTIVE TELEPHONE TECHNIQUES

Regular observance of the simple requirements of good telephone practice will help you make friends, bring in more business, and create goodwill for the salon.

To acquire skill in handling different situations and clients, you should study and practice the following effective telephone techniques:

1. Booking appointments by phone
2. Adjusting complaints over the phone
3. Answering price objections over the phone

BOOKING APPOINTMENTS BY PHONE

Whoever is assigned to handle salon appointments has an important responsibility. For this task, special qualifications and experience are required, such as:

1. Being familiar with all types of services and products available in the salon, and the prices to be charged
2. Being familiar with the quality of work done by each employee
3. Using judgment in giving assignments and being fair
4. Being accurate in recording name, service, and time when making appointments
5. Spacing appointments uniformly to permit the efficient functioning of the salon
6. Confirming appointments by telephone—A salon can lose a lot of business by cancelled appointments. There are clients who wait until the last minute to cancel or just do not show up for appointments. When this happens, the esthetician's time is lost because no one else has been booked to fill this time. It may be extra work for the receptionist, but it is a good policy to call the client the day before the appointment. The client should be told who is calling, and that it is a call to confirm his or her appointment. The client will appreciate the courtesy, and if he or she plans to cancel, will probably feel obligated either to do so immediately or to keep the appointment. If the appointment is cancelled, there is a better chance of filling the vacant time slot.
7. Time is money—When appointments are booked on the hour and a client is late (15 minutes or more), it puts the esthetician behind schedule with all the appointments for the day. In this case, the client should be told tactfully, that a step in the treatment will be shorter because other clients cannot be kept waiting past their appointment time. The client will make an effort to be on time for the next appointment. The client should understand that an esthetician has a time schedule and that loss of time is loss of money. The esthetician must also be considerate of the client's time and avoid running the treatment past the appointment time. If the client wishes to purchase products, service should be efficient and courteous. A client should never be ignored while employees engage in personal conversations in the salon or on the telephone. When more than one client is waiting to be served, it is courteous to pause, acknowledge the client who is waiting, and then serve the client as soon as possible.

First Aid

Emergencies arise in every line of business, and a knowledge of first aid measures is invaluable to the salon management and staff.

A physician (or emergency ambulance) should be called as soon as possible after any accident has occurred, both as a courtesy to the patient and as a protection to the salon.

For more information about emergency care, consult the latest edition of the First Aid Manual published by the American Red Cross.

> **Caution:** We suggest that you do *not* recommend any treatment for specific emergencies.

IN CASE OF EMERGENCY

Every salon should have information that may be needed in case of emergency posted or placed (in clear view) near the telephone. The owner of the salon or manager should have the names, addresses, and telephone numbers of employees on file in case of emergency. The file that is kept for regular clients should also have information that might be needed in case of emergency. The following information should be placed near the salon telephone:

Fire station

Police (local and state)

Emergency ambulance

Nearest hospital emergency room

Taxi service

Telephone numbers of persons and organizations that provide service

Also, a first-aid kit should be kept and employees notified where it is. With today's rapid-response paramedic system, your primary role in the event of emergency is to maintain calm and direct the situation as best as possible.

Utility service companies such as electricity, water, heat, air-conditioning, etc., should also be posted. Additional information that should be included are the names and telephone numbers of the owner and/or manager, custodian, and others who might need to be called if something goes wrong during his or her absence.

Each employee should know where exits are located and how to evacuate the building efficiently in case of fire or other emergencies. Fire extinguishers should be placed where they can be reached easily, and employees should know how to use them. A well-stocked first-aid kit should be kept within easy reach.

QUESTIONS DISCUSSION AND REVIEW

THE SALON BUSINESS

1. What are the three major building blocks of a business?
2. When getting started in a business, what two people should you select to help you with financial matters?
3. Give examples of fixed costs and variable costs.
4. What should you do before signing a lease?
5. List the different types of insurances needed for a salon.
6. What is the criteria when selecting employees for your business?
7. List ten needs to consider when planning a layout of a salon.
8. List the contributing factors to salon failures.
9. What are the highest expenses in a salon?
10. Why is the use of time so important in a salon?
11. Why is it important to keep accurate records of income and expenses?
12. Why is an organized inventory system used in the salon?
13. Explain the purpose of a service record card.
14. List the three types of ownership for a salon.
15. What should be included in an agreement when buying an established salon?
16. List important things to consider when going into business.
17. What can a salon gain with the use of good telephone habits and techniques?
18. What does the motto "Phone as you would like to be phoned to" mean?
19. When answering the salon telephone, what are the four basic rules?
20. Name three qualities of a good telephone personality.
21. What information should be kept in the salon in case of an emergency?

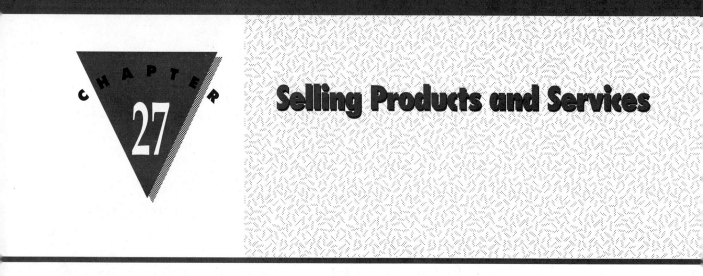

Selling Products and Services

LEARNING OBJECTIVES

After completing this chapter, you should be able to:

❶ Explain selling and why it's important to the salon.
❷ Discuss promotions and how they work for the salon.
❸ Discuss advertising and how to make it work for the salon.
❹ Discuss communication skills and why they are important.
❺ Demonstrate how to set up a retail display.

INTRODUCTION

To be successful—that is, to serve your clients well, to earn a good living, and to be recognized and respected as a professional—you must sell your services and products. From the outset, you must be aware that selling is a critical link in service between yourself and the client. Some estheticians shrink from the thought of themselves as salespeople. This is because they have a false, often stereotypical image of what selling is. If the word "sell" conjures up images in your mind of an obnoxious, fast-talking used car salesman in a plaid suit, relax. Nothing could be farther from the truth.

What Selling Is

Selling is *ethical*. It is how honest businesspeople provide good products and services to the people who need them.

Selling is *helping*. The best salespeople in any industry are sought out by their customers and clients. Why? Because these top performers work hard to understand their clients' needs, and then offer the goods or services that will satisfy them. In other words, they sell benefits, not simply products or services. And they don't push or wheel-and-deal; they advise. This approach, called **consultative selling**, should be the basis of your own sales philosophy.

Selling is a natural consequence of your *enthusiasm*, your *self-confidence*, and your *professionalism*. In a sense, people buy a relationship with a product or service, especially in a field as personal as esthetics. Your clients will be seeking products and services that satisfy their esthetic needs. They will look to you for guidance. If you are self-assured, enthusiastic, and professional, they will place their trust in you and purchase the products and services that you recommend.

Selling is *everybody's business*. Whether you work at the reception desk, answer a phone, take a class on new techniques, or give a facial, you are selling. Everything you do that has an impact on how well you serve your clients and on how good they feel when they have any contact with or visit your salon, is part of selling.

Promotions

In order to get noticed, you must do something special. That's why traffic cops use whistles: to be heard through the dull roar of traffic. In order to be heard above the dull roar of other businesses competing vigorously for consumer dollars, you must promote your business through the most effective means available. Without good promotion, sales would stagnate or decline, so it's imperative that you *promote* your business wisely and consistently.

SHORT-TERM BENEFITS OF PROMOTIONS

A promotion helps bring in clients right away and helps to get you through a lean period. If you are overstocked on certain products, it can help you clear out your inventory. (Remember that unsold inventory costs you money.)

Promotions also help *introduce clients to new products and services*. If you are introducing a new line of makeup or a new service such as aromatherapy, a promotion entices clients to experience this.

Promotions *increase your other business*, too. Suppose you introduce aromatherapy into your salon. Those clients who respond to the promotion will visit your salon. There, they will see other products displayed that they may need. They will talk to you about other concerns that they have. They will see your in-salon signage and advertising for other products and posters. In short, you will have more opportunities to serve them, and serving your clients is why you became an esthetician.

LONG-TERM BENEFITS   Over the long term, a consistent promotion schedule will keep your salon's name before your clients' eyes and in their thoughts. It will position your salon in their mind as a place that offers them value as well as service, a business that cares about them enough to always stay in touch and keep them informed about the goods and services they need.

TYPES OF PROMOTIONS   The kinds of promotions you do are limited only by your imagination and the type of image that you want to maintain. Following is a list of basic, tried-and-true promotions.

Gift-With-Service (GWS) or Gift-With-Product (GWP)   A client purchases a service or product at full price and receives a free gift, usually a professional product, with it. This is a very effective promotion because:

1. It is *cost-effective.* You pay much less for the product than you ordinarily charge the client for it.
2. It has a *highly perceived value.* The client receives a product worth much more to him or her than it costs you to provide.
3. It *introduces a new product* to a client who has not tried it, or it keeps your clients accustomed to the performance of a professional product.
4. Your supplier will often work with you on making gift-with-service or gift-with-product promotions work effectively for your salon, helping you to plan and promote, perhaps even providing you goods at a discount rate.

Discounts   Everybody loves a bargain! Judicious use of discounts will encourage clients to try new services or a new esthetician. You can also encourage people to come in during the slow hours of the day, so that your schedule is more evenly balanced.

Be careful, though. Too many sales will cheapen the value of a service; people will see the sale price as the "real" price.

Generally speaking, you should avoid discounting products. Instead, offer the gift-with-service or gift-with-product promotions as described above.

Client Referrals   Your most effective advertising and promotion vehicle is not the newspaper, nor is it radio, television, or direct mail. *Clients* have traditionally been the most powerful force for bringing in new clients to a salon. *Word-of-mouth* is the vehicle, and you should take full advantage of it. Here are two approaches to promoting your business through your present clientele.

1. *Referral:* Reward the existing client who refers a new client to your salon. Free product, free service, special merchandise—choose a gift that is meaningful to the referring client.
2. *Bring a Friend:* Offer a discounted price for those who bring a friend. For example, offer full price for the first person, half-price for the second; or two for the price of one. Of course, this offer is not limited to friends. It can be used effectively for Valentine's Day, Father's Day,

Mother's Day, etc. Use your imagination. The important thing is that the two people schedule their appointments together.

Holidays and Special Occasions

We just mentioned Father's Day and Mother's Day, but any holiday or special occasion is an opportunity to promote your business. Sit down with a calendar and look at all the days that are important in your community. Look beyond holidays such as Easter and the Fourth of July. What about graduation? What about prom night? What about back-to-school? Can you offer any products or services that fit well with those events? If you can, you have a great opportunity to help your business grow.

Cooperative Promotions

Notice all the businesses that are located close to yours. Do they attract the kind of customers you want for clients? If so, and if they are not competitors, you can try combining your promotional efforts with those businesses.

For example, if the clothing store located in a nearby mall has a clientele that you want to reach, you can try to arrange a cooperative promotion. The store will hand out coupons for your salon to their customers, and you will distribute store coupons to your clients. Your clients will appreciate the value, as will your co-promoter's customers.

Public Speaking

If you can get up in front of an audience and deliver a 15- or 30-minute lecture on better skin care, you have what it takes to build your business through public speaking. Women's clubs, service organizations, business organizations—all of these have meetings and often seek speakers.

Although the lecture should not be an advertisement for how great your salon is, when you address these groups, you position yourself as an expert, and you stimulate interest in your salon and in the services you provide.

Before contacting any of these, prepare a lively lecture on topics of interest. Make sure you have plenty of visuals—slides, posters, charts—that are both clear and helpful to what you will be explaining. Keep it upbeat, positive, and appropriate to the occasion (no skin disease lectures over lunch), and be sure to hand out your business card to everybody after each lecture.

Public Relations/ Public Service

When you do something good for the community—charitable work, for example—*take credit for it*. It will boost your business and it will raise the image of your profession in the eyes of the public.

If, for example, you donate a certain percentage of sales in 1 week to a worthy cause, or if you visit a nursing home to provide free or at-cost services, be sure the media knows about it well in advance. In the case of services performed in your salon, you may find that some people will sign up for the service strictly because of the cause. The cause will benefit as a result.

Also, your clients will think more highly of you if they know that you are "giving back" to your community. But they must know that you are doing it.

Advertising

Always keep in mind these two critical points about advertising:

1. It is expensive.
2. It works, if done correctly.

To make advertising pay off, you must plan carefully, choosing your approach and media to suit your needs. Here are some tips to help you make the most of this costly but effective business tool.

ESTABLISH YOUR BUSINESS GOALS

What kind of clients do you want visiting your salon? What age group? What income bracket? Housewives? Businesspeople? When you know the clientele you want to reach, you can plan an advertising campaign that appeals to their taste and needs.

Similarly, you must think about what image you want your advertising to reflect, because this is a critical part of your appeal to the clients you want to attract.

When you sit down to plan your advertising, think about which services and products you want to feature. Think about which hours you need to fill with appointments and which are already too full. Plan your advertising around this.

FOCUS AND CONSISTENCY

In order to achieve significant results, you must focus your efforts. Notice how major brands use advertising campaigns centered on certain characters or ideas. These campaigns can run for years, using the same slogans, the same characters, and very similar situations from one commercial or ad to the next. They concentrate their efforts in order to avoid confusing people about what the product is, what it stands for, and what it will do for them.

Focus your advertising efforts in the same way. Single out one or two features or benefits that you want to position in your clients' and potential clients' minds. Emphasize that in your advertising. If your clients are concerned about stress and toxins, emphasize the relaxing, detoxifying benefits of your services.

Consistency means that your advertising has consistent elements: a logo; frequency; an image; slogans or catchwords.

KEEP IT FRESH

While you want your advertising to be consistent, you also want it to be fresh. Running the same ad month after month will make your business look tired and stale. Change your approach. Change your offer. Change your promotion. Change the artwork. Your logo and a slogan can provide continuity. Your focus will provide integrity. Now you must add a little excitement by offering something new, something different.

K.I.S.S.　*Keep It Short and Simple.* Don't crowd your advertising with too many messages or too much information. Avoid complicated or confusing instructions. The major points should "jump out" at the reader or be immediately obvious.

Think of it this way: Your reader has 5 seconds to figure out why this ad is of interest to him or her. If that isn't immediately obvious in 5 seconds of glancing over an ad, change the ad so that it is.

THINK A CAMPAIGN, NOT AN AD　A campaign will bring *consistency, focus* and *organization* to your advertising. You will be able to budget more efficiently and with greater accuracy by having your advertising expenditures carefully plotted out.

Remember that advertising typically operates on a *cycle.* When you first begin to advertise, introducing yourself to your potential clients, people will respond to your advertising message. If you've sent a good, strong message, and your service delivers on your advertising promises, your business will grow.

Later, after you have reached the overwhelming majority of your intended audience, you will notice a marked decline (40 to 50 percent less) in response to your ads. The campaign has "matured." Keep tabs on expenditures and responses, because you want to make sure that your advertising is cost-effective.

The last phase of a campaign is its decline. Now you can choose between reaching out to a greater market or working on appealing more strongly to your present clients.

BE FLEXIBLE　Sometimes we fail. Or we don't succeed as well as we would like. If your advertising simply isn't generating the response you want, don't be afraid to sit down and rethink your entire strategy.

A word of warning: If at all possible, find a disinterested other person, one who knows about advertising but has no direct interest in how and where you spend your advertising dollars. For example, your radio ad salesperson will be predisposed to seeing you invest in radio ads; an inept ad agency will find fault with everything except themselves. Go outside for help, even if you must pay for it.

MEDIA　Television? Radio? Newspaper? Local magazine? Direct mail? Direct response? All of these? Some of these?

Choosing the right media can be a frustrating task. Choosing the wrong media is an expensive mistake. How do you choose?

The best advise is to think like your clients. Which newspapers do they read? Which magazines? Which television stations do they watch? Which radio stations do they listen to? Which mail offers do they respond to?

If you are already in business, you should poll your clients at least twice a year by having them fill out a short survey form. Ask them which newspapers and local magazines they read, which television and radio stations they favor (and at what times). Chart the responses, and then go with those newspapers, magazines, television stations, or radio stations that they favor. Why? Because that is where you will locate other clients like them. And the more specific, the better.

Here's an example: You poll your clients and find that 75 percent of them read the Sunday arts and entertainment section of the local paper. That is where you want to advertise. If they listen to a certain radio show on weekday mornings, that is your best bet. Remember, though, that you may be charged more for an ad if you want it to run at a particular time. Balance response against cost.

BE SELECTIVE

Being selective is part of being focused. Whether your ad appears in print or on the electronic media, you must always think "selective." The newspaper or television station may reach 120,000 people, but how many of those are close enough to your salon to be potential clients? How many of these are likely clients?

Radio is less expensive than television, and the format (easy listening, jazz, rock, talk, news, etc.) makes for a very selective audience. Again, you must think about how many listeners are potential clients.

Local magazines are more selective than newspapers, generally speaking. In fact, they may be too selective—reach too few people. They are usually more expensive than newspapers, and you need a longer lead time—sometimes as much as 2 or 3 months—to run an ad.

Direct mail is often seen as the most selective and efficient form of advertising for local businesses. It can be very expensive, often exceeding $1.00 per household, because you are paying for preparation, packaging, and postage, in addition to the cost of a list, generally purchased from companies that specialize in selling lists of postal addresses by zip code, profession, income, etc.

One form of direct mail, coupon packs or card decks, is very cost-efficient, typically offering a cost between 15¢ and 20¢ per household, including all costs. Because these are selected by zip code, you can be sure of reaching households only in those areas close to your salon. Be careful that your ad is not lost in a thick stack of cards, and that the ad or medium does not detract from the image you want to convey.

MEET WITH MEDIA REPRESENTATIVES

Meet with sales representatives from all the media that you are considering for advertising. Let each one make a presentation about how his or her medium can reach your intended audience, how efficiently, and at what cost. Resist any pressure to buy immediately.

Once you have all the details, go back to your business goals. See how the different media will help you reach those goals. Then decide on what is best for you.

YOUR ADVERTISING REFLECTS WHO YOU ARE

For many people your advertising will be their first impression of your salon. For that reason you want every ad to represent your salon at its very best. Generally speaking, it is unwise to insist on doing your own ads. Leave this to professionals.

Newspapers and radio stations typically have people on staff whose job is to help you with ad design, at no charge to you. Magazines expect camera-ready art work, or charge for their services to prepare an ad. Television stations also charge for writing and videotaping your commercials.

Freelancers or ad agencies are other alternatives for designing or writing ads or commercials. Look for those that have experience with doing ads for your type of business, and ask to see some of their work.

AD AGENCIES   An advertising agency can take charge of your advertising needs from start to finish. They will evaluate your needs, design a marketing plan and advertising strategy, plan your media purchases, and oversee the creation of your ads. Of course, these services are figured into their charges, but you are relieved of a great part of the burden if you use an agency to handle your advertising needs.

If you decide to use the services of an agency, seek out one that has experience with your size of business, and preferably with salon work. Contact several of them. Ask to see a sample of their work, and then choose the agency that meets your needs and where you feel most comfortable. They should provide you with a detailed and complete listing of costs before you sign any agreement for their services.

INVEST IN YOURSELF   Advertising and promotion are investments in your business. As we mentioned in the beginning, such expenditures are necessary if you want your business to grow and prosper.

How much should a salon invest? No definite answer exists. A business starting up in a crowded market (with plenty of competition) may spend as much as 10 to 12 percent of their budget on advertising. Others may invest 6 to 8 percent. Once the business is established, 2 to 3 percent is a normal expenditure for advertising.

Just remember that $1,000 of well-chosen, well-designed advertising beats $5,000 wasted on advertising to the wrong people, at the wrong time, in the wrong place. If your advertising is not working, don't just think about spending more; think about spending more wisely.

TRACK YOUR RESULTS   Unless you track the response to each advertising and promotional campaign, you cannot make objective, sound business decisions about its effectiveness. The better computer programs for businesses will allow you to track results and will generate reports with little effort on your part, but with or without a computer, you must keep track of the response.

All you need to track responses is a sheet of paper and a pen. At the top, write the name of the promotion. Divide the page into columns: client name, services purchased, total dollar amount, other purchases. Write in the information as the clients come in. Tally up the totals once a week, then compare this with the total cost of the advertising or promotion. Don't forget, though: Any promotion that brings in first-time clients is especially valuable because you will be seeing a greater return over the long-term, but only if you can retain that client's loyalty.

Interpersonal Communication Skills

Advertising and promotion bring people into the salon. Everything thereafter depends on you and on your staff. It is up to you to follow through all the way to the sales, so that your clients receive the products and services they need in order to look and feel their best.

Everything you think, say, and do, even your gestures and appearance, will influence how your clients react. You are the professional, the expert. You must not let your appearance or actions detract from that statement. Refer back to Chapter 1, because a *professional image is vital to good sales.*

DON'T SELL — CONSULT

As stated in the beginning of this chapter, effective selling means solving your clients' problems, using an approach called *consultative selling.* This approach begins by adopting an attitude of helpfulness and caring, so that you are attuned to the clients' needs. And consultative selling does not end with the sale. It is a *relationship* between client and esthetician, and is thus ongoing.

Here is a simplified approach to consultative selling.

Know Your Products and Services

Be completely knowledgeable about all the products and services you offer, not just in terms of what they are and what they do, but in terms of how they benefit the client. Know the advantages of your products over the "drugstore brands," always emphasizing the positive (your products) rather than the negative (the mass market remedies) (Fig. 27.1).

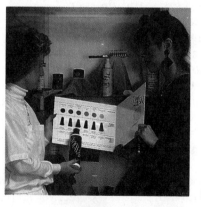

27.1 — Retail specialist

Listen

Begin by *listening* to your client. What does he or she need? Don't think in terms of products. Think in terms of *psychology.* Some people may need the self-confidence that having clear, healthy skin will give them. Others need the reassurance that they are taking the best possible steps for their overall health and appearance. Some want the direct benefits of de-stressing treatments. Others want to hold on to their youthful appearance.

It is up to you to listen for the client's concerns, and to hear what is unsaid as well as what is said. A person's major concerns will be heard time and again in their conversation. Listen for these themes, and you will know what people want you to know but cannot or will not tell you.

Analyze, Question, Probe   Ask your client questions about how he or she feels. Get a history of his or her experiences with this problem, when it is particularly bothersome, when it is not a concern.

Be Sensitive   Never make declarations about how your client feels. You may address the clinical problem, and here you should be definite, but always be sensitive to your clients' feelings. People are never more vulnerable than when they reveal their problems, so express concern and sympathy, then move on to the solutions.

Offer Benefits, not Products or Services   Your client does not want a product or a service. He or she wants the *benefits* that these will provide. Rather than saying, "We have an excellent exfoliation treatment," say, "This exfoliation treatment will clean your skin and it will look and feel healthier after just one treatment."

Experience Is Worth a Thousand Words   Benefits are better experienced than talked about. If you can offer a sample, this is an extremely effective way of introducing a product to a client. Similarly, promotions that offer new services or products at enticing prices or with added value (such as gift-with-service) get clients to sample services they would not have tried otherwise.

    You must also allow the client to *look*, *touch*, and *smell* the products that you use. Retail displays help, but even better is allowing the client to hold a product in the hand, smell it, read the label, ask questions about it, etc.

Close the Sale   Unless you *ask for the sale*, everything you've done up to that point—your education, your advertising, your promotion, your service—will be meaningless (Fig. 27.2). How do you ask?

1. *Let the client choose*, and restate the benefits along with any added value: "Both of these products will clear up that skin condition, and with either purchase you'll receive a free bottle of moisturizer that sells for $10.00. Which one would you like to take home with you?"
2. *Assume* that he or she wants the product(s) or services: "We have an opening next Tuesday, the 14th, at 4:30 P.M. I'll write you in right away."

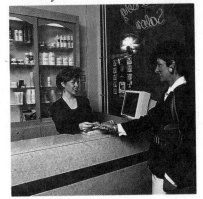

27.2—Closing the sale

THE TELEPHONE — ONE OF YOUR MOST IMPORTANT BUSINESS TOOLS

Think about it: Why would a person call your salon? Almost always the answer will be, *because he or she is interested in your business!* For that reason, the telephone should never be taken for granted. Learn how to use it well, and you will be rewarded with more business.

The Basics of Good Phone Communication

Be *courteous* when you answer the phone. If you are having difficulties or any sort of problem and the phone rings at the worst possible time, it is not the fault of the person calling you. Keep in mind that the person on the other end is making an effort to give you his or her business, and respond accordingly.

Cultivate a *clear, pleasant phone manner.* Smile: It will make a difference in the tone of your voice. Listen to yourself on a tape recorder, and work at eliminating any harsh or unpleasant vocal mannerisms.

Responding to Phone Inquiries

The best response to an inquiry is *information*, but not necessarily the information the caller asked for. Yes, you should answer the question, but try not to be limited by it.

For example, if a person calls asking about the price for a facial, avoid just giving the price. Become a consultant, just as you would with a client in the salon. Here is a good pattern for responding to price inquiries:

1. Answer that you have a variety of services available, each designed to meet specific needs.
2. Immediately begin asking questions to ascertain what the client's needs are. Be sure to ask for the caller's name right away, and respond with a cheerful hello and give your own name.

> **Note:** If you use the person's name several times during the first minute or so of conversation, you will be much more likely to remember it.

3. Mention any current specials or promotions that would be of interest to the caller.
4. Offer some advice and guidance. Suggest several courses of action that the client can take using your services and products. Emphasize the benefits that each service will provide, and stress the quality of the care and service your clients can expect in your salon.
5. Usually the client will ask for the cost at this point. Summarize each alternative (the service/product and benefits) and then the cost, starting with the most expensive one first.
6. If necessary, explain that just as a doctor won't diagnose patients over the phone, you need to consult with the client personally before recommending specific options.
7. Offer a specific time for the caller to come in for a consultation or service. If that is not a good time, offer another one. If that is not suitable, ask which time is good for him or her.

8. If the caller absolutely does not want to come in, but you sense some interest in your services, ask for a complete name, address, and phone number so that you can keep him or her informed about promotions and special events at your salon.

9. When you take your leave, be sure to thank the client for the call, and remind the client about the appointment, if appropriate. ("I'll see you next Wednesday, the 27th, at 4:00 P.M.") If the client did not schedule, invite him or her to call with any questions.

10. Those clients who make an appointment should receive a card thanking them for their interest in your salon and reminding them of the appointment time and date. Those who don't make an appointment should receive a thank-you card and an invitation to call back with any questions.

11. Write down all the information on a client record or a 5×7 card, so when the client does come in or calls back, you will be prepared for the questions.

CALLING TO PROMOTE, CHECK UP, SURVEY

You should call your clients to *follow up* on any home treatment plans, to *confirm appointments* and to *inform* them of promotions or events (such as a new service) that are of special interest to them, and to *poll* them on how satisfied they are with your services and products. Calling does take significant time and effort as well as organization, but it pays off in greater client loyalty, stronger sales, and fewer no-shows for appointments.

Calling Your Clients

1. Call at convenient times. Avoid meal times, early morning, or late in the evening, unless the client specifically indicates that he or she prefers being called at those hours.

2. Immediately identify yourself by name and salon and extend a warm greeting.

3. Take a moment to be personal. Ask about the children, the job—anything that is of importance to the client.

4. Get to the point. Explain the purpose of your call. If the client expresses sufficient interest, make an appointment immediately or offer to set aside some product for him or her to pick up on a certain date.

5. Keep your call brief. Thank the client and say goodbye as soon as you have taken care of business.

6. Use a list to keep yourself organized so that you don't call the same client twice or overlook a client.

7. Schedule your phone calling activities. That way you won't neglect to do it, and you can schedule it so that you do it in short intervals of 20 or 30 minutes.

If you still feel that calling your clients is not worthwhile, remember that old saying, "Out of sight, out of mind." Your business depends on your relationship with your clients, and relationships are built on contact and communication—the more, the better.

Retail Displays

Professional-looking displays are essential to good selling (Fig. 27.3). To look professional, here is what your displays should be:

1. Attractive and functional: Choose attractive display racks and furniture designed for the purpose.
2. Well-lit: Good lighting draws attention to the display.
3. Well-stocked: Show that you mean business. Keep the shelves well-stocked to show that the items are more than just an afterthought.
4. Stocked with a variety of products: Clients like having choices. The more choices they have, the more likely it is that they will make a purchase.
5. Well-organized and neat: Items should be grouped by category, with the front labels clearly visible and lined up, and the entire area should be spotless.
6. Visible: Place retail items where clients can see and touch them. Small displays in service areas can enhance the effect of the larger, main display in your reception area. Impulse-buy items such as jewelry or small boutique items should be located next to the cash register.
7. Supported by signage: Shelf-talkers, small signs, posters—use whatever is necessary to call attention to the products and entice the client to browse and ask questions.
8. Supported by people: Verbally call attention to the products—those that have been selling well, those that are particularly appropriate for the client's needs, new products, specialty products, etc. Be sure to describe in detail any products that you use, while you are using them and always in terms of their benefits. And always, always make professional recommendations for home care.

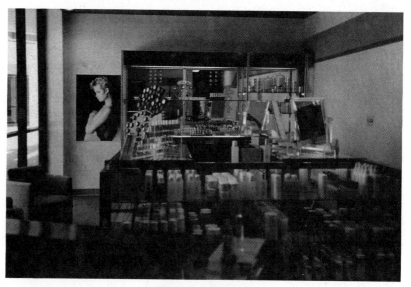

27.3—Retail displays

QUESTIONS   DISCUSSION AND REVIEW

SELLING PRODUCTS AND SERVICES

1. Explain consultative selling.
2. What can promotions do for your salon?
3. List two types of promotions.
4. What is your most effective advertising and promotion vehicle?
5. Explain cooperative promotions.
6. What are two critical points about advertising?
7. List some tips to help you make the most of advertising.
8. Why should you track your results when advertising?
9. List seven key points in consultative selling.
10. List the seven key points in phone surveying.
11. List the eight key points in retail displays.

Chapter 1
Your Professional Image

1. Hygiene is the branch of applied science that deals with healthful living.

2. Personal hygiene concerns the care taken by individuals to preserve health by following the rules of healthful living.

3. Public hygiene refers to the steps taken by the government to protect and promote public health.

4. The eight basic requirements for good personal hygiene are: (a) Take a daily bath or shower; (b) Brush teeth after meals; (c) Use a deodorant; (d) Keep clothing clean and neat; (e) Have regular medical and dental checkups; (f) Keep hair clean and well groomed; (g) Keep hands and nails clean and well groomed; (h) Follow a daily regimen of good diet, exercise, and adequate rest.

5. A thought may either stimulate or depress the functions of the body. Strong emotions, such as worry, anger, and fear, have a harmful effect on the heart, arteries, and glands. Mental depression weakens the functions of the organs, thereby lowering resistance of the body to disease.

6. The five basic rules for maintaining good posture are: (a) Carry the weight on the balls of your feet, not on the heels; (b) Keep your knees flexed; (c) Keep your shoulders back; (d) Hold your abdomen in; (e) Hold your head high.

7. The three rules for standing in the basic stance are: (a) Turn the left foot out at a forty-five degree angle; (b) Point the right foot straight ahead with the heel at the instep of the left foot; The right foot may also be placed several inches ahead of the left; (c) Keep both knees slightly flexed with the right knee bent inward.

8. Three benefits of correct posture are: prevention of fatigue, improved personal appearance, and improved functioning of the internal organs.

9. A good sitting posture is accomplished by: (a) Placing the feet on the floor directly under the knees; (b) Having the seat of the chair even with the knees; (c) Allowing the feet to carry the weight of the thighs; (d) Resting the weight of the torso on the thigh bones; (e) Making sure the chair is at the correct height; (f) Sitting well back in the chair; (g) Never slouching.

10. Lift with your back straight, pushing with the heavy thigh muscles, never the back muscles.

11. Six suggestions for hand and nail grooming are: (a) When you place your hands in harsh solutions, wear plastic or rubber gloves; (b) Use a protective hand cream or lotion after washing your hands and at bedtime; (c) Keep the cuticles pushed back; (d) Nail enamel, colored or clear, should never be smeared or chipped; (e) Nails should not be too long and never pointed; (f) If you bite or pick your nails, you must break this habit.

12. Three rules for the care of the feet are: (a) Wear shoes that fit correctly; (b) Keep toenails filed smooth; (c) Give the feet daily care, and medical attention as needed.

13. Four desirable qualities to cultivate in your personality are: (a) To have a healthy attitude toward life; (b) To display pleasant emotions; (c) Politeness toward others; (d) To have a sense of humor.

14. A pleasant sounding voice has a friendly, positive manner, that is clear and loud enough to be heard without being overwhelming.

15. Six good topics for conversation between an esthetician and a client are: (a) Client's personal interests, personal grooming, and cosmetic needs; (b) Client's own activities; (c) Fashions; (d) Literature; (e) Travel.

16. Topics to avoid when conversing with a client are: (a) Your own personal problems; (b) Religion; (c) Other client's poor behavior; (d) Your own financial status; (e) Poor workmanship of co-workers; (f) Your own health problems; (f) Information given to you in confidence.

17. Some ways to project professionalism are: (a) To be punctual; (b) To have a clean work area; (c) To be prepared for each client, and each question; (d) To genuinely care that each client receives the very best service and products possible.

18. Eight rules for treating a client as a V.I.P. are: (a) Be honest, but tactful; (b) Be alert, cheerful and enthusiastic; (c) Be patient and courteous; (d) Be orderly and punctual; (e) Be honest, dependable and loyal; (f) Be concerned about your clients' needs; (g) Be diligent about educating yourself, so that you can better serve your clients.

19. Ethics deals with the study and philosophy of human conduct, with emphasis on the determination of right and wrong.

20. Five rules for ethical behavior are: (a) Be honest, but tactful, with all your clients; (b) Treat all clients fairly, and with equal amounts of respect; (c) Be dependable in all your dealings with co-workers, clients, and others; (d) Take the initiative in solving problems for your clients and for your salon; (e) Practice the highest standards of professionalism at all times.

21. Develop a respectful relationship with them by knowing what their duties, rights and responsibilities are, and by always dealing with them on a professional level.

22. The esthetician must know the laws, rules, and regulations governing esthetics, and must comply with them.

Chapter 2
A History of Skin Care and the Use of Cosmetics

1. Coloring matter used in cosmetic practices has been made from a great number of natural substances. Some of these include: berries, clay, tree bark, saffron, flowers, nuts, herbs, leaves, animal and insect materials. In recent years, a wide range of colors have also been introduced synthetically.

2. Kohl is a powdered metallic substance (powder of antimony) that ancient Egyptians used as eye makeup to outline the eyes and darken the eyelids.

3. The Egyptians kept their skin lubricated by applying fragrant oils, lotions, or ointments.

4. From the Greek word "kosmetikos" meaning skilled in decorating.

5. Roman women used facials made of milk and bread and sometimes fine wine. Some facials were made of corn, flour and milk, and flour mixed with fresh butter.

6. During medieval times cosmetology and medicine were taught as combined subjects in English universities. Cosmetology and medicine were not officially separated until late in the 16th Century.

7. During the Renaissance period, women shaved off their eyebrows and the hairline to show a greater expanse of forehead. The bare brow was thought to give women a look of greater intelligence.

8. During the reign of Elizabeth I, formulas for lotions and facial masks were made from such ingredients as powdered eggshell, alum, borax and ground almond and poppy seeds. Milk, wine, butter, fruits, and vegetables were also used.

9. Makeup and elaborate clothing were discouraged during the Victorian Age (1837–1901).

10. During the 1930's, men and women were strongly influenced by the media (newspapers, magazines, radio, and motion pictures).

Chapter 3
Bacteriology

1. Bacteriology is the science or study of bacteria.

2. The practice of sanitary measures protects the student, the esthetician, and the client against pathogenic bacteria.

3. Bacteria are minute, one-celled micro-organisms found nearly everywhere.

4. Bacteria are also called micro-organisms, germs, and microbes.

5. Bacteria are too small to be seen with the naked eye. Fifteen hundred rod shaped bacteria barely reach across the head of a pin.

6. Non-pathogenic bacteria: non-disease producing, beneficial or harmless type. Pathogenic bacteria: disease producing and harmful type.

7. Parasites are bacteria that live on living matter. Saprophytes are bacteria that live on dead organic matter.

8. (a) Coccus—round shape; (b) Bacillus—rod shape; (c) Spirillum—corkscrew shape.

9. Staphylococci; streptococci.

10. Each organism divides in the middle, forming two daughter cells which grow to full size and then reproduce again.

11. A local infection, such as a boil, is confined to a small part of the body. A general infection, such as blood poisoning, results when bacteria or their poisons enter the bloodstream.

12. An infection is caused by an invasion of the body tissues by disease producing bacteria.

13. Staphylococcus and streptococcus.

14. Tuberculosis, virus infections, ringworm, and head lice.

15. One that may be transmitted from one person to another.

16. By the practice of personal hygiene, cleanliness and sanitation at all times.

17. Through the mouth, nose, eyes, and breaks or wounds in the skin.

18. (a) Unbroken skin; (b) Body secretions, such as perspiration; (c) White blood cells; (d) Antitoxins.

19. The ability of the body to fight and overcome certain diseases caused by germs and their poisons.

20. Natural immunity means natural resistance to disease. Acquired immunity is secured after the body has by itself overcome certain diseases, or by injections of serum.

21. A human disease carrier is a person who, although immune to the disease himself, can infect other persons with the germs of the disease. Two examples are diphtheria and typhoid fever.

22. Disinfectants, intense heat and ultra-violet rays.

Chapter 4
Sterilization and Sanitation

1. Sterilization is the process of making an object germ-free, by destroying all micro-organisms, both pathogenic and nonpathogenic.

2. Sanitation is the process of making objects clean and safe for use, to prevent the growth of germs and to reduce the risk of infectious disease.

3. Sterilization and sanitation are important to the esthetician because they deal with methods used either to prevent the growth of germs or to destroy them entirely.

4. An antiseptic is a chemical agent that kills or retards the growth of bacteria.

5. Asepsis is freedom from disease causing germs.

6. Sepsis is contamination due to pathogenic germs.

7. Three forms of heat sterilizing are boiling, steaming, and baking.

8. Disinfectants usually are stronger than antiseptics and must be used with caution.

9. Ultra-violet radiation, especially in the shorter wavelength, destroys most bacteria. Gamma ray radiation destroys microorganisms through the action of ionized particles.

10. A 25% solution of formalin, equivalent to 10% formaldehyde gas, is used to sanitize implements.

Chapter 5
Cells, Anatomy, and Physiology

1. The skin, the membranous tissue which covers the body, is the body's largest organ.

2. A cell is a minute portion of living substance consisting of protoplasm, which is living matter surrounded by a membrane and containing a nucleus, cytoplasm, and various organelles.

3. The cell contains the following structures: cell membrane, nucleus, cytoplasm, and centrosome.

4. When a cell reaches maturity, it reproduces by mitosis or indirect division.

5. Metabolism is a complex chemical process in which cells are nourished and supplied with the energy needed to carry on these many activities. The two phases of metabolism are: anabolism, which builds up cellular tissues and catabolism, which breaks down cellular tissue.

6. Body tissues are classified in five groups: (a) connective tissue supports, protects, and binds together other tissues of the body. Bone, cartilage, ligaments, tendons, and fat tissues are examples; (b) Muscular tissue contracts and allows movement in various parts of the body; (c) Nerve tissue transmits messages to and from the brain and controls and coordinates all body functions; (d) Epithelial tissue is the protective covering on body surfaces. It includes the skin, mucous membranes, linings of the heart, digestive and respiratory organs and glands; (e) Liquid tissue carries food, waste products, and hormones. This type includes the blood and lymph.

7. The skin is both a tissue and an organ.

8. The human body is composed of the following systems: Skeletal system—bones; Muscular system—muscles; Nervous system—nerves; Circulatory system—blood and lymph supply; Endocrine system—ductless glands; Excretory system—organs of elimination; Respiratory system—lungs; Digestive system—stomach and intestines; Reproductive system—reproduction.

9. Besides the teeth, bone is the hardest structure of the body.

10. There are 206 bones in the body.

11. (a) one occipital bone; (b) two parietal bones; (c) one frontal bone; (d) two temporal bones; (e) one ethmoid bone; (f) one sphenoid bone.

12. (a) one nasal bone; (b) two lacrimal bones; (c) two zygomatic bones; (d) two turbinal bones; (e) one vomer bone; (f) two palatine bones; (g) two maxillae bones; (h) one mandible bone.

13. The thorax, or chest, is an elastic bony cage made up of the breast bone, the spine, the ribs, and connective cartilage.

14. The clavicle and scapula are found in the shoulder.

15. The humerus is the largest bone of the upper arm.

16. The carpus is composed of eight bones.

17. The metacarpal bones are the long slender bones of the palm.

18. The function of the muscular system is to produce all the movements of the body.

19. Myology is the study of the structure, functions, and diseases of the muscles.

20. The cardiac is the heart muscle.

21. Muscles can be stimulated by: (a) chemicals—certain acids and salts; (b) massage; (c) electric current; (d) dry heat; (e) moist heat.

22. The direction of pressure in massage is usually performed from the insertion to the origin.

23. The muscles of the scalp are epicranius, occipitalis, frontalis, aponeurosis.

24. The muscles of the eyebrows are obicularis oculi and corrugator.

25. The muscle of the nose is the procerus.

26. The muscles of the mouth are quadratus labii superioris, quadratus labii inferioris, buccinator, caninus, mentalis, orbicularis oris, risorius, zygomaticus, and triangularis.

27. Neurology is the branch of anatomy that deals with the nervous system and its disorders.

28. The main purpose in studying the nervous system is to understand the effects various facial services have on the nerves, skin, and face and on the body as a whole.

29. The three main divisions of the nervous system are cerebrospinal, peripheral, and sympathetic.

30. The two types of nerves are sensory or afferent, and motor or efferent.

31. The brain is the largest mass of nerve tissue in the body.

32. Nerve fatigue can be caused by excessive mental or muscular work, resulting in an accumulation of waste products. Weariness, irritability, poor complexion, and dull eyes may be signs of nerve exhaustion.

33. Trigeminal or trifacial.

34. The blood vascular system consists of a closed system of vessels, including arteries, veins and capillaries, which carry blood from the heart to all parts of the body, and then back to the heart.

35. Arteries carry pure blood from the heart to the tissues.

36. White corpuscles, or leucocytes, destroy disease-causing germs.

37. The lymphatic system is the waste disposal and drainage system for the body tissues.

38. The endocrine system is the body's chemical control system.

39. The skin is considered part of the endocrine system because it produces Vitamin D.

40. Kidneys, liver, skin, intestines, and lungs are all part of the excretory system.

41. Oxygen is required to change food into energy.

42. Nose breathing is healthier than mouth breathing because the air is warmed by the surface capillaries, and the bacteria in the air is caught by the hairs that line the nasal passages.

43. It is important to the esthetician because of the effects nutrition and elimination have on keeping the skin healthy.

Chapter 6
Physiology and Histology of the Skin

1. The skin is a slightly moist, soft, strong, flexible covering of the body, and it is acidic.

2. A fine texture, healthy color, and free of blemishes.

3. The epidermis and dermis.

4. It is the outermost layer of the skin and the outer protective covering of the body.

5. (a) Stratum corneum (horny layer); (b) Stratum lucidum (clear layer); (c) Stratum granulosum (granular layer); (d) Stratum germinativum (deepest layer).

6. Stratum corneum.

7. Stratum lucidum.

8. Stratum granulosum.

9. Stratum germinativum.

10. The dermis is a highly sensitive and vascular layer of connective tissue. Within its structure are numerous blood vessels, lymph vessels, nerves, sweat glands, oil glands, hair follicles, arrector pili muscles, and papillae.

11. Papillary and reticular layers.

12. Papillae.

13. Fat cells, blood vessels, lymph vessels, oil glands, sweat glands, hair follicles, and arrector pili muscles.

14. It gives smoothness to the body, contains fat for use as energy, and is a protective cushion for the outer skin.

15. ½ to ⅔ of the entire blood supply in the body is distributed to the skin.

16. Blood and lymph nourish the skin.

17. Motor, sensory, and secretory nerve fibers.

18. The fingertips.

19. To arrector pili muscles attached to hair follicles.

20. The elastic fibers in the dermis.

21. In the basal layer.

22. They react to heat, cold, touch, pressure, and pain.

23. They regulate the excretion of perspiration from sweat glands, and control the flow of sebum to the surface of the skin.

24. After the skin is stretched, it regains its former shape almost immediately.

25. Loss of elasticity.

26. The coloring matter melanin, and the blood supply.

27. Protection, sensation, heat regulation, secretion, excretion, and absorption.

28. Blood circulation through the skin, and evaporation of sweat.

29. 98.6 degrees Fahrenheit.

30. Hair, nails, sweat glands, oil glands.

31. Sudoriferous or sweat glands, sebaceous or oil glands.

32. They consist of a coiled base and a tube-like duct, which forms a pores at the surface of the skin.

33. Over the entire area of the skin, more numerous on the palms, soles, forehead, and armpits.

34. They help to eliminate waste products in the form of sweat.

35. Heat, exercise, mental excitement, and certain drugs.

36. They consist of small sacs whose ducts open into the neck of the hair follicle.

37. Sebum, an oily substance.

38. It lubricates the skin and hair, keeping them soft and pliable.

39. Oil glands are found in all parts of the body, with the exception of the palms and soles.

40. The skin protects the body, regulates body heat, secretes, excretes, and absorbs.

Chapter 7
Disorders of the Skin, Dermatology, and Special Esthetic Procedures

1. To help prevent their spread, and to avoid more serious conditions.

2. To help prevent the spread of infection to others.

3. To safeguard his/her own and the public's health.

4. Dermatology is the study of the skin, its nature, structure, functions, diseases and treatment.

5. A skin specialist.

6. A structural change in the tissues caused by injury or disease.

7. An objective lesion can be seen (pimples). A subjective lesion can be felt (itching).

8. Macule, papule, wheal, tubercle, tumor, vesicle, bulla, and pustule.

9. Scale, crust, excoriation, fissure, ulcer, scar, and skin stain.

10. Any departure from a normal state of health.

11. (a) Blackheads; (b) Whiteheads.

12. A worm-like mass of hardened sebum obstructing the duct of the oil glands.

13. Acne is a chronic inflammatory disorder of the sebaceous (oil) glands.

14. Milia, acne, comedones, and seborrhea.

15. Bromidrosis—foul smelling perspiration. Anidrosis—lack of perspiration. Hyperidrosis—excessive perspiration. Miliaria rubra—prickly heat.

16. Dermatitis is a term used to denote an inflammatory condition of the skin.

17. An inflammation of the skin of acute or chronic nature. Its cause is unknown.

18. The lesions are round, dry patches covered with coarse, silvery scales.

19. On the scalp, elbows, knees, chest, and lower back.

20. It is a virus infection. Fever blister.

21. Lips, nostrils or other parts of the face.

22. Albinism is the absence of color pigmentation in the skin and hair.

23. Discolorations classified as naevus, commonly called a birthmark. Usually found on the neck and face.

24. Age, extremes of heat and cold, illness, diet, and medication.

Chapter 8
Chemistry for Estheticians

1. The science that deals with the composition structure and properties of matter, and how matter changes under different conditions.

2. The two branches of chemistry are inorganic and organic.

3. Substances that do not contain carbon are inorganic and substances that do contain carbon are organic.

4. Matter is anything that has mass and occupies space.

5. Liquids are shapeless, but readily take the shape of their containers. They cannot be compressed.

6. Gas is shapeless like liquids, but they expand easily, and are compressible.

7. An atom is the smallest part of an element that possesses the characteristics of the element.

8. Protons, neutrons, and electrons.

9. A molecule is the smallest particle of an element or compound that possesses all the properties of the element or compound.

10. An element is the basic unit of all matter. It is a substance that cannot be made by the combination of simpler substances, and the element itself cannot be reduced to simpler substances.

11. A compound is two or more elements combined chemically.

12. There are 105 known elements.

13. The four most important classes of compounds are oxides, acids, bases, and salts.

14. Matter can be changed in two ways; either through physical or chemical means.

15. (a) physical change: ice into water; (b) chemical change: soap is formed from the chemical reaction between an alkaline substance and oil or fat.

16. Odor, color, and taste.

17. Distilled or filtered water is used in most salon machines.

18. The pH of the skin's acid mantle ranges from 4.5 to 6 and is most often referred to as 5.5.

19. So it will have a softening effect on the skin, which makes it easier for the skin to absorb the beneficial ingredients in the moisturizer.

20. Water is a universal solvent.

21. A *dilute* solution contains a small quantity of solute in proportion to the quantity of solvent. A *concentrated* solution contains a large quantity of solute to solvent. A *saturated* solution will not dissolve or take up more of the solute than it already holds at a given temperature.

22. Oil-in-water and water-in-oil.

Chapter 9
Ingredient and Product Analysis

1. An esthetician should be familiar with ingredients in products he or she uses so the correct product is recommended for each client's skin.

2. *Active* works directly on the skin; *inactive* doesn't work on the skin but performs a function that helps the product, such as a preservative or stabilizer.

3. Ingredients may come from plants, animals, vitamins, or minerals, or may be synthesized from chemicals.

4. Chemically synthesized ingredients include alcohol and petroleum derivatives, such as mineral oil.

5. Chamomile or zinc oxide.

6. Humectants are substances that have the ability to attract water.

7. Algae products are used widely in face masks and other products to remineralize and revitalize the skin.

8. Collagen is a fibrous substance, derived from the placenta of cows.

9. Soaps, detergents, bath accessories, deodorants, antiperspirants, and depilatories.

10. When a substance is derived from or produced by nature.

11. Material that has been derived from something living, such as plants or animals.

12. To protect the consumer who may be allergic to certain ingredients, and provide information that will help the consumer when making a buying decision.

13. It can occur immediately or several days after the application of the preparation.

14. Hypoallergenic means that the product does not contain a fragrance.

15. Acne cosmetica is acne caused by cosmetics.

16. Consumer complaints are sent to the manufacturer, and a copy sent to the Food and Drug Administration Division of Cosmetic Technology, Washington, DC 20204.

Chapter 10
Nutrition and the Health of the Skin

1. Nutrition is the process by which food is assimilated and converted into tissue in living organisms.

2. Fats, carbohydrates, and proteins.

3. Protein, because it is the material that the body uses to build tissue, and replace and repair tissue as it is worn out or injured.

4. Crash diets are bad for the skin because when weight is reduced too fast, the skin will sag and wrinkle rather than gradually return to its former condition. The skin will also suffer from lack of proper nourishment.

5. Enzymes are substances that can bring about reactions that would not otherwise occur or that can speed up reactions that normally are very slow.

6. Water aids in digestion, carries waste materials from the body, helps form body fluids, sustains the health of all cells, and helps regulate body temperature.

7. Yes, a lack of Vitamin C over a period of time can cause scurvy. Pellagra is the result of a severe Vitamin B deficiency. Acne, eczema, psoriasis and dermatitis can also be caused from deficiencies.

8. Tobacco—nicotine affects the blood vessels and slows circulation. Alcohol—dilates the blood vessels; with heavy, regular intake, it may cause tiny blood vessels to burst in the white of the eyeball and beneath the skin. It can also contribute to dehydrated sagging skin.

9. Aspirin, penicillin, birth control pills, codeine, diet pills, barbiturates, and laxatives; also tranquilizers, amphetamines, marijuana, heroin or drugs of this type can all affect the skin.

10. Tearing eyes, nausea, headaches, hives, diarrhea, *or* constipation and upset stomach.

11. An allergist.

12. Milk, eggs, nuts, grains, chocolate, fish, shellfish, and some fruit and vegetables.

13. Vitamin E.

Chapter 11
Client Consultation and Skin Analysis

1. Because it may determine if he or she will return for future services, or recommend the salon to others.

2. Because the first contact that the client has with the salon is often by way of the telephone.

3. It should be immaculately clean and uncluttered; decor should be pleasant and furnished in good taste. A coordinated color scheme should be used throughout the salon. It is desirable to have an office or consultation room or combination of both that is separate from the treatment rooms.

4. A skin analysis is necessary to determine the condition of the skin and the proper treatments.

5. Yes, because of the treatments the skin is improving, and from change in season.

6. Normal, dry, mature *or* aging, oily, acne, couperose, and combination.

7. Yes, because if they are not using the proper products that are formulated for their skin type they then may be doing more harm than good to their skin.

8. An esthetician cannot make guarantees for a cure nor make exaggerated claims.

Chapter 12
Client Preparation and Draping

1. It shows the client that you are efficient, organized, and considerate.

2. They should be removed with a spatula; never should the fingers be dipped into any products.

3. The purpose of the head drape is to cover and protect the client's hair during the facial treatment.

4. The most popular types of head covering used in facial and beauty salons are cloth or paper towels.

5. Cotton and clean water from a metal, enamel, or plastic basin.

Chapter 13
Cleansing the Skin

1. Water soluble cleansing lotion is preferred when cleansing the face.

2. The facial chart helps the esthetician to identify movements as applied to various areas of the face during the application and removal of cleansers.

3. Cotton pads and facial sponges.

4. With a folded tissue and a small amount of cleansing lotion, start at the outside corner of lips and slide to the center; alternate the strokes on both sides of the mouth.

5. The eyebrow is lifted and the lashes gently cleansed with a wet cotton pad. Moist eyepads may be left on the eyes for a few minutes to soften mascara. It can then be wiped away with clean, moist cotton pads.

6. No, the water temperature should be kept comfortable for the clients so as not to shock or feel unpleasant.

7. Yes, whenever it won't interrupt the progress of the facial.

8. When removing a treatment mask.

Chapter 14
Techniques for Professional Massage

1. (a) Nourishes the skin and its structures and stimulates blood circulation; brings oxygen and carries away waste products; (b) Reduces fat cells in the subcutaneous tissue; (c) Increases the secretion of sebum and perspiration, which in turn opens pores; (d) Makes the skin softer and more pliable. It tones muscles and retards aging of skin; (e) Deplete excess fluids in tissues; (f) Strengthens, nourishes and tones muscle fiber; (g) Soothes and rests the nerves; (h) Appearance of the skin; (i) Sometimes relieves pain by helping tense muscles relax; (j) Loosens and clears away surface dead cells.

2. (a) Swedish massage—manipulates deep muscle tissue; (b) Accupressure massage—works with accupressure points on the body; (c) Shiatsu—combines stretching of limbs with pressure on accupressure points.

3. Reflexology is a therapeutic massage that manipulates areas on the hands and feet.

4. It is using essential oils, which penetrate the skin during massage movements and provide beneficial effects.

5. Using gentle pressure on the lymphatic system to move waste materials out of the body more quickly.

6. It will help to maintain control of your hands when doing fast or slow movements.

7. Everyday to improve hand mobility.

8. Effleurage, petrissage, friction, tapotement, and vibration.

9. Once or twice a month with proper home care.

10. The main purpose of massage #1 is to continue the cleansing process, help remove dead surface cells, and increase blood circulation.

11. Cold cream.

12. We do not use a penetrating cream with massage #1 because it could act as a vehicle in carrying dirt and makeup deeper into the pores.

13. The main purpose of massage #2 is to aid in the deep penetration of treatment creams and lotions, and to induce relaxation.

14. Oily skins benefit most from the Dr. Jacquet movement because its main purpose is to empty the oil ducts in the skin.

Chapter 15
Mask Therapy in Facial Treatments

1. Facial masks and packs are the same.

2. The primary purpose of a facial mask is to remove impurities from the skin. Facial masks are also soothing, toning, and calming to the skin.

3. A wax mask traps moisture beneath the mask so that it will not evaporate. Instead, the moisture is forced into the corneum layer of the skin where it plumps up fine lines.

4. Facial masks (after removal) make the skin feel clean, refreshed, smoother, and firmer.

5. A clay mask absorbs oil and debris from the skin, leaving it with a smoother, more even texture. It is also beneficial in removing inflammation.

6. A custom-designed mask is a mask that the esthetician prepares especially for the client. A custom mask may be prepared from a variety of ingredients such as fresh fruit, vegetables, herbs, eggs, milk, honey, herbs, and oils. It is up to the esthetician to determine the effects of certain ingredients on the client's skin and to choose the most beneficial ingredients.

7. The "peel-off" gel mask helps to hydrate the skin and remove dead, dry, flaky cells from the surface of the skin. The non-peel type gel mask is very hydrating to the skin and has a calming, soothing, and refreshing effect on the skin.

8. Gauze is used with some mask preparations that tend to slip or run off the face. The gauze holds the mask substance in place.

9. Preprepared commercial facial masks are easy to use, save time and are often more economical than custom-prepared masks.

10. Vitamin A used in a facial mask is said to have a softening effect on the skin; Vitamin C is used for its astringent qualities; Vitamin D is considered to be healing to the skin; and Vitamin E is used to soften and lubricate dry, rough skin.

11. Allantoin comes from the comfrey root and is used in cosmetics for its healing and soothing qualities.

12. The main purpose of a wax mask is to insure deep penetration of products into the skin. The warmth of the mask relaxes the skin. The wax mask leaves the skin moist, of good color, and superficial lines will often be diminished.

Chapter 16
Facial Treatments without the Aid of Machines

1. Because the salon you work in may not have a facial machine. As a professional, you should be able to perform this service.

2. Opens follicles, softens dead surface cells, helps stimulate the sebaceous glands, aids sweat glands in the elimination of toxins, increases circulation of blood, leaves skin feeling soft and glowing, and leaves the client feeling relaxed.

3. Wax mask or epidermabrasion.

4. Yes.

5. No, each area is treated for its particular problem.

6. Twice a week.

7. Disincrustation is a process that softens and emulsifies grease deposits and blackheads in the follicles.

8. (a) Do not use infrared lamps in treatment; (b) ice should not be used; (c) mild skin lotions, not astringent; (d) no strong massage movements.

9. Epidermabrasion.

10. The epidermabrasion treatment is not done on acne or couperose skin.

Chapter 17
Electricity, Machines, and Apparatus for Professional Skin Care

1. Estheticians use magnifying lamps to aid in detecting tiny imperfections when analyzing the skin. It is especially helpful when extracting blackheads and whiteheads, and cleaning out pimples.

2. Robert Williams Wood developed the Wood's lamp.

3. Thin dehydrated skin will appear purple under the Wood's lamp.

4. The benefits of the vaporizer are: (a) Softens dead surface cells; (b) opens pores; (c) soften deposits of grease,

blackheads, makeup, and dirt; (d) helps eliminate toxins; (e) temporarily softens superficial lines; (f) increases blood circulation; (g) improves cell metabolism.

5. The vapor nozzle should be set approximately 16 inches from the client's face.

6. 1 cup white vinegar to 1 quart of water.

7. To work cleansers into the skin more effectively and to slough off the dead surface cells.

8. With soap and water, then placing them in a bowl of alcohol for about 20 minutes.

9. (a) disincrustation to soften grease and sebum deposits; (b) iontophoresis to introduce water soluble treatment products into the skin.

10. When this current is passed through certain solutions containing acids and salts, and when galvanic current passes through the tissues and fluids of the body.

11. Negative pole—cathode; positive pole—anode.

12. The primary action of the high-frequency current is thermal or heat-producing.

13. Mushroom—face and neck; horse-shoe—neck; roller—face.

14. The benefits of high-frequency are: (a) stimulates circulation of blood; (b) increases glandular activity; (c) aids in elimination and absorption; (d) increases metabolism; (e) germicidal action; (f) generates heat inside the tissues; (g) aids in deeper penetration of product into the skin.

15. Three to five minutes.

16. Three methods of using the high-frequency current are: (a) direct current application; (b) indirect application; (c) general electrification.

17. A spray machine is used to suction out deeply embedded dirt, grease, and other impurities.

18. Another name for the spray machine is atomizer.

19. Achieves cleansing of the skin surface, and has a cool and soothing effect. It is used to flush out pores.

20. Dehydrated, mature, and couperose skin.

21. Oily and acne skin.

22. Protect the client's eyes; never surprise the client with the spray; test on client's hand the first time you use the spray. Drape a towel across client's shoulders, and spray approximately 20 inches away from client's face.

23. Do not use the electric mask if your client has a large percentage of broken capillaries.

24. An electrical current is a stream of electrons moving along a conductor.

25. A conductor is a substance that readily transmits an electrical current.

26. Fuses and circuit breakers.

27. The current delivered by most machines used for facial treatments is measured in milliamperes.

28. A polarity changer alters the direction of the current.

29. A rheostat regulates the strength of the current by means of a dial.

30. Examine cords regularly. Repair or replace worn cords to prevent short circuiting, electric shock, or fire.

31. Light therapy is a treatment using light rays.

32. Three forms of light rays used in salons are: (a) infra-red rays; (b) ultra-violet rays; (c) visible light.

33. Natural sunlight is composed of 8% ultra-violet, 12% visible, and 80% infra-red rays.

Chapter 18
Facial Treatments
with the Aid of Machines

1. The vaporizer, the brushing machine, the suction, and the electric mask are all helpful aids when giving a treatment for combination skin.

2. When giving a treatment for oily skin, machines help to soften dead cells and other debris. Follicles are opened and debris is cleansed away. Once the follicles are cleansed and unplugged, as in the extraction of blackheads, the sebum can flow more easily to the surface of the skin where it can be cleansed away.

3. When giving a treatment for oily skin with the use of machines, the Dr. Jacquet movements are performed following disincrustation in the oily areas and where there are open follicles and blackheads.

4. The client should be aware that acne cannot be cleared in one treatment. It is estimated that if an acne condition has persisted for less than a year, it will usually take about three months of treatments to clear the condition. If the acne condition has persisted for more than one year, three is added to the number of years the client has had acne. For example: if the acne has persisted for two years, it is estimated that it will take about five months to achieve results.

5. During the beginning of acne treatments the client may experience a "flare-up" or slight worsening of the condition. This is a sign that the infectious material is working its way to the surface of the skin.

6. When giving treatments for acne skin, it is important that the client follow a home care regimen. The client should not be mixing products or applying medications that may interfere with the salon treatments.

7. A sterilized needle or blood lancet may be used to prick a blemish when it is ready to be extracted.

8. Dry skin is classified as oil-dry (lacking sebum), dehydrated (lacking moisture), and mature (aging). Dry skin can be oil and moisture dry.

9. The warm wax mask is used on dry skin to aid in deep penetration of products.

10. Massage #1 and Massage #2 may be eliminated from the treatment for oily-blemished skin so that the esthetician can spend more time on the disincrustation and extraction of blackheads.

Chapter 19
Removing Unwanted Hair

1. Electrolysis is the process of removing hair permanently by means of electricity. The term "electrolysis" has become synonymous with both the multiple needle galvanic method and the more modern single needle shortwave method.

2. Epilation is the removal of hair by the roots. This is done by waxing, tweezing, and electrolysis.

3. Depilatories belong to the group of temporary methods for the removal of unwanted hair. There are physical (wax) and chemical (cream, paste, or powder) types of depilatories.

4. When hair is shaved, it will grow back with a blunt stubble.

5. The wax hair removal treatment is used to remove hair from large areas such as legs and arms.

6. When eyebrows are thick and unruly, shaping can be done faster by first waxing then plucking excess hair with a tweezer.

7. Wax is applied and removed in the direction of the hair growth.

8. It takes from 8 to 13 weeks for the hair to grow from the papilla to the surface of the skin.

Chapter 20
Enemies of the Skin, Aging Factors, and Cosmetic Surgery

1. Lines and wrinkles often start before mid-life but start to become more prominent after the age of forty. Lines and wrinkles are primarily due to loss of skin elasticity and the body's biological changes during mid-life.

2. Too much sun affects living cells and causes the skin to lose oil and moisture. This loss in turn, causes the skin to become lined and in some cases, leathery.

3. Sulfur-containing compounds are among the most common pollutants in the air. When this polluted air comes in contact with the skin, it is partially converted to sulfuric acid, which is dehydrating and deteriorating to the skin.

4. Excessive intake of alcohol dilates blood vessels and can weaken the walls of the capillaries. This can lead to a couperose condition.

5. When weight is lost too rapidly, the skin does not have time to adjust to the changes in the underlying facial tissues and muscles. This causes sagging and wrinkling of the skin.

6. Drugs may interfere with the intake of oxygen that the body needs for healthy cell growth. Drugs can cause allergic reactions and aggravate skin problems.

7. Chemical face peeling is a treatment that requires a specially formulated solution that when applied to the face, produces a peeling of the skin. This treatment should be done only by a qualified dermatologist or surgeon.

8. Dermabrasion is a treatment that is done with a special kind of apparatus that scours or sands away the surface layers of skin. This treatment is done only by qualified dermatologists and specialists.

9. The "canon" of beauty devised by the Greeks gave them an established rule of judgment as a means of determining ideal proportions of the human face and body. A working knowledge of the dimensional relationship between one facial feature and another helps us to appreciate the differences in individual faces.

10. Plastic or reconstructive surgery is especially beneficial to those individuals who have suffered injuries that have left them scarred or deformed in some way. Plastic surgery as cosmetic surgery also helps to restore an individual's confidence.

11. The medical name for face lift is rhytidectomy, the excision of wrinkles for cosmetic purposes.

12. Rhinoplasty is the medical name for nose surgery.

Chapter 21
Male Skin Care and Grooming

1. Men are becoming more aware of the need for healthy skin and for good grooming.

2. Men are more muscular than women, and are, therefore, stronger, larger, and have more endurance.

3. Women have more fatty tissue than men, and it is distributed differently. In women, fat is concentrated around the breast, hips and buttocks. In men, it is more evenly distributed.

4. Men's skin tends to be oilier because there are more sebaceous glands. It is also slightly thicker and coarser. Structurally, there is no difference.

5. Men usually wash their faces with a harsh bar soap, then lather on a shaving cream, shave, rinse quickly, and splash on an after shave lotion.

6. The salon can offer almost all of the same skin care and hair removal services to men as they do to women.

7. The salon should be more unisex in nature. It should be clean and attractive, well-equipped and staffed, but should not be too feminine. It should be a comfortable place for the male client.

8. Skin care products for men are almost identical to those for women, except they tend to be lighter and less complicated chemically. They also tend to be free of fragrances and perfumes.

9. The single most important aspect of male skin is facial hair. Shaving is a consideration in facial treatments, both because it tends to irritate the skin and because beard stubble can interfere with most of the steps in a facial treatment.

10. There are very few differences in treatment procedures for male skin and female skin. It may be necessary for the male client to shave before arriving at the salon for the facial. Since male skin tends to be oilier, those treatment steps designed for oily skin will be used more often.

Chapter 22
Esthetics and Aromatherapy

1. When essences and fragrances are used as a part of a facial or body treatment, the procedure is called aromatherapy, meaning to use aroma as a therapeutic aid.

2. Fragrances from herbs and plants have been used by people around the world. Almost all civilizations have produced cosmetic and treatment products which they have used for their therapeutic value. We find evidence of the use of fragrance in the Bible and in many ancient writings. Artifacts have also been discovered still bearing traces of the fragrances they contained.

3. The seven basic categories of fragrances are: (a) Floral; (b) Floral bouquet; (c) Oriental; (d) Modern blends; (e) Spicy blends; (f) Forest or woodsy blends; (g) Fruity blends.

4. Fragrances can evoke pleasant memories and increase a person's sense of well-being. Fragrance is often used to lessen depression and lethargy. Repulsive odors can make a person physically ill.

5. Aromatic essences are obtained in the following ways: (a) distillation—the use of steam or boiling water; (b) extraction by solvents—the use of a solvent such as ether or petroleum; (c) expression—a method where essential oils are pressed out of the substance; (d) enfleurage—fat is used to absorb the oils pressed from a fragrant substance; (e) maceration—substances are submerged in hot fat to obtain fragrant oils.

6. Three herbs that are valued for their antiseptic action are: clove, thyme, and sandlewood.

7. Musk from the musk deer, and civet oil from the civet cat are two of the most widely used natural (animal) fixatives used in the manufacture of fragrances.

8. Aromatic substances having an agreeable odor and stimulating qualities are: herbs and spices, such as nutmeg, rosemary, and sage. Substances known to be antiseptic are: thyme, peppermint, heather, and clove. Astringent substances are: witch hazel, alum root, comfrey root, and lemon. Substances with very stimulating qualities are: ginsing, spearmint, wintergreen, and sandlewood. Calming and soothing substances are: almond, camomile, jasmine, and marjoram. Cleansing substances are: lemon-grass, witch hazel, milfoil, and lovage root. Emollient substances are: almond, aloe, and olive leaves. Substances known for their healing qualities are: aloe, camomile, comfrey root, peppermint, and rosemary. Moisturizing substances are: orange blossoms, rose leaves, rose hips, camomile flowers, and white willow bark.

Chapter 23
Advanced Topics for Esthetics

1. New developments and products are constantly being introduced. Many of these offer significant business opportunities for the knowledgeable esthetician. Also, the esthe-

tician must be aware of and be able to discuss the topics with clients.

2. The esthetician must remember that he or she is not a medical doctor, and must be careful not to cross the thin line that separates the beauty and health care profession from the medical profession.

3. Phytotherapy is the use of herbs to treat disorders.

4. Although both are based on plant materials, phytotherapy uses any or all of the parts of the plant, while aromatherapy uses only the essential oils of the plant.

5. They detoxify or cleanse the body; they normalize or correct imbalances in the body; they build or strengthen the body.

6. Commercial preparations are safer and more effective than homemade preparations.

7. Reflexology is an energy-based system of massage that balances the inner organs of the body through manipulations on the hands or feet.

8. Reflexology works by applying pressure at the endpoint of each energy meridian in the body, thus correcting blockages in the meridians and rebalancing the system.

9. Unlike other techniques, such as lymphatic drainage massage, water therapies and body wraps, reflexology may be given as an added service during a facial treatment.

10. Lymphatic drainage massage is a structure-based system of massage that helps detoxify the body by moving waste materials through the lymphatic system.

11. Gentle pressure and stroking along the lymphatic channels increases the lymph flow and speeds up the natural detoxification process of the system.

12. While both are water therapies, thalassotherapy utilizes sea water or products from the sea, while balneotherapy uses fresh water.

13. Hydrotherapy tub treatments use jets of water and air bubbles to massage the lymphatic system, and the deeper tissues, while the client is immersed in water. The Scotch hose treatment is where the therapist sprays jets of hot water up and down the spine and main lymphatic channels of the client.

14. They are products from the sea and are rich in minerals and phytohormones. They are beneficial in remineralizing and revitalizing the skin.

15. Body wraps help improve circulation and elimination. They detoxify and temporarily recontour the body. They help reduce localized fatty deposits.

16. Plastic sheet materials are used when the treatment is for detoxification. They hold in heat, moisture, and help improve elimination and circulation. Contour tapes are cloth strips that are used for recontouring and reshaping the body.

17. Cellulite is the name given to localized, fatty deposits that accumulate around the hips, thighs, and buttocks. It consists of fat cells, water, and waste materials that form a semi-hard, gel-like mass under the skin.

18. Although cellulite treatments have been given in salons and spas for years, the medical community believes that cellulite does not exist. They believe cellulite is no more than ordinary fat, and can be eliminated through diet and exercise.

496 STANDARD TEXTBOOK FOR PROFESSIONAL ESTHETICIANS

19. A salon chemical peeling is a procedure in which a formula is applied to the skin that causes the epidermis to peel in the same way a deeply sun-burned skin would peel.

20. One of the major benefits of a salon chemical peeling is that it makes the skin produce biostimulins, a substance that helps the cells survive.

Chapter 24
Color Theory

1. Color psychology refers to color and its psychological associations. A person's choice of color is said to indicate something about his or her personality. For example: red indicates an outgoing personality while blue indicates a love for peace and quiet.

2. Melanin, hemoglobin, and carotenes.

3. Albinism is the lack of color in a person's skin, hair, and eyes.

4. Skin colors from lightest to darkest are described as follows: (a) white—with little or no color pigment; (b) light—creamy or pink undertones; (c) golden skin—skin with a yellow cast; (d) pink skin—skin with a flushed to florid cast; (e) tan skin—tan skin may have brown or yellow undertones; (f) olive skin—a deeper brown tone with a greenish cast; (g) brown skin—ranging from a light clear brown to deep brown, with varied undertones; (h) ebony—black skin that ranges from deep brownish black to almost jet black.

5. The three primary colors are red, yellow, and blue. By mixing any two primary colors in equal parts, you will obtain the secondary colors. For example: blue mixed with yellow produces green.

6. Intermediate or tertiary colors are formed by mixing a secondary color and a primary color in equal amounts. For example: the yellow (primary) and green (secondary) colors will produce the intermediate color known as yellow-green or chartreuse.

7. Hue is a color as the eye perceives it. For example: red is seen as red.

8. Value is the lightness or darkness of a color.

9. Bright colors advance and make the area covered appear larger. Dull, dark colors recede and make the area covered appear smaller.

10. Colors are classified as warm or cool. Some colors can be both warm or cool depending on the shade, tint, lightness, or darkness of the color.

11. Foundation should be selected to enhance the client's natural coloring.

12. Test the foundation color by applying a few dots to the client's jawline, blending it upward on the jaw and down onto the neck. There should be no line of demarcation.

13. The eyebrow pencil can be used to cover small scars and other imperfections in the eyebrows.

14. Brown, black, and charcoal are the most popular colors of eyeliners.

15. Eyecolor is used to enhance the beauty of the eyes, and to conceal imperfections.

16. The pencil or brush can be used to correct or change the natural outline of the lips, but should not be exaggerated.

Chapter 25
Professional Makeup Techniques

1. Applying makeup artistically, and to be able to interest the client in purchasing cosmetics.

2. Sales ability.

3. The main objective when applying makeup is to help the client, whether naturally attractive or not, to improve her appearance.

4. Direct overhead light will often flush out shadows that otherwise would be corrected by the makeup artist. The face tends to flatten in a prone position.

5. The ideal makeup mirror is one that resembles a theatrical makeup mirror. Bulbs surround the mirror on three sides only.

6. Cleanse thoroughly and use astringent to remove traces of stale makeup. Remove all eyecolor and lipcolor, and apply a small amount of moisturizer for protection.

7. The oval face, but all face shapes are attractive when makeup is applied.

8. Yes, makeup can be used to balance the features.

9. Waxing is the best method for removing extremely heavy eyebrows.

10. Brows should be tweezed in the direction that they grow.

11. Liquid foundation is the most popular because it gives good coverage, is easy to apply, and gives a healthy, natural look to the skin.

12. Cream or stick foundation is often used for theatrical makeup.

13. The cover-up cosmetic should match the foundation as closely as possible. Corrective makeup can be applied with fingers or brush, with edges of the cover-up cosmetic being blended into the foundation.

14. The most popular form of blush is the dry, brush-on type.

15. Blush should be so well-blended that it appears to be the woman's natural coloring.

16. Cream blush will give your client a softer and more natural look.

17. The eyeshadow color is often chosen to accentuate the client's eye color or to coordinate to match her clothing color.

18. Liner accentuates the eye, changes its shape, and makes the eyelashes appear thicker.

19. Mascara is used to make the lashes look thicker, longer, and darker.

20. Titanium dioxide.

21. Artificial lashes can be made of real or synthetic hair.

22. Surgical adhesive.

23. Yes, and it is advisable to give the client an allergy test before applying the lash.

Chapter 26
The Salon Business

1. Cost, revenues (sales), and profit.

2. A business accountant and a legal advisor.

3. (a) fixed costs: rent/mortgage, salaries, insurances, equipment leases; (b) variable costs: utilities, supplies, promotion, postage, taxes.

4. Before signing a lease you should review it with your attorney and accountant for advice.

5. Fire, liability, employee, theft, occupany, and equipment extended warranties.

6. General skill level, overall attitude, and personality.

7. (a) Maximum efficiency of operation; (b) adequate aisle space; (c) the flow of operational services toward the reception room with amenities such as: phone, coffee, magazines, and pleasant music; (d) enough space for each piece of equipment; (e) furniture, fixtures, and equipment chosen of the basis of cost, durability, utility, and appearance; (f) a color scheme that is restful and flattering to males and females, and young adult to senior groups; (g) a dispensary, and plenty of storage space; (h) a clean rest room containing toilet and basin; (i) proper plumbing, and sufficient lighting for satisfactory services; (j) air conditioning and heating.

8. (a) Inexperience in dealing with the public and with employees; (b) not enough capital to carry the business through until established, poor location, and overhead expenses that are too high; (c) lack of proper basic training; (d) business neglect and careless bookkeeping methods.

9. Salaries, rent, supplies, and advertising.

10. Depending on how it is used, it may spell either gain or loss.

11. Proper business records are necessary to meet the requirements of local, state, and federal laws regarding taxes and employees.

12. (a) To prevent overstocking; (b) prevent running short of supplies needed for services; (c) to help in establishing the net worth of the end of the year.

13. A service record card is used to record treatments given, and merchandise sold to each client. It is useful for suggestions and uniform services, which can result in increased sales.

14. Individual, partnership, and corporation.

15. (a) Correct identity of owner; (b) true representations concerning the value and inducements offered to buy the salon; (c) use of salon name and reputation for a definite period of time; (d) an understanding that the seller will not compete with the prospective owner within a reasonable distance from present location.

16. Capital, organization, banking, selecting location, decorating and floor plan, equipment and supplies, advertising, legal, booking system, cost of operation, management, office administration, insurance, methods of payment, compliance with labor laws, ethics, compliance with state cosmetology law, licensing.

17. Good telephone habits and techniques can increase business, and build up the salon's reputation.

18. Saying or doing the right thing, at the right time, and in the right manner.

19. (a) Display an interested, helpful attitude; (b) be prompt; (c) practice giving all necessary information to the caller; (d) be tactful.

20. (a) Clear speech; (b) correct speech; (c) pleasing tone of voice.

21. (a) Names, addresses, and phone numbers of employees; (b) first aid kit; (c) phone numbers of: fire station, police, emergency ambulance, nearest hospital emergency room, taxi service, telephone company, and utility service companies.

Chapter 27
Selling Products and Services

1. It is selling benefits, not just products or services; it is not pushing but advising the client.

2. Promotions can get you through a lean period by bringing in clients and introducing clients to new products and services.

3. Gift-with-service (GWS) or Gift-with-product (GWP).

4. Client referrals, word-of-mouth.

5. Combining your promotional efforts with businesses that are located close to yours.

6. It is expensive and it works, if done correctly.

7. (a) Establish your business goals; (b) focus and consistency in your efforts, and have consistent elements in your advertising; (c) keep it fresh; (d) K.I.S.S.—keep it short and simple; (e) think about a campaign, not an ad; (f) be flexible; (g) media—choosing the right media; (h) be selective; (i) meet with media representatives; (j) your advertising reflects who you are; (k) ad agencies—can help take charge of your advertising needs.

8. To determine its effectiveness.

9. (a) Know your products and services; (b) listen, analyze, question, probe; (c) be sensitive; (d) offer benefits, not products or services; (e) experience is worth a thousand words; (f) close the sale.

10. (a) Call at convenient times; (b) immediately identify yourself; (c) take a moment to be personal; (d) get to the point; (e) keep your call brief; (f) use a list to keep yourself organized; (g) schedule your phone calling activities.

11. (a) Attractive and functional; (b) well-lighted; (c) well-stocked; (d) stocked with a variety of products; (e) well organized and neat; (f) visible; (g) supported by signage; (h) supported by people.

Bibliography

The following list of books, periodicals, and video-cassettes are considered to be especially helpful to instructors and students of esthetics. It can serve as an additional source for the instructor's development of course and curriculum subject matter and instructional exercises. These selections also consider the specific needs of students who wish to supplement their readings of particular topics discussed in this book. All of the books and videos listed can be purchased directly from Milady/Delmar Publishers.

Books:

The Art and Science of Professional Makeup—Stan Campbell Place

Body Structures & Functions—Elizabeth Fong, Elvira B. Ferris, Esther G. Skelley

A Consumer's Dictionary of Cosmetic Ingredients—Ruth Winter

Electrolysis, Thermolysis and the Blend—Arthur R. Hinkel

Lesson Plans for Milady's Standard Textbook for Professional Estheticians

Management Tools for Cosmetology Education—Michele Johnson

Medical Terminology: A Programmed Text—Genevieve Love Smith, Phyllis E. Davis, Jean Tannis Dennerll

Milady's Illustrated Cosmetology Dictionary—Bobbi Ray Madry

Milady's Standard Workbook for Professional Estheticians

Milady's State Exam Review for Professional Estheticians

Modern Electrology: Excess Hair, Its Causes and Treatments—Fino Gior

Salon Management for Cosmetology Students—Edward J. Tezak

Science in Your Salon—Bronwyn Cozens

The Theory and Practice of Therapeutic Massage—Mark Beck

You and Your Clients: Human Relations for Cosmetology—Leslie Edgerton

Periodicals:

Dermascope Magazine (bi-monthly)
4447 McKinney Avenue
Dallas, Texas 75205
1-214-526-0752

Les Nouvelles Esthetiques (bi-monthly)
7, av. S. Mallarme
75017 Paris, France
(1) 43.80.06.47

Skin Inc. (bi-monthly)
P.O. Box 318
Wheaton, Illinois 60189
708-653-2155

Videocassettes:

Professional Skincare Techniques (8 videocassettes featuring Joel Gerson, author of *Milady's Standard Textbook for Professional Estheticians*) which includes:
Preparation for the Facial Treatment (#1)
Product Application and Cleansing Procedure (#2)
Basic Facial Massage (#3)
Massage No. 1—For Cleansing and Stimulating the Skin (#4)
Massage No. 2—For Product Penetration and Client Relaxation (#5)
Special Facial Treatment (#6)
Facial Treatment for Combination Skin without Machines (#7)
Facial Treatment for Combination Skin with Machines (#8)

NOTE: BOLDFACE entries are definitions.

Esthetician's Comprehensive Glossary

Compiled of words used in connection with esthetics, defined in the sense of anatomical, medical, electrical and esthetic relationship only. The key to pronunciation is as follows:

fāte, senáte, câre, ăm, finâl, ärm, ȧsk, sofa̬;
ēve, ĕvent, ĕnd, recênt, evẽr; īce, ĭll; ōld,
ōbey, ôrb, ŏdd, cônnect, sŏft, fōod, fŏot; ūse,
ṵnite, ûrn, ŭp, circûs; those.

A

abdomen (ăb-dō'mĕn): the belly; the cavity in the body between the thorax and the pelvis.

abducent nerve (ăb-dew'sunt): the sixth cranial nerve; a small motor nerve supplying the external rectus muscle of the eye.

abductor (ăb-dŭk'tẽr): a muscle that draws a part away from the median line (opp., adductor), i.e.: spreads the fingers.

abrasion (ȧ-brā'zhûn): scraping of the skin; excoriation.

abscess (ăb'sĕs): an enclosed cavity containing pus.

absorption (ăb-sôrp'shûn): assimilation of one body by another; act of absorbing.

accessory nerve (ăk-sĕs'ô-rē nûrv): spinal accessory nerve; eleventh cranial nerve; affects the sternocleido-mastoid and trapezius muscles of the neck.

acetic (ȧ-sĕt'ĭk): pertaining to vinegar; sour.

achroma (ay-kro'muh): color - complexion color; (absence of color).

acid (ăs'ĭd): 1) a substance having a sour taste; 2) a substance containing hydrogen replaceable by metals to form salts, and capable of dissociating in aqueous solution to form hydrogen ions; 3) having a pH number below 7.

acid balanced (ăs'ĭd băl'ânst): a condition of a cosmetic product where its acidity is the same as the acidity of the skin or hair.

acidic (ȧ-sĭd'ĭk): containing a high percentage of acid.

acidify (ȧ-sĭd'ĕ-fī): to make or become sour; to change into an acid.

acid mantle (ăs'ĭd măn't'l): the natural acidity of the skin or hair which helps to retard irritation or bacterial growth.

acidosis (ăs-ĭ-dō'sĭs): a condition in which there is an excess of acid products in the blood or excreted in the urine.

acid rinse (ăs'ĭd rĭns): a solution of water and lemon juice or vinegar.

acidum boricum (ăs'ĭ-dûm bôr'ĭ-kûm): boric acid.

acne (ăk'nē): inflammation of the sebaceous glands from retained secretion.

acne albida (ăl'bĭ-dȧ): milium; white-head.

acne artificialis (är-tĭ-fĭsh-ăl'ĭs): pimples due to external irritants or drugs internally administered.

acne atrophica (ȧ-trŏf'ĭ-kȧ): vulgaris in which the lesions leave a slight amount of scarring.

acne cachecticorum (kȧ-kĕk-tĭ-kôr-ûm): pimples occurring in the subjects of anemia or some debilitating constitutional disease.

acne cream (ăk-nē krĕm): a facial cream, containing medicinal substances or agents used in the treatment of acne.

acne hypertrophica (hī-pêr-trŏf'ĭ-kȧ): pimples in which the lesions on healing leave conspicuous pits and scars.

acne indurata (ĭn-dū-rä'tȧ): deeply seated pimples with hard tubercular lesions occurring chiefly on the back.

acne keratos (kĕr-ȧ-tō'sȧ): an eruption of papules consisting of horny plugs projecting from the hair follicles, accompanied by inflammation.

acne punctata (pŭnk-tä'tȧ): appear as red papules in which are usually found blackheads.

acne pustulosa (pŭs-tû-lō'sȧ): vulgaris in which the pustular lesions predominate.

acne rosacea (rô-zā'shē'ȧ): a form of acne usually occurring around the nose and cheeks, due to congestion, in which the capillaries become dilated and sometimes broken.

acne simplex (sĭm'plĕks): acne vulgaris, simple uncomplicated pimples.

acne vulgaris (vŭl-găr'ĭs): acne simplex; simple uncomplicated pimples.

acoustic (ȧ-kōos'tĭk): auditory; eighth cranial nerve; controlling the sense of hearing.

acute (ȧ-kūt'): attended with severe symptoms; having a short and relatively short course; not chronic; said of a disease.

additive (ăd'ĭ-tĭv): a substance which is to be added to another product.

adductor (ȧ-dŭk'tẽr): a muscle that draws a part toward the median line. i.e.: draws fingers together.

adenoma sebaceum (ȧ-dĕn-ō'mȧ sē-bā'sē-ûm): small tumor of translucent appearance, originating in the sebaceous glands.

adipose tissue (ăd'ĭ-pōs): fatty tissue; areolar connective tissue containing fat cells; subcutaneous tissue.

adrenal (ăd-rē'nâl): an endocrine gland situated on the top of the kidney.

adulterate (ȧ-dŭl'tẽr-āt): to falsify; to alter, make impure by combining other substances.

aesthetician (ĕs-thē't'sh-en): a specialist in aesthetics. ....also see esthetician.

aesthetics (ĕs-thĕt'ĭks): relating to or dealing with aesthetics or the beautiful........also see esthetics.

aeration (ȧ-ēr-ȧ'shûn): airing; saturating a fluid with air, carbon dioxide or other gas; the change of venous into arterial blood in the lungs.

afferent nerves (ăf'ĕr-ênt): convey stimulus from the external organs to the brain.

affinity (ȧ-fĭn'ĭ-tē): 1) inherent likeness or relationship; 2) chemical attraction; the force that unites atoms into molecules.

African (af'rĭ-kan) pertaining to Africa or its inhabitants.

agnail (ăg′nāl): hangnail.

albida, acne (ăl′bĭ-dă): whitehead; milium.

albinism (ăl′bĭ-nĭz′m): congenital leucoderma or absence of pigment in the skin and its appendages; it may be partial or complete.

albino (ăl-bī′nō): a subject of albinism; a person with very little or no pigment in the skin, hair or iris.

albumin (ăl-bū′mĭn): a simple, naturally-occurring protein soluble in water, coagulated by heat; found in egg white (ovalbumin), in blood (serum albumin), in milk (lactalbumin).

alcohol (ăl-kô-hŏl): a readily evaporating colorless liquid with a pungent odor and burning taste; powerful stimulant and antiseptic.

alkali (ăl′kâ-lī): an electropositive substance; capable of making soaps from fats; used to neutralize acids.

alkaline (ăl′kâ-lĭn): having the qualities of, or pertaining to, an alkali.

alkalinity (ăl-kâ-lĭn′ĭ-tē): the quality or state of being alkaline.

allantion (al-an′shŭn): used in cold creams, lotions and other cosmetics; prepared from uric acid.

allergy (ăl′ēr-jē): a disorder due to extreme sensitivity to certain foods or chemicals.

allergy test: a test to determine the existence or nonexistence of extreme sensitivity to certain things such as food or chemicals which do not adversely affect most individuals.

almond (ăl′mŭnd): the kernel or seed of the almond fruit.

almond oil: emollient; natural vegetable oil pressed from almonds; held to have most penetrating and softening power.

aloe (ă′lō): any chiefly African liliaceous plant of the genus Aloe, certain species of which yield a drug and a fiber; sap used to relieve and heal burns.

alopecia (ăl-ô-pē′shē-â): deficiency of hair; baldness.

alopecia areata (ăl-ô-pē′shē-â ā-re-ă′tă): baldness in spots or patches.

alternating (âl′tēr-nāt-ĭng): occurring in reciprocal succession.

alternating current (kŭr′ĕnt): a rapid and interrupted current, flowing first in one direction and then in the opposite direction.

alum, alumen (ăl′ŭm, ă-lū′mên): sulphate of potassium and aluminum; an astringent; used as a styptic.

ambergris (am-bēr′gris): secretion from the intestinal tract of the sperm whale found in tropical seas; used as a fixative in fragrances.

amino-acid (ăm′ĭ-nō): an important constituent of proteins.

amitosis (ăm-ĭ-tō′sĭs): cell multiplication by direct division of the nucleus in the cell.

ammonia (ă-mō′nē-ă): a colorless gas with a pungent odor; very soluble in water.

ammonium sulphide (ă-mō′nē-ŭm sŭl′fĭd): a combination of ammonia and sulphur.

ampere (ăm-pâr): the unit of measurement of strength of an electric current.

anabolism (ăn-âb′ō-lĭz′m): constructive metabolism; the process of assimilation of nutritive matter and its conversion into living substance.

analysis (ă-năl′ĭ-sĭs): a process by which the nature of a substance is recognized and its chemical composition determined.

anaphoresis (ăn-ă-fôr-ē′sĭs): the process of forcing liquids into the tissues from the negative toward the positive pole.

anatomy (â-năt′ō-mē): the study of the gross structure of the body which can be seen with the naked eye.

anesthetic (ăn-ĕs-thĕt′ĭk): a substance producing anesthesia.

angiology (ăn-jē-ŏl′ō-jē): the science of the blood vessels and lymphatics.

angioma (ăn-jē′ō-mă): a tumor formed of blood vessels and lymphatics.

angular artery (ăng′û-lăr): supplies the lacrimal sac and the eye muscle.

anidrosis, anhidrosis (ăn-ĭ-drō′sĭs): a deficiency in perspiration.

aniline (ăn′ĭ-lēn): a product of coal tar used in the manufacture of artificial dyes.

anode (ăn′ōd): the positive terminal of an electric force.

anterior (ăn-tē′rē-ēr): situated before or in front of.

anthrax (ăn′thrăks): malignant pustule, gangrenous corpuscle-like lesion.

antibiotic (ăn′tĭ-bī-ŏt′ĭk): used in treating certain infectious diseases.

antibody (ăn′tĭ-bôd-ē): a substance in the blood which builds resistance to disease.

antidote (ăn′tĭ-dōt): an agent preventing or counteracting the action of a poison.

antigen (an′ti-jen): any of several substances, such as toxins, enzymes, or foreign proteins, that cause the development of antibodies.

anti-perspirant (ăn-tĭ-pĕr-spĭ′rânt): a strong astringent liquid or cream used to stop the flow of perspiration in the region of the armpits, hands or feet.

antiphlogistic (an′-tee-flo-jis′tick): rducing or preventing fever or inflammation.

antiseptic (ăn-tĭ-sĕp′tĭk): a chemical agent that prevents the growth of bacteria.

antitoxin (ăn-tĭ-tŏk′sĭn): a substance in serum which binds and neutralizes toxin (poison).

Antoinette, Marie (ăn′twă-nĕtt): 1755-1793, Queen of France, wife of Louis XVI; known for extravagant beauty practices such as bathing in tubs of fresh strawberries and milk.

aorta (ā-ôr′tă): the main arterial trunk leaving the heart, and carrying blood to the various arteries throughout the body.

aponeurosis (ăp-ô-nū-rō′sĭs): a broad, flat tendon; attachment of muscles.

apparatus (ăp-ă-rā-tûs): a collection of instruments or devices adapted for a special purpose.

appendage (â-pĕn′dêj): that which is attached to an organ, and is a part of it.

approximately (ă-prŏk′sĭ-māt-lē): about; nearly; closely.

aqueous (ā′kwē-ûs): watery; pertaining to water.

aromatic (ăr-ô-măt′ĭk): pertaining to or containing aroma; fragrant.

arrector pili (ă-rĕk′tôr pī′lī): plural of arrectores pilorum.

arrectores pilorum (â-rĕk-tō′rēz pĭ-lôr′ûm): the minute involuntary muscle fibers in the skin inserted into the bases of the hair follicles.

arterioles (ar-′tir-e′ols): one of the small terminal twigs of an artery that ends in capillaries.

artery (ahr′tur-ee): a vessel that conveys blood from the heart.

arthritic (āhr-thrit′-ick): pertaining to or affected with arthritis; inflammation of a joint.

articulation (är-tĭk-û-lā′shŭn): joint; a connection between two or more bones, whether or not allowing any movement between them.

asepsis (ă-sĕp′sĭs): a condition in which pathogenic bacteria are absent.

aseptic (ă-sĕp′tĭk): free from pathogenic bacteria.

asphyxia (ăs′fĭk-sē-ă): a lack of oxygen, or excess of carbon dioxide in the body, causing unconsciousness.

asteatosis (ăs-tē-ă-tō′sĭs): a deficiency or absence of the sebaceous secretions.

asthma (az-′muh): a disease characterized by coughing or wheezing.

astringent (ăs-trĭn'jênt): a substance or medicine that causes contraction of the tissues and checks secretions.

athlete's foot: a fungus foot infection; epidermophytosis.

atmosphere (ăt'mos-fēr): the whole mass of air surrounding the earth.

atom (at'um): the smallest quantity that can exist and still retain the chemical properties of the element.

atomize (ăt-ō'mīz): to reduce to minute particles or to a fine spray.

atrium (ăt'rē-ŭm): pl., **atria** (-a): the auricle of the heart.

atrophy (ăt'rô-fē): a wasting away of the tissues of a part of or of the entire body from lack of nutrition.

auburn (ô'bûrn): a reddish brown color.

auditory (ô'dĭ-tô-rē): eighth cranial nerve; controlling the sense of hearing.

auricle (ô'rĭ-k'l): the external ear; one of the upper cavities of the heart.

auricular (ô-rĭk'û-lâr): pertaining to the ear or cardiac auricle.

auricularis (ô-rĭk'û-lâr'ĭs): a muscle of the ear.

auriculo-temporal (ô-rĭk'û-lô tĕm'pôr-âl): sensory nerve affecting the temple and pinna.

autonomic nervous system (ô-tô-nŏm'ĭk): the sympathetic nervous system; controls the involuntary muscles

avulsion (ā-vul-'shun): the forcible tearing or wrenching away of a part of the body.

axon (ăk'sŏn): a long nerve fiber extending from the nerve cell.

azulene (az'yoo-leen): anti-inflammatory agent; a concentrate extract of the camomile flower used for its highly soothing qualities.

B

bacillus (ba-sil'us): pl., **bacilli** (i): rod-like shaped bacterium.

bacteria (bak-te're-a): microbes, or germs.

bactericide (bak-te-ri-sid): an agent that destroys bacteria.

bacteriology (bak-te-re-ol'o-je): the science which deals with bacteria.

bacterium (bak-te're-um); pl., **bacteria** (-a): unicellular vegetable micro-organism.

baldness: a deficiency of hair; hair loss.

balm (bäm): an aromatic resinous substance used as a medicine or fragrance.

balneotherapy (bal-ne'o-ther-ah-py): scientific medical study of bathing and its effects.

barbituate (bar'bit-toor'it): a sedative or sleeping pill.

basal layer (bās'âl): the layer of cells at base of epidermis closest to the dermis.

base: the lower part or bottom; chief substance of a compound; an electropositive element that unites with an acid to form a salt.

beaker (bē'kĕr): a vessel of glass with a lip for pouring; used in chemical analysis.

beautician (bū-tĭsh'ân): one skilled in the art of beautifying the personal appearance.

beeswax (bēz'wăks): wax given out by bees, from which they make honeycomb; used in the making of some types of cosmetics.

benign (bē-nīn'): mild in character.

benzine (bĕn'zēn): an inflammable liquid derived from petroleum and used as a cleansing fluid.

benzoin (bĕn'zō-ĭn, zoin): a balsamic resin used as a stimulant, and also as a perfume.

bicarbonate of soda (bī-kär'bŏn-āt): baking soda; relieves burns, itching, urticarial lesions and insect bites; is often used in bath powders as an aid to cleansing oily skin.

bichloride (bī-klō'rīd): a compound having two parts or equivalents of chlorine to one of the other elements.

biocatalyst (bī'ō-kăt'ă-lĭst): a substance that acts to promote or modify some physiological process, especially an enzyme, vitamin or hormone.

biceps (bī'sĕps): having two heads; a muscle producing the contour of the front and inner side of the upper arm.

biochemistry (bī'ō-kĕm'ĭs-trē): the chemistry of living animals and plants; the study of chemical compounds and processes occurring in living organisms.

bioflavonoid (-'flā-vō-nōid): a biologically active flavonoid; also called Vitamin P.

biology (bī-ŏl'ō-jē): the science of life and living things.

blackhead (blăck'hĕd): a comedone; a plug of sebaceous matter.

bleach (blēch): to make lighter or white; to remove color or stains.

bleb (blĕb): a blister of the skin filled with watery fluid.

blemish (blĕm.'ĭsh): a mark, spot or defect on the skin.

blister (blĭs'tĕr): a vesicle; a collection of serous fluid causing a raised elevation of the skin.

blonde; blond (blŏnd): a person of fair complexion, with light hair and eyes.

blood (blŭd): the nutritive fluid circulating through the arteries and veins.

blood vascular system (văs'kû-lâr sĭs'tĕm): comprised of structures (the heart, arteries, veins and capillaries) which distribute blood throughout the body.

blood vessel (vĕs'ĕl): an artery, vein or capillary.

blue light: a therapeutic lamp used to soothe the nerves.

blusher (blŭsh'ĕr): a powdered rouge used as cheek color or for contour shading.

boil (boil): a furuncle; a subcutaneous abscess; it is caused by bacteria which enter through the hair follicles.

boiling point: 212° F. or 100° C.; the temperature at which a liquid begins to boil.

bond (bŏnd): 1) the linkage between different atoms or radicals of a chemical compound usually effected by the transfer of one or more electrons from one atom to another; 2) it can be found represented by a dot or a line between atoms shown in various formulas.

booster (boos'tĕr): oxidizer added to hydrogen peroxide to increase its chemical action; such chemicals as ammonium persulfate or percarbonate are used.

borax (bō'răks): sodium tetraborate; a white powder used as an antiseptic and cleansing agent.

boric acid (bō'rĭk ăs'ĭd): acidum boricum; used as an antiseptic dusting powder; in liquid form as an eyewash.

brachial artery (brā'kĭ-âl): the main artery of the upper arm.

brain (brān): that part of the central nervous system contained in the cranial cavity, and consisting of the cerebrum, the cerebellum, the pons, and the medulla oblongata.

bristle (brĭs'l): the short, stiff hair of a brush; short, stiff hairs of an animal, used in brushes.

brittle (brĭt'l): easily broken; fragile.

bromidrosis (brō-mĭ-drō'sĭs): perspiration which smells foul.

buccal nerve (bŭk'âl): a motor nerve affecting the buccinator and the orbicularis oris muscle.

buccinator (bŭk'sĭ-nā-tĕr): a thin, flat muscle of the cheek, shaped like a trumpet.

bulbous (bŭl'bûs): pertaining to, or being like a bulb in shape or structure.

bulla (boo'lă): a large bleb or blister.

C

calamine lotion (kăl'ă-mīn): zinc carbonate in alcohol used for the treatment of dermatitis in its various forms.

calcium (kăl'sē-ŭm): a brilliant silvery-white metal; enters into the composition of bone.

callous, callus (kăl'ŭs): skin which has become hardened; thick-skinned.

calorie (kăl'ō-rē): a unit of heat.

camomile (kăm-ō-mīl): plant having strongly scented foliage and flowers which are used medicinally; having characteristics of soothing the skin and slight bleaching powers.

camphor (kăm'fēr): a mild cutaneous stimulant; it produces redness and warmth and has a slightly anaesthetic nd cooling effect.

cancellous (kăn'sê-lŭs): having a porous or spongy structure.

caninus (kă-nīn'ŭs): the muscle which lifts the angle of the mouth.

capillary (kăp'ĭ-lâ-rē): any one of the minute blood vessels which connect the arteries and veins; hair-like.

carbohydrate (kär-bō-hī'drăt): a chemical containing carbon, hydrogen, and oxygen.

carbolic acid (kär-bŏl'ĭk): phenol made from coal tar; a caustic and corrosive poison; used in dilute solution as an antiseptic.

carbon (kär'bŏn): coal; an elementary substance in nature which predominates in all organic compounds and occurs in three distinct forms: black lead; charcoal, and lampblack.

carbon-arc lamp (kär'bŏn ärk lămp): an instrument which produces ultra-violet rays.

carbon dioxide (dī-ŏk'sĭd): carbonic acid gas; product of the combustion of carbon with a free supply of air.

carbonic acid (kär-bŏn'ĭk): a weak, colorless acid, formed by the solution of carbon dioxide in water, and existing only in solution.

carbonic gas (kär-bŏn'ĭk): carbon dioxide.

carbuncle (kär-bŭn'k'l): a large circumscribed inflammation of the subcutaneous tissue that is similar to a furuncle, but much more extensive.

carcinoma (kär-sĭ-nō'mă): cancer; a malignant new growth of epithelial or gland cells infiltrating the surrounding tissues.

cardiac (kär'dē-ăk): pertaining to the heart.

carotid (kă-rŏt'ĭd): the principal artery of the neck.

carpus (kär'pŭs): the wrist; the eight bones of the wrist.

cartilage (kär'tĭ-lăj): gristle; a non-vascular connective tissue softer than bone.

castile soap (kăs'tēl sōp): a fine, hard, white soap containing olive oil and other oils; originated in Castile, Spain.

castor oil (kăs'tēr): obtained from the castor bean. Used as a cathartic, a lubricant in eyedrops and some creams and pastes. Rarely used in cosmetics.

catabolism (kâ-tăb'ō-lĭz'm): chemical changes which involve the breaking down process within the cells.

catalyst (kăt'â-lĭst): a substance having the power to increase the velocity of a chemical reaction.

cataphoresis (kă-tăf-ō-rē'sĭs): forcing of medicinal substances into the deeper tissues, using the galvanic current from the positive towards the negative.

cathode (kăth'ōd): the negative pole or electrode of a constant electric current.

caucasian (kô-kā'-zhen): a member of the caucasoid division of the human species.

caustic (kôs'tĭk): an agent that burns and chars tissue.

caustic soda: sodium hydroxide.

cell (sĕl): a minute mass of protoplasm forming the structural unit of every organized body.

cell division: the reproduction of cells by the process of each cell dividing in half and forming two cells.

cellular (sĕl'û-lăr): consisting of, or pertaining to, cells.

cellulitis (sĕl'û-lī-tĭs): inflammation of connective tissue.

cellulose (sĕl'û-lōs): a carbohydrate, such as a vegetable fiber.

celsius (sel'sē-us): a temperature scale in which the freezing point of water at normal atmospheric prssure is 0° and the boiling point is 100°; the centigrade scale.

centigrade (sĕn'tĭ-grād): consisting of 100 degrees; one hundredth part of a circle.

centigrade scale (sĕn'tĭ-grād skāl): a temperature scale with the freezing point at (0) zero degrees and the boiling point at 100 degrees.

centimeter (sen'ti-mēter): in the metric system, the hundreth part of a meter.

centrosome (sĕn'trô-sōm): a cellular body which controls the division of the cell.

cerebellum (sĕr-ê-bĕl'ûm): the posterior and lower part of the brain.

cerebral (sĕr'ê-brâl): pertaining to the cerebrum.

cerebrospinal system (sĕr-ê-brô-spī'nâl sĭs'tĕm): consists of the brain, spinal cord, spinal nerves and the cranial nerves.

cerebrun (sĕr'ê-brûm): the superior and larger part of the brain.

certified color (sûr'tĭ-fĭd kŭl'ēr): a commercial coloring product used in cosmetics and hair coloring products.

cervical (sûr'vĭ-kâl): pertaining to the neck.

chamomile: (see camomile).

chap (chăp): to split, crack or redden the skin.

chemical change (kĕm'ĭ-kâl chānj): alteration in the chemical composition of a substance.

chemistry (kĕm'is-trē): the science dealing with the mutual reactions, and the phenomena resulting from composition of substances; the elements and their formation and decomposition of compounds.

chiropody (kī-rŏp'ō-dē): the art of treating minor diseases of the hands and feet.

chloasma (klō-ăz'mă): irregular large brown patches on the skin, such as liver spots.

chlorine (klō'rĭn, rēn): greenish yellow gas with a disagreeable suffocating odor; used in combined form as a disinfectant and a bleaching agent.

chlorophyll (klō'rô-fĭl): the green coloring matter found in plants.

cholesterin; cholesterol (kô-lĕs'tēr-ĭn; -ōl): a waxy alcohol found in animal tissues and their secretions; it is present in lanolin, and used as an emulsifier.

chromosome (krō'mō-sōm): tiny dark stained bodies found in the nucleus of the cell; transmits hereditary characteristics in cell division.

chronic (krŏn'ĭk): long-continued; the reverse of acute.

cicatrix (sĭ-kā'trĭks): pl., **cicatrices** (sĭk-ă-trī'sēz): the skin or film which forms over a wound, later contracting to form a sar.

cilia (sĭl'ĭ-ă): the eyelashes; microscopic hair-like extensions which assist bacteria in locomotion.

circuit (sûr'kĭt): the path of an electric current.

circulation (sûr-kû-lā'shûn): the passage of blood throughout the body.

citric acid (sĭt'rĭk): acid found in the lemon, orange, grapefruit; used for making a rinse.

clavicle (klăv'ĭ-k'l): collarbone, joining the sternum and scapula.

clay (klā): an earthy substance containing hydrous aluminum silicates, etc., and used for facial packs.

Cleopatra (klē'ō-pat'-ra): 69-30 B.C. Queen of Egypt; known for her beauty and the use of a wide variety of fragrances and cosmetics.

clockwise (klŏk'wīz): movements in the same direction as the hands of a clock.

coagulate (kō-ăg'ū-lāt): to clot; to convert a fluid into a soft, jelly-like solid.

coccus (kŏk'ŭs; pl., **cocci** (kŏk'sī): spherical cell bacterium.

cocoa butter (kō'kō): a hard, yellowish fatty substance obtained from cocoa seeds, used for making soaps, and cosmetics.

coconut oil (kō'ka-nut'): the oil derived from the dried meat of the coconut, used in cosmetics.

collagen (kŏl'ă-jĕn): a protein forming the chief constituent of the connective tissues and the bones.

collodion (kō-lō'dē-ŏn): a thick liquid used to form an adhesive covering.

cologne (ko-lōn): a toilet water consisting of alcohol scented with aromatic oils.

coltsfoot (kōlts'fŏŏt): an herb bearing yellow flowers that is used for medicinal purposes.

combustion (kŏm-bŭs'chŭn): the rapid oxidation of any substance, accompanied by the production of heat and light.

comedone (kŏm'ē-dōne): blackhead; a worm-like mass in an obstructed sebaceous duct.

comedone extractor (ĕks'trăk'tĕr): an instrument used for the removal of blackheads.

comfrey (kum'fre): a rough, hairy herb of the borage family; its root contains tannin.

communicable (kō-mū'nĭ-kă-b'l): able to be communicated; transferable.

compact tissue (kŏm'păkt): a dense, hard type of bony tissue.

complementary (kŏm'plē-mĕn'tĕr-ē): serving as a complement; completing.

complimentary (kŏm'plĭ-mĕn'tĕr-ē): an expression of admiration or something given free.

complexion (kôm-plĕk'shŭn): hue or general appearance of the skin, especially the face.

composition (kŏm-pō'zĭsh'ŭn): the kind and number of atoms constituting the molecules of a substance.

compound (kŏm'pound): a substance formed by a chemical union of two or more elements, and different from any of them.

compounds (kŏm'poundz): 1) made of two or more parts or ingredients; 2) in chemistry, a substance which consists of two or more chemical elements in union.

compress (kōm-prĕs): a cloth or pad sometimes medicated for applying moisture, cold, heat or pressure to a part of the body.

concentrated (kŏn'sĕn-trăt-ĕd): condensed; increasing the strength by diminishing the bulk.

conducting cords (kŏn-dŭckt'ĭng): insulated copper wires which convey the current from the wall plate to the client and operator.

conductor (kŏn-dŭk'tĕr): any substance which will attract or allow a current to flow through it easily.

configuration (kŏn-fĭg'ū-rā'shŭn): the arrangement and spacing of the atoms of a molecule.

congeal (kŏn-jēl): the change from a fluid to a solid state.

congenital (kŏn-jĕn'ĭ-tâl): existing at birth; born with.

congestion (kŏn-jĕs'chŭn): overfullness of the capillary and other blood vessels in any locality or organ; local hyperemia.

connecting cords (kŏn-ĕkt'ĭng kôrdz): the insulating strands of copper wires which join together the apparatus and the commercial electric current.

constitutional (kŏn-stĭ-tū'shŭn-âl): belonging to or affecting the physical or vital powers of an individual.

contagion (kŏn-tā'jŭn): transmission of specific diseases by contact.

contaminate (kŏn-tăm'ĭ-nāt): to make impure by contact.

contour (kŏn-tōŏr): the outline of a figure or body.

contraction (kŏn-trăk'shŭn): the act of shrinking, drawing together.

converter (kŏn-vûr'tĕr): an apparatus used to convert the direct current to alternating current.

coordinate (kō-ôr'de-nāt): to bring into harmonious relation or action.

corium (kō'rē-ŭm): the derma or true skin.

cornification (kŏr-nĭ-fĭ-kā'shŭn): the process of becoming a horny substance or tissue; a callosity.

cornstarch (kôrn'stärch'): starch made from corn; used primarily as a thickening agent or powder.

corpuscles, red (kôr'pŭs'lz, rĕd): cells in blood whose function is to carry oxygen to the cells.

corpuscles, white (whīt): cells in the blood whose function is to destroy disease germs.

corrosive (kô-rō'sĭv): something causing corrosion.

corrugations (kŏr-ū-gā'shŭns): alternate ridges and furrows; wrinkles.

corrugator supercilli (kŭr'ŭ-gā-tĕr sū-pĕr-sĭl'ī): draws eyebrows inward and downward, thus causing vertical wrinkles at the root of the nose.

cortisone (kor'ta-sōn): a powerful hormone extracted from the cortex of the adrenal gland and also made synthetically; used in the treatment of disease.

cosmetic (kŏz-mĕt'ĭk): of or relating to, or making for beauty, especially of the complexion.

cosmetic dermatology (kŏz-mĕt'ĭk dûr-mă-tŏl'ō-jē): a branch of dermatology devoted to improving the health and beauty of the skin and its appendages.

cosmetician (kŏz-mĕ-tĭsh'ân): one who is professionally trained in the use of cosmetics.

cosmetologist (kŏz-mĕ-tŏl-ō-jĭst): one skilled in the art of improving beauty.

cosmetology (kŏz-mĕ-tŏl'ō-jē): the science of beautifying and improving the complexion, skin, hair and nails.

counterclockwise (koun'tĕr-klŏk'wīz): movements in the opposite direction to the hands of a clock.

couperose (cōō'pĕr-ōs): a word used in the field of esthetics to describe a broken capillary condition of the skin.

cranium (krā'nē'ŭm): the bones of the head excluding bones of the face; bony case for the brain.

cream (krēm): a semi-solid cosmetic.

creosol (krē'ō-sōl): a colorless, oily liquid or solid derived from coal tar and wood tar and used as a disinfectant.

crest (krĕst): a ridge, line or thin mark made by folding or doubling; a scar may have a crest of scar tissue.

cross bonds (krŏs bŏndz): the bonds holding together the long chains of amino-acids, which compose hair; the bonds holding together the parallel chains of amino-acids to form hair.

current, alternating; A.C. (kŭr'ênt, ôl'tĕr-nāt-ĭng): an interrupted current.

current, D'asonval (d'-är'sôn-vâl): a high-frequency current of low voltage and high amperage.

current, direct; D.C. (dĭ-rĕkt'): an uninterrupted and even flowing current.

current, electric (ē-lĕk'trĭk): electricity in motion, or moving within a conductor.

current, faradic (fâ-răd'ĭk): an induced interrupted current whose action is mechanical.

current, galvanic (găl-văn'ĭk): a direct constant current having a positive and negative pole and producing a chemical reaction.

current, high-frequency; Tesla (hī-frē'kwên-sē; těs'lå): an electric current of medium voltage and medium amperage.

current, sinusoidal (sĭn-û-soi'dâl): an induced interrupted current somewhat similar to faradic current.

current strength (kûr'ênt strĕngth): the relation of the electromotive force to the resistance of the circuit.

cutaneous (kû-tā'nê-ûs): pertaining to the skin.

cuticle (kū'tĭ-k'l): the outer layer of the skin or hair.

cutis (kū'tĭs): the derma or deeper layer of the skin.

cuvette (kōō'vĕt): a specially designed bowl used to protect the client's body from spray during a facial treatment.

cylinder (sĭl'ĭn-dêr): a long circular body, solid or hollow, uniform in diameter.

cyst (sĭst): a closed, abnormally developed sac containing fluid, semi-fluid or morbid matter.

cytoplasm (sī'tô-plăz'm): the protoplasm of the cell body, exclusive of the nucleus.

D

dandruff (dăn'drŭf): pityriasis; scurf or scales formed in excess upon the scalp.

debris (dā-brē'): remains, rubbish.

decade (dek'ād): a period of ten years.

decimeter (des'a-mē'ter): in the metric system, the tenth part of a meter.

decompose (dē-kôm-pōz): to decay or rot; to separate into the constituent parts; to bring to dissolution.

degenerate (dē-jĕn'ér-āt): to pass from a higher to a lower type or condition.

degrease (dē-grēs'): to remove grease from.

dehydrate (dē-hī'drāt): to deprive of water or to suffer loss of water; to dry out.

deltoid (dĕl'toid): a muscle of the shoulder.

demarcation (dē-mär-kā'shûn): a line setting bounds or limits.

dendrite (dĕn'drīt): a tree-like branching of nerve fibers extending from a nerve cell.

deodorant (dē-ō'dĕr-ânt): a substance that removes or conceals offensive odors.

depilatory (dê-pĭl'å-tô-rē): a substance, usually a caustic alkali, use to destroy the hair; having the power to remove hair.

depressor (dē-prĕs'ér): that which presses or draws down; a muscle that depresses.

dermabrasion (dûr'muh-bray-'zhun): the removal of skin in varying amounts and depths by such mechanical means as revolving wire brushes or sandpaper, for the purpose of correcting scars.

dematitis (dûr-mǎ-tī'tĭs): inflammation of the skin.

dermatitis, contact: an inflammation of the skin caused by coming in contact with chemicals, dyes, etc., to which the individual may be allergic.

dermatitis, cosmetic: an inflammation of the skin caused by coming in contact with some cosmetic product to which the individual may be allergic.

dermatitis, occupational (ŏk-û-pā'shûn-âl): an inflammation of the skin caused by the kind of employment in which the individual is engaged.

dermatologist (dûr-mǎ-tŏl'ō-jĭst): one who understands the science of the treating of the skin, its structure, function and diseases.

dermatology (dûr-mǎ-tŏl'ō-jē): the science which treats the skin and its diseases.

dermatosis (dûr-mǎ-tō'sĭs): any disease of the skin.

dermis, derma (dûr'mĭs, dûr'mǎ): the layer below the epidermis; the corium or true skin.

detergent (dē-tûr'jĕnt): a compound or solution used for cleaning; an agent that cleanses the skin and hair.

deteriorate (dē-tē'rē-ôô-rāt): to make or to grow worse; to become impaired in quality; to degenerate.

dexterity (dĕks-tĕr'ĭ-tē): skill and ease in using the hands; expertness in manual acts.

diabetic (dī'a-bet'ĭk): one who has diabetes, a disease associated with deficient insulin secretion.

diagnosis (dī-ăg-nō'sĭs): the recognition of a disease from its symptoms.

dialysis (dī-ăl'ĭ-sĭs): the process of separating different substances in solution by diffusion through a moist membrane or septum; separation.

diaphoretic (dī'afa-ret'ik): producing perspiration.

diathermy (dī'ă-thûr-mē): a method of raising the temperature in the deep tissues, using high-frequency current.

dielectric (dī'e-lek'-trik): nonconducting; capable of sustaining an electric field.

diffusion (dĭ-fū'zhûn): a spreading out; dialysis.

digestion (dī-jĕs'chûn): the process of converting food into a form which can be readily absorbed by the body.

digits (dĭj'ĭts): fingers or toes.

dilator (dī-lā'tĕr; dĭ-): that which expands or enlarges.

dilute (dĭ-lūt'; dĭ-): to make thinner by mixing, especially with water.

dimension (dĭ-mĕn'shûn): any measurable extent, as length, breadth or thickness.

diminish (dĭ-mĭn'ĭsh): to make small or less; to reduce.

diphtheria (dĭf-thē-'rē-ǎ): an infectious desease in which the air passages, especially the throat, becomes coated with false membrane, caused by specific bacillus.

diplococcus (dī-plô-kŏk'ûs): bacteria exhibiting pairs.

diplomacy (di-plō'ma-sē): skill or tact in dealing with others.

disease (dĭ-zēz'): a pathologic condition of any part or organ of the body, or of the mind.

disinfectant (dĭs-ĭn-fĕk'tânt): an agent used for destroying germs.

dispensary (dĭs-pĕn'så-rē): a place where medicines or other supplies are prepared and dispensed.

dispersion (dĭs-pûr'shôn): 1) the act of scattering or separating; 2) the incorporation of the particles of one substance into the body of another, comprising solutions, suspensions and colloid solutions.

distill (dĭs-tĭl'): to extract the essence or active principle of a substance.

drape (drāp): to arrange or cover with cloth.

dsychromis (dīz'krō-mĭs): abnormal pigmentation of the skin.

duct (dŭkt): a passage or canal for fluids.

E

eczema (ěk'zē-mǎ): an inflammatory itching disease of the skin.

edema (ě-dē'ma): an abnormal accumulation of clear watery fluid in the lymph spaces of the tissues.

efferent (ěf'ĕr-ênt): motor nerves conveying impulses away from the central nervous system.

effleurage (ě-flū-razh'): a stroking movement in massage.

Egyptian (ē-jĭp'shân): pertaining to Egypt, its people or their culture.

elasticity (ē-lăs'tĭs'ĭ-tē): the property that allows a thing to be stretched, and to return to its former shape.

electricity (ē-lĕck'trĭs'ĭ-tē): a form of energy which when in motion, exhibits magnetic, chemical or thermal effects.

electrode (ê-lĕk′trōd): a pole of an electric cell; an applicator for directing the use of electricity on a client.

electrologist (ê-lĕk-trŏl′ō-jĭst): proposed term for a person versed in electrology, and who may, in addition, be skilled in applying the science.

electrology (ê-lĕk-trŏl′ō-jē): science in relation to electricity.

electrolysis (ê-lĕk-trŏl′ĭ-sĭs): decomposition of a chemical compound or body tissues by means of electricity.

electrolyte (ê-lĕk-trō-līt): any compound which, in solution, conducts a current of electricity and is decomposed by it.

electron ((ê-lĕk′trŏn): an extremely minute corpuscle or charge of negative electricity, the smallest known to exist.

electrophoresis (i-lek′trō-fa-rē′sis): the slow movement of the electrically charged colloidal particles, dispersed in a fluid when under the influence of an electric field.

electropositive (ê-lĕk′trō-pŏz′ĭ-tĭv): relating to or charged with positive electricity.

electro-static (ê-lĕk′trō-stăt′ĭk): pertaining to static electricity.

element (ĕl′ê-mĕnt): 1) a simple substance which cannot be decomposed by chemical means, and which is made up of atoms which are alike in their peripheral electronic configurations and in their chemical properties; 2) any one of the 103 ultimate chemical entities of which matter is believed to be composed.

elevation (ĕl-ĕ-vā′shŭn): raised above the normal level.

Elizabethan (i-liz′-a-bē′then): pertaining to Elizabeth I of England and/or her era.

embryo (em′brē-ō): the first stages of development.

embryonic extracts: extracts of any living thing in its earliest stage of life. e.g. chicken embryo used in live cell therapy.

emolient (ê-mŏl′yĕnt): an agent that softens or soothes the surface of the skin.

emphasize (em′fa-sīz): to give emphasis to; to make prominent or important.

emulsifier (ê-mŭl′sĭ-fĭ-ēr): a substance, as gelatin, gum, etc., for emulsifying a fixed oil.

emulsion (ê-mŭl′shŭn): a product consisting of minute globules of one liquid dispersed throughout the body of a second liquid.

end bonds (peptide bonds) (pĕp′tĭd): the chemical bonds which join together the amino-acids to form the long chains which are characteristic of all proteins.

endocrine (ĕn′dô-crĭn): any internal secretion or hormone.

environment (ĕn-vī′rŭn-mĕnt): surrounding conditions; influences or forces which influence or modify.

enzyme (ĕn′zīm): a substance which induces a chemical change in other substances without undergoing any change itself.

epidemic (ĕp-ĭ-dĕm′ĭk): common to many people; a prevailing disease.

epidermis (ĕp-ĭ-dûr′mĭs): the outer layer of the skin.

epilation (ĕp-ĭ-lā′shŭn): the removal of hair by the roots.

epithelium (ĕp-ĭ-thê′lē-ûm): a cellular tissue or membrane, with little intercellular substance, covering a free surface or lining a cavity.

eponychium (ĕp-ô-nĭk′ê-ûm): the extension of cuticle at base of nail-body.

eruption (ê-rŭp′shŭn): a visible lesion of the skin due to disease, marked by redness or papular condition or both.

erythema (ĕr-ĭ-thê′mă): a superficial blush or redness of the skin.

erythematous (ĕr-ĭ-thĕm′ă-tûs): abnormal redness of the skin caused by a congestion of capillaries.

erythrocyte (ĕ-rĭth′rō′sĭt): a red blood cell; red corpuscle.

esophagus; oesophagus (ê-sŏf′ă-gûs): the canal leading from the pharynx to the stomach.

essence (es′ans): the extract of a plant or food containing the distinctive properties of the plant or food in a perfume.

essential (ĕ-sĕn′shâl): important in the highest degree.

essential oils: any of a class of volatile oils that import the characteristic odors to plants and are used in perfumes and flavorings.

ester (ĕs′tēr): an organic compound formed by the reaction of an acid and an alcohol.

esthetic (ĕs-thĕt′ĭk): sensitive to art and beauty; showing good taste; artistic.

esthetician (ĕs-thê′tĭ-shûn): a specialist in or devotee of esthetics; one who works to clean and beautify the skin (also aesthetician).

esthetics (ĕs-thĕt′ĭks): a branch of philosophy pertaining to or dealing with the forms and nature of beauty; judgment concerning beauty (also spelled aesthetics).

estrogen (ĕs′trō-jĕn): any of various substances that influence estrus or produce changes in the sexual characteristics of female mammals.

ethics (eth′icks): principles of good character and proper conduct.

ethmoid (ĕth′moid): resembling a sieve; a bone forming part of the walls of the nasal cavity.

ethnic (eth′nik): belonging to or distinctive of a particular racial, cultural division of human kind.

etiology (ê-tē-ŏl′ō-jē): the science of the causes of disease.

evaporation (ê-văp-ô-rā′shŭn): change from liquid to vapor form.

excoriation (ĕks-kō-rē-ā′shŭn): act of stripping or wearing off the skin; an abrasion.

excrete (ĕks′krēt): to separate (waste matter) from the blood or tissue and eliminate from the body as through the kidneys or sweat glands.

excretion (ĕks-krē′shŭn): that which is thrown off or eliminated from the body.

exhalation (ĕks-hà-lā′shŭn): the act of breathing outward.

expel (ĕks′pĕl): to force out, to eject or dislodge.

extensibility (ĕks-tĕn-sĭ-bil′ĭ-tē): capable of being extended or stretched.

extensor (ĕks-tĕn′sôr): a muscle which serves to extend or straighten out a limb or part.

extract (ĕks′trăkt): to withdraw by physical or chemical process; a product prepared by extracting.

extremity (ĕks-trĕm′ĭ-tē): the distant end or part of any organ; a hand or foot.

exudation (ĕks-û-dā′shŭn): act of discharging from the body through pores as sweat, moisture or other liquid.

eye-brow (ī′brow′): the arch of small hairs growing on the bony ridge over the eyes.

eye-lash (ī′lăsh′): one of the stiff curved hairs growing from the edge of the upper and lower eyelids.

eye-shadow: a cosmetic applied on the eyelids to accentuate their brilliance.

F

facial (fā′shâl): pertaining to the face; the seventh cranial nerve.

facial treatment (fā′shâl trēt′mĕnt): a cosmetic treatment applied to the face and neck which is generally applied for preventive or corrective purposes and for the general enhancement of skin and muscle tone.

Fahrenheit (fä'rên-hĭt): pertaining to the Fahrenheit thermometer or scale; water freezes at 32° F. and boils at 212° F.

fat (făt): a greasy soft solid material found in animal tissue.

fatty acid (făt'ē ăs'ĭd): an acid derived from the saturated series of open chains of hydro-carbons.

favus (fā'vŭs): a contagious parasitic disease of the skin with crusts.

felon (fĕl'ŭn): paronychia of the nail.

fermentation (fûr-mĕn-tā'shŭn): a chemical decomposition of organic compounds into more simple compounds, brought about by the action of an enzyme.

fetid (fĕt'ĭd): having a foul smell; stinking.

fever (fē'vĕr): rise of body temperature.

fever blister (fē'vĕr blĭs'tĕr): an acute skin disease characterized by the presence of vesicles over an inflammatory base; herpes simplex.

fiber (fī'bĕr): a slender, threadlike structure that combines with others to form animal or vegetable tissue.

fibrin (fī'brĭn): the active agent in coagulation of the blood.

fibrous (fī'brŭs): containing, consisting of like fibers.

filter (fĭl'tĕr): anything porous through which liquid is passed to cleanse or strain it.

fission (fĭsh'ŭn): reproduction of bacteria by cellular division; any splitting or cleaving; atomic f.: the splitting of the neutrons of an atom in two main fragments.

fissure (fĭsh'ûr): a narrow opening made by separation of parts; a furrow; a slit.

fixative (fĭk'sä-tĭv): serving to render permanent or fixed.

flabbiness (flăb-ē'nĕs): lacking resilience or firmness.

flaccidity (flă(k)-sĭd'ĭt-ē): lacking normal or youthful firmness; lacking vigor or force.

flagella (flă-jĕl'ă): slender whip-like processes which permit locomotion in certain bacteria.

flexible (flĕk'sĭ-b'l): able to adjust to change; pliant; adaptable.

flexor (flĕk'sôr): a muscle that bends or flexes a part or a joint.

florid (flŏr'ĭd): flushed with red.

fluorescent (floo'ôr-ĕs'n't): an ability to emit light after exposure to light, the wave length of the emitted light being longer than that of the light absorbed.

foamer (fō'mĕr): a substance which creates an excessive amount of foam.

follicle (fŏl'ĭ-k'l): the depression in the skin containing the hair root.

foreign (fôr'in): belonging to a characteristic of, or derived from another country, region or society.

formaldehyde (fôr-măl'dè-hīd): a pungent gas possessing powerful disinfectant properties.

Formalin (fôr'mă-lĭn): a 37% to 40% solution of formaldehyde.

formula (fôr'mū-lă): a prescribed method or rule; a recipe or prescription.

foundation (foun-dā'shŭn): (base) a cream used as a base for make-up or make-up base.

fragrance (frā'granse): a pleasant scent; sweet odor.

freckle (frĕk'l): a yellow or brown spot on the skin; lentigo.

free edge: part of the nail body extending over the fingertip.

frequency (frē'kwên-sē): the number of complete cycles per second of current produced by an alternating current generator; standard frequencies are 25 and 60 cycles per second.

friction (frĭk'shŭn): the resistance encountered in rubbing one body on another.

frontal (frŭn'tâl:) in front; relating to the forehead; the bone of the forehead.

Fuller's earth (fool'ĕrz ûrth): an absorbent clay often used as a foundation for packs and masks.

fulling (fool'ĭng): a massage movement in which the limb is rolled back and forth between the hands.

fumigate (fū'mĭ-gāt): disinfect by the action of fumes.

fundamental (fûn-dă-mĕn'tâl): essential, basic rule or principle.

fungus (fŭn'gŭs): a vegetable parasite; a spongy growth of diseased tissue on the body.

furuncle (fū-ûrn'k'l): a small skin abscess (boil).

fuse (fūz): to liquify by heat; a special device which prevents excessive current from passing through a circuit.

fusion (fū'zhŭn): the act of uniting or cohering.

G

galvanic current (găl-văn'ĭk kŭr'ênt): a direct and continued silent current having a positive and a negative pole; named for Galvani (1737-1798).

ganglion (găn'glē-ŏn): pl., **ganglia** (-ă): bundles of nerve cells in the brain, in organs of special sense, or forming units of the sympathetic nervous system.

gastric juice (găs'trĭk): the digestive fluid secreted by the glands of the stomach.

gauge (gāj): to estimate, appraise or judge.

gauze (gôz): a thin, open-meshed cloth used for dressings.

gel (jĕl): comprised of a solid and a liquid which exist as a solid or semi-solid mass.

gelatine (jĕl'â-tĭn): the tasteless, odorless, brittle substance extracted by boiling bones, hoofs and animal tissues used in various foods, medicines, etc.

gene (jēn): the utlimate unit in the transmission of hereditary characteristics.

genes: chromosomes by which hereditary characters are transmitted and determined.

generator (jĕn'ēr-ā-tĕr): one that generates, causes or produces.

genetic (jĕ-nĕt'ĭk): the genesis or origin of something.

genitalia (jen'a-ta'-lē'a): pertaining to the reproductive organs.

germ (jûrm): a bacillus, a microbe; an embryo in its early stages.

germicide (jûr'mĭ-sīd): any chemical, especially a solution that will destroy germs.

germinative layer (jûr-mĭ-nā'tĭv): stratum germinativum; the deepest layer of the epidermis resting on the corium.

ginseng (jĭn'sĕng): an herb native to China and North America, having a root of aromatic and stimulant properties.

gland (glănd): a secretory organ of the body.

glandular (glăn'dû-lâr): pertaining to a gland.

globule (glŏb'ūl): a small, spherical droplet of fluid or semi-fluid material.

glossopharyngeal (glŏs-ô-fă-rĭn'jē-âl): pertaining to the tongue and pharynx; the ninth cranial nerve.

glucose (gloo'kōs): a thick syrup containing dextrose, maltrose and dextrin.

glycerin; glycerine (glĭs'ĕr-ĭn): sweet, oily fluid used as an application for roughened and chapped skin; used also as a solvent.

glycogen (glī'kō-jĕn): animal starch.

gonorrhea (gŏn-ô-rē'ă): a contagious venereal disease, due to the presence of the gonococci bacteria in the genetal tract.

gram (grăm): the basic unit of mass or weight in the metric system.

granules (grăn'ūlz): small grains; small pills.

granulosum (grăn-û-lōs'ûm): granular layer of the epidermis.

gravity (grăv'ĭ-tē): the effect of the attraction of the earth upon matter.

great auricular (grāt ô-rĭk′û-lär): a nerve affecting the face, ear, neck and parotid gland.

greater occipital (ŏk-sĭp′ĭ-tâl): sensory and motor nerve affecting the back part of the scalp.

Greek (grēk): pertaining to Greece, its people, language or culture.

green soap (grēn sōap): a soft soap made from linseed oil and the hydroxides or potassium and sodium, used in the treatment of skin diseases.

gristle (grĭs′l): cartilage.

grooming (grōōm′ĭng): to make neat or tidy.

ground wire (ground wīr): a wire which connects an electric current to a ground (waterpipe or radiator).

H

hacking (hăk′ĭng): a chopping stroke made with the edge of the hand in massage.

hair bulb (hâr bŭlb): the lower extremity of the hair.

hair coloring: artificially changing the color of the hair; dyeing brows and lashes.

hair density: the number of hairs per square inch on the scalp or body.

hair follicle (fŏl′ĭ-k′l): the depression of the skin containing the root of the hair.

hair papilla (hâr pă-pĭl′ă): a small, cone-shaped elevation at the bottom of the hair follicle.

hair pilus (pī′lŭs): a slender threadlike outgrowth on the body.

hair root: that part of the hair contained within the follicle.

hair shaft (shăft): the portion of the hair which projects beyond the skin.

hair, superfluous (sŭ-pûr′flōō-ûs): unwanted or excess hair, usually found on the faces of women; see: hirsuties.

hair texture (tĕks′tŭr): the general quality of hair, as to coarse, medium or fine; the feel of the hair.

halitosis (hăl-ĭ-tō′sĭs): offensive odor from the mouth; foul breath.

Hebrew (hē′brōō): a member of that group of semitic peoples claiming descent from the house of Abraham; Israelite; Jew.

helix (hē′lĭks; hĕl′ĭks): the fleshy tip of the ear (ear lobe).

hematocyte (hĕ′mă-tō-sīt): a blood corpuscle.

hemoglobin; haemoglóbin (hē-mō-glō′bĭn): the coloring matter of the blood.

hemorrhage (hĕm′ô-râj): bleeding; a flow of blood.

herb (hûrb): a plant without woody tissue that withers and dies away after flowering; valued as seasoning, medicine or used in scents.

heredity (hĕ-rĕd′ĭ-tē): the inborn capacity of the organism to develop ancestral characteristics.

herpes (hûr′pēz): an inflammatory disease of the skin having small vesicles in clusters.

herpes simplex (sĭm′plĕks): fever blister; cold sore.

hexachlorophenol (hĕks-ă-klō-rō-fē′nŏl): white, free flowing powder, essentially odorless; used as a bactericidal agent in antiseptic soaps, deodorant products, including soaps and various cosmetics.

high-frequency (hī-frē′kwĕn-sē): violet ray; an electric current of medium voltage and medium amperage.

highlight (hī′līt): adding brightness or lustre to the skin or hair by artificial means.

hirsute (hûr-sūt, hĕr-sūt′): hairy; having coarse, long hair; shaggy.

histology (hĭs-tŏl′ō-jē): the science of the minute structure of organic tissues; microscopic anatomy.

hives (hīve′z): urticaria; a skin eruption.

Hodgkin's Disease (hoj′kinz): a generally fatal disease characterized by progressive enlargement of the lymph nodes, lymphoid tissue and spleen.

homogeneous (hō-mōj′ē-nûs): having the same nature or quality; a uniform character in all parts.

homogenizer (hō-mōj′ĕ-nīz-ĕr): serving to produce a uniform suspension of emulsions from two or more normally immiscible substances.

hormone (hôr′mōn): a chemical substance formed in one organ or part of the body and carried in the blood to another organ or part which it stimulates to functional activity or secretion.

horny (hôr′nē): composed of or resembling horns.

humectant (hew-meck′tānt): a substance used to retain moisture.

humerus (hū′mĕr-ûs): the bone of the upper part of the arm.

humidity (hew-mid′i-tee): moisture; dampness.

hydrate (hī′drāt): a compound formed by the union of water with some other substance.

hydro (hī′drō): a prefix denoting water, hydrogen.

hydro carbon: any compound composed only of hydrogen and carbon.

hydrogen: the lightest element; it is an odorless, tasteless, colorless gas found in water and all organic compounds; h. acceptor: a substance which, on reduction, accepts hydrogen atoms from another substance called a hydrogen donor.

hydrogen bond (physical bond): that bond formed between two molecules when the nucleus of a hydrogen atom, originally attached to a florine, nitrogen or oxygen atom of a second molecule of the same or different substance.

hydrogen peroxide (hī′drō-jĕn pĕr-ŏk′sīd): a powerful oxidizing agent; in liquid form it is used as an antiseptic and for the activation of lighteners and hair tints.

hydrophilic (hī-drō-fĭl′ĭk): capable of combining with or attracting water.

hydrotherapy (hī′drō-′thĕr-ă-pē): the scientific use of water in the treatment of disease.

hygiene (hī′jēn): the science of preserving health.

hygroscopic (hī-grō′skōp-ĭk): readily absorbing and retaining moisture.

hyoid (hī′oid): the "u" shaped bone at the base of the tongue.

hyper (hī′pĕr): a prefix denoting excessive; above normal; above; beyond.

hyperemia (hī′pĕr-ē′mē-ă): the presence of an excessive quantity of blood in a part of the body; congestion.

hyperhidrosis, hyperidrosis (hī′pĕr-ĭ-drō′sĭs): excessive sweating.

hyper-sensitivity (hī-pĕr-sĕn-sĭ-tĭv′ĭ-tē): unusually affected by external agencies or influences to which a normal individual does not react.

hypertrophy (hī′pĕr-trō′fē): abnormal increase in the size of a part or an organ; overgrowth.

hypoglossal (hi′pô-glō′sâl): the twelfth cranial nerve; motor nerve to base of tongue.

hyponychium (hī-pō-nĭk′ē-ûm): the portion of the epidermis upon which the nail-body rests under the free edge.

I

ichthyosis (ĭk-thē-ō′sĭs): a skin disease in which the skin becomes rough with diminished sweat and sebaceous secretion; fish skin disease.

idiosyncrasy (ĭd-ē-ô-sĭn′kră-sē): characteristic peculiarity of habit or structure; susceptibility, peculiarity to the individual due to the action of certain drug or cosmetic ingredients or diet.

imbrication (ĭm-brĭ-kā′shŭn) cells arranged in layers overlapping one another; found in cuticle layer of hair.

immerse (ĭ-mûrs): to plunge into; dip; submerge in a liquid.

immunity (ĭ-mūn'ĭ-tē): freedom from, or resistant to disease.

impetigo (ĭm-pê-tī'gō): an eruption of pustules which soon rupture and become crusted, occurring chiefly on the face around the mouth and nostrils.

implement (ĭm'plê-mênt): an instrument or tool used to do a specific work.

impurity (im-pyōor'it-ē): containing something offensive or contaminating; tainted.

incense (in'sens): an aromic substance that gives off an agreeable odor when burned; gums and spices.

incision (ĭn'sĭzh'ăn): a cut; a division of soft parts made with a knife.

incite (in-sīt): to spur to action; urge on; stir up; instigate.

incubation (ĭn-kû-ba'shûn): the period of a disease between the implanting of the contagion and the development of the symptoms.

indelible (in-del'i-bel): incapable of being blotted out or effaced; not easily erased.

index (ĭn'dĕks): the forefinger; the pointing finger.

Indian (in'dē-an): a citizen of India; an American-Indian and other natives.

induce (in-dōōs'): to cause to act; to convince; persuade; prevail on.

infection (ĭn-fĕk'shûn): the invasion of the body tissues by disease germs.

infection, general: the result of the disease germs gaining entrance into the blood stream and thereby circulating throughout the entire body.

infection, local: confined to only certain portions of the body, such as an abscess.

infectious (ĭn-fĕk'shûs): capable of spreading infection.

inflammation (ĭn-flă-mā'shûn): the reaction of the body to irritation with accompanying redness, pain, heat, and swelling.

influenza (ĭn-flōō-ĕn'ză): a contagious epidemic catarrhal fever, with great prostration and varying symptoms of sequels; grippe.

infra-orbital (ĭn-fră ôr'bĭ-tâl): below the orbit; a sensory and motor nerve affecting the cheek muscles, nose, and upper lip.

infra-red: rays pertaining to that part of the spectrum lying outside of the visible spectrum and below the red rays.

infra-trochlear (trŏk'lē-âr): sensory nerve affecting the skin of the nose and the inner muscle of the eye.

infusion (in-fyōo'zhan): a liquid extract obtained by infusing or soaking a substance in water.

ingredient (ĭn-grē'dē-ĕnt): any one of the things of which a mixture is made up.

ingrown hair (ĭn'grōn hâr): a wild hair that has grown underneath the skin, which may cause an infection.

ingrown nail (ĭn'grōn nāl): the growth of the nail into the flesh instead of toward the tip of the finger or toe, which may cause an infection.

inhalation (ĭn-hă-lā'shûn): the inbreathing of air or other vapors.

inoculation (ĭn-ŏk-û-lā'shûn): the process by which protective agents are introduced into the body.

inorganic (ĭn-ôr-găn'ĭk): composed of matter not relating to living organisms.

insanitary; unsanitary (ĭn-săn'ĭ-tâ-rē; ŭn-): not sanitary or healthful; injurious to health; unclean.

insoluble (ĭn-sŏl'û-b'l): incapable of being dissolved or very difficult to dissolve.

insulator (ĭn'sû-lā-tēr): a non-conducting material or substance; materials used to cover electric wires.

intensity (ĭn-tĕn'sĭ-tē): the amount of force or energy of heat, light, sound, electric current, etc. per unit area; the quality of being intense.

intercellular (ĭn-tĕr-sĕl'û-lär): between or among cells.

intestine (ĭn-tĕs'tĭn): the digestive tube from the stomach to the anus.

involuntary muscles (ĭn-vŏl'ûn-tâ-rē): function without the action of the will.

iodine (ī'ô-dĭn): a non-metallic element used as an antiseptic for cuts, bruises, etc.

ion (ī'ŏn): an atom or group of atoms carrying an electric charge.

ionization (ī-ŏn-ĭ-zā'shûn): the term used in facial treatments to aid in the absorption of cosmetic products into the skin, until the use of electric current, high frequency current.

iris (ī'rĭs): the colored, muscular, disk-like diaphragm of the eye which regulates the pupil or opening in the center.

irreversible (ĭr-ê-vĕr'sĭ-bl): not capable of being reversed.

irritability (ĭr-ĭ-tâ-bĭl'ĭ-tē): readily excited or stimulated.

iron (ī'ûrn): element found mainly in the hemoglobin of the red cell.

J

jack (jăk): a metallic connecting device provided with spring clips to which the wires of a circuit may be attached, and into which a plug may be inserted.

jaundice (jôn'dĭs): a morbid condition characterized by yellowness of the eyes, skin and urine, constipation, loss of appetite and general languor.

jet (jĕt): a sudden spurt or gush of liquid or gas emitted from a narrow orifice, such as water from a garden hose.

joint: a connection between two or more bones.

jowl: the hanging part of a double chin; lower cheeks and jaw.

jugular (jōō'gû-lâr): pertaining to the neck or throat; the large vein in the neck.

K

kaolin (kā-ê-lĕn): a fine, white clay that is used in ceramics or a refraction.

keloid (kē'loid): a skin disease marked by whitish indurated patches surrounded by a pinkish or purplish border; a fibrous growth arising from irritations and usually a scar.

keratin (kĕr'ă-tĭn): a fiber protein characteristic of horny tissues: hair, nails, feathers, etc.; it is insoluble in protein solvents and has a high sulfur content.

keratinization (kĕr'ă-tĭn-ĭ-zā'hûn): the process of being keratinized.

keratoma (kĕr-ă-tō'mă): a callosity: a horny tumor; an acquired thickened patch of the epidermis.

keratosis (kĕr-ă-tō'sĭs): any disease of the epidermis, especially one marked by the presence of circumscribed over growths of the horny layer; callous or keratoma.

kermes (ker-'meez): dried insect matter of a purplish-red color; used in medicine and as a dye.

kilogram (kil'e-gram): in the metric system, a thousand grams.

kilometer (kil'a-me'ter): in the metric system, a thousand meters.

kilowatt (kĭl'ô-wŏt): one thousand watts of electricity.

knead (nēd): to work and press with the hands as in massage.

kohl (kōl): a preparation used to darken the edges of the eyelids.

kyphosis (kī-fō'sĭs): backward curvature of the spine; humpback.

L

labii (lā-bē-ī): of or pertaining to the lip.

labium (lā'bē-ûm); pl., **labia** (-ă): lip.

laceration (lăs'ěr-ā'shŭn): a tear of the skin or tissue.

lancet (lăn-cět'): a small, sharp and very pointed, double edged surgical blade used by estheticians and physicians to pierce a papule.

lanolin (lăn'ŏŏ-lĭn): purified wool fat.

lanugo (lă-nū'gō): the fine hair which covers most of the body.

larynx (lăr'ĭnks): the upper part of the trachea or wind pipe; the organ of voice production.

lateral (lăt'ěr-âl): on the side.

lather (lath'ěr): froth made by mixing soap and water.

latissimus dorsi (lă-tĭs'ĭ-mŭs dôr'sī): a broad, flat superficial muscle of the back.

lecithin (lĕs'ĭ-thěn): emulsifying agent; lowers surface tension between oils and water, hence aiding absorption through skin.

lentigo (lĕn-tī'gō); pl., **lentigines** (lĕn-tī-jǐ'nēz): a freckle; circumscribed spot or pigmentation in the skin.

lesion (lē'zhŭn): a structural tissue change caused by injury or disease.

lesser occipital (lĕs'ěr ŏk-sĭp'ĭ-tâl): the nerve supplying muscles at the back of the ear.

lethargy (leth'ar-jē): a state of sluggish inaction, indifference, of dullness.

leucocyte (lū'kŏ-sīt): a white corpuscle; white blood cell.

leucoderma (lū-kŏ-dûr'mă): abnormal white patches on the skin; absence of pigment in theskin.

leuconychia (lū-kŏ-nĭk'ē-ă): a whitish discoloration of nails; white spots.

lichen (lī'kěn): a dry, papular eruption of the skin.

ligament (lĭg'ă-mĕnt): a tough band of fibrous tissue, serving to connect bones, or to hold an organ in place.

light therapy (līt thěr'ă-pē): the application of light rays for treatment of disorders.

lipids (lĭp-ěds): any of various substances that are soluble in nonpolar organic solvents.

lipophilic (lĭp-ō-fĭl'ĭk): having an affinity or attraction to fat and oil.

lipstick (lĭp'stĭk): a paste-like cosmetic, usually in the form of a small cylinder, used to color the lip; also called lipcolor.

liquefy (lĭk'wě-fī): to reduce to the liquid state; said of both solids and gases.

liquor cresolis compound (lĭk'ěr krē-sōl'ĭs kŏm'-pound): a powerful germicide.

litmus paper (lĭt'mŭs): a blue coloring matter that is reddened by acids and turned blue again by alkalies.

liver spots (lĭv'ěr spŏts): the discolorations of chloasma.

lobe (lōb): a branch extending from a body; ear lobe.

lock-jaw (lŏk'jôw): tetanus; specifically trismus; a firm closing of the jaw due to tonic spasm of the muscles of mastication.

lordosis (lôr-dō'sĭs): inward curvature of the spinal column resulting in an abnormal hollow in the back.

lotion (lō'shŭn): a liquid solution used for bathing the skin.

louse (lous); pl., **lice** (līs): pediculus; an animal parasite infesting the hairs of the head.

lubricant (lū'brĭ-kânt): anything that makes things smooth and slippery, such as oil.

lucidum (lū'sĭ-dŭm): the clear layer of the epidermis.

lumbar (lum'bar): pertaining to or situated near the loins; a lumbar vertebra, nerve or artery.

lung (lûng): one of the two organs of respiration.

lunula (lū'nŭ-lă): the half-moon shaped area at the base of the nail.

lymph (lĭmf): a clear yellowish or light straw colored fluid, which circulates in the lymph spaces, or lymphatics of the body.

lymphagial (lim-fan'jē-al): pertaining to the lymphatic vessels.

lymphatic system (lĭm-făt'ĭk): consists of lymph flowing through the lymph spaces, lymph vessels, lacteals, and lymph nodes or glands.

Lysol (lī'sōl): a trade name; a disinfectant and antiseptic; a mixture of soaps and phenols.

M

macroscopic (măk-rō-skŏp'ĭk): visible to the unaided eye.

macula (măk'ū-lă); pl., **maculae** (-lē): a spot or discoloration level with skin; a freckle; macule.

magnetism (măg'ně-tĭz'm): the power possessed by a magnet to attract or repel other masses.

magnify (măg'nĭ-fī): to increase the importance of; to exaggerate.

makeup (māk'ŭp): the way in which one is dressed, painted for a part in a play; cosmetics applied to the face.

malar (mā'lăr): of or pertaining to the cheek; the cheek bone.

malformation (măl-fôr-mā'shŭn): an abnormal shape or structure; badly formed.

malignant (mă-lĭg'nânt): resistant to treatment; growing worse, occurring in severe form; a tumor recurring after removal.

malnutrition (măl-nū-trĭsh'ûn): faulty or inadequate nutrition; undernourished.

malpighian (măl-pĭg'ē-ân): stratum mucosum; the deeper portion of the epidermis.

mandible (măn'dĭ-b'l): the lower jaw bone.

mandibular nerve (măn-dĭb'ū-lăr): the fifth cranial nerve which supplies the muscles and skin of the lower part of the face.

manganese (măn'gă-nēs): a grayish-white, metallic chemical element which rusts like iron, but is not magnetic.

manicure (măn'ĭ-kūr): the artful care of the hands and nails.

manifest (măn'ĭ-fěst): to prove; to evidence; to reveal; show; display.

manipulation (mă-nĭp-ū-lā'shŭn): act or process of treating, working or operating with the hands or by mechanical means, especially with skill.

mantle (măn't'l): nail mantle, the fold of the skin into which the nail is lodged.

marijuana (mâr'ă-wă'nă): the dried leaves and flower tops of this plant, which yield a narcotic smoked in cigarettes.

mascara (măs-kă'ră): a preparation used to darken the eyelashes.

mask (măsk): a special cosmetic formula used to beautify the face.

massage (mă-säzh'): manipulation of the body by rubbing, pinching, kneading, tapping, etc., to increase metabolism, promote absorption, relieve pain, etc.

masseter (mă-sē'těr): chewer; one of the muscles of the jaw used in mastication.

mastication (măs-tĭ-kā'shŭn): the act of chewing.

matrix (mā'trĭks): the formative portion of a nail.

matter (măt'ěr): a substance that occupies space and has weight.

matured (mă-tūrd): fully developed.

maxilla (măk-sĭl'ă): upper jaw bone.

maxillary (măk'sĭ-lă-rē): pertaining to the jaws.

measles (mē'z'lz): an acute contagious disease marked by fever and other constitutional disturbances, usually in children, with inflammation of the respiratory mucous membrane and a general red papular eruption.

medulla (mē-dŭl'ǎ): the marrow in the various bone cavities; the pith of the hair.

melanin (mĕl'ǎ-nĭn): the dark or black pigment in the epidermis and hair, and in the choroid or coat of the eye.

melanophore (mĕl-ân'ō-fôr): a pigment cell containing melanin.

membrane (mĕm'brān): a thin sheet or layer of pliable tissue, serving as a covering.

menopause (mĕn'ō-pôz): physiological cessation of menstruation.

mental nerve: a nerve which supplies the skin of the lower lip and chin.

mentalis (mĕn-tā'lĭs): the muscle that elevates the lower lip, and raises and wrinkles the skin of the chin.

metabolism (mē-tăb'ō-lĭz'm): the constructive and destructive life process of the cell.

metacarpus (măt-ă-kär'pǔs): the bones of the palm of the hand.

metallic salts (mē'tăl-ĭk sôlts): a compound of a base and an acid.

metatarsus (mĕt-ă-tär'sǔs): the bones which comprise the instep of the foot.

meter (mē'tĕr): an instrument used for measuring.

microbe (mī'krōb): a micro-organism; a minute one-celled animal or vegetable bacterium.

micrococcus (mī-krō-kŏk'ǔs): a minute bacterial cell having a spherical shape.

micro-organism (mī'krō-ôr'gân-ĭz'm): microscopic plant or animal cell; a bacterium.

microscope (mī'krō-skōp): an instrument for making enlarged views of minute objects.

mildew (mil'dōō): a disease of plants or a moldy coating that can appear on walls, fabrics, etc. Usully occurs in damp areas.

milliampere (mĭl-ē-ăm-pâr): one thousandth of an ampere.

milliamperemeter (mē'tĕr): an electrical instrument which registers the amount of current required for a given treatment.

miliaria rubra (mĭl-ē-ā'rē-ă rōōb'rǎ): prickly heat; burning and itching usually caused by exposure to excessive heat.

milium (mĭl'ē-ûm); pl., **milia** (-ǎ): a small whitish pearl-like mass due to a retention of sebum beneath the epidermis; a whitehead.

millimeter (mĭl'ĭ-mē-tĕr): one thousandth of a meter.

mineral (mĭn'ĕr-âl): any inorganic material found in the earth's crust.

mineral oils: cheaper oils usually used in cosmetics; cleanses and lubricates.

mineral salts: salts derived from an inorganic chemical compound.

minimize (mĭn'ĭ-mīz): to reduce to the smallest possible degree.

mink (mingk): a semiaquatic mammal, common to North America; valued for its fur; oil from the glands of the mink is used in some cosmetics.

mint (mĭnt): any of several aromatic herbs used as a flavoring, etc.

miscible (mĭs'ĭ-b'l): the property of certain liquids to mix with each other in equal proportions.

mixture (mĭks'tūre): a preparation made by incorporating an insoluble ingredient in a liquid vehicle; sometimes used to identify an aqueous solution containing two or more solutes.

modifier (mŏd'ĭ-fī-ĕr): anything that will change the form or characteristics of an object or substance.

moisturize (moist'ûr-ize): to make moist with water or other liquids.

mole (mōl): a small brownish spot on the skin.

mold (mōld): to form into a particular shape.

molecule (mŏl'ē-kūl): the smallest unit of any substance having all the properties of the substance.

mongoloid (mŏn-gō'loid): pertaining to or belonging to a major ethnic division of the human species; characterized by yellowish skin, slanting eyes, straight hair, broad nose and high cheekbones.

monilethrix (mō-nĭl'ē-thrĭks): beaded hair; a condition in which the hairs show a series of constrictions, giving the appearance of a string of fusiform beads.

monochromatic (mon'a-krō-mat'ik): having only one color; a color scheme based on one color in varying degrees of lightness or darkness.

monoxide (mŏn'ŏk-sīd): an oxide containing a single atom of oxygen in each molecule.

mordant (môr'dânt): a substance, such as alum, phenol, aniline oil, which fixes the dye used in coloring.

morphology (môr-fŏl'ō-jē): the branch of biology which deals with structure and form; it includes the anatomy, histology and cytology of the organism at any stage of its life history.

motile (mō'tĭl): having the power of movement, as certain bacteria.

motor nerves (mō'tĕr): carry impulses from nerve centers to muscles for certain motions.

mould (mōld): to form or to shape into a definite pattern.

mucous membrane (mū'kûs mĕm'brān): a membrane secreting mucous which lines passages and cavities communicating with the exterior.

multicellular (mŭl-tĭ'sĕl-ō-lâr): having many cells.

muscle (mŭs'l): the contractile tissue of the body by which movement is accomplished.

muscle tone: the normal degree of tension in a healthy muscle.

musk (mŭsk): a secretion with a penetrating odor, obtained from the male musk deer, and used in making perfume and in medicine.

muslin (mŭz'lĭn): any of several plain-weave cotton fabrics of varying fineness.

mutilate (myōō'ta-lāt): to maim, injure or damage an important part or parts.

myology (mī-ŏl'ō-jē): the science of the function, structure, and diseases of muscles.

N

naevus; nevus (nē'vûs); pl., **naevi; neve** (-vī): a birthmark; a congenital skin blemish.

nail (nāl): unguis; the horny protective plate located at the end of the finger or toe.

nail-bed: that portion of the skin on which the body of the nail rests.

nail-grooves: the furrows on the sides of the nail upon which the nail moves as it grows.

nail matrix (mā'trĭks): the portion of the nail-bed extending beneath the nail-root.

nail-root: located at the base of the nail, imbedded underneath the skin.

nail-wall: folds of skin overlapping sides and base of the nail-body.

nape (nāp): the back of the neck.

narcotic (när-kŏt'ĭk): a drug which in moderate doses relieves pain, but in poisonous doses produces stupors and convulsions.

naris (nā'rĭs); pl., **nares** (-rēz): a nostril.

nasalis (nâ-zā'lĭs): a muscle of the nose.

natural năt'ū-răl: not artificial.

necrosis (nĕk-rō'sĭs): the death of cells surrounded by living tissue.

negative (nĕg'ă-tĭv): the opposite of positive; expressing denial.

neoplasm (nē'ō-plăz'm): a new growth or tumor.

nerve (nûrv): a whitish cord, made up of bundles of nerve fibers, through which impulses are transmitted.

nervous (nûr'vŭs): easily excited or agitated.

neuritis (nū-rī'tĭs): inflammation of nerves, marked by neuralgia.

neurology (nū-rŏl'ō-jē): the science of the structure, function and pathology of the nervous system.

neuron (nū'rŏn): the unit of the nervous system, consisting of the nerve cell and its various processes.

neurosis (nū-rō'sĭs): a functional nervous disorder.

neutral (nū'trăl): exhibiting no positive properties; indifferent; in chemistry, neither acid nor alkaline.

neutralization (nū-trăl-ĭ-zā'shŭn): a chemical reaction between an acid and a base.

neutralizer (nū'trăl-zī-ẽr): an agent capable of neutralizing another substance.

neutron.. ('n (y) u-'tran): an uncharged elementary particle that has a mass nearly equal to the proton.

nevi, neavi, nevus: a colored spot in the skin, usually congenital.

nicotine (nĭk-ō-tēn): a poisonous alkaloid; the active principles of tobacco.

nit (nĭt): the egg of a louse, usually attached to a hair.

nitrate (nī'trāte): an oxidizing agent.

nitric acid (nī'trĭk): concentrated acid employed as a caustic.

nitrite (nī'trīte): a reducing agent; sodium nitrite is used as a sanitizing agent and acts as an anti-rusting agent.

nitrogen (nī'trō-jĕn): a colorless, gaseous element, tasteless and odorless, found in air and living tissue.

nodule (nŏd'yūle): a small, circumscribed solid elevation that usually extends into the deeper layers of the skin.

non (nŏn): a prefix denoting not.

non-conductor (kôn-dŭk'tẽr): any substance that resists the passage of electricity, light or heat towards or through it.

non-pathogenic (păth-ō-jĕn'ĭk): non-disease producing; growth promoting.

non-striated (strī'āt-ĕd): involuntary, smooth muscle which functions without the action of the will.

nordic (nôr'dĭk): pertaining or eblonging to the caucasian ethnic division of humankind; distributed mainly in Northwestern Europe.

normal (nôr'mâl): regular; natural.

nucleus (nū'klē-ŭs); pl., **nuclei** (-ī): the active center of cells.

nutrient (nū'trē-ēnt): nutritious.

nutrition (nū-trĭsh'ŭn): the process of nourishment.

O

obese (ō-bēs'): extremely fat; overweight.

objective (ŏb-jĕk'tĭv): pertaining to an object of action or feeling.

oblique (ŏb-lēk'; lĭk); **obliquus** (us): slanting or inclined.

obsolete (ŏb-sō-lēt'): old; gone out of date.

occipital (ŏk-sĭp'ĭ-tâl): the bone which forms the back and lower part of the head.

occupational disease (ŏk-û-pā'shŭn-âl): due to certain kinds of employment, in which contact with chemicals, dyes is involved.

oculist (ŏk'û-lĭst): a specialist in diseases of the eyes.

oculomotor (ŏk'û-lō-mō'tẽr): third cranial nerve; controlling the motion of the eye.

oculus (ŏk'û-lŭs); pl., **oculi** (-lī): the eye.

oestrogene ('estregen): a female hormone.

ohm (ōm): a unit of measurement used to denote the amount of resistance in an electrical system or device.

Ohm's law (ōmz lô): the simple statement that the current in an electric circuit is equal to the pressure divided by the resistance.

oil: a greasy liquid whose sources are from animals, plants and minerals.

oily skin (oil'ē skĭn): skin that is excessively oily due primarily to the over activity of the sebaceous glands.

ointment ('oint-mônt): a fatty, medicated mixture used externally.

oleic acid (ō-lē'ĭk): an oily acid used in making soap and ointments.

olfactory (ŏl-făk'tō-rē): relating to the sense of smell; first cranial nerve, the special nerve of smell.

olive oil (ŏl'ĭv oil): a light yellow oil pressed from olives; used in food preparation and cosmetics.

onychatrophia (ŏn-ĭ-kă-trō'fē-ă): atrophy of the nails.

onychauxis (ŏn-ĭ-kôk'sĭs): enlargement of the nails.

onychia (o-nĭk'ē-ă): inflammation of the matrix of the nail with pus formation and shedding of the nail.

onychoclasis (ŏn-ĭ-kō-klā'sĭs): breaking of the nail.

onychocryptosis (ŏn-ĭ-kō-krĭp-tō'sĭs): ingrowing nail.

onychogryposis (ŏn-ĭ-kō-grī-pō'sĭs): denotes enlargement with increased curvature of the nail.

onycholysis (ŏn-ĭ-kŏl'ĭ-sĭs): loosening of the nail without shedding.

onychomycosis (ŏn-ĭ-kō-mī-kō'sĭs): refers to any parasitic disease of the nails.

onychophagy (ŏn-ĭ-kŏf'ă-jē): the habit of eating or biting the nails.

onychophosis (ŏn-ĭ-kŏf-ō'sĭs): growth of horny epithelium in the nail-bed.

onychophyma (ŏn-ĭ-kŏf-ī'mă): a morbid degeneration of the nail.

onychoptosis (ŏn-ĭ-kŏp-tō'sĭs): falling off of the nails.

onychorrhexis (ŏn-ĭ-kō-rĕk'sĭs): abnormal brittleness of the nails with splitting of free edge.

onychosis; onyshonosus (ŏn-ĭ-kō'sĭs; ŏn-ĭ-kō-nō'sûs): any disease of the nails.

onyx (ŏ'nĭks): a nail of the fingers or toes.

opaque (ō-pāk'): impervious to light rays; neither transparent nor translucent.

optic (ŏp'tĭk): second cranial nerve; the nerve of sight; pertaining to the eye, or to vision.

orangewood stick: a stick made of orangewood used in manicuring the nails.

orbicularis oculi (ôr-bĭk-û-lā'rĭs ŏk'û-lī): orbicularis palpebrarum; the ring muscle of the eye.

orbicularis oris (ō'rĭs): orbicular muscle; muscle of the mouth.

orbit (ôr'bĭt): the bony cavity of the eyeball; the eye-socket.

organic (ôr-găn'ĭk): relating to an organ; pertaining to substances derived from living organisms.

organism (ôr'găn-ĭz'm): any living being, either animal or vegetable.

oriental (ôr'ē-en'tal): pertaining to the Orient; Eastern; an inhabitant of Asia; an Asian.

orifice (ŏr'ĭ-fĭs): an opening; a mouth.

origin (ŏr'ĭ-jĭn): the beginning; the starting point of a nerve; the place of attachment of a muscle to a bone.

oris (ō'rĭs): pertaining to the mouth; an opening.

os (ŏs): a bone.

oscillation (ŏs-ĭ-lā'shŭn): movement like a pendulum; a swinging or vibration.

osmidrosis (ŏs-mĭ-drō'sĭs; ŏz-): bromidrosis; foul smelling perspiration.

osmosis (ŏs-mō'sĭs; ŏz-): the passage of fluids and solutions through a membrane or other porous substance.

osseous; osseus (ŏs′ê-ûs): bony.

osteology (ŏs-tê-ŏl′ô-jê): science of the anatomy, structure and function of the bones.

ounce (ouns): a unit of measure of weight; one-sixteenth of a pound.

outline (out′līn): the line that defines a shape; the outline of an eye, etc.

ovary (ō′vă-rê): one of the two reproductive glands in the female, containing the ova or germ cells.

ovular (ō′vû-lăr): egg-like in shape.

oxidation (ŏk-sĭ-dā′shŭn): the act of combining oxygen with another substance.

oxygen (ŏk′sĭ-jĕn): a gaseous element, essential to animal and plant life.

oxygenation (ŏk′sĭ-jê-nā′shŭn): saturation with oxygen, noting especially the aeration of the blood in the lungs.

oxymelanin (ŏk′sĭ-mĕl′ă-nĭn): a compound formed by a combination of an oxidizing agent with the dark melanin (color) pigments in the hair; (generally found in the red to yellow shades).

ozone (ō′zōn): a form of oxygen used as a disinfectant.

P

pack (păk): a special cosmetic formula used to beautify the face.

palatine bones (păl′ă-tĭn): situated at the back part of the nasal depression.

pallid (păl′ĭd): of a pale or weak appearance; lacking in color.

palmar (păl′măr): referring to the palm of the hand.

papaya (pä-pä′ya): a yellow nutritious melon type fruit.

papilla, hair (pă-pĭl′ă): a small cone-shaped elevation at the bottom of the hair follicle in the dermis.

papillary layer (păp′ĭ-lä-rê): the outer layer of the dermis.

papule (păp′ūl): a pimple; a small, circumscribed elevation on the skin containing no fluid.

para (păr′ă): see para-phenylene-diamine.

paraffin (păr′ă-fĭn): a translucent, waxy mixture used in facial masks.

parasite (păr′ă-sīt): a vegetable or animal organism which lives on or in another organism, and draws its nourishment therefrom.

parasiticide (păr-ă-sĭt′ĭ-sīd): a substance that destroys parasites.

parietal (pă-rī′ê-tăl): pertaining to the wall of a cavity; a bone at the side of the head.

paronychia (păr-ō-nĭk′ê-ă): felon; an inflammation of the tissues surrounding the nail.

parotid (pă-rŏt′ĭd): near the ear; a gland near the ear.

patch test: see predisposition test.

pathogenic (păth-ô-jĕn′ĭk): causing disease; disease producing.

pathology (păth-ŏl′ô-jê): the science of the nature of disease.

pectin (pĕk′tĭn): a class of carbohydrates contained in a variety of fruits and vegetables; used to set, thicken, or jell substances.

pectoralis (pĕk-tô-rā′lĭs): a muscle of the breast.

pedicure (pĕd′ĭ-kūr): care of feet and toe nails.

pellagra (pĕ-lăg′rä): a skin affliction with digestive disturbances, followed by scaling or peeling of the skin, and nervous and mental disorders.

penetration (pĕn-ê-trā′shŭn): act or power of penetrating.

penicillin (pĕn′ĭ-sĭl′ĭn): a powerful antibiotic found in the mold fungus penicillium and produced in several forms for the treatment of a wide variety of infections.

peptide (pĕp′tĭd): a compound of two or more amino-acids containing one or more peptide groups; continuous filaments in the case of fiber protein or keratin.

peptide bonds: see end bonds.

percarbonate (pĕr-kär′bô-nāt): quantity of salts or esters of carbonic acid.

percussion (pĕr-kŭsh′ŭn): a form of massage consisting of repeated light blows or taps of varying force.

perfume (pĕr′fūm): a fluid preparation, as of the essence of flowers, used in scenting.

pericardium (pĕr-ĭ-kär′dē-ŭm): the membranous sac around the heart.

peripheral nervous system (pĕ-rĭf′ĕr-âl): consists of the nerve endings in the skin and sense organs.

permeable (pûr′mê-ă-b'l): permitting the passage of liquids.

peroxide of hydrogen (pĕr-ŏk′zĭd hĭ′drô-jĕn): a powerful oxidizing agent; in liquid solution it is used as an antiseptic; used in tinting and lightening treatments.

perspiration (pûr′spĭ-rā′shŭn): sweat; the fluid excreted from the sweat glands of the skin.

persulfate (pĕr-sŭl′fāt): a sulfate which contains more sulfuric acid than the ordinary sulfide.

petrissage (pĕt-rĭ′säj): the kneading movement in massage.

petrolatum (pĕt-rô-lā′tûm): petroleum jelly; vaseline; a purified, yellow mixture of semi-solid hydrocarbons obtained from petroleum.

petroleum (pê-trô′lê-ûm): an oily liquid coming from the earth and consisting of a mixture of hydrocarbons.

petroleum jelly (pê-trô′lê-ûm): a translucent semi-solid; a protective, nonpenetrable lubricant.

pH: symbol for potential hydrogen concentration; the relative degree of acidity or alkalinity.

pH number: a measure of the degree of acidity or alkalinity of a solution.

phalanx (fā′lănks); pl., **phalanges** (fă-lăn′jēz): the long bone of the finger or toe.

pharmacologist (fär-ma-kōl′ô-jĭst): one versed in the science of the nature and properties of drugs.

pharynx (făr′ĭnks): the upper portion of the digestive tube, behind the nose and mouth.

phenol (fē′nōl): carbolic acid; caustic poison; in dilute solution is used as an antiseptic and disinfectant.

phoresis (fô-rē′sĭs): the process of introducing solutions into the tissues through the skin by the use of galvanic current.

phosphates (fŏs-fāt): a salt of ester of a phosphoric acid.

phosphorus (fŏs′fôr-ûs): an element found in bones, muscles and nerves.

phyma (fī′mă); pl., **phymata** (fi′ma-ta): a circumscribed swelling on the skin, larger than a tubercle.

physics (fĭz′ĭks): the branch of science that deals with matter, motion, light, heat, electricity, sound and mechanics.

physiognomical (fĭz-ĭ-ŏg-nŏm′i-câl): pertaining to the design of hair style or makeup to the facial features of the client.

physiology (fĭz-ê-ŏl′ô-jê): the science of the functions of living things.

picealis (pĭs-ê-ă′lĭs): a type of acne caused by an allergy to tar products.

pigment (pĭg-mênt): any oragnic coloring matter, as that of the red blood cells, the hair, skin, iris, etc.

pigmentation (pĭg′mên-tā′shŭn): the deposition of pigment in the skin or tissues.

pilus (pī′lûs); pl., **pili** (-lī): hair

pimple: any small, pointed elevation of the skin; a papule or small pustule.

pituitary (pĭ-tū′ĭ-târ-ê): a ductless gland located at the base of the brain.

pityriasis (pĭt-ĭ-rī'ă-sĭs): dandruff; an inflammation of the skin characterized by the formation and flaking of fine branny scales.

pityriasis capitis simplex (kăp'ĭ-tĭs sĭm'plĕks): a scalp inflammation marked by dry dandruff or branny scales.

pivot, hair shaping (pĭv'ŏt): the exact point from which the hair is directed in forming a curvature or shaping.

placenta (pluh-sen'tuh): the organ on the wall of the uterus to which an embryo is attached by means of the umbilical cord; the embryo receives its nourishment from the placenta.

placenta-extract (pluh-sen'tuh-eck'stract): a vascular organ serving as nourishment for the fetus.

plasma (plăz'mă): the fluid part of the blood and lymph.

plastic surgeon (plăs'tĭk sûr'jŭn): a surgeon who builds up or molds tissue or repairs physical skin defects; plastic surgery; plastic operations.

platelets (plāt'lĕts): blood cells which aid in the forming of clots.

platysma (plă-tĭz-mă): a broad, thin muscle of the neck.

pledget (plĕj'ĕt): a compress or small, flat mass of lint, absorbent cotton, or the like.

plexus (plĕk'sŭs): a network of nerves or veins.

pliability (plī-ă-bĭl'ĭ-tē): flexibility.

plug (plŭg): to stop or close; as inserting a plug; a plugged follicle.

pneumogastric (nū-mū-găs'trĭk): relating to the lungs and stomach.

pneumogastric nerve (nū-mō-găs'trĭk nûrv): vagus nerve; tenth cranial nerve.

polarity (pō-lăr'ĭ-tē): the property of having two opposite poles, as that possessed by a magnet or galvanic current.

pollex (pŏl'ĕks): the thumb.

pollutant (pa-loo'tant): any of various noxious chemicals and refuse materials that impair the purity of water, soil or the atmosphere.

polyhedral (păl-i-'he-dral): having more than six sides.

polypeptide (pŏl-ē-pĕp'tīd): strings of amino-acids joined together by peptide bonds, the prefix "poly" meaning many.

pomphus (pŏm'fŭs): a whitish or pinkish elevation of the skin; a wheal.

pore (pôr): a small opening of the sweat glands of the skin

porosity (pō-rŏs'ĭ-tē): ability of the hair to absorb moisture.

porous (pō'rŭs): having many pores.

positive (pŏz'ĭ-tĭv): affirmative; not negative; the presence of abnormal conditions; having a relatively high potential in electricity.

posterior (pŏs-tē'rē-ĕr): situated behind; coming after or behind.

posterior auricular (ô-rĭk'ū-lăr): a nerve which supplies muscles in the posterior surface of the ear.

potassium hydroxide (pô-tăs'ē-ŭm hī-drŏk'sīd): a powerful alkali, used in the manufacture of soft soaps.

potassium permanganate (pĕr-măn'gâ-nāt): a salt of permanganate acid; used as an antiseptic and deodorant.

practitioner (prak-tish'en-ar): one who practices an art or profession.

precipitate (prē-sĭp'ĭ-tāt): to cause a substance in solution to settle down in solid particles; to decrease solubility.

predisposition (prē-dĭs-pô-zĭsh'ŭn): a condition of special susceptibility to disease; allergy.

predisposition test (prē-dĭs-pô-zĭsh'ŭn tĕst): a skin test designed to determine an individual's over-sensitivity to certain chemicals (patch test, allergy test, skin test).

primary colors (prī-mă-rē kŭl'ĕrz): pigments or colors that are fundamental; red, yellow and blue are the primary colors in pigments.

primary hair: the baby fine hair that is present over almost the entire smooth skin of the body.

prism (prĭzm): a transparent solid with triangular ends and two converging sides; it breaks up white light into its component colors.

procedure (prō-sē'jĕr): a manner of proceeding or acting in any course of action.

procerus (prō-sē'rŭs): muscle that covers bridge of the nose.

progesterone (prō-jes'ta-rōn): a female hormone.

prognosis (prŏg-nō'sĭs): the foretelling of the probable course of a disease.

promulgate (prō-mul'gāt): to make known or to announce officially and formally.

pronate (prō'nāt): to bend forward.

pronators (prō-nā'tôrs): the muscles which turn the hand inward so that the palm faces downward.

properties (prŏp'ĕr-tēz): the identifying characteristics of a substance which are observable; a peculiar quality of anything; i.e., color, taste, smell, etc.

prophylaxis (prō-fĭ-lăk'sĭs): prevention of disease.

protection (prō-tĕk'shŭn): the act of shielding from injury.

protein (prō'tē-ĭn): a complex organic substance present in all living tissues, such as skin, hair and nails; necessary in the daily diet; also present in skin and hair conditioners.

proteolytic (prō'-tē'ō-lĭt'ĭk): an organic substance which breaks down protein to form simple substances.

protoplasm (prō'tô-plăz'm): the material basis of life; a substance found in all living things.

protozoa (prō-tô-bō'ă): subkingdom of animals, including all the unicellular animal organisms.

prutitis (proot'ĭ-tĭs): itching produced by contact with cold water.

psoriasis (sô-rī'ă-sĭs): a skin disease with circumscribed red patches, covered with adherent white silver scales.

psychology (sī-kŏl'ô-jē): the science of the mind and its operation.

puberty (pū'bĕr-tē): the period of life in which the organs of reproduction are developed.

pulmonary (pŭl'mô-nâ-rē): relating to the lungs.

pulsate (pŭl'sāt): to move with rhythmical impulses.

pulverize (pul've-rīz): to reduce to powder or dust, as by crushing.

pumice (pŭm'ĭs): hardened volcanic substance, white or gray in color, used for buffing in manicuring; also called pumice stone.

puncture (pungk'cher): to pierce with a sharp point.

pungent (pun'jent): a keen, penetrating odor.

purification (pū-rĭ-fĭ-kā'shŭn): the act of cleaning or removing foreign matter.

pus (pŭs): a fluid product of inflammation, consisting of a liquid containing leucocytes and the debris of dead cells and tissue elements.

pusher (poosh'ĕr): a steel instrument used to loosen the cuticle from the nail.

pustule (pŭs'tūl): an inflamed pimple containing pus.

Q

quadratus (kwŏd-rā'tŭs): a square shaped muscle; a muscle of the lower jaw.

quadratus labii inferiores (kwŏd-rā'tŭs lā'bē-ī ĭn-fe-rē-ŏr'ĭs): a muscle of the lower lip.

quadratus labii superioris (kwŏd-rā'tŭs lā'bē-ī sû-pē' rē-ôr'ĭs): a muscle of the upper lip.

quarantine (kwŏr'ân-tēn): the isolation of a person to prevent spread of a contagious disease.

quaternary ammonium compounds (quats) (kwă-tēr' nä-rē ă-mō'nē-ŭm kŏm'poundz): a group of compounds of organic salts of ammonia employed effectively as disinfectants.

quince seed (kwĭns sēd): the dried seed of Pyrus Cydonia which yields a mucilage used in the making of hand lotion.

quinine (kwī'nĭn): enters into the composition of many hair lotions in small quantities; its effect is slightly antiseptic.

R

rabies (rā'bĭ-ēz): an acute infectious disease of dogs, wolves, and other animals, corresponding to hydrophobia in human beings.

radial nerve (rā'dê-ăl): a nerve which affects the arm and hand.

radiation (rā-dē-ā'shûn): the process of giving off light or heat rays.

radius (rā'dē-ûs): the outer and smaller bone of the forearm.

rash (răsh): a skin eruption having little or no elevation.

reconstruction (rē'kŏn-strŭkt'shûn): the act of reconstructing, or state of being reconstructed.

rectifier (rĕk'tĭ-fī-ēr): an apparatus to change an alternating current of electricity into a direct current.

rectus (rĕk'tûs): in a straight line; the name of small muscles of the eye.

reddish cast: a tinge of red.

refined (rē'fīnd): free from impurities; cultivated; polished.

regeneration (rē-jĕn'a-rā'shûn): the renewal or reproduction of cells, tissues, etc.

regimen (rĕg'ĭ-mĕn): a systematized course of action (also called regime); a daily routine or regimen.

rejuvenate (rē-jōō've-nāt): to make young or vigorous again.

Renaissance (rĕn-e-'säns): the revival of the arts in Europe, marking the transition from medieval to modern history.

reproductive (rē-prô-dŭk'tĭv): pertaining to reproduction or the process by which plants and animals give rise to offspring.

reservoir (rez'ar-vwôr): a basin, either natural or artificial for collecting or containing a supply of water.

residue (rĕz'ĭ-dū): that which remains after some part is taken away.

resilient (rê-zĭl'ĭ-ĕnt): elastic.

resin (rĕ'zĭn): a mixture of organic compounds used in some cosmetics.

resistance (rē-zĭst'âns): the difficulty of moisture or chemical solutions to penetrate.

respiration (rĕs-pĭ-rā'shûn): the act of breathing; the process of inhaling air into the lungs and expelling it.

respiratory system (rē-spĭr'â-tô-rē): consists of the nose, pharynx, larynx, trachea, bronchi and lungs which assist in breathing.

restorative (re-stōr'ă-tĭv): to restore to an original state; repair; rebuild.

rete (rē'tê): any interlacing of either blood vessels or nerves.

reticular layer (rê-tĭk'û-lâr): the inner layer of the corium.

retina (rĕt'ĭ-nă): the sensitive membrane of the eye which receives the image formed by the lens.

reversible (rē-vērs'ĭ-b'l): capable of going through a series of changes in either direction, forward or backward, as a reversible chemical action.

rhagades (răg'ă-dēz): cracks, fissures or chaps on the skin.

rheostat (rē'ō'stăt): a resistance coil; an instrument used to regulate the strength of an electric current.

rickettsia (rĭk-ĕt'sĕ-ä): a type of pathogenic microorganism, capable of producing disease.

ringworm (rĭng'wûrm): a vegetable parasitic disease of the skin and its appendages which appears in circular lesions and is contagious.

rinse (rĭns): to cleanse with a second or repeated application of water after washing; a prepared rinse water.

risorius (rĭ-zôr'ē-ûs): muscle at the side of the mouth.

rolling (rōl'ĭng): a massage movement in which the tissues are pressed and twisted.

Roman (rō'man): pertaining to or characteristic of modern or ancient Rome or its people.

root (rōōt): in anatomy, the base; the foundation or beginning of any part.

rosacea acne (rō-zā'shē-ă): an eruption on the cheeks and nose due to congestion.

rose water (rōz): water tinctured with the essential oil of roses; free of irritants.

rotary (rō'tă-rē): circular motion of the fingers as in massage.

rouge (rōōzh): a cosmetic used to color the skin (especially the cheeks) pink or red in color.

S

saccular (săk'ū-lâr): consisting of little sacs, such as oil glands.

sachet (sà-shā'): a perfumed bag or pad.

saffron (săf'rŏn): orange colored stigmas of the crocus plant, used as an herb in cookery and for coloring purposes.

salicylic acid (săl-ĭ-sĭl'ĭk ăs'ĭd): white crystaline acid, used as an antiseptic.

saline (sā'lĭn): salty; containing salt.

saliva (să-lī'vă): the secretion of the salivary glands; spittle.

sallow (săl'ō): a yellowish hue or complexion.

salt (sôlt): in chemistry, the union of a base with an acid.

sanitary (săn'ĭ-tâ-rē): pertaining to cleanliness in relation to health; tending to promote health.

sanitation (săn-ĭ-tā'shûn): the use of methods to bring about favorable conditions of health.

sanitize (săn'ĭ-tīz): to make sanitary.

saprophyte (săp'rō-fīt): a microorganism which grows normally on dead matter, as distinguished from a parasite.

saturate (săt'ū-rāt): to cause to become soaked or completely penetrated with moisture or a substance; that which has absorbed all it can hold.

sauna ('sau-ne): sauna vapor bath.

scab (skăb): a crust formed on the surface of a sore.

scabies (skā'bĭ-ēz): a skin disease caused by an animal parasite, attended with intense itching; the itch.

scale (skāl): any thin plate of horny epidermis; regular markings used as a standard in measuring and weighing.

scar (skär): a mark remaining after a wound has healed.

scarf skin: epidermis.

science (sī'ĕns): knowledge duly arranged and systematized.

sclera (sklĭr'a): the hard, white fibrous outer coat of the eyeball, continuous with the cornea.

scurf (skûrf): thin, dry scales or scabs on the body, especially on the scalp; dandruff.

sebaceous cyst (sĕ-bā'shŭs sĭst): a distended, oily or fatty follicle or sac.

sebaceous glands: oil glands of the skin.

seborrhea (sĕb-ō-rē'ă): an oily condition caused by the over-action of the sebaceous glands.

seborrhea oleosa (ō-lē-ō'să): excessive oiliness of the skin, particularly of the forehead and nose.

seborrhea sicca (sĭk'ă): an accumulation on the scalp of greasy scales or crusts, due to over-action of the sebaceous glands; dandruff or pityriasis.

seborrheic (sĕb-ō-rē'ĭk): seborrheal; pertaining to the over-action of the sebaceous glands.

sebum (sē'bŭm): the fatty or oily secretions of the sebaceous glands.

secondary color (sĕk'ŭn-dă-rē): second in order; secondary colors are combinations of two primary colors. Example: red and yellow (primary colors) mixed together create orange (a secondary color).

secondary hair: the stiff, short, coarse hair found on the eyelashes, eyebrows and within the openings or passages of the nose and ears.

secretion (sē-krē'shŭn): a product manufactured by a gland for a special purpose.

senility (sē-nĭl'ĭ-tē): quality or state of being old.

sensation (sĕn-sā'shŭn): a feeling or impression arising as the result of the stimulation of an afferent nerve.

sensitivity (sĕn-sĭ-tĭv'ĭ-tē): the state of being easily affected by certain chemicals or external conditions.

sensory nerve (sĕn'sō-rē nûrv): afferent nerve; a nerve carrying sensations.

sepsis (sĕp'sĭs): the presence of various pus-forming and other pathogenic organisms, or their toxins, in the blood or tissues; septicemia.

septic (sĕp'tĭk): relating to or caused by sepsis.

septum (sĕp'tŭm): a dividing wall; a partition.

serratus anterior (sĕ-rā'tŭs ăn-tē'rē-ôr): a muscle of the chest assisting in breathing and in raising the arm.

sewerage (sū'ăj): the waste matter, solid and liquid, passing through a sewer.

shaft (shăft): slender, stem-like structure; the long, slender part of the hair above the scalp.

shaping (shāp'ĭng): the process of shaping and thinning the hair of the head and eyebrows.

sheath (shēth): a covering enclosing or surrounding some organ.

shock (shŏk): a marked lowering of the vital activities from an injury or operation; a blow to the feelings.

shortwave (shŏrt'wāv): a form of high-frequency current used in permanent hair removal.

silicone (sĭl'ĭ-kōn): various compounds used as lubricants, and in some other types of cosmetic preparations.

sinus (sī'nŭs): a cavity or depression; a hollow in bone or other tissue.

skeletal muscles (skĕl'ē-tăl): muscles connected to the skeleton.

skeleton (skĕl'ē-tûn): a bony framework of the body.

skin (skĭn): the external covering of the body.

skin texture: the general feel and appearance of the skin.

skull (skŭl): the bony case or the framework of the head.

slip (slĭp) a smooth and slippery feeling imparted by talc to face powder.

slippage (slĭp'âj): the shifting and changing of position of the sulphur bonds.

slough (slŭf): to separate, as dead cells from living tissues; to discard.

small pox (smôl pŏks): an eruption, first papular, then pustular, resulting in the production of pock marks.

smaller occipital (ŏk-sĭp'ĭ-tăl): sensory nerve affecting skin behind the ear.

soap (sōp): a compound of fatty acid, derived from fats and oils, chemically combined with an alkaline base; used as a cleansing agent.

sodium (sō'dē-ŭm): a metallic element of the alkaline group.

sodium bicarbonate (bī-kär'bŏn-āt): baking soda; it relieves burns, bites; is often used in bath powders as an aid to cleansing oily skin.

sodium carbonate (kär'bŏn-āt): washing soda; used to prevent corrosion of metallic instruments when added to boiling water.

sodium lauryl sulfite (lô'rêl sŭl'fīt): a metallic element of the alkaline group, in white or light yellow crystals; used in detergents.

sodium perborate (pĕr'bō-rāt): a compound, formed by treating sodium peroxide with boric acid; on dissolving the substance in water, peroxide of hydrogen is generated; used as an antiseptic.

sodium sulphite (sŭl'fīt): a soft, white metallic salt of sulphurous acid.

softening (sŏf'ĕn-ĭng): to make soft; less harsh.

solar (sō'lâr): pertaining to the sun.

solubility (sŏl-ŭ-bĭl'ĭ-tē): the extent to which a substance (solute) dissolves in a liquid (solvent) to produce a homogeneous system (solution).

soluble (sŏl'û-b'l): able to be dissolved.

solute (sŏl'ūt): the dissolved substance in a solution.

solution (sō-lū'shŭn): the act or process by which a substance is absorbed into a liquid.

solvent (sŏl'vĕnt): an agent capable of dissolving substances.

soothing (sōō'thĭng): tending to soothe; having a sedative effect.

souffle (sōō'flă): to make light and frothy and fixed in that condition by heat.

spatula (spăt'û-lă): a flexible, knife-like implement for handling creams and pomades, etc.

spectrum (spĕk'trŭm): the band of rainbow colors produced by decomposing light by means of a prism.

spermaceti (spûr-mă-sĕt'ē): an animal product (wax) obtained from the sperm whale; used to give body to creams.

sphenoid (sfē'noid): wedge-shaped; a bone in the cranium.

sphere (sfēr): a ball or globular body.

spherical (sfēr'ĭ-kăl): relating to or having the shape of a sphere.

spinal accessory (spī'nâl ăk-sĕs'ō-rē): eleventh cranial nerve.

spinal column (kŏl'ŭm): the backbone or vertebral column.

spinal cord (kôrd): the portion of the central nervous system contained within the spinal or vertebral canal.

spinal nerves: the nerves arising from the spinal cord.

spine (spīn): a short process of bone; the backbone.

spiral (spī'răl): coil; winding around a center, like a watch spring.

spirillum (spī-rĭl'ûm); pl., **spirilla** (-ă): curved bacterium.

spore (spôr): a tiny bacterial body having a protective wall to withstand unfavorable conditions.

squama (skwā'mă): an epidermic scale made up of thin, flat cells.

stabilized (stā'bĭ-līzd): made stable or firm, preventing changes.

stabilizer: see fixative.

stable (stā'b'l): in a balanced condition; not readily destroyed or decomposed; resisting molecular change.

stain (stān): an abnormal skin discoloration.

staphylococcus (stăf-ĭ-lō-kŏk´ŭs): cocci which are grouped in clusters like a bunch of grapes; found in pustules and boils.

starch (stärch): a white odorless, tasteless granular or powdery complex carbohydrates.

static (stăt´ĭk) **electricity:** a form of electricity generated by friction.

steamer (stēm´ẽr), **facial:** an apparatus used in place of hot towels for steaming the scalp or face.

stearic acid (stē-ăr´ĭk): a white, fatty acid, occurring in solid animal fats and in some of the vegetable fats.

steatoma (stē-ă-tō´mă): a sebaceous cyst; a fatty tumor.

steatosis (stē-ă-tō´sĭs): fatty degeneration; adiposis.

steep (stēp): to soak in a liquid, as for softening or cleansing.

sterilization (stĕr-ĭ-lĭ-zā´shŭn): the process of making sterile; the destruction of germs.

sterno-cleido-mastoideus (stŭr´nō-klī´dō-măs-toid´ē-ŭs): a muscle of the neck which depresses and rotates the head.

stimulation (stĭm-ū-lā´shŭn): the act of arousing increased functional activity.

stomach (stŭm´ŭk): the dilated portion of the alimentary canal in which the first process of digestion takes place.

stratum (strā´tŭm); pl., **strata** (-a): layer of tissue.

stratum corneum (kôr´nē-ŭm): horny layer of the skin.

stratum germinativum (jŭr-mĭ-nā´tĭv-ŭm): the deepest layer of the epidermis resting on the corneum.

stratum granulosum (grăn-ū-lō´sŭm): granular layer of the skin.

stratum lucidum (lū´sĭ-dŭm): clear layer of the skin.

stratum mucosum (mū-kō´sŭm): mucous or malpighian layer of the skin.

streptococcus (strĕp-tō-kŏk´ŭs): pus-forming bacteria that arrange in curved lines resembling a string of beads; found in erysipelas and blood poisoning.

striated (strī´āt-ĕd): marked with parallel lines or bands; striped; voluntary muscles.

stroking (strōk´ĭng): a gliding movement over a surface; to pass the fingers or any instrument gently over a surface; effleurage.

strontium sulphide (strŏn´shē-ŭm sŭl´fīd): a light gray powder capable of liberating hydrogen sulphide in the presence of water; used as a depilatory.

styptic (stĭp´tĭk): an agent causing contraction of living tissue; used to stop bleeding; an astringent.

subcutaneous (sŭb-kū-tā´nē-ŭs): under the skin.

subcutis (sŭb-kū´tĭs): subdermis; subcutaneous tissue; under or beneath the corium or dermis; the true skin.

subdermis (sŭb-dûr´mĭs): subcutis or subcutaneous tissue of the skin.

subjective symptom (sŭb-jĕk´tĭv sĭmp´tŭm): sensed by the individual and not by the examiner.

submental artery (sŭb-mĕn´tăl är´tẽr-ē): supplies blood to the chin and lower lip.

substance (sŭb´stăns): matter; material.

suction machine (sŭk´shŭn): a small machine that is used to glide over the skin and draw out waste material from the open follicles.

sudamen (sū-dā´mĕn); pl., **sudamina** (sū-dăm´ĭ-nă): a disorder of the sweat glands with obstruction of their ducts.

sudoriferous glands (sū-dôr-ĭf´ẽr-ŭs glăndz): sweat glands of the skin.

sulfite (sŭl´fīt): any salt or sulfurous acid.

sulfonated oil (sŭl´fŏn-āt´ĕd): an organic substance prepared by reacting oils with sulphuric acid; has an alkaline reaction and is miscible with water; used as a base in soapless shampoo.

sulphide (sŭl´fīd): compound of sulphur with another element or base.

sulphur (sŭl´fŭr): a chemical element whose compounds are used in lightening, in hair preparations and in medicine.

sulphur bonds: sulphur cross bonds in the hair, which hold the chains of amino-acids together in order to form a hair strand.

supercilium (sū-pẽr-sĭl´ē-ŭm); pl., **supercilia** (-ă): the eyebrow.

superficial (sū-pẽr-fĭsh´ăl): pertaining to or being on the surface.

superfluous (sū-pẽr´flōō-ŭs): excessive; more than is wanted or needed.

suppuration (sŭp-ū-rā´shŭn): the formation of pus.

supraorbitan (sū-pră-ôr´bĭ-tăl): above the orbit or eye.

supra-trochlear (sū-pră-trŏk´lē-ăr): above the trochlea or pulley of the superior oblique muscle.

susceptible (sŭ-sĕp´tĭ-b´l): capable of being influenced or easily acted on.

suspension (sŭ-spĕn´shŭn): a mixture of a liquid and insoluble particles which have a tendency to settle on standing.

sweat (swĕt): see perspiration.

sympathetic nervous system (sĭm-pă-thĕt´ĭk): controls the involuntary muscles which affect respiration, circulation and digestion.

symptom (sĭm´tŭm): a change in the body or its functions which indicates disease.

symptom, objective (sĭmp´tŏm ŏb-jĕk´tĭv): that which can be seen, as in pimples, pustules, etc.

symptom, subjective (sŭb-jĕk´tĭv): can be felt, as in itching.

synthetic (sĭn-thĕt´ĭk): any man-made substance; nylon, rayon, etc.

syphilis (sĭf´ĭ-lĭs): a chronic, infectious venereal disease.

system (sĭs-tĕm): a group of organs which especially contribute toward one of the more important vital functions.

systematic (sĭs-tĕm-ăt´ĭk): proceeding according to a system or regular method.

systemic (sĭs-tĕm´ĭk): pertaining to a system or to the body as a whole.

T

tactile corpuscle (tăk´tĭl kôr´pŭs´l): tough nerve endings found within the skin.

tag: in cosmetology: an appendage or growth on the skin.

talc (tălk): a soft mineral that is a basic magnesium silicate to use, whitish, greenish, or grayish with a soapy feel.

talcum powder (tăl´kŭm): a fine powder used as a dusting agent for the relief of chapped skin.

tannic acid (tăn´ĭk): a plant extract used as an astringent.

tannin (tăn-ĕn): any of various soluble astringents; dyeing; the making of ink.

tapotemet (tă-pŏt-măn): a massage movement using a short, quick slapping or tapping movement.

tapping (tăp´ĭng): a massage movement; striking lightly with partly flexed fingers.

tartaric acid (tär-tă-rĭk): a colorless crystalline acid compound.

technician (tĕk´nĭ´shăn): an individual trained and expert in a special skill or subject.

temple (tĕm´p´l): the flattened space on the side of the forehead.

temporal bone (tĕm´pō-răl): the bone at the side and base of the skull.

temporalis (tĕm-pō-rā´lĭs): the temporal muscle.

tendon (tĕn´dŏn): fibrous cord or band connecting muscle with bone.

tensile (tĕn'sĭl): capable of being stretched.

tension (tĕn'shŭn): stress caused by stretching or pulling.

tepid (tĕp'ĭd): neither hot nor cold; lukewarm.

terminology (tĕr-mĭ-nŏl'ŏ-jē): the special words or terms used in science, art or business.

tertiary (tûr'shē-er'ē): third in point of time, number or degree; a tertiary color is achieved by mixing a secondary color (ex. green) and a primary color (blue) in equal amounts; blue and green create a turquoise color.

tetanus (tĕt'â-nŭs): a disease with spasmodic and continuous contraction of the muscles; lockjaw.

textometer (tĕks-tŏm'ĕ-tĕr): a device used to measure the elasticity and reaction of the hair to alkaline solutions.

texture (tĕks'cher): apparent surface structure such as fabric; thick or thin as in a cosmetic.

texture of hair: the general quality as to coarse, medium or fine; feel of the hair.

texture of the skin: the general feel and appearance of the skin.

thallium (thă'lĭ-ûm): a bluish-white metallic element, the salts of which have been used for epilation; thallium is highly toxic to humans.

theory (thē'ar-ē): a plan or scheme existing in the mind only; a speculative or conjectural view of something.

therapeutic lamp (thĕr-ă-pū'tĭk): an electrical apparatus producing any of the various rays of the spectrum; used for skin and scalp treatments.

therapy (thĕr'ă-pē): the science and art of healing.

thermal (thûr'măl): relating to heat.

thermostat (thûr'mŏ-stăt): an automatic device for regulating temperature.

thinning, hair: decreasing the thickness of the hair where it is too heavy.

thio (thĭ'ō): see ammonium thioglycolate.

thioglycolic acid (thī-ō-glī'kŏ-lĭk): a colorless liquid or white crystals with a strong unpleasant odor, miscible with water, alcohol or ether; (used in permanent wave solutions, hair relaxers and depilatories).

thorax (thō'răks): the part of the body between the neck and the abdomen; the chest.

thrombocyte (thrŏm'bō-sīt): a blood platelet which aids in clotting.

thyme (tĭm): a small plant of the mint family; used in seasoning food and in some cosmetic preparations.

thymol (tĭm'ŏl): a crystalline phenol of aromatic odor and antiseptic properties found especially in thyme.

thyroid gland (thī'roid): a large, ductless gland situated in the neck.

tincture (tĭnk'tūr): an alcoholic solution of a medicinal substance.

tincture of benzoin (tĭnk'tūr bĕn'zō-ĭn, -zoin): a protective antiseptic astringent used in healing of erupted skins.

tinea (tĭn'ē-â): a skin disease, especially ringworm.

tissue (tĭsh'ū): a collection of similar cells which perform a particular function.

tissue, connective (kŏ-nĕk'tĭv): binding and supporting tissue.

titanium dioxide (tĭ-tā'nē-ûm dī'ŏk-sīd): a white crystalline powder used in the manufacture of paints, cosmetics, etc. to give better coverage; especially useful in foundations, cover sticks, mascara, lipstick and nail polish.

titian (tĭsh'ĕn): a reddish, yellow color used by the artist Titian, a Venetian painter of the fourteenth century; the color is found in certain modern day cosmetics such as lipcolor and cheek color.

toluene diamine (tŏl'ū-ēn dī-ăm'ĭn): a colorless liquid, obtained from a coal tar product, used as a solvent and also in a drug designed to increase the amount of bile secreted.

tone (tōn): healthy functioning of the body or its parts.

tonic (tŏn'ĭk): increasing the strength or tone of the system.

toxemia (tŏk-sē'mē-ă): form of blood poisoning.

toxin; toxine (tŏk'sĭn; -sēn): a poisonous substance of undetermined chemical nature, elaborated during the growth of pathogenic micro-organisms.

trachea (trā'kĕ-ă; tră-kē'ă): windpipe.

trait (trāt): a distinguishing feature or quality of character.

tranquil (trang'kwil): quiet, calm; free from agitation.

tranquilizer (trang'kwal-ī'zer): any of a class of drugs having the properties of reducing nervous tension and anxiety.

translucent (trăns-lū'sênt): somewhat transparent.

transformer (trăns-fôr'mĕr): used for the purpose of increasing or decreasing the voltage of the current used; it can only be used on an alternating current.

transverse facial (trăns-vûrs'): an artery supplying the skin, the parotid gland and the masseter muscle.

trapezius (tră-pē'zē-ûs): muscle that draws the head backward and sideways.

triangularis (trī-ăn-gû-lā'rĭs): a muscle that pulls down the corner of the mouth.

triceps (trī'sĕps): three headed.

trichology (trĭ-kŏl'ŏ-jē): the science of the care of the hair.

trichonosus (trĭk-ō-nō'sûs): any disease of the hair.

trichophytosis (trĭ-kŏf-ĭ-tō'sĭs): ringworm of the skin and scalp due to growth of a fungus parasite.

trichosis (trĭ-kō'sĭs): abnormal growth of hair.

trifacial (trī-fā'shâl): the fifth cranial nerve; also known as the trigeminus nerve.

trigeminal (trī-jĕm'ĭ-nâl): relating to the fifth cranial or trigeminus nerve.

true skin: the corium.

trypsin (trĭp'sĭn): an enzyme in the digestive juice secreted by the pancreas; trypsin changes proteins into peptones.

tubercle (tū'bĕr-k'l): a rounded, solid elevation on the skin or membrane.

tumor (tū'mĕr): a swelling; an abnormal enlargement.

turbinal; turbinate (tûr'bĭ-nâl; -nāt): a bone in the nose; turbinated body.

Tutankhemen (tōōt'ăngk-ä'min): fourteenth century B.C. Egyptian pharoah.

tweezers (twēz'ĕrz): a pair of small forceps to remove or extract hair.

typhoid fever (tī'foid): an acute infectious fever caused by the typhoid bacillus and characterized by severe intestinal disturbances, red spots on the chest and abdomen.

tyrosine (tī-rō'sĭn): an amino-acid widely distributed in proteins, particularly in casein.

U

ulcer (ŭl'sēr): an open sore not caused by a wound.

ulna (ŭl'nă): the inner and larger bone of the forearm.

ultra-violet (ŭl'tră-vī-ō-lĕt): invisible rays of the spectrum which are beyond the violet rays.

unadulterated (ŭn-ă-dŭl'tĕr-āt-ĕd): pure.

undertone (ŭn'dĕr-tōn): a subdued shade of color; a color upon another color through which the underlying color can be seen.

unguentum (ŭn-gwĕn'tûm); pl., **unguenta** (-ă): a salve or ointment.

unguium, tinea (ŭn'gwē-ûm tĭn'ē-ă): ringworm of the nails.

unit (ūn′ĭt): a single thing or value.

United States Pharmacopeia (U.S.P.) (fär-mȧ-kô-pē′yȧ): an official book of drug and medicinal standards.

unique (yōō-nēk′): being the only one of its kind; unusual; rare.

unsaturated (un-sach′ărȧ′tid): containing less of a solute required for equilibrium, as a solution.

unstable (ŭn-stā′b'l): liable to fade.

urea (ū-rē′ȧ): a diuretic; also employed externally in treating infected wounds; occurs as colorless to white crystals or powder; soluble in water.

V

vaccination (văk-sĭ-nā′shûn): inoculation with the virus of cowpox, or vaccina, as a means of producing immunity against small pox.

vaccine (văk′sĭn; sēn): any substance used for preventive inoculation.

vacuum (văk′ū-ûm): a space from which most of the air has been exhausted.

vagus (vā′gŭs): pneumogastric nerve; tenth cranial nerve.

vapor (vā′pĕr): the gaseous state of a liquid or solid.

vaporizer (vā′pa-rī′zer): a device for converting a substance into vapor for use on the skin; sometimes used to produce vapor for inhalation.

varicose veins (văr′ĭ-kōs): swollen or knotted veins.

vascoconstrictor (văs-ô-kŏn-strĭk′tēr): a nerve which, when stimulated, causes narrowing of blood vessels.

vascular (văs′kŭ-lăr): supplied with small blood vessels; pertaining to a vessel for the conveyance of a fluid as blood or lymph.

Vaseline (văs′ĕ-lĭn): a tradename; petrolatum; a semisolid greasy or oily mixture of hydro-carbons obtained from petroleum.

vasodilator (văs-ô-dĭ-lā′tēr): an agent that induces or initiates vasodilation.

vein; vena (vē′nȧ): a blood vessel carrying blood toward the heart.

vena cava (kā′vȧ): one of the large veins which carries the blood to the right auricle of the heart.

venereal (vē-nē′rē-âl): a disease contacted by sexual relations with an infected person.

ventilate (vĕn′tĭ-lāt): to renew the air in a place.

ventricle (vĕn′trĭ-k'l): a small cavity; particularly in the heart.

vermin (vûr′mĭn): parasitic insects, as lice and bedbugs.

verruca (vĕ-rōō′kȧ): a wart; a growth of the papillae and epidermis.

vertebra (vûr′tĕ-brȧ; pl., **vertebrae** (-bre): a bony segment of the spinal column.

vesicle (vĕs′ĭ-k'l): a small blister or sac; a small elevation on the skin.

vibrator (vī′brȧ-tēr): an electrically driven massage apparatus causing a swinging, shaking sensation on the body, producing stimulation.

Victorian (vik-tôr′ē-an): of or relating to Queen Victoria or her reign (1837-1901); prudish, narrow, conventional.

violet-ray (vī′ô-lĕt rā): high frequency; Tesla; an electric current of medium voltage and medium amperage.

virgin hair: normal hair which has had no previous lightening or tinting treatments.

virus (vī′rŭs): poison; the specific poison of an infectious disease.

viscid vĭs′ĭd): sticky or adhesive.

viscosity (vĭs-kŏs′ĭ-tē): 1) resistance to change of form; 2) a resistance to flow that a liquid exhibits; 3) the degree of density, thickness, stickiness and adhesiveness of a substance.

viscous (vĭs′kŭs): sticky or gummy.

visible (vĭs′ĭ-b'l) **rays:** light rays which can be seen; are visible to the eye.

vitamin (vī′ta-min): any of a group of complex organic substances found in minute quantities in most natural foodstuffs.

vitiligo (vĭt-ĭ-lī′gō): milky-white spots on the skin.

volatile (vŏl′ȧ-tĭl): easily evaporating; diffusing freely; not permanent.

volt (vŏlt): the fractional unit of electromotive force.

voltage (vŏl′tȧj): electrical potential difference expressed in volts.

voluntary (vŏl′ûn-tĕ-rē): under the control of the will.

vomer (vō′mĕr): the thin plate of bone between the nostrils.

vulnerable (vŭl′nēr-ȧ-b'l): capable of receiving injury.

W

wart (wôrt: verruca.

water (wô′tĕr) **hard:** water containing certain minerals; does not lather with soap.

water softener: certain chemicals, such as the carbonate of phosphate of sodium, used to soften hard water to permit the lathering of soap.

water soluble (wô′tĕr sŏl′ū-b'l): any substance that dissolves in water.

wattage (wŏt′ȧj): amount of electric power expressed in watts.

wen (wĕn): a sebaceous cyst, usually on the scalp.

wheal (whēl): a raised ridge on the skin, usually caused by a blow, a bite of an insect, urticaria, or sting of a nettle.

whitehead (whīt′hĕd): milium.

wind pipe (wĭnd pīp): trachea.

witch hazel (wĭch hā′z'l): an extract from the bark of the hamanelis shrub, widely used as an astringent, after shave lotion, and as a remedy for sprains and bruises.

World War II (1939-1945): an armed conflict between major nations of the world.

wrinkle (rĭnk′l): a small ridge or a furrow.

X

xanthoma (zăn-thō-mă): a skin disease characterized by the presence of yellow nodules or slightly raised plates in the skin.

xanthoma palpebrarum (zăn-thō-mă păl-pê-brā′rûm): a form of skin disease which may be treated with an electric needle.

xanthoelanous (zăn-thō-mĕl′ăn-ûs): having a yellow skin and black hair.

Y

yeast (yēst): a rich source of vitamin B.

Z

zinc oxide (zĭnk): a white pulverulent compound used as a pigment, and in medicine; also used as a mild antiseptic and astringent.

zinc sulphate (sŭl′fāt): a salt often employed as an astringent, both in lotions and creams.

zinc sulphocarbonate (zĭnk sŭl-fô-kär′bôn-āt): a fine white powder having the odor of carbolic acid; used as an antiseptic and astringent in deodorant preparations.

zygomatic (zī-gô-măt′ĭk): pertaining to the malar of cheekbone.

zygomaticus (zī-gô-măt′ĭ-kŭs): a muscle that draws the upper lip upward and outward.